Health, Illness, and Medicine in Canada

FOURTH EDITION

Juanne Nancarrow Clarke

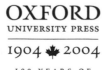

OXFORD

UNIVERSITY PRESS

1904 ❦ 2004

100 YEARS OF
CANADIAN PUBLISHING

OXFORD
UNIVERSITY PRESS

70 Wynford Drive, Don Mills, Ontario M3C 1J9
www.oup.com/ca

Oxford University Press is a department of the University of Oxford.
It furthers the University's objective of excellence in research, scholarship,
and education by publishing worldwide in

Oxford New York

Auckland Bangkok Buenos Aires Cape Town Chennai
Dar es Salaam Delhi Hong Kong Istanbul Karachi Kolkata
Kuala Lumpur Madrid Melbourne Mexico City Mumbai Nairobi
São Paulo Shanghai Taipei Tokyo Toronto

Oxford is a trade mark of Oxford University Press
in the UK and in certain other countries

Published in Canada by Oxford University Press

National Library of Canada Cataloguing in Publication

Clarke, Juanne N. (Juanne Nancarrow), 1944–

Health, illness, and medicine in Canada/Juanne Nancarrow Clarke.– 4th ed.

Includes bibliographical references and index.
ISBN 0-19-541901-4

1. Social medicine–Canada.   I. Title

Cover Design: Brett Miller
Cover Image: *Dare to Age Well!* CD, Health Canada (2001). Reproduced with the permission
of the Minister of Public Works and Government Services Canada, 2003.

1 2 3 4 5 — 08 07 06 05 04

This book is printed on permanent (acid-free) paper ∞.
Printed in Canada

Contents

List of Figures

List of Tables

List of Boxes

Preface

As we face the twenty-first century, significant changes in the medical care system and in the health of the population loom on the horizon. Perhaps the most basic change confronting Canadians today is the withering away of a universal medical care system. As federal transfer payments continue to decrease and the responsibility for medical care shifts to the provinces, the likelihood grows of inequality in the availability of services across the nation. Universal medical care has never been as threatened as it is today, as Canada shifts to the political right in the context of economic globalization. Unless there is a dramatic alteration in direction, inequality in medical services among provinces, between the rich and the poor, among racialized and ethnic groups, and between women and men will continue to grow.

Many argue that this crisis in the provision of allopathic medical care will have positive effects on the health of the population. The argument is that as the near-monopoly in allopathic medical care is weakened, complementary and alternative care strategies will grow in their availability for the population. In fact, already about 40 per cent of the US and Canadian populations use alternative or complementary health care. To the extent

that the current medical care crisis destabilizes the hegemonic status of allopathic medicine and, in turn, other types of health care take up positions as possible health-care strategies for Canadians, this crisis in medical care must be seen as an opportunity.

Health promotion and disease prevention now predominate in the developing medical ideology of the federal government. To the extent that these strategies individualize health problems that result from social-structural inequalities and 'blame the victim', they have met with criticism. Focusing on individual choice with respect to prevention issues such as seat-belt use, quitting smoking, moderation in alcohol consumption, low-fat diets, and exercise obscures the social, cultural, and structural constraints within which choice operates.

The deleterious effects of numerous social and economic arrangements appear to be unabated in spite of widespread environment-related policy changes. Changes that the citizenry takes part in on an individual basis, such as paper, metal, glass, and cardboard recycling and reducing and reusing whenever possible, have only a minor effect in an industrial and corporate context where environmental controls compete with profitability. Major environmental challenges, such as chlorinated water and the pervasive use of bleach in manufacturing, the widespread use of pesticides, herbicides, and fertilizers in agriculture, and the use of nuclear energy, continue to affect the health of the population and threaten to do so in the future.

Many have noted that sociology is approached from four different perspectives: structural-functional, conflict, symbolic interactionist, and feminist. Each of these is based on different assumptions, asks different questions, and uses different methods and rules of evidence. This book is organized into three major sections. The first part, Chapters One and Two, addresses some theoretical and methodological issues. Chapter One discusses the theory behind each of the four sociological perspectives and provides an illustration of each perspective as applied to a concrete study. Chapter Two examines the methodology employed by each perspective in studying health-related problems, including concepts such as causality, objectivity, and reliability, and each is illustrated by concrete examples. Chapter Two ends with a discussion of the criticisms that have been levelled at each methodology.

The second part of the book, Chapters Three to Eight, explores the meaning and measurement of health and illness from these four different sociological perspectives. Chapter Three examines Canadian mortality in historical and cross-cultural contexts. It examines questions such as: What are the chief causes of death in Canada today? What were the chief causes of death 150 years ago? Why has the difference between male and female mortality rates increased over time?

Chapter Four examines the impact on health of environmental, occupational, and other health and safety issues, as well as violence in society. It asks questions such as: What are the major threats to the environment? What do we know about their impact on the health of the population? Are the health effects of environmental degradation spread equally across Canada and throughout the global community? What occupations are safe? Is shift work bad for our health? Does violence affect the health of Canadians?

Chapter Five focuses on the impact of unequal social status on the health of the population. In particular, it looks at the effects of age and gender. Questions such as the following are asked: Are older people more likely to be sick or just more likely to be medicalized? Which sex lives a longer and more disabled life? Which sex lives a shorter lifespan? Do men and women get sick from and die from different or similar diseases?

Chapter Six examines two other aspects of inequity in the social system—class and race/ethnicity. Pertinent questions include: Is there evidence of class differences in morbidity and mortality? Do people of different race/ethnic backgrounds experience different health and life changes?

Chapter Seven looks at the social and psychological antecedents to illness and disease and considers such questions as: What is the relationship between stress and illness? Can the loss of a loved one lead to serious illness? Is the inability to express anger sometimes implicated in the onset of cancer? Can social support minimize the effects and shorten the duration of an illness?

Chapter Eight concerns the experience of illness and answers questions such as: How do epilepsy, cancer, or multiple sclerosis affect the everyday life of the patient and family members? Do diseases have social meanings?

The third part of the book deals with the social construction of medical research and practice and the organization of the medical care system. It addresses questions such as: Does a universal medical care insurance scheme guarantee universal accessibility? Why has the number of malpractice suits increased? What is the impact of the increasing number of female doctors? What is the fate of idealism in medical school?

Chapter Nine discusses the social basis of

medical science and medical research. It also examines some strategies of lay resistance to conventional medicine. Questions asked include: Is allopathic medical practice entirely based on the findings of traditional medical science research? Is medical science objective? Are new medical technologies necessarily better? When and why do people sometimes resist medical prescriptions and diagnoses?

Chapter Ten examines the relationship between medicine and religion in cross-cultural and historical contexts. It considers questions such as the following: Is medicalization increasing? ('Medicalization' may be defined as a tendency for more and more of human social life to be considered relevant to medicine.) Is medical practice an art or a science? Do physicians act as moral entrepreneurs? What sort of ethical dilemmas do doctors face as they do their work?

Chapter Eleven examines the history of universal medical care insurance in Canada. What is the impact of universal medical insurance on class-based differences in health status? What is the future of extra-billing? What role did Tommy Douglas play in the foundation of Canada's universal medical care system?

Chapter Twelve examines medical practice as an occupation, and seeks to answer such questions as: Is medicine a profession? What is a profession? How do doctors handle mistakes? What is medical culture?

Chapter Thirteen considers two major criticisms of the contemporary medical system—the dominance of one type of medical care system and sexism. It examines questions such as the following: How prevalent is chronic illness? What is the likely impact of the aging of the population on the medical care system? What is sexism? What is patriarchy? Why are most nurses women and most doctors men?

Chapter Fourteen describes other health-care providers—nurses and midwives. Typical questions are: What is the importance of Florence Nightingale for nursing work today? What are the consequences of the bureaucratic work organization of the hospital on the work of nurses? What is the status of the midwife in Canada?

Chapter Fifteen examines the place of complementary and alternative health care in Canadian and other Western industrialized societies. In-depth examinations of two alternative forms of health care, chiropractic and naturopathy, are included.

Chapter Sixteen examines the pharmaceutical industry as one component of the medical-industrial complex. It considers questions such as: How does the pharmaceutical industry maintain its position as one of the lowest-risk and highest-profit industries in Canada today? What is the role of doctors and pharmacists in prescribing drugs? Which Canadians are most likely to use mood-altering drugs?

Acknowledgements

Many people have contributed to this fourth edition, first of all my students, who have asked questions, shown enthusiasm, and made suggestions for the inclusion of new material. Several students helped specifically with aspects of the book. Here I would like to thank Sara Harris and Jackie De Silva. Colleagues here at Laurier and at universities across the country have supported the previous editions and suggested and encouraged new directions. I would especially like to thank authors of three helpful reviews of the text: Catherine Chiappetta, McMaster University; Maureen Goutier, University of Alberta; and Rebecca Sutherns, University of Western Ontario.

As always, I am grateful to Wilfrid Laurier University for the opportunities to do such writing as a part of teaching in a very busy sociology department. Also, the Office of Research at Laurier provided some funds for an undergraduate assistant through a student fellowship. Megan Mueller and Phyllis Wilson at Oxford University Press have been greatly helpful and supportive in this and other writing projects. Finally, Richard Tallman, the fine editor for Oxford, has helped enormously, especially at the final stages, by noticing a myriad of small details and larger questions of substance and meaning that needed to be attended to before publication.

Part I   **Sociological Perspectives**

Chapter 1

Ways of Thinking Sociologically about Health, Illness, and Medicine

Learning Objectives

- There are many different approaches to doing sociology.
- In this book we have divided these into four different theories: structural-functional, conflict, symbolic interactionist, and feminist.
- Each perspective involves a fundamentally different paradigm or way of seeing the important issues in sociology as well as some distinct methodological strategies.
- Structural-functionalism, based on the work of Émile Durkheim, sees society as a system of interlocking and functional parts.
- Conflict theory, from the work of Karl Marx, is concerned about the documentation of injustice.
- Symbolic interactionism, based on the writing of Max Weber, sees sociology as the study of social action insofar as it is socially meaningful.
- Feminist theory is much more recent, dating from the latter part of the last century. Women's lives are at the centre of this paradigmatic approach. The work of the contemporary Canadian sociologist, Dorothy Smith, exemplifies this approach.

Introduction

Almost all of us have been sick at some time in our lives. When do we acknowledge that we are sick? Is it when we stay in bed for a day or two? Perhaps it is when we feel a pain but take a pill and go on with the day as planned? Or perhaps we may not truly claim sickness unless we go to the doctor to find a name for the unusual way we feel? Whatever our view, all of us experience illness in a social context: we recognize it because we have developed a vocabulary that allows us to talk about it with others in our immediate circle or in the larger social world; we learn what to do about it as we interact with others, with friends and families, at times with the formal medical system, and with our society through such media as television or magazines.

Are you aware of the relationship between sickle-cell anemia and ethnicity? Do you know the reason for that relationship? Unemployment is often followed by ill health. What might the

Table 1.1   Examples of Topics within the Sociology of Medicine and of Health and Illness

Sociology of Medicine	Sociology of Health and Illness
The organization of the medical care system	The distribution of disease and death
The profession of medicine (and auxiliary and competing health-care professionals)	Disease and death in socio-historical context
Alternative health-care providers	Socio-demographic explanations for disease and death
The financing of medical care	Class, patriarchy, and sexism as explanations for disease and death
The medico-industrial complex	
Class, patriarchy, and sexism and the organization of medical care	Socio-psychological explanations for disease and death
The health-promotion industry	Experiencing and talking about disease and death
The development and perpetuation of medical discourse and ideology	Ways people construct or label certain signs as symptoms of disease
	Environmental conditions and health, occupational health, safety issues, and health consequences

sociological explanations of such a finding be? Are most types of morbidity and mortality inversely related to income? That is, is it statistically correct to say that the lower the income, the higher the rates of sickness, disability, and death? These are the sorts of questions asked in the sociology of health and illness. To provide a working definition, the *sociology of health and illness* seeks to describe and explain the social causes and consequences of illness, disease, disability, and death; to show the ways lay people and professionals alike constitute or construct their categories of disease and illness; and to portray the ways that illness affects and is affected by social interaction among various people or institutions. Table 1.1 lists examples of topics studied in this area of sociology.

When we think that we are sick, what do we do? Some of us treat ourselves with our favourite home remedies such as bed rest and tea or chicken soup. Some of us seek advice from friends or family members. Some of us visit our general practitioner, a medical specialist, or a pharmacist.

A few head off to the emergency room of the nearest hospital. A few others seek alternative health care such as homeopathy, acupuncture, or Ayurvedic medicine. When you seek the advice of a doctor, do you think you would receive better medical care from a physician who works in a fee-for-service setting or from one on a salary paid by the state, a corporation, or a clinic? Do practitioners in group practice provide better care than those in practice on their own? Does the Canadian government have adequate drug safety procedures to protect Canadians against another drug disaster such as thalidomide? Why does the universal medical insurance scheme provide guaranteed funds for medical practitioners but only limited funds for chiropractors, and generally none for naturopaths or other alternative health-care providers? Did the moratorium on the use of breast silicone implants result from new scientific or medical knowledge or consumer organizing and lobbying?

The *sociology of medicine* is the study of the ways the institutionalized medical system constructs what it deems to be illness out of what it recognizes as signs and symptoms, and constitutes its response to such 'illness' through the treatments it prescribes (see Table 1.1). This field of sociology examines and offers explanations for such topics as the varying types of medical practice and medical discourse, the ideology and organization of medicine, different ways of financing medical care, the structure and operation of the hospital, and the occupational worlds of the nurse and the doctor. It also attempts to explain the relationships among the different types of medical care and the importance of the medical care system in the context of the culture and the political economy of the state.

Sociologists study the social world from a variety of perspectives. Depending on their perspective, they focus on some aspects of social life and ignore others, and ask different questions and use different ways to answer them. As you might expect, these varied sociological perspectives are manifest in the sociology of health and illness and of medicine. Sociologists have approached these fields with different or even contradictory assumptions. At times different sociologists have described or analyzed an aspect of illness or medicine from such widely differing points of view that they appear to be discussing different phenomena. There is some agreement that the various perspectives can be distilled into four distinct paradigms. It is now conventional to call these perspectives structural-functional theory, conflict theory, symbolic interactionist theory, and feminist theory. Table 1.2 outlines the principal characteristics of each approach.

Structural Functionalism

Structural functionalism dominated North American sociology for many years. It has been the reigning paradigm, the 'normal' science of the discipline (Kuhn, 1962). Most sociological studies published in North America have adopted this perspective. Auguste Comte (1798–1857), who first gave the name of sociology to the science of society, thought that sociology's goal was to better society so that it might become orderly and progressive. He might be called the godfather of sociology. Émile Durkheim (1858–1917) provided both the theoretical and methodological model for structural functionalism. Durkheim defined sociology as a science of social facts. Social facts, he said, were to be treated and studied as if they were real, external to individuals, and yet capable of constraining and directing human behaviour and thought. The subject matter of sociology was the knowledge of these social facts and their impact on human behaviour. Constrained by the external world, human beings, in Durkheim's view, were predictable and controllable through the power of norms that exist in their own right, aside from their manifestations in individuals.

Sociology in the Durkheimian tradition is often called structural functionalism. It assumes that the proper level of study for the sociologist is the society or the system. The social system is said to be composed of parts, institutions that function to maintain order in the social system. Just as the organs in the human body are inextricably tied to one another and function as interrelated parts, so, too, are the parts or the institutions of society—the family, the economy, the polity, and the educational, welfare, military, and medical care systems. All these institutions operate interdependently to keep the society functioning. It is the problem of maintaining a good working order in society that motivates theorizing and research in this sociological perspective.

Structural-functional theory is often associated with a positivist methodology. Positivists view sociology as a science in the same way that physicists view physics as a science. Positivists assume that social scientists both should and can remain objective and value-free while observing, recording, and measuring external social facts. Just as the natural sciences seek universally true causal explanations of relationships in the natural world, so do positivist sociologists in the social world. As well, since positivists believe that social facts are to be treated as real and external, they tend to rely on data that are assumed to be objective, collected from interviews and questionnaires administered to individuals in survey research, and analyzed and organized to reflect the probability of the occurrence of certain behaviours among a certain aggregate or group of individuals.

Five things distinguish *structural functionalism* from conflict theory, symbolic interactionism, and feminist theory. They are the assumptions (1) that sociology aims to discover and to explain the impact of social facts on human behaviour, attitudes, or feelings; (2) that social facts are to be treated as things that are real and external to human actions, and that determine human behaviour; (3) that social facts can be seen in aspects of the social structure such as the norms that guide behaviour, in social institutions such as the family or the economy, and in social behaviours such as those in relationships between the sexes, in marriage, or at work; (4) that sociology is a science that seeks to describe the world in a series of universal causal laws; and (5) that this science considers that human behaviour is objectively and quantitatively measurable through methods such as experiments and survey research.

One of the most influential contributions to medical sociology from a structural-functional point of view is Talcott Parsons's work on the sick role (Parsons, 1951: 428–79). To understand Parsons's sick role, it is necessary to understand that each individual plays a number of roles in society. Roles arise out of the institutions with which the individual is associated. For example, an individual will likely play some of the following family roles—daughter, son, mother, father, niece, nephew, and a whole series of in-law roles. An individual may also play a variety of work roles, neighbourhood roles, friendship roles, and so on. All roles reflect something of the intermeshing of the individual in society. The idea of role is a pivotal one in conceptualizing the relationship between the individual and society.

Parsons's main concern was to describe the processes that maintain societal institutions. His notion of the sick role should be looked at in this context. Sickness could lead to societal breakdown resulting from the inability of the sick to fulfill their necessary social roles, such as parenting, maintaining a home, and working in the paid labour force. Therefore sickness must be managed, and must be accorded a special role. However, this legitimation is only temporary and is contingent on the fulfillment of certain obligations by the individual who claims the sick role. There are four components to the sick role. The first two are rights, the second two are duties. Both the rights and duties of the sick role must be fulfilled if the equilibrium of society is to be maintained.

(1) The sick person is exempt from 'normal' social roles.

The sick individual has a legitimate excuse for missing an exam or a major presentation at work, for staying in bed all day and neglecting household chores, or for staying home from work. The length of the exemption depends on the severity of the illness. In order to win exemption, the individual may need formal, medical acknowledgement. The sick person may have to obtain an official medical diagnosis and even a medical certificate as proof of illness. Exemptions from examinations, for instance, generally require a formal written note from a physician.

(2) The sick person is not responsible for his or her condition.

The sickness must be the result of an accident or other circumstances beyond the control of the individual if that person is to be accorded the sick role. Thus, the individual is not to be blamed or punished. Influenza, a cold, and a broken leg are considered the results of misfortune, not of personal will or desire. Therefore, sympathy rather than blame is considered the appropriate reaction of others.

Table 1.2   The Four Central Sociological Perspectives

	Structural Functionalism	Conflict Theory	Symbolic Interactionism	Feminist Theory
Exemplar Model of subject matter	**Émile Durkheim** Society is a social system of interlocking and interrelated parts or institutions.	**Karl Marx** Society is a system of classes.	**Max Weber** Society is composed of selves who make their social lives meaningful through interaction.	**Dorothy Smith** Understanding social organization, structure, power, and knowledge from women's perspective.
Model of the subject matter in process	Institutions perform (dys)functions that are both manifest and latent in the interest of the (dis)continuation of the social system in equilibrium.	Power groups with contradictory purposes, based on their relationship to the basic economic structures.	Selves create reality anew from situation to situation in interaction with others.	Women's selves are tied to the relations of ruling. Feminist research has change as one of its goals. It emphasizes the empowerment of women along with the transformation of a patriarchal social system.
Ways of doing sociological analysis	System explainable and predictable through a series of 'if x . . . then y' causal statements; x and y are social facts.	Power groups are understandable from a committed stance examining the conflicts in historical context.	Selves' world views and symbols arise out of interaction and are made understandable through process of interpretive, empathetic understanding—*verstehen*.	All methods of data collection may be used but a collaborative approach (between researcher and subjects of research) is advocated. Triangulation is suggested. Language is gender appropriate or neutral.
Objectivity/ subjectivity	Necessary to be objective and to study the social world objectively.	Value-committed perspective necessary.	Acknowledgement of the inevitability of contextual reflexivity of knower and known.	Quite often focuses on/begins with women's experience. Impossible to be objective. Therefore important to clarify standpoint and acknowledge reflexivity.
Image of human nature	Human beings believe, think/feel, and do as the result of external constraining forces.	Human beings are alienated from self, others, and meaningful work, and need the liberation that would come from revolutionary change.	Human beings continually construct reality as they interact with others in their social worlds.	Differences by class, gender/power, sexual orientation, dis/ability limit generalization about human nature (Clarke, 1992b).

(3) The sick person should try to get well.

The person who is given the legitimacy of the sick role is duty bound to try to get well. Sick role exemption is only temporary. If an individual does not want to get well or does not try to get well then the sick role is no longer considered legitimate. Thus, if a person has received a diagnosis of pneumonia, he or she must do what the doctor orders. If not, the legitimacy of the sick label deteriorates into the shame of such a label as 'foolish', 'careless', or 'malingerer'.

(4) The sick person should seek technically competent help and co-operate with the physician.

The duties associated with the sick role also require that the ill person seek 'appropriate' medical attention and comply with the treatment provided. For example, a person with AIDS who refuses both to accept medical care and to change certain sexual or drug-use habits would not be accorded the rights of the sick role but could be subject to legal punishment.

From the viewpoint of Parsons, illness is a form of deviance. It is a potential threat to the social system unless it is managed for the benefit of the social system. Medicine is the institution responsible for providing legitimation and justification and for bringing the sick back to wellness or 'normality'. Medical institutions can be seen as agents of social control in much the same way that religious institutions and the criminal justice system are.

Parsons's formulation of the sick role was primarily theoretical: it was not based on extensive systematic empirical investigation. Empirical analysis subjects his definition of the sick role to a number of criticisms. Some of these criticisms will be examined in the following sections.

(1) The sick person is exempt from 'normal' social roles.

The extent to which a person is allowed exemption depends on the nature, severity, and longevity of the sickness, and also on the characteristics and normal social roles of the person. A short and self-limiting burn on the fingers merits only temporary, minimal exemptions from life roles. On the other hand, multiple sclerosis, a chronic and degenerative disease, allows extensive exemptions.

The university student's sick role is mostly informal. Most professors do not take attendance; students can avoid the library for weeks on end without any formal notice being taken; they can stay in bed half the day and stay out half the night. These things are the student's own responsibility. It is only at the time of regularly scheduled deadlines for papers, presentations, and examinations that universities typically take any official notice of the student's actions. At these times the student may need to adopt the sick role formally by obtaining official legitimation from a physician.

(2) The sick person is not responsible for her or his condition.

This belief varies depending on the nature of the condition and the circumstances through which the person is believed to have acquired the condition. The sick person may be held responsible for having a cold, for instance, if he or she stayed out overnight and walked miles in the freezing rain without a jacket. The notion of stress that is prevalent today has an aspect of blame attached to it—that is, people who succumb to disease because they have been overworked or worried may be chastised for having failed to take preventive action. One of the implications, in fact, of the recent emphases on health promotion through lifestyle change (giving up smoking, drinking alcoholic beverages, and so on) is that people who do not change may be more likely to be held responsible for lung cancer or cirrhosis, for example, or the person with AIDS may be blamed for his or her sexual habits. In addition, a number of diseases are thought to reflect on the moral and social worth of the individual, and when an individual succumbs to these diseases he or she is blamed by virtue of the stigma attached.

There is considerable evidence that even though the specific causes of particular cancers are not known, there is a way in which the person with the disease is sometimes blamed for succumbing. For instance, the person with adult-onset diabetes may be held responsible if he/she is overweight. Several social researchers have noted the way that a person diagnosed with HIV/AIDS is often thought to be at fault because of a 'nefarious' lifestyle or 'immoral' sexual choices (Altman, 1986; Sontag, 1989; Radley, 1999). Crandall and Moriarty (1995) asked people to examine case histories representing 66 illnesses and to rate the illnesses according to a number of dimensions. They found that the diseases that were most likely to lead to social rejection, i.e., to be stigmatized, were those (1) that were believed to be under personal onset control and (2) that were most severe. They did not find that gender, age, or ethnicity had an impact. Clarke's study of women with cancer found that respondents sometimes talked of how friends and even some family members seemed to reject them after their cancer diagnosis. Some spoke of people walking to the other side of the street rather than stopping to converse. Some talked of being avoided by their husbands. Some perceived discomfort in their doctor's inability to relate to them once the cancer was discovered (Clarke, 1985: 121). Even daughters experience some stigma and isolation as the result of others' knowledge of their mothers' diagnosis (Clarke, 1995).

Epilepsy, leprosy, mental illness, and venereal disease are other stigmatizing diseases (Schneider and Conrad, 1983; Markowitz, 1998). In a sense, people with such discrediting or discreditable diseases are not given the social legitimacy of the sick role (Goffman, 1963). In fact, the negative associations of some diseases have caused discrimination and exile. Such stigma heightens both physical and emotional pain. Even when they are not held materially responsible, people are sometimes held morally responsible (Williams, 1998).

(3) The sick person should want to get well.

There are illnesses from which people cannot or are not expected to recover. People are expected to adjust to such illnesses. A so-called 'terminal' illness is a case in point. Patients are not granted legitimacy for wanting to get well once they have been diagnosed with a terminal illness. In fact, if people continue to want to get well when they have been diagnosed as terminal, they are often criticized because they may be said to be denying reality. Similarly, people with a whole range of chronic illnesses are not expected to want to get well, but rather to adapt to daily limitations and disabilities.

(4) The sick person should seek technically competent help and co-operate with the physician.

The dominant medical care system is that of allopathic medicine. Allopathic medicine treats disease by trying to create a condition in the body that is opposite to or incompatible with the disease state. While this medical care system still claims a monopoly on the right to provide treatment and thus to legitimate sickness, there are competing medical systems with varying and growing degrees of legitimacy. In 1990, 34 per cent of Americans reported that they used at least one unconventional method of medical therapy in the previous year (Eisenberg et al., 1993). By 1997, 42 per cent of Americans used at least one alternative therapy in the previous year (Eisenberg et al., 1998). In 1997, 42 per cent of those polled by a Canadian national polling organization said they used alternative treatments (*Canada Year Book*, 1999: 109). Most did not inform their allopathic doctor of this. Some, such as midwifery, have grown in their acceptance as rightful alternatives to conventional medicine. Moreover, allopathic medical practice is the subject of growing critical analysis by consumer interest groups, particularly the women's health movement. Critical evaluations of such things as unnecessary surgery, side effects from taking pre-scribed drugs, and unnecessary medical interven-tion in childbirth raise the possibility that co-operation with physicians may not always be the most efficacious road to good health. The determination of which profession is the techni-cally competent one becomes quite problematic in this context.

In spite of the critical problems raised above, the sick role concept is important in medical soci-ology. Parsons was the first to note explicitly that there are ways in which medical practice, its ide-ology, and its associated medical institutions serve to fulfill social control functions for the society. A number of sociologists since Parsons have exam-ined and critiqued the social control functions of medicine. Szasz (1969), Freidson (1970), Zola (1975), Illich (1976), and Conrad and Schneider (1980) are just some of those who have expressed concern about medicine's powers of social control. The concept of medicalization has been used to describe this process. Behaviours once considered illegal or immoral and thus under the jurisdiction of judicial or religious institutions are more and more likely to be seen as medical problems requir-ing diagnosis and treatment, and thus come under the jurisdiction of the medical care system. Some argue that medicine has established a jurisdiction far wider than that merited by its demonstrated ability to provide a 'cure' (see Freidson, 1970, for a theoretical discussion).

Although Parsons's sick role concept has, as Freidson says, provided 'a penetrating and apt analysis of sickness from a distinctly sociological point of view' (1970: 228), it must be evaluated critically. As a generalization, its empirical appli-cability is seriously limited. Criticisms have been levelled at Parsons's sick role because of its lack of attention to differences in the degree of legitima-tion given to patients of differing age, gender, class, or ethnic background. Furthermore, differ-ent types of illnesses provide different degrees of legitimacy to the sick person. The allopathic doc-tor described by Parsons is only one of several

alternatives available today. Indeed, as noted ear-lier, complementary or alternative medicine is used by a growing number of people. Doctors themselves differ in their practice according to class, gender, age, and ethnic background, among other things. Moreover, numerous alternative healers compete with the allopathic physician for the right to be seen as the appropriate practition-er for care.

While positivism is the research methodolo-gy most closely associated with the structural-functional perspective, all positivists are not structural functionalists. Parsons's sick role is peripheral to a great deal of medical sociology in the positivist tradition. Contemporary positivists study human health behaviours as both inde-pendent and dependent variables. An examina-tion of the impact of a diagnosis, e.g., of cystic fibrosis, on the family of the ill person treats health behaviour related to the diagnosis as the independent variable. On the other hand, when the impact of income level on the incidence of disease is studied, human health behaviour becomes the dependent variable.

Today, positivists, following Durkheim, assume that the social structure has a constrain-ing impact on individuals. Social structural posi-tions (social facts) determine individual thoughts, behaviours, feelings, and, in this case, health and illness, medical utilization, professionalization, and so on. Changes in one institution, such as the family, necessitate changes in other institutions, such as the medical care system. Such changes, according to the positivists, can be described in a series of causal laws of the 'if x then y' variety. The underlying assumption of this perspective is that a complete understanding of social facts will explain all that needs to be explained about human beings. Research along these lines exam-ines the effects of such things as gender, class, educational level, family type, marital status, age, rural/urban background, religious affiliation, religiosity, and political ideology on such (dependent) health-related variables as health ex-

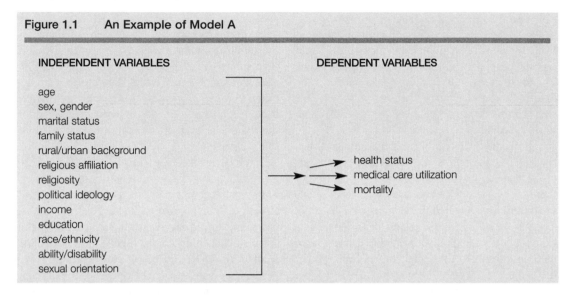

Figure 1.1   An Example of Model A

INDEPENDENT VARIABLES   DEPENDENT VARIABLES

age
sex, gender
marital status
family status
rural/urban background
religious affiliation   health status
religiosity   medical care utilization
political ideology   mortality
income
education
race/ethnicity
ability/disability
sexual orientation

periences, death rates, health lifestyles, and utilization of medical care. Research that considers
health and medical variables as dependent variables is here called Model A (see Figure 1.1).

A prosaic example of the logic of this
research would be a statement such as this: the
health status of a certain aggregate, e.g., students
at university, is a function of the distribution of
such personal characteristics as the age, gender,
marital and family status, class, and ethnic background of the students. Thus, for example, one
hypothesis might be that female students will
have a poorer health status than male students.
This might be explained further as follows:
female students are more likely to have part-time
jobs than male students, and students who have
part-time jobs are more likely to become ill.

Other positivists change this causal order
and treat the health-related aspects as the independent variables. They examine the impact of
the experience of illness on the social structure.
They study the ways that such independent variables as health status, death rate, and utilization
of medical care alter social structural conditions
such as socio-economic status, educational level,
religiosity, marital and family status, and

rural/urban background. We call this Model B
(see Figure 1.2).

An example of the logic of this research
would be a statement such as the following: the
religiosity of a given aggregate of people is a function of the mortality rate in the community and
the medical care use rate. More specifically, it
might be hypothesized that when there is a high
death rate in a society people tend to turn to religious ways of understanding the world and life
hereafter.

Summary

Several examples of theory and research have
demonstrated the basic principles of structural
functionalism. The goal of sociology, from this
perspective, is to discover and explain the place
of social facts in human behaviour, attitudes, or
feelings. It aims to do this through scientific
methods that seek to uncover universal causal
laws based on quantitative analysis of 'objective'
social phenomena. Such empirical analyses are
implicitly part of the larger theoretical analysis,
which concerns the functions performed by various parts of the social system for the maintenance
of that social system.

Figure 1.2   An Example of Model B

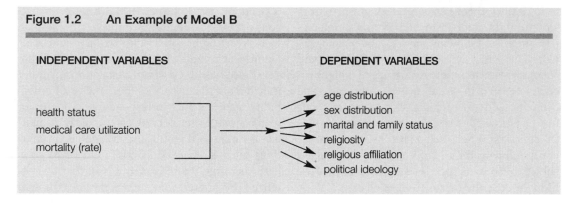

INDEPENDENT VARIABLES

health status
medical care utilization
mortality (rate)

DEPENDENT VARIABLES

age distribution
sex distribution
marital and family status
religiosity
religious affiliation
political ideology

Conflict Theory

Conflict theory has had a much less dominant role in the development of sociology in North America. It has provided and does still provide a radical critique of the more conservative aspects of the mainstream of structural-functional sociology and of the economic and social arrangements found in society. In conflict theory, all social arrangements, all sociological theories, and all sociological methods have political and economic bases and consequences. Conflict theory tends to focus on class/gender power relations and dynamics. Research topics, methodological approaches, and commitment to the use of findings all reflect the political and economic interests of the researcher.

The model of this paradigm is the work of Karl Marx (1818–83). Marx was directly involved in the analysis of and the organization for changes in his society. The author of numerous books, he was the leader of the First Communist International in Europe during the nineteenth century, and was also a busy and effective investigative journalist. He asserted that human thought and behaviour were the result of socioeconomic relations, and that both were alterable for human and social betterment. Believing that human beings could change their social order, Marx worked towards human liberation through a social and economic revolution.

Society, according to Marx, has historically been composed of a constantly varying balance of opposite forces that generate change through their ongoing struggle. The motivating force behind this continuous struggle is the way in which people interact with one another as they attempt to obtain their livelihood. Marx described the various modes of production with their corresponding types of social relations that occurred in consecutive historical periods, including primitive communal societies, slave societies, and feudal and capitalist economic systems. He described each of these periods of human history as a period of struggle between classes. The class struggle is related to the means of production, e.g., the land or the factory, because members of one class own the means of production and members of the other class sell their labour for cash. For Marx, an end to conflict was both possible and desirable in a communist state in which all citizens owned the means of production.

In their study of sociology, conflict theorists use information from a variety of sources, but it tends to have a historical and critical focus. As with structural functionalism, the level of analysis is the social system, because ultimately the system must be changed and a new one established. What is distinct about some conflict theorists is that they may also be activists. Some see injustice everywhere, and some try to alleviate it.

Conflict theory can be distinguished from structural functionalism and symbolic interactionism in the following ways: (1) the sociologist's work is to discover and document injustice (and sometimes to attempt to change it); (2) all knowledge is rooted in social, material, and historical contexts; and (3) sociological research methods must acknowledge social, economic, and historical contexts. When the conflict theorist is particularly influenced by Marx's analysis, the primary subject of study is social classes, because they are thought of as the means to effect change.

Sociology from the perspective of conflict theory is generally thought to involve the documentation of injustice for the purpose of understanding its origins and causes in a historical and socio-political context. The analysis usually focuses on recurrent patterns and the dynamics of power relations between social classes or between the sexes. Social injustice is everywhere, and medical institutions are no exception.

A long tradition of scholarship documents the ways in which health and illness are related to unequal social arrangements. Marx's collaborator, Friedrich Engels, in *The Condition of the Working Class in England* (1845), showed how the working and living conditions that resulted from early capitalist production had negative health effects. Engels described how capitalism introduced mechanization on farms, resulting in a mass of unemployed rural workers who were forced to migrate to the cities to make a living. Capitalists in the city, driven to make a profit, kept their labour costs low, and thus the working classes could afford only very cheap shelter and food. The great slums that resulted were the perfect breeding grounds for the diseases endemic to such living conditions: rickets, tuberculosis, typhoid, scrofula, and other infectious diseases. Thus ill health was related to the living conditions of the working class and the material conditions of capitalism (Navarro, 1986).

Advanced monopoly capitalism and globalization more than a century and a half later

(O'Connor, 1973; Turner, 1987) have generated considerably different but equally troublesome working/living conditions for workers and their families. Standards of living have improved in the developed world. However, tremendous inequity is evident in the disparities in mortality and morbidity statistics and corresponding standards of living around the globe. Contemporary capitalism is dominated by huge international corporations such as General Foods, General Motors, IBM, Microsoft, and Exxon and is further characterized by attempts to increase profit through worker productivity, new time-saving technologies, and expansion into the less-developed countries (both for production and for markets). Profits are increased by getting the workers and, increasingly, new technologies to produce more in the same time period, and by decreasing wages. As a result there is a continuous contradiction between the needs of the workers for a good living wage, good working conditions, adequate time for rest and relaxation, and meaningful, satisfying work on the one hand, and the needs of the capitalists for expansion and profit on the other.

Vincente Navarro (1976) is one of the foremost of contemporary conflict theorists of medical sociology. He explains that there is a contradictory relationship between capitalism, which is an economic system fuelled by the profit motive, and the health needs of the population. At times the need to make a profit requires that workers labour, live, and eat in unhealthy and unsafe environments. For example, the US National Cancer Institute estimates that 86 per cent of all cancer mortality is the result of (preventable) lifestyle, occupational, and environmental factors (Epstein, 1993: 26; 1994).

The manufacture, sale, and tax level of cigarettes illustrate the way that the need for corporate profits and state tax revenues may outweigh the desire for good health. The tobacco industry has maintained a successful profit margin by opening up new markets in spite of anti-smoking sentiments and some no-smoking legislation. In Canada, for example, the market has expanded into the younger age groups and women (Cunningham, 1994). People generally do not begin smoking as adults. The highest rate of initiating the smoking habit is among young people, especially young women. So successful have advertising campaigns directed towards the young been that Joe Camel is as recognizable to an average six-year-old as Mickey Mouse (Cunningham, 1994). Though laws prohibit the sale of cigarettes to minors, they are rarely enforced, and even when they are enforced the fines are so low that they are virtually useless. Similarly, in the interests of profit, as the overall rates of cigarette smoking are declining in the developed world, they are rapidly increasing in developing countries around the globe.

According to Navarro (1976) there are two main goals of contemporary capitalism: the concentration of capital and the growth of the state. The state intervenes in the health sector to promote capitalist goals. Some of the ways in which this occurs are, first, that the class structures of society are reproduced within the medical sector, so that the distribution of functions and responsibilities of occupational groups within the medical care system mirrors the class, ethnic, and gender hierarchies within the other sectors of capitalist society. Second, the medical system has a bourgeois ideology of medicine that regards both the cause and the cure of illness as the responsibility of the individual. Health itself becomes a commodity with a certain value within the marketplace. Thus, the capitalist medical model is a politically conservative model; it directs attention away from the social-structural causes of ill health, such as gender, 'race', class, occupation, and environmental degradation. Third, the state supports alienation when people are not free to choose alternatives to physicians, such as chiropractors, naturopaths, masseuses, or dieticians. The state provides full financial support for only one type of medical service—that

provided by the allopathic practitioner. Today with globalization many would argue that states have actually given away much of their power of governance to international capital through multinational corporations.

The state also uses strategies to exclude conflicting ideologies from debate and discussion. One example, cited by Navarro, is the emphasis on the individual causation of disease for research funding. Such viewpoints exclude analysis of the processes through which class origins, environmental pollutants, occupational hazards, and working conditions are significant causes of ill health.

A sociological analysis by Hilary Graham in *Women, Health and the Family* (1984) illustrates research in the conflict perspective. Although Graham's research was carried out in Great Britain, it raises questions for all societies regarding the home health-care work roles of women and the consequences of economic impoverishment for the health of families. Graham analyses the impact of poverty and the manifold effects of the relative scarcity of resources such as transportation, housing, fuel, food, and health care in the home on the health status of family members.

Health-care work in the home is composed of four elements. First is the provision of healthy conditions in the home. This involves the maintenance of a warm and clean home with sufficient space for rest and relaxation for all family members, sufficient and adequately nutritious foods, and clean water. Home health care also involves managing social relations and meeting emotional needs for the optimal mental health of family members. The second element is nursing the sick: much of the work of caring for the sick child or adult, and for elderly or disabled people, falls on the shoulders of the women in the home. Furthermore, increasing deinstitutionalization of the mentally, chronically, and acutely ill increases the level of intra-family responsibility. Nursing the sick is often a very time-consuming and exhausting job. It involves sleepless nights, heavy lifting, preparation of complicated menus, administering medicines, coping with bandages, and the like. A third element is teaching about health, including such things as modelling good health habits and giving instruction on diet, hygiene, and exercise. The fourth and final aspect of home health-care work is mediating with outsiders such as doctors and hospitals, making visits to clinics, talking with a social or public health worker, or getting advice from an expert in a health-related area, such as nutrition.

Graham documents the existence of class differences in home health-care work and in mortality and morbidity rates. She notes the consistently inverse relationship between class and some of the most sensitive indicators of a nation's health: stillbirths, prenatal mortality, neonatal mortality, postnatal mortality, and infant mortality rates. In each case the higher social classes have far lower mortality rates than those in the lower social classes. Babies with low birth weights are much more likely to become sick and die than babies with high birth weights. Women who bear babies with low birth weights generally live in poor households and lack safe and adequate nutrients. In Canada, even today, there is wide variation across the country in infant mortality rates (*Canada Year Book*, 2001: 135).

These class differences in outcomes among infants are mirrored in the morbidity statistics for children and adults. Accidents, the largest single cause of childhood death, are probably one of the best indicators of an unsafe, inadequately supervised environment: the accident rate increases sharply among the lower social classes. Kronenfeld et al. (1997), using a survey research methodology with a sample of 1,247 young mothers, found that such parental resources as income and education were associated with better safety behaviours in respect to their children. Class was positively associated with safety behaviours such as leaving a child alone in the house, hiring babysitters younger than 13 years of age, leaving a child alone in the bathtub, using an approved car seat, and a child's wearing a safety helmet while bicycling. Poorer families are more likely to suffer from other environmentally related causes of the death of children, such as respiratory diseases. The incidence of infections and parasitic illnesses is also class-related. There is some evidence that the mortality rate for childhood cancer is inversely related to class. One study compared the mortality rate of children with cancer whose parents received 'welfare' support in the Aid to Families with Dependent Children program to the mortality rate when parents were self-sufficient and not dependent on the state. These researchers found that the average death rate was 2.8 times higher among the children whose families received financial aid (Nelson, 1992). In contrast, there is no documented relationship between social class and the incidence of childhood diseases without known environmental, nutritional, or other material causes.

Samuel S. Epstein is an epidemiologist with an expertise and a lengthy list of publications on the occupational and environmental causes of cancer. In an analysis of the policies of the National Cancer Institute he documented the high incidence of preventable cancer deaths and the minimal research investment of the NCI in understanding these preventable deaths. He noted that 17 per cent of the $2 billion budget for 1992 of NCI research initiatives went to research into primary cancer prevention; 1 per cent of the total appropriations were dedicated to research into occupational cancers (Epstein, 1993: 24). The rest of the monies were directed towards diagnosis and treatment. He attributes the bias towards research on diagnosis and treatment to the lack of expertise on occupational and environmental carcinogens within the National Cancer Advisory Board—even though this situation violates the National Cancer Act, which stipulates 'that no fewer than 5 members shall be individuals knowledgeable in environmental carcinogens' (ibid., 19). In addition to the failure to include people with such backgrounds on the board, the NCI is further compromised by institutionalized conflicts of interest. As Epstein says, 'for decades the war on cancer has been dominated by powerful groups of interlocking professionals and financial interests, with the highly profitable drug development system at its hub—and a background that helps explain why "treatment", not prevention, has been and still is the overwhelming priority' (ibid., 20).

As a particular case, Epstein cites the conflicts among board members of the Memorial Sloan-Kettering Cancer Center in New York. Included among the overseers of this major cancer treatment and research centre are directors, board chairmen, and presidents of major pharmaceutical and medical technology corporations. In addition, Epstein documents similarly impressive and powerful directorships and other important ties with various multinational industrial corporations, such as Exxon, Philip Morris, Texaco, Nabisco, General Motors, Algoma Steel, and Bethlehem Steel. Even the media, including the New York Times Corp., Reader's Digest, Warner Communications, and CBS, are involved (ibid., 22–3). He asks whether men (usually they were men) with industrial and pharmaceutical interests can reasonably be expected to support research that might criticize and challenge their products. It is no wonder, argues Epstein, that cancer research focuses on diagnosis and treatment to the relative exclusion of prevention.

Summary

Two examples of conflict theory have demonstrated its basic principles. These are that (1) the purpose of sociology is the documentation and analysis of injustice resulting from such factors as class, race, gender, and power; (2) knowledge is never objective but always dependent on its social, material, and historical context; and (3) understanding conflicting social and economic forces is essential for an understanding of all the other conditions of social life.

Symbolic Interactionist Theory

What is the meaning of illness? Does cancer have the same meaningful impact when it happens to an 80-year-old man or woman as when a 17-year-old child is diagnosed with it? What are the processes through which the slow onset of Alzheimer's comes to be noted by family, friends, and the patient? How do families work through their changing understanding of the uncertainty and then the certainty of the death of one of their members? How does the self-identity of the person with AIDS change once he or she has received the diagnosis? How do others change in the ways that they relate to the person with AIDS? These are the sorts of questions asked in the symbolic interactionist perspective.

Max Weber provided a relevant definition of sociology: 'a science which attempts the interpretive understanding of social action in order thereby to arrive at a causal explanation of its course and its effects' (1947: 88). There are two crucial elements in this statement, each of which exemplifies an aspect of Weber's work. First, social action, as defined by Weber, meant action to which the individual attached subjective meaning. Second, the sociologist, while looking for what Weber calls causal explanation, was actually directed to interpret empathetically the meaning of the situations from the viewpoint of the subject.

Symbolic interactionist sociologists study how the subjective definitions of social reality are constructed and how this reality is experienced and described by the social actors. Human beings create their social worlds. As W.I. Thomas said, if a situation is defined as real, it is real in its consequences (Martindale, 1960: 347–53).

The paradox here is that, just as the subjects who are being studied are busy defining reality for themselves, so, too, are the researchers. Thus, the symbolic interactionist is faced with the problem, when collecting data, of intersubjectivity or reflexivity, that is, that the data are given a subjective slant both by the people being studied and by the researcher.

The sociological researcher must be aware of his or her own processes of attaching subjective meanings just as he/she studies the subjective meanings of the subjects of study. The symbolic interactionist researcher must also face a second problem: that the research act itself creates and changes meanings and processes. From the perspective of symbolic interactionism it is impossible to gather objective data. All social reality is subjectively defined and experienced and can be studied only through the subjective processes of social researchers.

Empathetic understanding, or what has come to be called, following Weber, *verstehen*, is the desirable methodological stance of the researcher. Generally, sociologists adopting this stance collect data by observing social action in close participation with the subjects or by long, unstructured interviews. The level of analysis is not of the system but rather of individual interaction with others, the mind or the self, and meaning. This is microanalysis. The structural-functional and conflict theories, because they focus on systems, are macro analyses.

There are three assumptions characteristic of this perspective: (1) sociology is a science whose purpose is to understand the social meanings of human social action and interaction; (2) reflexivity or intersubjectivity, rather than objectivity or critical analysis, characterizes the relationship between the subject and the researcher; and (3) rich, carefully detailed description and analysis of unique social situations from the perspective of the subjects under investigation is typical of symbolic interactionist research.

The sociological problem to be understood and explained in the symbolic interactionist tradition is the meanings that individuals see in the actions of themselves, of others, of institutions, and so on (Weber, 1968). Analysis of society demands different methods from those used to describe and explain the natural world. It requires methods that attempt to grasp the motives and meanings of social acts. Sociology is

a science that must deal with the subjective meanings of events to social actors.

A good example of work in this perspective is the study of the meaning of the diagnosis of epilepsy within the lives of a sample of people with this disease. *Having Epilepsy* (Schneider and Conrad, 1983) is based on long, semi-structured interviews with a number of people who have been diagnosed with epilepsy. The authors make the point that it is important that sociologists provide an antidote to medical research. It is crucial, they note, to distinguish between disease and illness. Disease is the pathology of the human body; illness is the meaning of the experience associated with a given pathology. In this research the subjects were selected for study because they have epilepsy. However, they live most of the time without the symptoms of the disorder being present. They go about their daily activities, eating, dressing, working, cooking, cleaning, visiting, enjoying leisure and social activities, unrestrained and unconstrained by an awareness of their disease.

Medicine attempts to understand the nature and cause of disease and to formulate methods for its treatment. One of the tasks of the sociologist is to describe the impact of disease and diagnosis on the individual's self and on his or her relationships with others. As Schneider and Conrad say: 'We cannot understand illness experiences by studying disease alone, for disease refers merely to the undesirable changes in the body. Illness, however, is primarily about social meanings, experiences, relationships, and conduct that exist around putative disease' (1983: 205).

Schneider and Conrad suggest that one of the most pervasive aspects of epilepsy is a continuing sense of uncertainty. From the earliest stages of pre-diagnosis and throughout the illness, a sense of uncertainty is a defining quality of this and other chronic conditions. People with epilepsy, as do those with cancer, Alzheimer's disease, or multiple sclerosis (just a few of the chronic conditions to which this analysis is relevant), at first wonder what is happening to their bodies or their minds. They wonder whether or not to take this or that small sign of change as a symptom of a disease. They wonder whether it is a symptom of a serious or a minor disease.

Once diagnosed, they wonder how severe their illness will become and whether they will live for long or only for a short time. They ask whether they will be seriously debilitated or only mildly affected. Relationships are altered. Others respond to this sense of uncertainty with their own confusion about the disorder and its likely course. Not only does relating to the self become tinged with ambiguity arising from dealing with change, but so, too, does relating to others become unclear. The lack of easy, honest, open, and straightforward communication is frequently seen as one of the most painful aspects of the disorder. Cancer patients, for instance, have said that the difficulties of communication (born of uncertainty) are frequently even more painful than the disease or its treatment (Dunkel-Schetter and Wortman, 1982).

Chronic illnesses give rise to several sources of uncertainty. First of all, there is ontological uncertainty. Self-identity arises from interaction with the self (identity and body) and others. When a part of this interactive mix is altered, for instance, when the taken-for-granted health of the body is called into question, so is the self. And so people, when confronted with a disease, disability, or accident, may ask questions such as: Why me? Why not me? Why now? Why this disease? Who am I now that I am a cancer patient? Will I still be a husband/wife/lover? Will I be able to continue working? Will my friends continue to be friends?

Another source of uncertainty surrounding some chronic illnesses is the fact that they are poorly understood both by the medical profession and by the patient and significant others. There is a general lack of knowledge about the probable prognosis of some chronic illnesses. Some chronic diseases receive a considerable

amount of press; others receive very little. Some are well understood by the lay public; most are not. Some have been diagnosable for many, many years. Others, such as Alzheimer's, are relatively recent diagnoses. For some, the norms of possible remissions, plateaus, and disease exacerbations have long been charted. The short history of others means that there are few standards for what to expect.

Epilepsy is a disease with a long history. Like venereal disease and leprosy, and more recently cancer and now AIDS, epilepsy is a disorder that is believed to reflect not just the state of the physical body, but also the moral character of the person. At times the person with epilepsy has been considered to be divine, at other times satanic. At various times and places seizures have been understood as signs both of prophetic ability and of madness.

Chronic illness requires symptom control. This is particularly necessary when the symptoms can be highly disruptive, as in diabetes, which can exhibit diabetic reaction or coma; or in colitis, which may involve unexpected evacuation; or in epilepsy, if there is a grand mal seizure. Symptom control can involve following the doctor's orders. It can also involve non-medical procedures such as biofeedback, hypnosis, diet change, meditation, exercise, relaxation, vitamin therapy, and others. Managing medical regimens does not necessarily mean following the medical rules. Instead, people often manage their medicines according to their own values, habits, activities, relationships, and side effects.

People with epilepsy control their drug use in such a way as to moderate the number and severity of seizures to a level with which they feel comfortable. Doctor's orders are only one of several sources of information upon which people with epilepsy choose to base their use of medication. Drug use patterns develop as an outcome of a complex of self-perceived considerations such as (1) the meaning of the seizure to the subject, (2) the personal view of the effectiveness of the drug,

(3) the personal estimation of the costs of side effects, (4) the desire to test whether the epilepsy is still present, (5) the wish to avoid having others recognize that one has epilepsy, and (6) the need to protect oneself from seizures in particular situations (Schneider and Conrad, 1983).

Relationships within the family and with significant others are also profoundly affected as people work out how to live with a chronic condition. Interaction with employers and employees may be altered. Recreation patterns change. People may need to reorganize their time in order to manage the disease. As interpersonal adjustments are made, revisions to the concept of self frequently are required as the person copes with illness over time.

The work of Schneider and Conrad exemplifies the symbolic interactionist approach to understanding behaviour in health and illness. Through the presentation of quotations from the subject interspersed with sociological analysis, the authors have provided a work with relevance to others in similar health circumstances, to their families, to health-care workers who deal with people with such diagnoses, and to the academic sociological community. Research such as this often has an orientation that can be applied to patients and workers in the health-care field.

Strauss uses a similar methodology, this time explaining the world of the health-care provider, in her study of the caregivers of patients with Alzheimer's disease (1987). It is very difficult to provide a deep, qualitative analysis of the experience of the person who develops this disease. Alzheimer's disease is degenerative, and it affects the mind. At its onset the individual experiences minor symptoms that may be attributed (both by the person himself or herself and by significant others) to the natural course of aging, to an emotional upset, or to a physical illness. But as time goes on the person with Alzheimer's may become more and more forgetful, confused, easily angered, irritable, restless, and agitated. Judgement, speech, and concentration are affected.

Eventually people with this disease may become totally unable to care for themselves.

As Alzheimer's progresses it becomes more and more difficult for the patient to describe his or her experience. A study based on the world views of Alzheimer's patients would thus be very difficult. On the other hand, talking to the person taking care of the patient with Alzheimer's is useful and important for two reasons. In the first place, these people are in the next best position to describe the life of the person with Alzheimer's because they are most closely involved on a daily basis. Second, the role of the caregiver is an under-researched area. As we have noted (see Graham, 1984), home health care has been largely ignored.

Alzheimer's may be one of the most difficult illnesses to deal with. Its course is uncertain and erratic. Caring for the patient can be emotionally and physically exhausting; at a certain point in the course of the disease, an adult may have to be cared for in much the same way as one would care for a helpless infant. The pre-diagnosis stage may be the most difficult time of all. At this stage the family members, as well as the future patient, often know that something is intermittently wrong and yet do not know what it might be. One woman explained her experience of the pre-diagnosis stage as follows: 'Joe was coming home later from work a lot and I would ask him to be a little more considerate and call the next time and he would just yell back at me and we usually just ended up fighting' (Strauss, 1987: 13).

The early stages are characterized primarily by uncertainty. Sometimes behaviours are interpreted as those of normal aging; other times the same behaviours are thought to indicate a serious problem: 'Mom thought dad was just getting miserable and stubborn just like other old people. So it was hard to convince her that dad had a problem and needed help' (ibid., 17). Some of the early symptoms of Alzheimer's are quite similar to some of the common stereotypes of old age. They include short-term memory loss, crankiness, and confusion. The early pre-diagnosis stage is difficult. Patients struggle to manage their symptoms and modify and manage their personal habits. As the disease progresses and symptoms persist and increase, medical advice is often sought.

Diagnosis, however, also involves a difficult and ambiguous process. There are no tests that conclusively prove the presence of Alzheimer's in the sick person. As a result, many caregivers are left with a sense of uncertainty regarding the diagnosis. One of Strauss's respondents talks about this: 'It was a negative diagnosis . . . . she had a thyroid treatment. But it didn't seem to help her mental capacities. Then he sent her to another doctor to see if he could find anything else that could be causing it—but he couldn't. Therefore, it must be Alzheimer's they said' (ibid., 31). And another caregiver said, 'He was never officially diagnosed. After six months of struggling along . . . I said Dr Jones, is it hardening of the arteries or Alzheimer's? All he said was "a little of both." That's as far as any diagnosis went' (ibid., 32).

Once the diagnosis is made, however tentatively, the family caregivers move into a new stage of adaptation. The confusion involved in dealing with an undiagnosed Alzheimer's patient gives way to the fear of inheriting or passing on the disease. One of Strauss's respondents put this fear as follows: 'I've read a lot about Alzheimer's and I feared what lay ahead for him. But my greatest fear was that it was in the genes and it has the tendency to be inherited. But when Jake got it, I became concerned about the grandchildren and the children getting it' (ibid., 35). For some, and in some ways, the diagnosis was finally a relief: 'The diagnosis of Alzheimer's, well, it's like anything. You really don't want to accept it. But at least you do know and you're not hunting anymore. In some ways, it was a relief' (ibid., 36).

A recent paper in the journal *Health* (Payne-Jackson, 1999) illustrates that this methodology is of continuing significance in medical sociology. Payne-Jackson's study documents the differences in the meanings or explanatory models attached to adult-onset diabetes by doctors and patients in Jamaica. This research reinforces the finding that 'biomedical' and 'folk' models of illness are often quite different from one another. Payne-Jackson draws a number of conclusions in her work. Among them is the following pragmatic policy suggestion:

> If doctors hope to be more successful in treating their patients it will be necessary for them to discern how they are being understood and attempt to work with the variations of the models patients actually hold as their life circumstances change. (Ibid., 1999: 38)

Summary

Some examples of symbolic interactionist theory have demonstrated its basic principles. These are that (1) symbolic interactionism is characterized by close attention to the meaningful interaction of social actors; (2) the understandings the subjects of study have of their own situations become the object of investigation; (3) portrayal of the world views of the respondents in their own language is the desired outcome of such research.

Feminist Theory

Feminist theory and feminist methods have grown rapidly in the past two decades. A number of journals are now dedicated to feminist studies in many fields of scholarship. The social sciences, in particular, have been challenged and critiqued as having been male-stream in subject matter, research strategies, and theoretical assumptions. A whole new field called Women's Studies has emerged and become institutionalized in universities, with undergraduate majors and master's and doctoral degrees (Reinharz, 1992; Richardson and Robinson, 1993; Smith, 1993; Stanley and Wise, 1993). Numerous new journals have been established and books have been written and published on all aspects of social life from this perspective. There is a way in which, following Betty Friedan's *The Feminine Mystique*, the women's health movement can be seen as a major impetus to feminist scholarship and policy. The organization of women in the late sixties and seventies for abortion reform, following the liberalization of sexual norms and mores that accompanied the widespread prescription of the birth-control pill, was a crucial step in the second wave of the women's movement in the twentieth century. The women's health movement led to a radical critique of the patriarchal, allopathic medical care system and practice as exemplified by such monumental publications as *Our Bodies, Our Selves* (Boston Women's Health Collective, 1996).

A major theme in a feminist analysis of health has been a criticism of the medicalization of women's lives. Much of this analysis has focused on the dominance of the medical care system, medical practitioners, and the medical constructions of knowledge with regard to reproductive issues such as birth control and childbirth (Oakley, 1984), PMS (Pirie, 1988), and menopause (McCrea, 1983; Kaufert and Gilbert, 1987; Walters, 1991). Others have explained women's (poor) health as a result of social structural inequities, such as class (Doyal, 1979), participation in the labour force (Tierney et al., 1990), or familial and domestic roles (Graham, 1984). Nevertheless, as Vivienne Walters (1992) argues, little research had been done on women's views of their own health problems. To address this lack Walters interviewed 356 women over 21 years old in a community-based survey about their views of their own main health problems and the health-related worries, experiences, and perceptions of women in Canada. The findings of this study stand as a challenge to the widespread understanding and bases of health policy. Whereas key informants for Health Canada have indicated that women's chief health problems were related to their reproductive system, women themselves considered, when asked an unprompted question, their main problems to be

stress (19.7 per cent), arthritis (14.9 per cent), overweight (9.6 per cent), back problems (9.0 per cent), migraines/chronic headaches (8.1 per cent), and blood pressure (8.1 per cent). Only 10.1 per cent of women said that they didn't have any health problems.

Stress, the most important health concern of women, was often associated with family and work responsibilities and worries about money and violence. These issues, while resulting in health concerns, are not best addressed by the medical care system. Nor is it of much value to direct health-related research dollars towards understanding, minimizing, or eliminating these concerns. This example of feminist health research demonstrates several of its basic principles. It begins with the experience of women and asks them to articulate their own views of the issues. It relies on a combination of qualitative and quantitative data collection methods. It challenges the definitions provided by the powerful (in this case, major state health policy and funding bodies).

Summary

Feminist theory and research can be distinguished by several fundamental principles. (1) By virtue of gender, men and women occupy different places in the social structure and live in distinct yet overlapping cultures. (2) Men tend to dominate in all institutions in society. They tend to have more power, more money, and more access to all types of resources. (3) Sociology, including the sociology of health, illness, and medicine, has historically reflected male dominance with respect to subject matter and styles of theorizing and research. (4) Feminist researchers theorize, problematize, describe, and explain the social world so that women and gender are always central foci. More recently, feminists have also realized their own myopia and argue for the necessity of paying attention to class, 'race'/ethnicity, ability/disability, and sexual orientation as fundamental social categories along with gender.

These concerns with gender, class, ethnicity, and so on, while not yet theorized adequately, are increasingly well informed by feminist theory (Coburn and Eakin, 1993).

Sociology of Health in Canada

Much of the literature referred to in this book is based on Canadian populations, but much also is based on populations of other countries—particularly of Great Britain and the United States. The authors cited, too, are primarily from Canada, but also from other countries. The book in sum has general relevance, especially in the components concerned with the sociology of health. In an updated version of a paper first published in *Health and Canadian Society*, Coburn and Eakin (1998) reviewed Canadian literature in this field and drew some interesting conclusions. The authors argued that this subdiscipline, the sociology of health, illness, and medicine, has, to a large extent, mirrored the overall disciplinary trends. On the one hand, the emphasis on applied work parallels the central preoccupations of the discipline, particularly in the US. On the other hand, the growing emphasis on theoretical analysis and development plays a larger role in Canadian work. American work has more frequently focused on socio-psychological variables, such as stress, health locus of control, health behaviour models, and social support, and has tended to use survey research methods. US medical sociology also has leaned towards a more applied approach. Mechanic (1993) evaluated the field in the US and drew the conclusion that there is a shortage of structural and critical analysis. Canadian sociology, as Brym and Fox (1989) have argued, has moved its emphasis from culture to power. Moreover, it has often taken a critical or political-economy approach.

Still, according to Coburn and Eakin (1998: 629), there is room for substantial improvement in health sociology in Canada. It covers a 'wide territory' (ibid.) and 'helps us escape from perspectives which view health and illness as explainable simply as direct responses to changing health care "needs"'. But 'there is much description and measurement, little explanation or theory. . . . The whole is seldom seen as more than a sum of its parts.'

Summary

(1) Illness is experienced in a social context: we learn to think and talk about it with a vocabulary that others share and we learn what to do about it through interactions with family and friends, the formal medical system, and the media.

(2) The sociology of health and illness describes and explains the social causes and consequences of illness, disease, disability, and death. The sociology of medicine is the study of the institutionalized medical recognition of and response to illness.

(3) Sociologists use four main perspectives to study the social world: structural-functional theory, conflict theory, symbolic interactionist theory, and feminist theory. Each of these paradigms has different assumptions about the social world and therefore different ways of understanding it.

(4) Structural-functional theory was first discussed by Émile Durkheim. Its goal is to understand the social causes of social facts; it does this by studying the causal relationships among institutions. The parts of society are inextricably bound together to form a harmonious system. Human beings are constrained by the external world and they are therefore predictable and controllable through the knowledge of social facts.

(5) The origin of the conflict perspective is attributed to Karl Marx. Conflict theorists study competing groups within societies through history. The basic competing forces are the different classes. Conflict theorists are committed to the description and documen-

tation of injustice through the understanding of economic arrangements and their impact on other conditions of social life. In the conflict perspective, it is argued that health and illness are related to the unequal social arrangements found in capitalist, patriarchal societies.

(6) Symbolic interactionist theory is based on the definition of sociology given by Max Weber. Symbolic interactionists attempt to understand the subjective meanings and causes that social actors attribute to events.

The meaning social actors give to their diseases affects their self-concepts and their relationships with others.

(7) The feminist perspective provides a critique of sociology and a corrective to its narrow, neglectful, or biased representations. It attempts to remedy inequities in gender, class, 'race', disability, sexual orientation, and so on.

(8) The sociology of health in Canada is influenced by disciplinary trends in Canadian sociology as a whole.

Questions for Study and Discussion

1. Some people find that when they go away to university, particularly during the first year, they are likely to drink alcohol and to become drunk more often than they had done in the past. Which theories help to explain such behaviours and help you to understand them?

2. Several of your roommates have been taking anti-depressant drugs given to them by the health services doctors at the university health clinic. They do not appear to be taking them appropriately but rather in handfuls when they say they feel depressed or stressed. How would the theories discussed in this chapter help to explain this situation?

3. Male and female students not only tend to enrol in different disciplines, they also tend to use health services at different rates and for different issues. How might the four theories presented in this chapter be used to explain this phenomenon?

4. HIV/AIDS is much more prevalent among people who belong to the economically poorer groups in society. How might this be explained from each theoretical perspective?

5. Power is always an endemic feature of human social interaction. Do any of the theories help us to understand this? Which ones? How?

Suggested Readings

Coburn, David, and J. Eakin. 1998. 'The Sociology of Health in Canada', in Coburn et al. (1998: 619–34). Critical overview of the status of the sociology of health in Canada.

Epstein, Samuel S. 1993. 'Evaluation of the National Cancer Program and Proposed Responses', *International Journal of Health Services* 23, 1: 15–44 Full of detailed documentation regarding the National Cancer program.

Graham, Hilary. 1984. *Women, Health and the Family*. Brighton, Sussex: Wheatsheaf Books. Wonderful, rich

description and analysis of women's home health-care work and how it varies in different social classes.

Kuhn, Thomas. 1962. *The Structure of Scientific Revolutions*. Chicago: University of Chicago Press. Excellent, logically rendered and detailed description of his theory of science.

Navarro, Vincent. 1976. 'Social Class, Political Power and the State and Their Implications for Medicine', *Social Science and Medicine* 10: 437–57. Critical analysis of the dynamics of class in the health-care system.

Parsons, Talcott. 1951. *The Social System*. Glencoe, Ill.:

Free Press. Classic statement of structural functionalism.

Schneider, Joseph, and Peter Conrad. 1983. *Having Epilepsy: The Experience and Control of Illness*. Philadelphia: Temple University Press. Excellent example of symbolic interactionism that describes living with chronic disease—epilepsy.

Sontag, Susan. 1989. *AIDS and Its Metaphors*. Markham, Ont.: Penguin Books. Beautiful, historical, rich description of metaphors and meanings associated with the disease.

| *Ways of Studying Health, Illness, and Medicine Sociologically*

Learning Objectives

- Sociology is done using different methodologies, depending on the theoretical perspective chosen.
- Positivism is based on physics and other natural sciences. It is the method usually chosen within the structural-functional perspective.
- Conflict theory is less concerned about methods per se than are the other theoretical perspectives. It does, however, include an examination of the historical roots of oppression and inequity.
- Symbolic interaction theorists tend to use qualitative methods. They reject the proposed objectivity of the positivists in favour of the assumption that studying human beings involves interaction, meaning, and reflexivity.
- Feminist theorists use all sorts of methods but they highlight the centrality of gender (and class, ethnicity, ability/disability, etc.) in understanding social life, organization, and patterns.

Introduction

How do we come to know what we know? What do we understand to be the most important sociological questions concerning health or medicine? In fact, how do we conceptualize health, illness, and medicine? What assumptions do we make about the nature and essential characteristics of proof in any sociological study? Is sociology a science? Is the scientific approach to knowledge always the best approach? Each of the perspectives discussed in Chapter One encompasses a different picture of the relevant subject matter for the field, a different set of assumptions about the nature of proof, a different strategy for the collection and analysis of the data.

The purposes of this chapter are to describe and analyze critically the methodologies used in the construction of knowledge in the four theoretical paradigms: structural functionalism, conflict theory, symbolic interactionism, and feminist theory. Just as the previous chapter described and illustrated each perspective, this chapter will discuss the ways of knowing and the methods of proof adopted by each perspective. It will clarify the limitations and strengths, the presuppositions, and the consequences of each perspective's methodological strategies.

Positivism

The methodology most often associated with structural functionalism is positivism. Positivism is distinguished by three fundamental presuppositions: (1) sociology is a science that seeks to describe the social world in a series of universal causal laws; (2) this science sees human behaviour as objectively measurable through such methods as survey research and experimental designs; and (3) social facts are to be treated as things because they determine human social behaviour and attitudes through the norms that regulate human behaviour.

Much of the sociology of medicine falls within this paradigm, including studies of (1) who seeks medical services (from doctors, hospitals, etc.), and how frequently; (2) what role is played by such social factors as social norms for defining mental and physical illness; (3) how important social support from family and friends is in preventing, minimizing, or helping to adjust to illness; and (4) what role the quality of life—work, recreation, community, physical activity, occupational conditions—plays in the health and well-being of people. Essentially, positivist studies analyze the relationships between social facts and various sorts of health-related variables.

The two fundamental models of analysis in this paradigm were described in Chapter One. In the first, the one we have called Model A, health-related variables are dependent. For example, there is a well-documented finding that women are more likely to be ill than men; gender is considered the independent variable and illness is considered the dependent variable—the one that is being explained. In the second, Model B, the health-related variable is the independent variable and the study would be concerned with the impact of differences in health on a social factor. Examples of Model B research might be stud-

ies that examine the impact of changes in health status, such as serious illness, on income level. Here are just a few of the many socio-psychological and demographic variables that may be selected for study: age, sex, gender role, marital and family status, ethnicity, race, social class, occupation, education, social support, and beliefs about the disease and its curability. It must be emphasized that the preceding list is not by any means inclusive.

In these models of research, a variable can be causal in one study and caused in another. However, before *causal connections* can be determined and verified, at least four conditions must be met. They are:

1. that there is an association between the variables;
2. that there is evidence that one variable precedes the other in a time sequence;
3. that other, potentially intervening, variables can be eliminated;
4. that the relationship makes theoretical sense.

Furthermore, causal relationships may involve more than two variables at a time. Such complex modelling of the relationship between independent and dependent variables is called multivariate analysis; when causal ordering is tested, it is called path modelling. Path modelling involves assumptions about the time sequence of a number of variables that either affect the dependent variable directly or affect other variables and through them the dependent variable. Figure 2.1 illustrates the theoretical logic of path modelling.

In the illustration each arrow is meant to indicate a direct causal connection (e.g., gender causes or has an effect on quality of housing). The model in Figure 2.1 suggests that illness can be conceptualized as the end result of a chain of variables that operate together. There are both direct relationships and indirect relationships. An example of a direct relationship is the one between gender and working conditions. For

Figure 2.1   Hypothetical Path Model

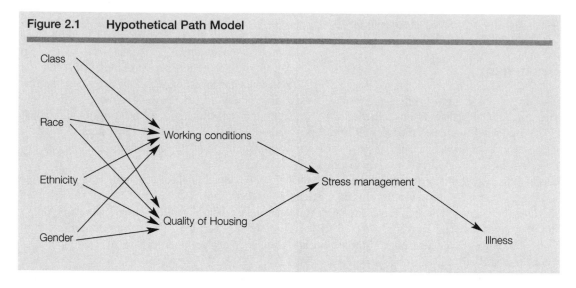

instance, it might be hypothesized that women are paid less than men for full-time work. An example of an indirect relationship is one between class and stress management: for example, it might be hypothesized that members of the working class tend to have longer working hours and therefore less time available to learn or use stress-management techniques.

Epidemiology

Epidemiology, the study of the causes and distribution of disease, is one example of a positivist methodology. Some argue that epidemiology is not a type of sociology. To the extent that the purpose of epidemiology is to understand disease patterns in order to minimize or alleviate their effects, it is not sociology. However, to the extent that social labelling of disease, social relations, and social-structural positions of people are considered relevant subjects for the analysis of *disease incidence* (the number of new cases of a disease in a given period of time) and *prevalence* (the number of cases of disease in a population), then it can be considered to be an example of one use of sociology.

Epidemiological investigation began in the last century when the prevalent diseases seemed to be contagious and infectious diseases. Patterns of human contact were obviously relevant in studying the incidence of these diseases. The discovery of bacteria and their connection with disease raised hopes that clear and observable cause and effect relationships would be found in all diseases. There are several interesting, classic examples of early 'epidemiological' work. Sir John Snow is said to have done the first epidemiological research when he noted that a good proportion of the people who became ill with cholera had drunk water from the same water pump. Later, Sir Percival Pott discovered that scrotal cancer was prevalent among chimneysweepers. Further investigation led him to the conclusion that the extensive bodily exposure to soot, which was a necessary part of the work of the chimneysweeper, was implicated in the development of cancer in the scrotum.

One of the most important contemporary examples of epidemiological research concerns AIDS—acquired immune-deficiency syndrome. The following is a brief illustration of some of the methodologies involved in the epidemiological investigation of this disease. In this case, AIDS is the dependent variable. It is the causes of AIDS,

Box 2.1   Severe Acute Respiratory Syndrome (SARS)

With globalization there is increased concern about the potentially devastating effects of any new contagious disease becoming epidemic. One recent example of a new disease, which was quickly identified and brought under a relative degree of international control, is the syndrome now called severe acute respiratory syndrome or SARS. On 12 March 2003 the World Health Organization (WHO) issued a global alert about cases of atypical pneumonia. By 16 March the new health concern had a name, SARS, and by 17 March WHO was already beginning to coordinate an international effort to identify and treat SARS. On 22 March the SARS virus was isolated and a new and reliable diagnostic test was found. As of 14 May 2003 the worldwide total of SARS cases was 7,628 and the number of deaths was 587. As a result of the highly effective tracking and public health preventative measures put in place, by 6 May the incidence of new cases worldwide seemed to have ceased. The speed at which international efforts appear to have been effective is particularly important given the severity and the high rate of fatality of 14–15 per cent associated with SARS.

Source: World Health Organization, at: <www.who.int/csr/sars/country/2003-05-14/en/print.hcml>.

the independent variables, that are being sought. As you will see as you read through the following case study, the first issue in the epidemiological analysis was the definition of the strange new disease syndrome that was later called AIDS. In all positivistic research, one of the first and most important steps is the accurate, precise, valid, and reliable description of each of the relevant variables.

In the late spring of 1981, several doctors in Los Angeles noticed what seemed to be a surprising medical mystery. In the previous six months they had among them treated five young men with pneumocystic carinii pneumonia (PCP). This was a very rare infection. Even more unusual was the finding that all these men had other 'opportunistic infections', which had normally only been seen in organ-transplant patients whose immune systems had been intentionally depressed to aid the body's adoption of the new organ. All five men were homosexual. The doctors reported these unusual circumstances in the 5 June 1981 issue of the *Morbidity and Mortality Weekly Report* (MMWR) published by the Centers for Disease Control (CDC) in Atlanta, Georgia. At about the same time, a New York doctor called the CDC about an unusual number of cases of Karposi's sarcoma (KS). The 3 July 1981 issue of MMWR reported that 26 cases of Karposi's sarcoma had been diagnosed in New York and California in the previous 30 months. All 26 men were homosexual, their ages ranging from 26 to 51. Four also had PCP. Eight died within two years of the diagnosis of KS.

In reaction to these remarkable findings, the CDC established an epidemiological research program designed to investigate systematically the prevalence and incidence of PCP and KS and to look for any possible explanatory patterns. They chose to examine hospital records, tumour registries, and the records of medical doctors in certain cities selected because of their differing proportions of homosexuals. Next they interviewed as many patients as possible, using fairly wide-ranging interview schedules, during which they gathered information about the patients' lifestyles, sexual behaviour, drug use, and medical history. It was quickly discovered that most of the patients used 'poppers', such as amyl and butyl nitrates, as sexual stimulants.

The researchers designed a case-control study to compare diseased and healthy homosexuals in order to identify risk factors. With 20-page questionnaires as guides, the investigators studied 50 homosexual men with the illness(es) and 120 healthy homosexual men. The 60–90-minute interviews covered medical histories, drug use, sexual behaviour, occupation, travel, family history, and other lifestyle issues. In addition, the researchers collected various types of biological specimens for comparison.

After months of detailed analysis, these findings were noted: the diseased men (1) had more sexual partners; (2) were more likely to frequent bathhouses; (3) had histories of syphilis and hepatitis; and (4) were more frequent users of marijuana and cocaine. 'Poppers' seemed equally popular in both groups. The major conclusions of the study were that (1) the disease could be transmitted through the blood or semen; (2) patients tended to engage in frequent, anonymous sex; and (3) these sex practices often produced abrasions that exposed them to small amounts of blood, semen, and feces.

A year after the first questions about this new disease were raised, 216 cases had been reported to the CDC: 84 per cent were male homosexuals, 9 per cent were intravenous drug users, 2 per cent were Haitians, and 5 per cent were women. Eighty-eight of the patients had died. The common cause had yet to be discovered. Some thought that it was a new virus, others believed 'poppers' to be the cause, and yet others favoured a theory of overload to the immune system. The Haitian background of some of the diseased did not fit into any theory. Later the syndrome was found in hemophiliacs and in a 20-month-old boy who had received a blood transfusion from an AIDS patient. Still later, female sexual partners of AIDS patients and children of at-risk group members were found with the disease. As knowledge of the types of people found to suffer from AIDS grew, so, too, did the incidence grow—astonishingly quickly.

Looking for the causes of AIDS also involved the search for an accurate, precise, working definition of the disease. The operating definition that was developed included three criteria: (1) the patient must be under 60 years old and (2) have a specific diagnosed disease, such as PCP or KS, suggesting an underlying cellular immune deficiency, and (3) the disease had to occur without the presence of an immune deficiency that could be ascribed to another factor. Epidemiological research verified that there was no incidence of a disease fitting these characteristics until 1978 (Devita et al., 1985).

The process of tracing the development of AIDS and isolating causal factors is still continuing. Researchers today are concerned not only with documenting the spread of the disease, but also with predicting it. Increasingly, complicated statistical models are being developed to help predict the future of AIDS.

In addition, a number of methodological problems limit the potential predictive power of any model, no matter how complex. First, there seem to be a number of somewhat different AIDS epidemics happening at the same time, in different places, with somewhat different spread patterns, with different specific associated diagnoses, and so on. Second, there appear to be two periods when an individual is highly infectious: one shortly after the disease is contracted, another when he or she begins to show symptoms. Third, the length of time a person can have the disease before symptoms are observed is unknown. Fourth, reporting rates vary tremendously among different cultural groups, medical systems, public health regions, and so on. Fifth, changes in the spread of the disease, and thus the risk of getting it, are dependent on choices, most especially about sexual behaviour, that individuals make today, tomorrow, and thereafter. All these are influenced by a myriad of social structures, such as economics, politics, family practices, and gender. All may change in response to changes in any of these social structures. Epidemiological research into AIDS, therefore, has been and continues to be a very complicated and multi-faceted procedure.

The above case study provides an illustration of epidemiology, one type of positivistic research. Recent research on the spread of AIDS demonstrates a more theoretically based *historical materialist epidemiology*. The focus of this research is compatible with conflict theory. This approach assumes the primacy of economic conditions and practices in the explanation of health outcomes. In an attempt to understand the rapidity of the spread of AIDS in Africa, Hunt (1989) related its incidence to the ways in which people in eastern, southern, and central Africa make a living. In particular, he investigated the impact of the migratory labour system, which is accompanied by long absences of workers from their families, increased family breakdown, and an increased number of sexual partners. These patterns have historically resulted in recurrent epidemics of heterosexually based sexually transmitted diseases. Now these labour force demands are associated with a higher incidence and prevalence of HIV and AIDS. Here AIDS is primarily a heterosexually based disease and has been called Type II AIDS. Type II AIDS, characterized by a 1:1 ratio (male to female), is the typical 'type' in less-developed countries. By contrast, in the developed world Type I AIDS, with a much higher proportion of men, predominates. In Canada, incidence was 18.4 cases per 100,000 in men as compared with 1.2 per 100,000 in women in 1998. Among children it was 0.4 cases per 100,000 in 1994 as compared to 0.2 in 1985 (Frank, 1996: 6). As will be discussed in Chapter Three, however, the incidence is growing more rapidly among women than among men in Canada. Moreover, in Canada the disease is predominant among men who have sex with men although this pattern, too, is changing. Hunt (1989) is among those who argue that policies related to globalization maintain the dependence of the developing world on the developed world and are fundamental to the epidemic spread of Type II AIDS in the less-developed countries.

Table 2.1 summarizes the assumptions of positivistic science.

Conflict Theory

Have you ever been ill because you lacked nutritious food, a warm place to live, or clean, comfortable, and adequate clothing? Have you ever developed a cold because your family couldn't afford boots to keep your feet warm and dry in the snow and cold of the winter? Have you ever developed emphysema because you worked with asbestos in a factory producing fire-retardant fabrics? Have you ever had a lung disease because you smoked cigarettes? Have you ever known someone who was killed in a car accident because of excessive alcohol consumption? Have you ever had an allergic reaction to a prescribed drug such as penicillin? Do you know anyone who has suffered from the effects of thalidomide, DES (the drug diethylstilbestrol), or valium? Have you ever had unnecessary surgery? Have you ever eaten contaminated food and suffered food poisoning? Have you ever suffered ill health because you lacked clean drinking water?

All these health problems are related to unequal social arrangements that are present in North America and in other parts of the world. Social conflict theory predicates behavioural patterns on power differences in society resulting from class, gender, and other inequities: the poor, women, Native people, etc. have unequal access to rewards and to health-promoting resources. The poor are more likely to be ill than the rich. They have a shorter life expectancy than those with more resources. People in less-developed countries are more likely to suffer the effects of malnutrition, of impure drinking water, and of fatal infectious diseases than are people in developed countries. Women are more often prescribed addictive drugs such as valium and other mood-altering pharmaceuticals for their problems than are men. Men have been more likely to smoke cigarettes and to suffer such repercussions

Table 2.1	Methodological Assumptions of Positivist Social Science
Objectivity	Social science can be as objective as physical science and should be modelled on the physical sciences.
Generalizability	One of the most important goals of social science is to generalize and thereby to describe the world in a series of 'if x then y' causal laws.
Validity: Construct	It is possible to design measures that accurately and briefly describe sociological concepts.
Validity: Internal	It is possible in any social scientific research design to say with a degree of surety that 'x' is the probable cause of 'y'.
Validity: External	It is possible to select a sample so that generalization from the sample to the total population is accurate with a known but limited amount of error.
Reliability	It is possible for the same research to be completed in different settings and by different researchers and with essentially the same findings.
Causality	It is possible to demonstrate probable causal relationships between social science variables.
Adequacy	The data collected adequately describe and explain the phenomenon under investigation.
Data Collection Strategies	The usual data collection strategy involves survey research with either a questionnaire or an interview, either administered in person or over the telephone. Experimental laboratory research is sometimes done.
Quantification	The incidence of sociological phenomena can be quantified in statistical data.
Probability	Analysis is based on assumptions of probability, not determinism, i.e., hypotheses are put forward as probabilities.

as a higher mortality rate from lung cancer than women, though the incidence of women who smoke is increasing dramatically. Women are more likely than men to fall ill from any number of causes throughout their lives. Men are more likely than women to die from homicide, suicide, and motor vehicle accidents. People who stand in different positions in the social structure have correspondingly different levels of health and different rates of health-care use.

What methods are used to demonstrate and explain findings such as those above? What responsibility does the researcher have to attempt to change the sorts of injustice he/she is committed to discovering? The methods used by conflict theorists can be distinguished from those of structural functionalism and symbolic interactionism in the following ways. Conflict theorists

tend to believe that: (1) sociological research—indeed, all knowledge—is limited by the perspective derived from the place in the social system of those who develop knowledge and those who receive and interpret it; (2) research should be comparative and historical in scope; (3) it is impossible for research to be objective; and (4) understanding inequalities arising from class and gender differences is the foremost purpose of such research.

Several examples of research within this perspective will be presented in illustration. One is a general analysis of medicalization: the tendency for more and more areas of people's behaviour to be subject to medical intervention as an outgrowth of industrialization. This analysis also involves a critique of the growing power of the medical care system and its institutions to affect the lives of individuals, groups, and societies.

Ivan Illich has offered an influential critique of medicalization in *Limits to Medicine* (1976). His argument is that contemporary medical practice is *iatrogenic*, that is, it creates disease and illness even as it provides medical assistance. Three sorts of iatrogenesis are isolated and explained.

[It is] clinical, when pain, sickness, and death result from the provision of medical care; it is social, when health policies reinforce an industrial organization which generates dependency and ill health; and it is structural, when medically sponsored behaviour and delusions restrict the vital autonomy of people by undermining their competence in growing up, caring for each other and aging. (Illich, 1976: 165)

Clinical iatrogenesis, that is, injury and/or disability that results directly from the work of the doctor in the hospital or in the clinic, is the first problem addressed by Illich. Addictions to prescribed drugs, the side effects of prescribed drugs, harmful drug interactions, and suicide resulting from prescribed medication are specific examples of clinical iatrogenesis. Thalidomide, prescribed in the 1950s and 1960s in West Germany, Canada, and elsewhere to women with a history of miscarriage, resulted in untold tragedy when numerous children were born without limbs. DES (diethylstilbestrol), again prescribed (in the 1950s) to women with obstetric problems, has been found to result in thousands of cases of ovarian and cervical cancer in the daughters of those who used DES, and in other cancers in their sons. Unnecessary hysterectomies have caused extensive emotional, marital, and other social problems for the women who have undergone this procedure, as well as for their family members and significant others. Breast silicone implants have been found to be associated with numerous and various deleterious health outcomes (Rachlis and Kushner, 1993). Today, millions receive chemotherapy, radiation, and/or surgery as treatment for a variety of cancers. However, such treatments are often felt by the patients to be more painful than the disease itself. Those for whom a cure is effective may feel that the cost is worth the pain. On the other hand, those who are not cured, and whose lives can only be extended for a limited period, may regret having submitted to such treatments as chemotherapy. The spread of HIV/AIDS and hepatitis C through blood transfusions from Canada's blood supply is one of our most recent widely known examples of clinical iatrogenesis. These are just a few of the troubles that occur in an over-medicalized clinical practice.

In the developing world, sanitation, unsafe drinking water, malnutrition, and insufficient and/or dangerous birth control measures are the major health problems. However, large parts of the health budgets of poor nations are spent on drugs that do little to alleviate any of these problems. Substantial expenditures for pharmaceuticals by less-developed countries minimize and prevent expenditures for clean water, the development of a good agricultural base, and the promotion of safe and inexpensive birth-control devices and practices.

Social iatrogenesis is evident in the impact of medicine on lifespans. Medical and technological intervention begins at birth and ends with the care of the aging and dying. There are medical specialties to deal with pregnancy and childbirth (obstetrics), childhood (pediatrics), adult women (gynecology), the elderly (geriatrics), and the dying (palliative care). The presence of medical specialists to deal with various normal stages of the human lifespan is symbolic of the trend towards the medicalization of life and the increasing addiction of modern people to medical institutions.

The most onerous example of medicalization is the growing dependence on care in Western industrialized societies. The huge growth in spending on medical treatment, on hospitalization, and on pharmaceuticals is just one example of this. The earlier success of medicalization has played a part in the generation of the 'risk' society. 'In this view, risks are increasingly globalized and generalized in ways which are seen as out of the individual's control, bolstering the social and political significance of scientific institutions and expert knowledge represented by, for instance, medicine' (Howson, 1998: 196). Who in modern society is not aware of the myriad risks associated with just living? Air, water, and land pollution compete with fatty diets, botulism and dangerous bacteria in food, pesticide residues, excess alcohol consumption, and even sunshine as things we have to 'watch out for'. Public health policies are frequently based on 'prevention', which is really early detection. Examples such as screening for breast, cervical, testicular, and prostate cancer leap easily to mind. Such surveillance increases the development of 'risk consciousness'. Avoiding risks and maintaining health have become moral imperatives (Lupton, 1995; Howson, 1998).

Considerable evidence suggests that pharmaceuticals are often prescribed to people for social and psychological problems. Women consistently receive more prescriptions for tranquilizers than men do. Moreover, women in the middle and older age groups are at highest risk. Over a period of some 19 months in Saskatchewan, researchers noted that one in seven of the population received a prescription for diazepam (the generic name for valium). Yet research has found that the majority of those who used tranquilizers explained that they needed the valium because of a variety of societal, familial, and occupational demands and expectations rather than physical need (Cooperstock and Lennard, 1979). Women's very bodily shape and appearance have become medically diagnosable by plastic surgeons who recently instituted a new disease category—small breast syndrome. Cosmetic surgeons now offer designer vaginas. Naomi Wolfe in *The Beauty Myth* (1991) says that medical discourse tells women that beauty is, in fact, the equivalent to good health.

By *structural iatrogenesis* Illich means the loss of individual autonomy and the creation of dependency. The responsibility for good health has been wrested from the individual as a result of the imposition of the medical model—the prevalence of medical institutions and medical practitioners. Pain, suffering, disease, and death are important experiences for all human beings. They can encourage the development of service, compassion, and connectedness with others. But medical bureaucracy and technology minimize the possibilities for the fertile development of family and community-based models of care. The medical model and its institutions usurp individual initiative and responsibility and thus destroy humanism and spiritual development. In sum, in Illich's view, we rely excessively on medical care and this overdependence has many destructive consequences for people and their communities. To correct this problem he advocates the deprofessionalization and debureaucratization of medical practice, and the maximization of individual responsibility. Self-care, autonomy, and self-development should be the guiding principles.

Navarro, a leading Marxist critic of medicalization, takes issue with Illich's explanation. Whereas Illich's main foe appears to be the bureaucratic organization and growth in the numbers of medical practitioners and medicine-related industry, Navarro (1976) argues that medicine is a mere pawn in the hands of a much greater power—the power of the state directed through the dominant class. The health industry in the United States is neither administered nor controlled by medical professionals. Members of the corporate class (the owners and managers of financial capital) dominate in health and other important spheres of the economy. The upper middle class (executive and corporate representatives of middle-sized enterprises and professionals, primarily corporate lawyers and financiers) have major influence in the health delivery sector of the economy through the pharmaceutical/medical device, medical insurance, and medical organizations for service delivery industries.

Together these groups comprise less than 20 per cent of the health-care providers, yet they control most of the health institutions. The majority of those involved in health care (about 80 per cent) have no control over either the production or consumption of health services.

David Coburn is one of Canada's foremost medical sociologists working in the tradition of conflict theory. He argues that while the power of the state has been more or less visible at various times, the state has had and continues to have considerable power in the determination of the degree of medical dominance. The process of state-professional activities, he notes, has been altered by universal health care. Once the state began to finance health insurance plans, the relations between it and medicine and other health occupations changed. The state began to 'directly affect medical dominance through its attempts to rationalize health care' (Coburn et al., 1997). The numerous debates among doctors and nurses and the provinces and federal government attest to the conflicts that continue in these arenas. Medical organizations, however, are not only influenced and constrained by state policies but also by the public at large and their wishes. Recently, the College of Physicians and Surgeons in Ontario was severely criticized for ignoring the sexual abuse of patients by physicians. At the same time, medical dominance is declining, because of the growth of its competitors in the complementary and alternative medical field and an increase in power of the state: 'We argue that the state in Ontario is increasingly controlling both the context, and more indirectly, the content of medical care. Physician fees, incomes, number and modes of representation have all been affected' (ibid., 1997: 18).

The writings of Illich, Navarro, and Coburn et al. illustrate conflict methodology. A position is taken with regard to injustice, and then documentation of the injustice is found in both historical and other available evidence. Another type of conflict research uses a more positivistic methodology, including questionnaires and interviews as well as available statistics, to document injustice. Some of the studies of class and illness described in Chapter Four and elsewhere in this book illustrate this aspect of conflict methodology.

A persistent theme in the criticism of health and medical care is that sickness has societal origins. Some social arrangements generate the potential for disease and death. Certain social structural positions determine the likelihood of the type of illness or disease and the incidence of death. Social class, age, gender, race, ethnicity, and region are all correlated with particular health and illness profiles. People who differ in social background have differing rates of various types of illness, of illness in general, and of mortality. When the explanation for this inequity focuses on capitalism, it is usually Marxist; when it focuses on gender relations, the explanation is usually feminist. In either instance, the focus on inequity and the type of explanation offered make this research an example of conflict theory rather than of structural functionalism.

The common theme in conflict research, as outlined in Table 2.2, is that it is impossible to do objective research, and that historical analysis of power/class/gender relations provides an appropriate scheme for understanding the true dynamics of social relations.

Symbolic Interactionism

Symbolic interactionist sociology can be thought of as sociology from the inside. Its focus is on the world views and the meanings given to reality by the subjects of study. Definitions and understandings of social circumstances made by social actors are the topic of analysis. Several characteristics distinguish the methods of symbolic interactionist sociology. All are based on the assumption that a science of human subjects must take into account the particular character of unique social actors embedded in discrete situations. Therefore, symbolic interactionism consid-

Table 2.2	Methodological Assumptions of Conflict Theory
Value Commitment	Rather than seeking objectivity, the conflict theorist believes that sociologists must discover, document, and record recurrent patterns and dynamics of power/class/gender relations both because they have no choice (members of a society are committed to the ongoing action of the society) and because they believe that this is the morally correct position.
Historical Specificity	Rather than looking for generalizations, conflict theorists assert the necessity of understanding the unique features of the particular situation in its socio-historical context as an example of these recurrent patterns of power/class/gender relations.
Validity: Construct	Formal tests of validity are considered irrelevant. Researchers, it is assumed, of necessity study what they claim they are studying.
Validity: Internal	Formal statistical tests of causal relationships are not always necessary. Rather, logical meaningfulness may be the relevant criterion of causality.
Validity: External	The conflict theorist assumes that inequities based on power/class/gender relations are ubiquitous, yet analyzes the components separately in each historical situation.
Ethical Concerns	The primary importance in the research of the conflict theorist is the commitment to such ethical and humanitarian principles as justice and equality.
Data Collection	The usual sources of data are historical documents. As well, the conflict theorist may use other data collection methods, including surveys, statistical data, and methods such as unstructured interviews and participant observation that provide subjective and descriptive data.
Objectivity	Objectivity is not possible. Knowledge cannot be separated from the power/class/gender relations of the researcher and the subjects.
Quantification	While numerical data may be used to document an argument, they are not always considered necessary.

ers that: (1) sociology is a science whose purpose is to understand the social meanings of human social action and interaction; (2) reflexivity or intersubjectivity, rather than objectivity, characterizes the relationship between the subject and the researcher because human subjects construct meanings out of social contexts, or to some extent, create each situation anew; (3) rich, carefully rendered, intimate detail, description, and analysis of unique situations are the ultimate goal of study within this paradigm.

Research within this perspective is often based on intensive participant observation of a medical setting (for classic empirical examples, see Scully, 1980; Sudnow, 1967; Fisher, 1986; Goffman, 1963), long, unstructured interviews (see, e.g., Schneider and Conrad, 1983), or close analysis of language in context (Raffel, 1979). Other work is essentially autobiographical, such as that of Rose Weitz (1999), who described her experience and that of her family when her brother-in-law was severely burned and later died in an occupational accident, and Arthur Franks (1991), who told his own story of his diagnoses with heart disease and then cancer. What is common to these methods is the focus on the world views of the subjects of study. When the method is participant observation, a number of possible roles can be taken by the researcher, depending on whether she/he gives precedence to the observer role or the participation itself. These are: (1) complete observer, (2) complete participant, (3) observer as participant, and (4) participant as observer. When a hypothesis is to be tested by participant observation (or other inductive research strategies), the conditions of proof are very exacting. Called negative case analysis, this mode of proof requires that every single piece of evidence must support the hypothesis (Judd et al., 1991). As the data are collected, the researcher must make an effort to find a negative example, and if one is found, must revise the hypothesis accordingly. This form of proof to confirm a hypothesis uses deterministic logic based on the assumption that a variable must always cause or be associated with another variable. Deterministic logic contrasts with the probabilistic logic of positivism, which merely asserts the probability that the two variables are associated.

The data collected within this perspective are usually qualitative rather than quantitative. Positivism, in particular, is usually very exacting in its use of numerical data because these are used in sophisticated statistical analysis. However, symbolic interactionism tends to use numerical data for descriptive rather than analytic purposes. But data more usually consist of detailed descriptions of events and lengthy quotations, frequently from the subject of study.

A central justification for the use of the symbolic interactionist paradigm in sociological research is the focus on *meanings*. A study of the conceptualization of meanings in the process of adapting to a cancer diagnosis and subsequent treatment illustrates this approach. The research is based on qualitative interviews with 38 people diagnosed as having cancer (Fife, 1994). Among the meaningful impacts of the disease were those that related specifically to self-meaning. These included: the loss of personal control, threats to self-esteem or self-worth, and change in body image. The loss of personal control is illustrated by the following comments: 'You just have to put yourself in their hands and trust them to do their best for you'; 'the most difficult thing about having cancer is never knowing when it's over with. There's no way to "close the book".' The loss of self-worth is seen in such comments as: 'I feel

like, you know, like I'm not much good to anybody anymore' and 'I'm not the person that I was and that hurts me quite a bit.' It is notable, however, that changes in self-esteem are not always negative and can be quite positive, as the following shows: 'I feel that maybe I'm a stronger person for having gone through cancer so far. I have sort of taken charge, emotionally I think I'm stronger and I can cope with anything now' (ibid., 312, 313). Changes in body image that may result from both the treatment and the disease are another issue. Consider, for example, the comments of a 51-year-old male police officer with lung cancer: 'Going to work without my hair was one of the hardest things I have ever had to do in my life. It marks you as someone with cancer' (ibid., 313).

Research within the symbolic interactionist tradition often acknowledges the existence of reflexivity—the interaction between the researcher and the subject. The notion of reflexivity is based on the assumption and realization that it is impossible for human beings to 'study' other human beings with complete objectivity. This is true particularly in a situation where a researcher is interviewing, observing, or relating directly to research participants. Thus, in field research or participant observation the researcher is inevitably faced with being marginal to the ongoing interaction being observed, as well as being inextricably bound up in the dynamics of the scene under observation. Access to one side of a conflict, for example, often prevents access to another side.

Such marginality—the experience of belonging neither entirely in the shoes of the researcher nor entirely in the shoes of the subjects—is an inevitable dilemma for the field researcher (Shaffir et al., 1980). 'Going native', or becoming a member of the social group that one is studying, is always a potential problem in fieldwork when the researcher becomes deeply involved. On the other hand, at the minimum, a certain degree of closeness is necessary for the researcher

Table 2.3	Methodological Assumptions of Symbolic Interactionist Social Science
Reflexivity	Social researchers interpret the sayings and behaviour of their subjects from the subject's own perspectives and within the context of the researcher's own perspective. The researchers are affected by the needs and expectations of their subjects and the subjects' knowledge of the data collection process, and at the same time, they change the subjects' understanding. Thus it is impossible to measure human social behaviour objectively.
Ethical Concerns	Just as it is impossible to study human social action as if it were the action of so many atoms, molecules, neutrons, and protons, so it is impossible not to change the social situation that is the subject of the analysis.
Generalizability	While the method of analytic induction, one of the operating logics of this perspective, claims universality, most research in this paradigm is based on the specificity of human social action.
Causality	Causality is recognized in this perspective as a subject of study, e.g., 'I believe I have cancer because I sinned against God', rather than the 'if x . . . then y' causality of positivism.
Proof	The most stringent criterion of proof is sometimes required within this perspective— negative case analysis.
Validity	Validity is always hampered by intersubjectivity, but the depth and detail of the description of the data and their 'meanings' are considered important criteria.
Reliability	This is considered less important than validity because it is assumed that different researchers would be researching different situations and would therefore have (at least somewhat) different findings.
Scope of Analysis	The symbolic interactionist sociologist is generally content to describe the social world of a small population of people in rich complexity and detail.
Advocacy	Some symbolic interactionists view their work as advocacy (e.g., Millman, 1977; Scully, 1977). Others fervently argue for the value of knowledge for its own sake.

to be able to describe the world as it looks to the subjects of research. Gaining access or getting close to subjects and to their social world is also a significant challenge in fieldwork. Whether to introduce oneself as a social researcher, a historian, a social worker, or in some other role is a question that must be addressed and answered before the research begins. Learning how to spend time with the subjects; determining the desired depth or intimacy of the involvement; becoming aware of the language, habits, and locations of the subjects; and deciding which section of the community or institution to contact first: these are among the issues faced by field researchers. When leaving the field and presenting research findings, participant observers and others who develop close relationships with their research participants must consider a number of ethical questions: What are the responsibilities of the researcher to the community and the people in it? How can the anonymity of the subjects be guaranteed when the results of the study are reported? How can the sociologist be assured that the research will not cause harm to any of the participants? Does the researcher have a responsibility to try to improve the situations of the subjects? (ibid.).

Symbolic interactionism is a qualitative method based on the assumption that the meanings people attach to social actions must be the subject matter of the discipline. Table 2.3 highlights the basic features of this methodology.

Feminist Theory/Methodology

Are the worlds of men and women different? In what ways? Do men and women relate to their bodies differently? Do their doctors? Are women more likely to be involved in the domestic health sphere? Do they spend more hours in household-based work and family caretaking? And are such differences complicated by ethnicity, class, and power? Are women more likely to be prescribed mood-altering drugs? Do black women, while having a lower morbidity rate from breast cancer, have a higher mortality rate from breast cancer? Do poorer people live shorter lives? Do those with less power suffer more illness? These are the types of questions addressed within this perspective. Feminist methodologies and their logical corollaries in relation to ethnicity, class, and power are built on the observation of two features of gender organization—differentiation and inequity. Feminists argue that the institution of medicine operates to maintain the subordinate position of women in a patriarchal society. Indeed, medicine's dominance, in this view, maintains and constrains women's experience by providing a male medical conceptualization of and vocabulary for women's bodies and their functioning.

Feminist methods often transform positivist methods by critiquing such issues as objectivity, the purposes for research, and the like. They are based on a number of challenges to positivism (Clarke, 1992). The first is from the work of sociologists in the interactionist and ethnomethodological traditions. This work has emphasized how individuals as social actors continually create social reality as they interact with other social actors. From this perspective it became clear that the 'meaning' of an event varied, depending on the viewpoint (structural and cultural positions) of the social actor. The second challenge to positivism was from the work of Thomas Kuhn (1962), who demonstrated that science is not best represented as the continual accumulation of truths in the search for the ultimate causal explanations of the social and physical world. Rather, Kuhn represents the history of science as a history of growth and development in one hegemonic tradition followed by a challenge to this tradition. Thus, the development of science could be understood as consisting of revolts against findings, methods, and other aspects of scientific convention rather than simply the accumulation of truths. Third, the findings of quantum physics in the twentieth century emphasized the impossibility of an objective outside observer because of the profound universal interconnection of the subject and the object. Fourth is the challenge of the second wave of the women's movement in the second half of the twentieth century. The medical profession was among the first of the institutions challenged by the new feminism. Childbirth reform, including more 'natural' childbirth, home birth, and midwifery, and safe, accessible abortion have been among the issues fought for by the feminist movement as women seek to control their own bodies. Current legislation and public consciousness about (and in opposition to) violence against women, sexual assault, and harassment are some of the current issues in the struggle of women to reclaim their bodies.

Feminist research generally, in keeping with the fundamental principles elucidated above, focuses on gender as a significant social category worthy of extensive analysis. Equally important, research usually asks women to describe their own experiences and their own viewpoints regarding health issues. Currie (1988) takes issue with an exclusive focus on women's personal experience, which has characterized some versions of feminist research at the expense of social structural explanations. Instead of promoting a single focus on women's experience, she argues that feminist research should follow the course of inductive theorizing and theory-testing based on women's views and their interpretations of their experiences. In her work on reproductive decision-making, Currie noted that when women discussed their decision-making regarding whether they would have children or not their explanations could at first be considered to be private troubles or personal issues. For instance, when a woman says that she doesn't want children because they're too expensive she is making a statement about private troubles. However, these 'private troubles' can easily be understood as the result of social structural limitations due to, for example, workplace and family organization, support structures, and pay scales. Bridging the gap between structural and personal issues allows social scientists to see how solutions to opportunities and constraints are individually negotiated.

Pirie (1988) critiques current theory in medical sociology that emphasizes the patriarchal nature of the medical system and its dominance of women's experience of their bodies. She asks how it is that some women more than others, and women at some times but not others, may adopt or reject a medical definition of reality. Noting illnesses about which there is at least some dispute, such as premenstrual syndrome, she questions the processes whereby some conditions acquire medical legitimacy while others may not. To compensate for the overemphasis on structural influences on women's medicalization, Pirie argues for further analysis of '(1) the productional activities of dominant groups with commercial and or political self-interests in medical labelling; (2) the productional activities of those adopting the label; and (3) the cultural pathways or determinants which predispose the collective adoption of some illness categories, and not others' (ibid., 629). In other words, first Pirie advocates sociological research on strategies used by doctors and medical device and pharmaceutical industries to persuade the laity of the existence of certain diseases and of appropriate treatments for these diseases. Second, she suggests a new line of sociological research on how women come to adopt medical definitions of reality, with varying degrees of skepticism and acceptance. Third, she argues for studies of cultural forces, such as the

mass media, and how they work to promote the legitimization of some illnesses but not others.

Research done by feminists shares aspects of all of the previous research traditions. Those whose method is explicitly feminist often prefer a combination of conflict and symbolic interactionist approaches. Following Dorothy Smith (1987), they try to understand social structure and culture from the standpoint of women. More recently, feminists have added race, class, sexual orientation, and ability/disability as problematics to be raised in all feminist research.

Table 2.4 lists the assumptions of feminist social science.

Summary

(1) For the most part, structural functionalism uses positivism as its methodology. The social world is described using a series of universal causal laws: human behaviour is seen as objectively measurable, and social facts are treated as things. Most of medical sociology falls within this paradigm.

(2) An example of positivist methodology is epidemiology—the study of the causes and distribution of disease. A clear and observable cause and effect relationship is sought in order that the disease may be defined and the spread of the disease documented and predicted. Much of AIDS research is carried out in this way.

(3) A positivist methodology claims to be objective, and describes the world with a series of causal laws. It assumes that accurate measures can be designed to describe sociological concepts and that it is possible to say with certainty that 'x' is the cause of 'y'. It assumes that it is possible to generalize from a sample to the population as a whole and that the same research can be completed in different settings with different researchers. It also assumes that the data collected will adequately describe and explain the phenome-

Table 2.4	Methodological Assumptions of Feminist Social Science
Objectivity	It is impossible to be objective in social research. Therefore it is important to be as clear as possible about the biases that are brought to any research study. The continual necessity of reflexivity in research is acknowledged.
Generalizability	Class, gender, race, and power differences between researcher and subjects limit generalizability.
Subjectivity	Often focuses on women's experiences and/or their own viewpoints.
Subject Matter	Gender is always an important component of the investigations.
Language	Uses gender-neutral language where appropriate and specifies actual gender when relevant.
Data Collection Methods	All methods are used but a collaborative approach between research and subjects of research is advocated. Triangulation is suggested.
Purpose	Feminist research has change as one of its goals. It emphasizes the empowerment of women along with the transformation of patriarchal social structures.

Source: Adapted from Clarke (1992b).

non under investigation and that it is possible to demonstrate causal relationships between social science variables. Questionnaires and interviews are typically used for data collection.

(4) Conflict theorists do not attempt to be objective or to generalize. Formal tests of validity are considered to be irrelevant and formal tests of causal relationships superfluous. Components of injustice are analyzed uniquely in each situation, and conflict theorists maintain a commitment to ethical and humanitarian principles. Historical documents are the usual source of data, but many other methods of data collection are used.

(5) The symbolic interactionist perspective focuses on the meanings that the subjects of study attach to reality. Data collection methods traditionally used are participant observation, long unstructured interviews, and qualitative content analysis.

(6) A difficulty that many researchers have while doing participant observation is that they must empathize with their subjects yet remain objective observers. 'Going native' poses a potential problem in maintaining at least a degree of objectivity for those involved in fieldwork. Ethical considerations are also a concern.

(7) Researchers studying women's health and medical care have used all of the research traditions explicated. Those whose work adopts an explicitly feminist methodological perspective are distinguished by explicit attention to a primary focus on the standpoint of women in society and culture.

(8) Recently, feminists have argued for the necessity of problematizing not only gendered standpoints but those pertaining to 'race', class, sexual orientation, and ability/disability.

Questions for Study and Discussion

1. How would you design a study if you were interested in documenting the global crisis in HIV/AIDS?

2. When is epidemiology relevant to sociology and when is it not?

3. What methods do you think make most sense in trying to understand the experience of chronic illness, the incidence of chronic illness, class and chronic illness, and gender differences in chronic illness? Why? Which is the most useful method for the purposes of changing social and health policy?

4. Hilary Graham analyzes women's home health-care work. Can you relate her findings to your own family? To what extent do they not fit your experience?

5. How might you design a study to investigate iatrogenesis in the contemporary practice of medicine?

Suggested Readings

Coburn, David, Susan Rappolt, and Ivy Bourgeault. 1997. 'Decline vs. Retention of Medical Power Through Rest Ratification: An Examination of the Ontario Case', *Sociology of Health and Illness* 19, 1: 1–22. This is a tightly argued critical discussion about the state of interaction within the medical system.

Frank, Arthur. 1991. *At the Will of the Body*. Boston: Houghton Mifflin. Translated into many languages, this book has superbly captured an experience of two different catastrophic illnesses from both the personal and the social/cultural perspectives.

Hunt, Charles W. 1989. 'Migrant Labour and Sexually Transmitted Disease: AIDS in Africa', *Journal of Health and Social Behavior* 30: 353–73. An excellent research article on HIV/AIDS transmission in sub-Saharan Africa.

Illich, Ivan. 1976. *Limits to Medicine*. Toronto: McClelland & Stewart. A beautifully argued critique of medicalization from the perspective of a Roman Catholic social thinker and philosopher.

Rachlis, Michael, and Carol Kushner. 1994. *Strong Medicine: How to Save Canada's Health Care System*. Toronto: HarperCollins. Written by an activist and allopathic physician and a journalist, this is a highly accessible critique of the Canadian health-care system.

Wolf, Naomi. 1990. *The Beauty Myth*. Toronto: Vintage Books. A passionate expression of strong opinions critical of the cultural expectation regarding women as objects of beauty.

| *Part II* | **Sociology of Health and Illness** |

The next six chapters of the book illustrate each of the theoretical perspectives in the sociology of health and illness. Chapter Three describes some of the changes in mortality and morbidity in Canada over the past century and a half and some reasons for these changes. It also explores the importance of such things as nutrition, clean water, birth control, and immunization in the health of the population in early Canada and in the developing world today. It discusses various 'causes' of contemporary mortality and morbidity. Chapter Four describes environmental and occupational health and disease in the context of Canadian society as a whole. The analysis in these chapters is not unified by a single theoretical framework. These two chapters examine the operation of institutions at the level of society through discussion of such variables as food availability and quality (and thus, implicitly, the institutions that provide such food, as well as occupational health and safety in farming). Therefore, the analysis can be considered descriptive in the positivist tradition. Its critical focus also makes it compatible with conflict theory.

Chapter Five discusses the relevance of age and gender to health, illness, and death. Chapter Six examines the inequities of social class and ethnicity and their impact on differing levels of morbidity and mortality. Each of these is examined in regard to differing life expectancy among different groups. When the analysis deals with variables such as age, gender, class, and ethnicity as aspects of the social system and their relationships to human behaviour, and uses a variety of explanations for the relationships, it would be considered structural-functional. When the analysis focuses on a single prime economic determinant such as capitalism, as it does at the end of Chapter Four, it can be seen as an example of conflict theory. Chapter Seven, while it deals with the functions of the social system in a positivist way and is thus compatible with structural functionalism, focuses on the social-psychological behaviour of the individual and its relationship to illness and death. Chapter Eight is symbolic interactionist in that its focus is on the description of the illness experience from the perspective of the subjects, both people who are ill and others associated with them. Feminism as a theoretical perspective is woven through the chapters but the discussion of gender and health in Chapter Five is the most directly concerned with this paradigm.

Table II.1 provides an overview of many of the factors to be considered in explaining the health of a population. Disease and death are seldom the result of isolated conditions or incidents. Death rates, and most deaths, are the result of complex causes, including the *direct cause of death* (which may be, in the case of cancer, for instance, starvation); the *underlying cause*, which in this case might be the growth of malignancies; *the bridging cause,* which might be the malfunctioning of the stomach resulting from malignant growth so that food

Table II.1   Conditions Affecting Life Expectancy

Predisposing Conditions	Generating Conditions	
History (A) wars famine epidemics	**Social-Structural Position within a Society (B)** age sex marital and family status class education level occupation rural/urban location religion religiosity region ethnicity 'race'	**Socio-Psychological Conditions (C)** stress experience and stress management type A or B behaviour sense of coherence gender role expectations
Ecological/Geographical Conditions natural disaster (earthquake, tornado, heat wave)		**Lifestyle Conditions (D)** smoking habits seat-belt use alcohol consumption rate sexual behaviour drug use and abuse
Environmental quality and quantity of water quality of air quality and quantity of foodstuffs (nutrition) safety: roads, airways, waterways, transportation vehicles, workplace, home, tools, equipment birth control		**Existential Factors (E)** the meaning of the illness experience of illness
Medical immunization antibiotics other chemotherapy surgery, radiation		
Societal Structure political-economic system cultural values		

cannot be absorbed; *contributing causes,* which might include smoking and excess alcohol ingestion; *predisposing conditions,* which might be air pollution resulting from a certain industrial process; and *generating conditions,* which might be the economic position of the worker who had no choice but to work in an asbestos mine. However, this empirical complexity is obfuscated by the 'simplification' required by death certification. Thus, the meaning and interpretation of causes of death is variable.

This table lists a number of different groups of causes of death. It also considers causes at the individual level under the heading of existential factors. The next chapters will examine some of these causes in detail. Others are not dealt with because of space limitations and/or because of lack of research. Generally speaking, Chapters Three and Four focus on (A) and, to a limited extent, (B); Chapters Five and Six focus on (B) and, to a limited extent, (A); Chapter Seven focuses on (C) and (D); and Chapter Eight focuses on (E).

Definitions and measurements of disease, illness, and health are complex and debatable. Disease is determined in a number of ways: *self-reporting,* which includes asking respondents to describe their own state of health; *clinical records*, which include the records of physicians as well as *hospital statistics*; and *physical measurements*, which include such things as blood pressure readings and tests of tissue pathology. Each of these may record a disease state at a different level of development or potential acknowledgement (e.g., a Pap smear may indicate evidence of precancerous or cancerous tissue before either the physician or the 'patient' would be able to notice its occurrence). None of these three can be considered a 'true' or 'objective' way to determine illness. In combination, however, they may point to 'true disease' (or some other condition).

In addition to understanding disease causation, students of sociology are interested in questions regarding the meaning and social construction of disease and the differentiation among disease, sickness, and illness (see Chapter Eight for further discussion of this issue). Finally, sociologists are critical of the 'validity' of official statistics regarding both disease and death.

Chapter 3 | *Disease and Death: Canada in International and Historical Context*

Learning Objectives

- Life expectancy in Canada has increased substantially over the past 150 years.
- Whereas life expectancy rates used to be similar for men and women, today women live significantly longer lives.
- Medical interventions have played a small part in increased life expectancy.
- More important have been changes such as better hygiene and better quality and availability of food and birth control.
- In a global context inequities among the nation-states are the most significant cause of differences in mortality rates.
- To understand global health patterns it is necessary to understand such living conditions as: poverty; food security; water availability, access, and quality; violence (including interpersonal violence and wars); the position of women; birth control; comprehensive health care, including primary, secondary, and tertiary prevention; and immunization.
- The causes of sickness and death in the developed world, including Canada, are 'diseases of civilization', degeneration, and aging such as cancer and heart disease.
- Today in Canada poverty continues to be a very important cause of morbidity and mortality, along with cigarette, alcohol, and excess sugar, fat, and calorie consumption and a relative lack of exercise.

What are the major causes of death in Canada today? What were the major causes of death in Canada a century ago? What is the average life expectancy in Canada today? How long did Canadians live on average when your grandparents were children, or 150 years ago? How important has medicine been to the increase in life expectancy over the last century or so? You have probably heard that penicillin is a wonder drug. What was the importance of penicillin in the overall improvement of the health of the nation? What about other 'wonder drugs'? How important have immunizations been in the extension of life for the average Canadian?

Life Expectancy

The average life expectancy for men and women has varied considerably through thousands of epochs and in many different types of social and economic structures. For example, the average life expectancy of late Ice Age hunter-gatherers about 11,000 years ago has been estimated to have been approximately 38 years (Eyer, 1984). According to available records and estimates, the average life expectancy in Europe varied between 20 and 40 years from the thirteenth to the seventeenth centuries (Goldscheider, 1971). In Canada, too, there have been wide variations in life expectancy. In 1831 the average for Canadians is estimated to have been 39 years. Females born in 1996 can expect to live for about 81.45 years, while males can expect to live for about 75.69 years. This is an increase of 16.69 years for males and 20.45 years for females since 1920–2 (Statistics Canada, 1998). Canada's life expectancy is among the highest in the world.

Against this optimistic picture must be set the fact that the gap between the life expectancy for men and women in Canada is very wide. Furthermore, this life expectancy gap has widened since 1931, when it was about 2.1 years, to the present, when it is about six years. In effect, mortality declines over this period have benefited females to a greater extent than males.

Such dramatic changes in life expectancy as have occurred in the past 100–150 years in Canada (and elsewhere in the developed world) can be explained by a whole host of factors. One description of the process is epidemiological transition (Omran, 1979), which is based on the theory of *demographic transition*. Simply put, this idea suggests that as the economy changes from low to high per capita income, there is a corresponding transition from high mortality and high fertility to low mortality and low fertility.

Changes in the patterns of disease occur in three distinct stages: the Age of Pestilence and Famine, the Age of Receding Pandemics, and the Age of Degenerative and Man-Made Diseases (ibid.).

The *Age of Pestilence and Famine* is characterized by socio-economic conditions in which communities are traditional, economically underdeveloped with a low per capita income, and generally agrarian. Women usually have low status, the family is extended, and illiteracy is high. The high mortality rate is largely attributable to famine and infectious diseases. The *Age of Receding Pandemics* is characterized by a decrease in epidemics and famine and a consequent decline in the mortality rate. At this point the fertility rate continues to be high, resulting in a 'population explosion'. The fertility rate then begins to decline as people begin to live longer and to die of emerging industrial and degenerative diseases such as cancer, stroke, and heart disease. This characterizes the *Age of Degenerative and Man-Made Diseases* (these terms are Omran's). This description provides an outline of stages, but not an explanation.

What factors are responsible for the overall decline in mortality rate and the increase in life expectancy in the developed world? McKeown (1976) has offered an explanation based on studies of the decline in mortality in Britain (and supported by findings for Sweden, France, Ireland, and Hungary) over the last few hundred years. First, the decline in the mortality rate was almost entirely due to a decline in infectious disease. Second, the decline in infectious disease was largely the result of three basic changes: (1) improvements in nutrition, (2) improvements in hygiene, and (3) increasing control of disease-causing microorganisms. Improvements in birth control were also a factor. Infant and early childhood mortality is usually one of the most sensitive indicators of the health of a nation.

A second study by McKeown and Record (1975) spanning the period 1901–71 showed that this increase in overall life expectancy was the result of conditions in the twentieth century very similar to those described above for previous centuries. Improved nutrition accounted for about half the increase, and better hygiene, resulting in fewer

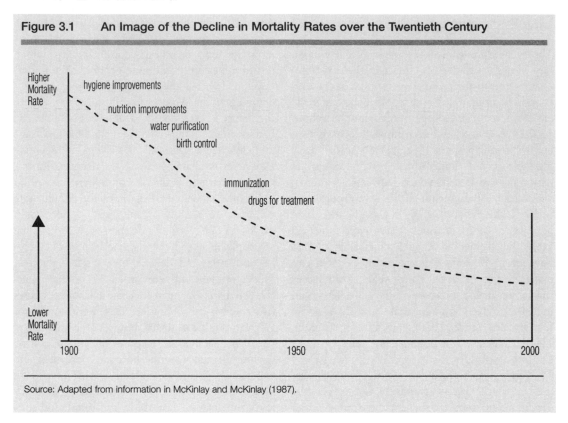

Figure 3.1   An Image of the Decline in Mortality Rates over the Twentieth Century

Source: Adapted from information in McKinlay and McKinlay (1987).

water- and food-borne diseases, accounted for about one-sixth of the improvement. Immunization and medical therapy were together responsible for about one-tenth of the increased life expectancy (see Figure 3.1). Recent research, based on 1988 data, evaluated the contemporary importance of medicine, as compared with various socioeconomic resources, for infant mortality rates in 117 industrialized, 'developing', and underdeveloped countries (Kim and Moody, 1992). Using GNP, energy consumption, daily caloric supply per capita, percentage of population enrolled in secondary education, urbanization, and safe water supplies as indicators of socio-economic status (SES), and comparing their effects to those of health resources (i.e., population per physician, nurse, hospital bed) on infant mortality rates, Kim and Moody noted that the contribution of medical resources to the health of the population is small as compared to socio-economic resources.

There are tremendous country-to-country discrepancies in the mortality rate. In Canada the infant mortality rate, one of the most sensitive indicators of the health of a nation, has dropped significantly as a result of better nutrition and living standards for the mother and baby, coupled with improved prenatal and postnatal medical care (*Canada Year Book*, 1994: 131). With the exception of Japan, Canada has had the most significant drop in infant mortality rates in the last 35 years (see Table 3.1 and Figure 3.2). In 1995, the infant mortality rate for Canada was 6.1 per 1,000 as compared to 27.3 per 1,000 in 1960 (Statistics Canada, *Selected Infant Mortality, 1921–90*; Statistics Canada, 1995). In 1901, 134 of every 1,000 infants (about one in seven) died in the first year of life; in 1997,

Table 3.1   Infant Mortality Rates,* Canada, Provinces, and Territories, 1975–1997

Year	Canada	Nfld**	PEI	NS	NB	Que.	Ont.	Man.	Sask.	Alta	BC	Yukon	NWT
1975	13.7	17.3	19.2	16.2	15.5	11.8	12.8	15.1	17.8	14.9	14.4	24.5	35.7
1976	13.0	15.6	14.4	13.8	14.2	11.7	12.4	15.6	14.3	14.3	13.8	22.3	34.7
1977	12.4	10.3	18.8	11.6	13.4	12.4	11.3	16.6	15.1	11.1	13.5	13.9	29.4
1978	12.0	13.4	7.6	11.9	11.8	11.8	11.4	13.7	14.3	11.4	12.7	11.2	23.3
1979	10.9	11.4	10.9	11.9	11.4	10.5	10.3	13.0	11.5	11.4	11.3	16.0	27.3
1980	10.5	11.8	11.2	10.9	10.9	9.8	9.5	11.5	11.3	12.6	11.0	18.9	22.3
1981	9.6	10.8	13.2	11.5	10.9	8.5	8.8	11.9	11.8	10.6	10.2	14.9	21.5
1982	9.1	10.8	7.8	8.6	10.5	8.8	8.3	9.1	10.5	9.8	9.9	20.9	16.1
1983	8.5	10.6	8.4	9.3	10.7	7.7	8.0	10.4	10.1	8.4	8.8	18.5	20.8
1984	8.1	9.2	8.2	7.8	7.8	7.3	7.6	8.7	9.4	9.6	8.6	13.5	17.3
1985	8.0	11.8	4.0	7.9	9.6	7.3	7.3	9.9	11.0	8.0	8.1	10.8	16.7
1986	7.9	8.5	6.7	8.4	8.3	7.1	7.2	9.2	9.0	9.0	8.5	24.8	18.6
1987	7.3	7.9	6.7	7.4	7.0	7.1	6.6	8.4	9.1	7.5	8.6	10.5	12.5
1988	7.2	10.9	7.1	6.5	7.2	6.5	6.6	7.8	8.3	8.3	8.4	5.8	10.3
1989	7.1	9.1	6.2	5.8	7.1	6.8	6.8	6.6	8.1	7.5	8.2	4.2	16.2
1990	6.8	10.3	6.0	6.3	7.2	6.2	6.3	8.0	7.6	8.1	7.5	7.2	12.0
1991	6.4	7.8	6.9	5.7	6.1	5.9	6.3	6.4	8.2	6.7	6.5	10.6	12.2
1992	6.1	7.1	1.6	6.0	6.3	5.4	5.9	6.8	7.3	7.2	6.2	3.8	16.7
1993	6.3	7.8	9.1	7.1	7.2	5.7	6.2	7.1	8.1	6.7	5.7	7.9	9.6
1994	6.3	8.2	6.4	6.0	5.4	5.6	6.0	7.0	8.9	7.4	6.3	2.3	14.6
1995	6.1	7.9	4.6	4.9	4.8	5.5	6.0	7.6	9.1	7.0	6.0	12.8	13.0
1996	5.6	6.6	4.7	5.6	4.9	4.7	5.7	6.7	8.4	6.2	5.1	0.0	12.2
1997	5.5	5.2	4.4	4.4	5.7	5.6	5.5	7.5	8.9	4.8	4.7	8.4	10.9

*The infant mortality rate is calculated as the number of deaths of children less than one year of age per 1,000 live births.
**The totals for Newfoundland are estimated for 1975 and for 1985 through 1990.

Source: Statistics Canada, Catalogue no. 82F0075XCB.

5.5 (a decrease from 1995 of 0.5) per 1,000 or approximately one in 82 did not live to their first birthday (*Canada Year Book*, 2001). This compares positively to the US, where the corresponding figure is 9.1 per 1,000 (Fuller, 1998: 149). In Alberta, however, where the welfare and health system has undergone radical restructuring in recent years, the infant mortality rate in some rural areas has grown to 10.6 (ibid., 164). It is also important to note that the death rate for infants in the Aboriginal community is twice the general Canadian rate. This is mostly as a result of sudden infant death syndrome and respiratory diseases and pneumonia, among other causes, and becomes even higher after the newborn phase (*Canada Year Book*, 2001). Still today, globally, millions of infants and children under five die every year as a result of such preventable health problems as diarrhea, acute respi-

Table 3.2   Life Expectancy: Selected Countries Around the World

| Country | Probability of Dying (per 1,000) | | | | Life Expectancy at Birth (years) | |
| | Under Age 5 | | Ages 15–59 | | | |
	Males	Females	Males	Females	Males	Females
Afghanistan	252	249	437	376	44.2	45.1
Canada	6	5	101	57	76.0	81.5
Costa Rica	18	15	131	78	73.4	78.8
Cuba	9	8	143	94	73.7	77.5
Czech Republic	6	6	174	75	71.5	78.2
Denmark	7	5	129	82	74.2	78.5
Democratic Rep. of the Congo	218	205	571	493	41.6	44.0
Germany	6	5	127	60	74.3	80.6
Malawi	229	211	701	653	37.1	37.8
Mexico	31	25	180	101	71.0	76.2
Mozambique	227	208	674	612	37.9	39.5
Rwanda	219	199	667	599	38.5	40.5
Switzerland	6	6	99	58	76.7	82.5
United Kingdom	7	6	109	67	74.8	79.9
United States	9	8	147	84	73.9	79.5
Zambia	170	156	725	687	39.2	39.5

Source: *The World Health Report 2001:* <http://www.who.int/whr/2001/main/en/pdf/annex.en.pdf>.

ratory disease, measles, tetanus, and malaria (UNICEF, 1990). (See Table 3.2.)

The following section will discuss the ways that some socio-economic and cultural factors affect health and longevity in a global context. The major causes of death among infants, children, and adults around the world today are preventable and could be eliminated with relatively minor and inexpensive interventions. Such measures would, of course, eliminate a great deal of suffering over and above these particular deaths. It is also important to note that the grief-stricken families and communities, as well as those children who do not die but suffer from all of the same diseases, are not counted in the statistical picture presented here.

Death, Disease, and Disability in Global Context

Poverty and Inequality
Both the overall level of income and the relative income of a people have a major impact on health. Income level is the context for all of the other ele-

Box 3.1 Politics and Dependency: Cuba and the Dominican Republic

Cuba and the Dominican Republic are similar in regard to language, religion, geographic location, and size, but they have very different medical systems and health care. In Cuba, health care is socialized and therefore universally available, centrally planned, and standardized both by physicians and for all citizens. Rural health care is as excellent as that in the cities. Prevention is valued. The overall health of Cubans is good.

By contrast, the health care in the Dominican Republic is unequally distributed. The poor and the rural people have little access. There are serious shortages of medical supplies. High-technology curative care for the rich is emphasized. This private system produces physicians of widely differing levels of training. The overall health of the people is comparatively poor.

Schwabe (1995) explains the difference between the health of the populations of the two countries by reference to their degrees of dependency. The hypothesis tested and not rejected by the comparison between Cuba and the Dominican Republic is that the relationships among nations

around the globe are reproduced internally in a nation's economic, social, and political relations. Inequalities among nations parallel inequalities within nations. This is especially the case with dependent nations. Schwabe contrasts degree of dependency in Cuba and the Dominican Republic. Cuba, on one hand, has experienced massive decreases in dependency since the revolution in 1959. This has been accompanied by an increase in autonomy with respect to internal decisions. Its ties to the former USSR have been less exploitive than the ties between the US and the Dominican Republic. In sum, Cuba has been able to be more autonomous than the Dominican Republic. This has had long-term positive effects for the economy and the level of internal equality. The Dominican Republic is more dependent on other nations. Its economy is oriented towards exports and less focused on internal needs. More than 50 per cent of its assets are US-owned. Much of the land is owned by an elite few.

There have been significant changes in Cuba with the disintegration of the Soviet Union and the dramatic decline in aid. Thus this study needs to be repeated.

ments of daily life, including work, education, food, shelter, water, hygiene, and sanitation. Poverty is also often associated with political powerlessness and marginalization. While the economic growth of a whole country is not necessarily associated with better health for all, economic decline usually affects the standard of living and, consequently, the health of many. This is due to the fact that the health costs of an economic recession tend to fall most heavily on those who were least well off to start with (*Beyond Adjustment*, 1993). Public policies regarding income security are also associated with infant mortality rates. On the basis of international comparative data, Wennemo

(1993) concluded that: (1) relative income inequality within a country seemed more important than overall level of economic development in the country with respect to infant mortality rates; and (2) the level of unemployment and the availability of unemployment and family and social security benefits were related to infant mortality rates. Figures 3.2 and 3.3 indicate infant mortality rates for Canada and OECD countries. Other comparative and contemporary analyses reinforce the primacy of socio-economic conditions to health and life expectancy (Wnuk-Lipinski and Illsley, 1990; Raphael, 2001). Navarro (1992) surveyed the health conditions of the world's population,

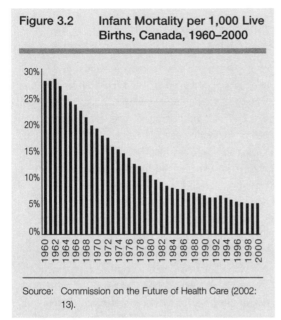

Figure 3.2   Infant Mortality per 1,000 Live Births, Canada, 1960–2000

Source: Commission on the Future of Health Care (2002: 13).

Figure 3.3   Infant Mortality per 1,000 Live Births, OECD Countries, 2000

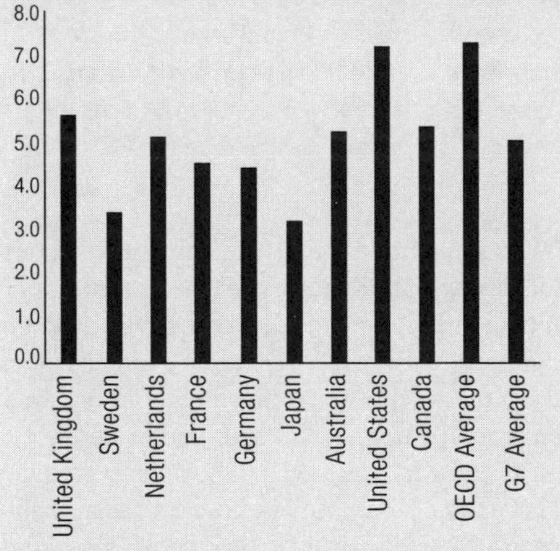

Note: Figures for Canada and the United States are for 1999.

Source: Commission on the Future of Health Care (2002: 13).

continent by continent, and showed how, contrary to current Western beliefs, socialism and socialist forces with their tendency towards class equalization have been, for the most part, better able to improve health conditions than capitalism. This finding tends to be true both in the developed and in the developing world.

Food Security

The availability of an adequate amount of nutritious food is fundamental to the health of a population. Experimental field studies have demonstrated that improvements in nutrition, particularly in the quantity and quality of the protein component, have a much larger impact on morbidity and mortality than any other public health or medical measure (see Eyer, 1984). Over 800 million people presently lack adequate nutrients for daily life, while 3 billion people lack essential micronutrients such as iodine, vitamin A, and iron. 'These deficiencies lead to poor physical and cognitive development as well as to lowered resistance to illness, brain damage, blindness and even death' (World Health Organization, 1997: 1B). More than half of the deaths occurring each year in the developing world are associated with malnutrition.

Nutrient deficiency in women is an even more prevalent and significant problem than in men. Globally, women work almost 65 per cent of the total hours worked and in return earn 10 per cent of world income and own 1 per cent of the world's property. Because women have less income, they have less access to adequate nutrients (Zabolai-Csekme, 1983). However, because women bear and breast-feed babies, they have a greater need for calories. The low standard of nutrition among women is pivotal, too, for the health of their offspring. In brief, underweight babies are born to women who suffer nutritional inadequacies. Underweight babies are more likely to die as infants and to suffer from any one of a number of diseases, as well as intellectual and physical disabilities.

Box 3.2   The Debt Crisis and Childhood Illness

Every day 40,000 children die from malnutrition and other preventable causes, particularly diarrheal diseases, measles, tetanus, whooping cough, and pneumonia. Those causes of death are simple to prevent, and to do so would be relatively inexpensive. Also, the death rates for children in less-developed countries are considerably higher than in the developed world. UNICEF has estimated that full immunization would cost $1.50 per child. Oral rehydration kits, which could prevent diarrheal deaths, cost approximately 10¢ each. Antibiotics, to combat pneumonia, cost about $1.00 per child. A co-ordinated program dedicated to combatting childhood malnutrition and death would cost only about $2.5 billion a year worldwide.

High rates of childhood death persist in underdeveloped countries although they have diminished somewhat. There are a number of explanations for this situation: urbanization, fertility rates, development itself, foreign investment, foreign control, and foreign exploitation of the environment and people for financing by the developed world. Today one of the chief causes of the persistence of childhood disease is the global debt crisis. The developing nations are heavily in debt to governments and financial institutions in the developed world. Consequently, the international financial community now requires that borrowers implement severe austerity measures (including government spending cuts and wage freezes) before they can obtain new loans on restrictive outstanding debts. Domestic austerity measures, also known as 'structural adjustments', are intended to increase efficiency and save resources to repay foreign debt. The result is the allocation of fewer resources for immunization, general health maintenance, prenatal care, nutrition, urban development, and other programs with direct impacts on children's health.

The Physical and Social Environment

The availability of a sufficient amount of clean drinking water is another crucial factor in health. Available statistics indicate that three out of five people (and an even greater proportion among the poor) in developing countries do not have access to safe drinking water. Yet numerous fatal and debilitating chronic illnesses are spread by unsanitary water. Two of the most prevalent are cholera and dysentery. Diarrheal disease is the single greatest killer of children in the developing world (*Beyond Adjustment*, 1993). Its prevention depends on changes in water supply, hygiene, and sanitation. Yet the infrastructure developments necessary for adequate improvements are extensive. They include drainage systems for the disposal of human and animal wastes, access to potable water, and water for irrigation.

The devastating effects of unclean water have nowhere been as dramatic as in death rates among babies in the underdeveloped countries who were fed by 'instant' infant formula that had to be mixed with water (for an overview, see Box 3.3). The export of infant formula to the developing world was responsible for a widespread increase in infant mortality from a specific source. Not only were babies made sick by being given contaminated water, but also, lacking adequate information (either because of illiteracy or because mixing directions were not available) or lacking sufficient income to purchase adequate amounts of formula, mothers were often diluting the formula so extensively that babies were dying of starvation.

Safety, Security, and Stability

Personal safety is of great concern, particularly in times of heightened national tensions. Civil war

Box 3.3   Infant Formula Feeding: The Crisis in the Developing World

In the early 1980s a crisis occurred in the developing world over the seemingly innocuous question of how best to feed infants. Starting in 1969, a new market for infant feeding formula was developed in Third World countries. It was regarded as a wise and humane move that would extend the lives of many of the millions of children in the Third World who died annually as a result of malnutrition. Advertising and promotion for infant feeding formula quickly became successful. Free samples donated by the companies manufacturing the formula were given to women who had just given birth. In the Third World, feeding babies formula rather than breast milk was very quickly taken to be a symbol of mother love and responsibility, because formula was associated in the minds of Third World peoples with the successful middle and upper classes in the Western world. A number of unexpected negative consequences resulted.

(1)   When women used the free samples given to them at the birth of their babies, their own milk supply would dry up and breast-feeding would become impossible.

(2)   When women went home with their babies, they were often ill-prepared to continue with the infant feeding formula for a variety of reasons.

   (a)   Formula was frequently unavailable in the small villages and communities, and as women's breast milk had dried up, the babies starved to death.

   (b)   When the formula was available, there were often no instructions on how to use it, the mothers were illiterate, or the instructions were in a language the mothers could not read. Thus many women mixed the formula with too much water, so that the nutrients in the mixture were inadequate for the baby's growth.

(c)   Generally, the formula was sold in powdered form, to be mixed with water. Frequently, the water source was polluted, resulting in unnecessary illnesses and death.

(d)   The bottles used for feeding the babies should have been sterilized. Many Third World mothers were unable to sterilize the bottles because they lacked clean water, a heat source, or a chemical sterilizing agent.

(e)   Aside from the problems enumerated above, one other fact stands out: breast milk is actually better for babies because it passes important immunities from mother to offspring. In the developing world, babies breast-fed for less than six months are five to ten times more likely to die than those breast-fed for a longer period.

When the dangers of infant formula became clear to the Western world, the companies manufacturing infant formula were boycotted, especially Nestle's, which held more than 50 per cent of the world's market. A World Health Organization conference called in 1979 initiated the adoption of a code to govern infant formula sales. Its aim was:

the provision of safe and adequate nutrition for infants; by the protection and promotion of breast feeding, and by ensuring the proper use of breast milk substitutes . . . on the basis of adequate information through appropriate marketing and distribution.

The infant formula companies agreed to support the code. While the extent of the problem declined, there were, and continue to be, numerous violations of the code. This is an ongoing problem.

Sources: 'A Boycott over Infant Formula', *Business Week*, 12 Apr. 1979, 137–40; Zabolai-Csekme (1983); World Health Organization (1981).

and international warfare and violence in communities, workplaces, and the home are all threats to fundamental safety. As local and international inequities grow, so, too, do violence and war. Consequently, death, disability, and disease can be expected to increase. Violence has increased dramatically around the world. 'During 1993, at least 4 million deaths (8 per cent of the total) resulted from unintentional or intentional injury, including 300,000 murders' (World Health Organization, 1997: 63). Those at risk of violence are more likely to be females, children, adolescents, old people, the homeless, the unemployed, migrants, refugees, members of visible ethnic minorities, the chronically ill and mentally disabled, and victims of war. In both the developing and developed world, 20 to 40 per cent of the deaths of young men aged 15–34 result from suicide or homicide. In the US alone, 65 people are murdered daily and 600 are wounded in acts of violence (ibid.).

The Position of Women

For a number of reasons the position of women in a society has a significant impact on the health of the people. In a worldwide context women's health is considerably poorer than that of men. This is particularly true in the developing world. The lifetime chance of maternal death is considerably lower in North America than in Africa. Ninety-nine per cent of the half-million who die annually in childbirth are from developing countries. Almost half of the billions of women in developing countries are malnourished; millions suffer from iodine deficiency or are blind because of vitamin deficiency. Poverty, malnutrition, illiteracy, level of education, and access to medical care all contribute significantly to women's health status worldwide. Women's reproductive and sexual health is also often seriously compromised by the lack of availability of contraception or abortion, cultural practices such as genital surgery (see Box 3.4), sexual inhibitions, and absent, distant, and/or male doctors. Discrimination that

results in feeding boys more and better food than girls and the greater proportion of female babies suffering infanticide are also significant problems. Violence—both sexual and non-sexual assault—is another major issue for women's health worldwide, as indicated in Box 3.5 (Koblinsky et al., 1993). Two of the most important interventions possible for the improvement of a nation's health are the education and increased paid employment of women.

Birth Control

Effective birth control is another important cause of the mortality rate. In developing countries such as India, Indonesia, Mexico, Brazil, Nigeria, and Morocco, the average woman has seven to eight live births and approximately five additional pregnancies that end in miscarriage (Hammer, 1980). Too many pregnancies, or pregnancies spaced too closely together, are a threat to the health of the mother and the child for a number of reasons (*Health and the Status of Women*, 1980). In the first place, when the pregnancy is unwanted, women may seek illegal abortions, which are extremely dangerous. In Latin America, for instance, illegal abortions are said to account for between one-fifth and one-half of all maternal deaths. Second, because of malnutrition, women's bodies may be undernourished and small, their pelvises misshapen, and they may experience fatigue during pregnancy and a difficult delivery. Third, pregnancy itself takes a toll on a woman's body because nutrients are needed for the baby as well as the mother. During pregnancy large increases in calories, vitamins, and minerals are required, including more iron, vitamin B12, and folic acid, especially during the last trimester of pregnancy. Fourth, because energy is used up during pregnancy, rest, especially in the last trimester, is important. Most women in developing nations, however, do not have the leisure to take the necessary rest. Fifth, childbirth itself, because of the lack of sanitation, prenatal care, or emergency medical services, is responsi-

Box 3.4　　Female Circumcision or Genital Mutilation?

The two terms used in the title reflect something of the contrasting views about this procedure (Kowser and Silver, 1994). Some argue that female genital surgery is mutilation, others that it is beautification. Some say it is a form of violence against women done to maintain their subordinate status and to control their reproduction. There are (at least) three different types of procedures: circumcision, where the hood of the clitoris is cut; excision, where the clitoris and all or part of the labia minora are cut; and infibulation, which includes cutting the clitoris, labia minora, and at least part of the labia majora. The two sides of the vulva are then sutured to obliterate the vaginal area except for a small opening for passage of urine and menstrual blood. The size of the opening is that of a corn kernel.

Infibulation prevents female sexual pleasure and assures the faithfulness of women to their husbands. It reinforces the male's right to control and dominance and the female's dependence. Women's attractiveness may depend on infibulation. In Somalia, for example, virtually 100 per cent of young girls between 4–10 years of age undergo infibulation. Little girls know that it's essential to their marriageability and thus want to have it done. It is also associated with gift-giving for the girls. Never having seen it occur, they may be unaware of the pain. The procedure is not only painful, however, but may also be dangerous because the tools used are often unhygienic and the stitching may be done with silk, catgut, or even thorns. Girls may have their legs bound together for a period of weeks to ensure the build-up of scar tissue. Sexual intercourse is forever after likely to be painful and even dangerous for infibulated women.

ble for a much higher rate of maternal mortality in the developing nations than in the developed nations. Some of the most prevalent causes of childbirth-related deaths are postpartum hemorrhage, which occurs when a woman has anemia, and sepsis (infection), which occurs because of inadequate sanitation or because of hypertensive disorders of pregnancy.

Infectious and parasitic diseases result from nutritional inadequacies and polluted water. Vulnerability to such diseases is increased by a high birth rate. Much of the dramatic decline in mortality in the last century or so in the developed world, including Canada, is the result of the drop in death rates from infectious or parasitic diseases. To a large extent, this decrease is the result of rising standards of nutrition and improvements in sanitation and birth control, resulting in a 'favourable trend in the relationship between some micro-organisms and the human host' (McKeown and Record, 1975: 391). As has been discussed, the less-developed countries are far behind in standards of nutrients, clean drinking water, sanitation, and birth control.

Comprehensive Health Care

Comprehensive health care, although relatively ineffective without such fundamentals as adequate food and clean water, is also an important factor in good health. Health care, both in the developed and in the developing world, can be divided into three types. These are sometimes called three levels of prevention. They are primary, secondary, and tertiary health care. Primary health care emphasizes equitably distributed prevention through community development and education. Environmental issues may also be addressed. Secondary health care is directed towards disease treatment in hospital and community via various (usually Western-style) medical practitioners. Tertiary care especially occurs in a teaching hospital attached to a university and

Box 3.5   The Global Health Burden of Rape

A review of numerous studies from all around the globe documents the prevalence of rape and the correspondingly widespread health effects. One way of conceptualizing the health effects is in terms of DALY, or disability-adjusted life years. According to the *World Development Report— 1993: Investing in Health* (World Bank, 1993), rape and domestic violence are major causes of disability and death, especially among women in their reproductive years. The report estimates that one in every five years lost (either by death or disability) results from gender-based victimization in the developed economies. In the developing world the health burden resulting from rape and domestic violence is about the same but because of the overall disease profile the percentage attributable to gender-based victimization is smaller. On a global basis the health burden of gender-based victimization (9.5 million DALY) is comparable to HIV (10.6 million DALY), tuberculosis (10.9 million DALY), sepsis during childbirth (10 million DALY), all cancers (9.0 million DALY), and cardiovascular disease (10.5 million DALY).

The health consequences discussed include psychological distress, socio-cultural impacts, and somatic consequences. Psychological distress may last throughout the lifetime of the woman who has been raped. The symptoms can be diverse and extensive. In North America they have been conceptualized by the psychiatric profession as a type of PSTD—post-traumatic stress disorder. Survivors of rape and violence are 'more likely to have received several psychiatric diagnoses during their adult life including major depression, alcohol abuse/dependence, drug abuse/dependence, generalized anxiety, and obsessive compulsive disorder'.

Socio-cultural effects are the effects that spread beyond the suffering of the individual woman and lead non-victimized women to change their behaviour and restrict movements out of fear. Surveys done in countries around the world indicate that many women consider the fear of rape a major stress in their lives. In some countries women who have been raped may be doubly abused. For instance, in parts of Asia and the Middle East, consequences of rape may include being divorced by one's husband, ostracized by one's family, or even killed by family members to cleanse the family honour. Rape can lead the victim to commit suicide or to be the victim of an 'honourable' murder. Physical illnesses that are disproportionally diagnosed among women who have been raped include chronic pelvic pain, arthritis, gastrointestinal disorders, headaches, chronic pain, psychogenic seizures, premenstrual symptoms, and substance abuse. For example, women in the United States who have been victims of rape (or other crimes) report more symptoms of illness across virtually all bodily systems and perceive their health less favourably than non-victimized women. There are also numerous reproduction-related issues that may result from rape: pregnancy, sexually transmitted diseases, including AIDS, future high-risk sexual behaviours, and loss of self-esteem.

Source: Koss, Heise, and Russo (1994).

---

has a side emphasis on health promotion. Primary health care is still the most efficacious with respect to positive health outcomes in both the developed and the developing worlds.

Immunization

Immunization makes an important contribution to the health of a population, although its importance appears to have been overemphasized.

Box 3.6   The Growth in Global Inequality

Global inequity has been growing over the past half-century or so. In the 1960s the richest one-fifth of the world's population earned 30 times the income of the poorest one-fifth. By 1997 the richest earned 74 times the income of the poorest (UNDP, 1999, as cited in Moss, 2002). Not only is inequality growing among nations of the world but also within nations. Countries such as Canada, Australia, the United Kingdom, the United States, and Sweden have grown in internal inequity. In fact, Sweden, previously one of the most equitable countries in the world, is now one of the most unequal (Moss, 2002). It is now widely accepted that global structural adjustment designed to enable the poor nations to pay their debts to the rich nations has led to greater inequality than prior to structural adjustment policies. In stark contrast, the richest countries of the world have gotten even richer.

The burden of global inequality falls most heavily on women around the world. Yet the legal position of women has in many ways improved. Almost all of the countries of the world have signed the Convention for the Elimination of All Forms of Discrimination Against Women (CEDAW). The major exceptions as of 1999 were Afghanistan and the United States (ibid.). Gender equity is now a cornerstone of economic and other development projects around the globe. In fact, the Canadian International Development Agency is widely thought to have one of if not the best gender equity screening processes for development. It has become a model for the rest of the world. Gender equity has repeatedly been shown to be associated with lower fertility and better health for women and children as well as overall economic development. Gender equity seems to be important both at the level of the public economy and in the intra-household context. Intra-household equity in decision-making and allocation of resources, as well as education for girls and women, is now seen as a form of human capital investment. The balance of power in the household is presently viewed as an analytic criterion on a par with social and economic equity (Moss, 2002: 650).

McKinlay and McKinlay (1977), using American data since about 1900, show that most of the decline in mortality from the infectious diseases prevalent in 1900 (about 40 per cent of the deaths in 1900 were attributable to infectious diseases) was the result of public health measures such as water purification and improvements in nutrition and birth control. Data for tuberculosis, typhoid, measles, scarlet fever, polio, whooping cough, influenza, diphtheria, and pneumonia demonstrate that the significant decline in mortality for each disease came before the introduction of the vaccine or drug to treat it. Significant declines in mortality preceded medical treatment of each disease.

Serious infectious and bacterial diseases have all but disappeared in the developed world (with the notable exception of AIDS). They persist in the developing world. But while immunization and medical measures may have made a relatively minor contribution to the decline of mortality in the developed world, they are, along with improvements in public health, nutrition, and sanitation, essential in the developing world, where only 10 per cent of all children receive protection from measles, tuberculosis, whooping cough, polio, tetanus, and diphtheria. Five million children still die from these diseases, and an additional five million are disabled annually. Even in Canada immunization is not universally available to infants and children. Between 5 and 15 per cent of Canada's children are not receiving adequate immunization for potentially fatal and disabling diseases such as polio, diphtheria, and measles.

Death, Disease, and Disability in Canadian Society

The chief causes of death in Canada today are heart disease, cancer, and accidents. In 1995, cancer and heart disease accounted for more than half of all deaths in Canada. Stroke was the third leading cause of death at 7.4 per cent. For the second consecutive year cancer deaths were more common than those due to heart disease. The proportion of deaths from heart disease has decreased by about 30 per cent over the past quarter-century or so (*Canada Year Book*, 1994). This is a reverse of the historical tradition. Still, heart disease is responsible for the loss of 277,000 person years of life, or 24 per cent of the total potential years of life lost in Ontario (ibid.). If the aging of the population is considered and death rate is age-standardized, cancer deaths actually fell from 188.3 per 100,000 population in 1994 to 184.9 in 1995. The case is similar for heart disease, with the rate per 100,000 decreasing from 184.4 to 179.9. The suicide rate grew, however, to 13.3 per 100,000 in 1995 as compared to 12.7 in 1994. The suicide rate is considerably higher in Quebec (19.0) and Alberta (16.7). AIDS deaths in Canada in 1996 numbered 1,306; by 2001 fewer than 500 people died of AIDS in Canada (http://www.whobarcelona.info/AIDS2002/Canada_En.pdf). (See Table 3.3.)

Accidents and violence are particularly prevalent among 15–24-year-old men—they are approximately twice as common as a cause of death among this age group as among the general population (*Canada Year Book*, 2001). Contrary to commonly held beliefs, however, the rate of violent and accidental death decreased by 27 per cent from 1980 to 1990. Still, unintentional injuries were responsible for 19 per cent of the overall potential years of life lost among Canadians (ibid.).

Table 3.3   Leading Causes of Death Changed Dramatically during the Twentieth Century

	Rate per 100,000
1921–5	
All causes	**1,030.0**
Cardiovascular and renal disease	221.9
Influenza, bronchitis, and pneumonia	141.1
Diseases of early infancy	111.0
Tuberculosis	85.1
Cancer	75.9
Gastritis, duodenitis, enteritis, and colitis	72.2
Accidents	51.5
Communicable diseases	47.1
1996–7	
All causes	**654.4**
Cardiovascular diseases (heart disease and stroke)	240.2
Cancer	184.8
Chronic obstructive pulmonary diseases	28.4
Unintentional injuries	27.7
Pneumonia and influenza	22.1
Diabetes mellitus	16.7
Hereditary and degenerative diseases of the central nervous system	14.7
Diseases of arteries, arterioles, and capillaries	14.3

Note: Disease categories not identical over time. Rates in 1996–7 are age-standardized.

Source: Statistics Canada, *Canadian Social Trends*, catalogue no. 11–008. (Winter 2000): 13.

Heart disease, cancer, and accidents are called the diseases of civilization or diseases of affluence, or what Omran (1979) has called 'man-made' diseases. Their causes are different from those of the diseases of development. Food

Box 3.7   Estimates of Potential Effects of Prevention or Early Detection of Cancer Incidence

According to research for the Cancer and Palliative Care Unit of the World Health Organization,* a portion of cancer cases in Canada are potentially preventable, given current knowledge of risk factors. Lifestyle choices, such as smoking and diet, in particular, have been identified as the predominant determinants of human cancer.

The percentage of cancer cases that are potentially preventable was derived by comparing age-standardized cancer rates in Canada to those of countries where populations were largely Caucasian, and where cancer rates for different sites were lowest. It provides an indication of the effect that would be achievable if Canadians were to have the same lifestyle as people in the countries compared.

Cancer site	Action	Percentage of cancer incidence potentially preventable
Lung	Eliminate smoking Reduce occupational exposure to carcinogens	60%
Prostate	Reduce fat consumption	78%
Breast	Reduce fat and increase vegetable consumption Reduce obesity (postmenopausal women) Screen women aged 50 to 69	70%
Colorectal	Reduce fat and increase vegetable consumption	77%
Lymphoma	Reduce exposure to herbicides and pesticides	86%
Bladder	Eliminate smoking and reduce dietary cholesterol Reduce occupational exposure to carcinogens	73%
Body of the uterus	Reduce obesity Benefit from the protective effect of oral contraceptives (women aged 20 to 54)	82%
Stomach	Reduce nitrite in cured meats and salt-preserved foods, and increase fruit and vegetable consumption	52%
Leukemia	Reduce exposure to radiation and benzene	70%
Oral	Eliminate smoking and reduce alcohol consumption Increase fruit and vegetable consumption	68%
Pancreas	Eliminate smoking Reduce sugar and increase vegetable consumption	64%
Melanoma of the skin	Reduce unprotected exposure to sunlight	77%
Kidney	Eliminate smoking Reduce fat consumption	67%

Cancer site	Action	Percentage of cancer incidence potentially preventable
Brain	Reduce occupational exposure to carcinogens	70%
Ovary	Reduce fat consumption	
	Benefit from the protective effect of oral contraceptives (women aged 20 to 54)	53%
Cervix	Eliminate smoking	
	Encourage use of barrier contraceptives	
	Screen women aged 20 to 69	62%

*A.B. Miller, 'Planning Cancer Control Strategies', *Chronic Diseases in Canada* (Health Canada, 1992).

Source: Belliveau and Gaudette (1995).

security and lack of clean water and birth control are no longer problems for most people in most of the developed world. Rather, socio-economic inequity within developed societies, lifestyle, and environmental, work-related, and other factors are important in explaining Canada's present mortality rates. Figure 3.4 illustrates the downward trend in infant mortality in Canada, while Box 3.8 discusses the impact of obesity and eat-

ing disorders on the health of Canadians.

The mortality statistic, called PYLL or potential years of life lost, sheds a particularly useful light on causes of death for men and women of all ages in one year. Assuming life expectancy to be 75 years, PYLL shows the average number of potential years of life lost among all Canadians who die before 75 years of age. PYLL is a valuable statistic for examining 'premature death'. It gives

Figure 3.4   Life Expectancy at Birth and Infant Mortality

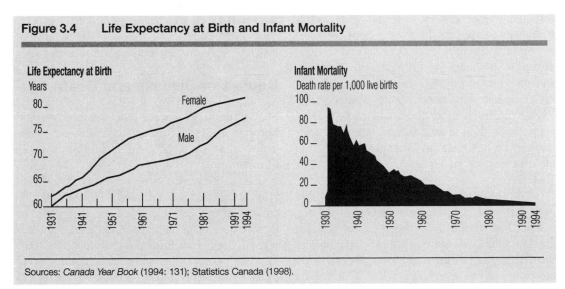

Sources: *Canada Year Book* (1994: 131); Statistics Canada (1998).

Box 3.8   Obesity and Eating Disorders

The rates of obesity in both adults and children are growing in Canada. One-third of Canadian boys and 27 per cent of Canadian girls were overweight in 1996. These figures are almost three times higher than they were in 1981. The rates of obesity in children have grown even more dramatically in the same period of time. Today, 10 per cent of boys and 9 per cent of girls are considered obese. These figures represent an increase of 500 per cent since 1981. This is much more than a concern about the aesthetics of overweight. Obesity in children is associated with higher rates of a myriad of disease conditions including higher blood pressure, abnormally high blood cholesterol levels, and associated cardiovascular problems. Some children may have the beginnings of arthritis and Type 2 diabetes (adult-onset diabetes). Obesity is implicated in deaths from a variety of causes.

What is going on? What are the sociological reasons for these dramatic changes in body size? How have lifestyles changed? How has the social and physical environment changed? What is the role of television? Of computerized games? Of cutbacks in support for team sports? What is the importance of the relative absence of swimming pools, skating rinks, and community athletic centres? How relevant are the increasing costs of sports equipment and access to arenas, ski hills, and pools? Why are poor children more likely to be overweight than children who are from families with more material resources? How important is the widespread availability coupled with the relative inexpensiveness of 'junk' food such as fat- and salt-laden chips? What role do fast-food restaurants play?

Source: John Demount, 'Growing Up Large', *Maclean's*, 5 Aug. 2002, 20–6.

---

heavier weight to deaths that occur at an early age than to deaths that occur late in life. Several contrasts are apparent when we compare PYLL with the leading causes of overall death. While malignant neoplasms have long been the most important PYLL, they have been second to heart disease as the cause of overall death. Accidents and suicides are a much more important cause of PYLL than overall death. Suicides and accidents are also a much more important cause of PYLL among men than among women, accounting for three and a half times as many potential years of life lost among males as among females (see Table 3.4).

The most important causes of death differ from the most important causes of PYLL. Of significant importance in the major causes of death are smoking, excessive alcohol consumption, diets rich in fat, sodium, and sugar, and stress. Of great importance in potential years of life lost are occupational and environmental hazards, lack of health and safety legislation or non-enforcement of existing legislation, risk-taking behaviour such as drinking alcoholic beverages and driving, lowered social cohesion and social capital, overall inequity, and impoverishment within society.

Causes of Disease and Death

Marc Lalonde, who at the time was the Canadian Minister of Health under Pierre Trudeau, published what was to be a significant health policy document in 1974. In it he broadened the explicit causes of disease beyond those confined to a biomedical model (see Chapter Thirteen for discussion of models of disease) and distinguished three causes of mortality: self-imposed, environmental, and biological host factors. By self-imposed factors Lalonde meant such things as (1) excessive alcohol consumption, (2) smoking, (3)

Table 3.4   Potential Years of Life Lost, by Cause of Death, 1997

	All causes	Neoplasms	Accidental deaths	Suicides	Perinatal mortality	Congenital anomalies	Respiratory diseases	Diseases of the heart	Cerebrovascular diseases	Other causes
					years					
All ages	1,019,155	303,060	193,502	102,080	459	13,362	29,992	34,962	27,901	213,840
1–4	30,485	3,417	9,849	—	201	3,819	1,407	1,139	268	10,385
5–9	19,750	3,938	8,125	—	125	1,250	438	563	188	5,125
10–14	23,000	3,335	9,085	2,933	58	1,150	633	978	288	4,543
15–19	60,638	4,515	30,030	13,703	—	1,313	893	1,260	210	8,715
20–4	61,513	4,703	29,735	13,918	48	998	1,188	1,235	95	9,595
25–9	57,843	6,970	21,590	12,070	—	978	850	2,083	765	12,538
30–4	75,750	10,800	23,625	14,513	—	900	1,313	3,563	1,163	19,875
35–9	92,820	21,158	19,565	14,560	—	683	1,690	8,125	2,730	24,310
40–4	107,828	33,440	15,978	11,825	28	715	1,980	13,970	3,300	26,593
45–9	116,438	43,695	10,868	9,225	—	653	3,330	20,025	4,118	24,525
50–4	118,510	51,538	7,228	5,215	—	333	3,693	23,765	4,480	22,260
55–9	111,100	52,338	4,225	2,600	—	325	4,238	24,038	3,888	19,450
60–4	95,168	43,103	2,595	1,193	—	203	4,943	22,238	4,028	16,868
65–9	48,315	20,113	1,005	328	—	45	3,400	11,983	2,383	9,060

Note: Potential years of life lost are calculated by taking the median age in each age group, subtracting from 70, and multiplying by the number of deaths in that age group disaggregated by sex and cause of death.

Source: Statistics Canada, Catalogue no. 82F0075XCB.

Box 3.9   The Horrors of War

Not only are millions of people wounded, killed, maimed, and raped as a result of wars, but the consequences of being in a war can be extremely problematic for survivors. Western governments are now realizing the potential for returning soldiers to suffer from a variety of types of psychological problems including post-traumatic stress disorder. In the summer of 2002, as the first Canadian soldiers to do a tour of duty in the war in Afghanistan came home, the Canadian government decided to send the 850 or so men and women who had fought in the deserts around Kandahar for six months to Guam on the way home to Canada. Here they rested and were given reintegration training, including group and individual counselling, to help them readjust to their lives in Canada, to their families and friends, and to the roles and responsibilities they had to resume in Canadian society (Radway, 2002: A7). At the same time the spouses and partners of the deployed soldiers had a series of workshops and counselling available to help them (and their children) adjust to life without their partners and to prepare them for their homecoming.

In the same day that a newspaper reported on this, a different paper reported on the murders of four women at a North Carolina army base. Their soldier husbands had killed three of these women after they had returned from fighting in Afghanistan. Two of the men killed themselves after killing their wives. The other two were arrested and charged. The first murder occurred when a soldier shot his wife and then himself two days after he had returned from Afghanistan. The next victim was strangled and the husband hid her body. The same day another murder-suicide was discovered. This one involved a soldier who had not been in Afghanistan.

Are these murders the result of the experiences that soldiers undergo as they do their work? Are they signs of post-traumatic stress disorder? Canadian Forces officials became resensitized to the issues facing returning soldiers recently when General Romeo Dallaire returned from 'peacekeeping' and spoke openly about the continuing effects of his experiences on his life (Bricker, 2002: A3).

Sources: Jon Bricker, 'Four Killings Bring Horrors of War Home', *National Post*, 27 July 2002., A3; Scott Radway, 'Soldiers easing back to normal life', *Globe and Mail*, 27 July 2002, A7.

drug abuse, (4) nutritional inadequacies such as overconsumption of sugar or fat, (5) lack of exercise or recreation, and overwork, (6) careless driving and failure to wear seat belts, and (7) promiscuity and sexual carelessness. Environmental factors include physical factors, such as contaminated water, acid rain, and air pollution; socio-economic factors such as urbanization and working conditions, including inadequate health and safety measures on the job. Finally, host factors are the result of individual biological heritage or genetics. The following sections will examine 'self-imposed' factors.

The Impact of Alcohol

Alcohol ingestion appears to affect health in paradoxical ways. On the one hand, excess consumption is known to be associated with morbidity and mortality through alcoholism, cirrhosis, malnutrition, accidents, obesity, suicide, and homicide. On the other hand, moderate drinking appears to have a beneficial impact on health. While most Canadians drink alcohol, the proportion who drink is declining (Single et al., 1996). In 1993, according to the General Social Survey, 74 per cent of Canadians over 15 years of age drank at least one alcoholic beverage in the

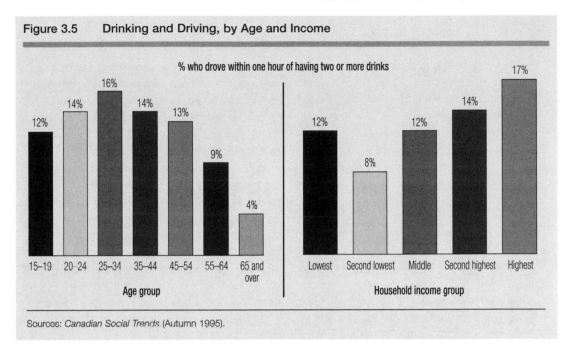

Figure 3.5   Drinking and Driving, by Age and Income

% who drove within one hour of having two or more drinks

Age group

Household income group

Sources: *Canadian Social Trends* (Autumn 1995).

year of the survey. This proportion is fewer than the 84 per cent in 1978 and the 78 per cent in 1989. Over the period 1978–93, Canadians both stopped drinking and failed to take it up at a higher rate. Heavy drinking has also become less common. Young people (20–4) continue to be the group most likely to have consumed alcohol (85 per cent in 1993). The proportion who drink declines as people age (Table 3.5). Men are more likely to consume alcohol than women—overall, 78.3 per cent of men consumed alcohol and 69.3 per cent of women in 1996 (Statistics Canada, 1997). Men also drink more frequently and more heavily. Those with some post-secondary education were more likely to drink than those with less education, as Box 3.10, which discusses drinking on college campuses, would appear to indicate. The higher the income group, the more likely it is that alcohol is consumed (88 per cent of those in the highest income group as compared to 63 per cent of those in the lowest income group). Driving while under the influ-

ence of alcohol is more common among the younger and more affluent (see Figure 3.6). Two thousand people died of cirrhosis of the liver (usually a direct result of overconsumption of alcohol) in 1997 and 35 per cent of all fatal car accidents in Canada involved alcohol (*Canada Year Book*, 2001). (See Tables 3.5, 3.6, and 3.7.)

Impact of Cigarette Smoking

Cigarette smoking is recognized as the leading cause of preventable death in Canada (Villeneuve and Morrison, 1995). There are still about seven million smokers in Canada. In 1999 about 27 per cent of men and 23 per cent of women smoked (ibid.). These figures constitute a decline for men (from 54 per cent) and for women (from 28 per cent) since 1966. A number of policies have been introduced (and then some have been retracted) to decrease the amount of cigarette smoking. Some successes have been noted. Between 1994–5 and 1996–7, 10 per cent of those who smoked quit and only 2 per cent of

Box 3.10   Alcohol on Campus

How often do you go to the pub? How do you feel about it? Is it fun for you or is it just something to do with your friends who seem to want to go 'pubbing'? Most universities seem to have at least one pub on the campus. Others have pubs in nearby towns and cities. Drinking alcohol is a major social activity for many young people in university and college today.

Many people are concerned about the amount and the frequency of alcohol consumption on campuses across the country. It appears to be normative on most campuses to go to the pub regularly, even weekly, as well as on 'special' occasions as a part of celebrations such as 'frosh week'. Students say that they drink to enhance their social activities and to 'break the ice' in a new social situation (Syre, 1997). Stress reduction and celebrating milestones in the school year (e.g., finishing a test or a paper and

exams) are among the other reasons students say they consume alcohol. As well as such personal and peer-based reasons, many universities institutionalize alcohol consumption as a regular part of campus life by including it in college-sponsored activities such as orientation week and residence socials. The presence of bars on campus and their centrality as meeting places for students off campus as well as in residences implicitly supports some degree of alcohol consumption. Cheaper beer prices, careless checking of age and identity cards, and the linking of alcohol with other forms of entertainment such as music are all ways to increase its consumption.

This sometimes becomes a problem. For example, students have died from over-indulging. What other issues do you think are important in considering drinking on campus?

Source: Thomas R. Syre, 'Alcohol and Other Drug Use at a University in the Southeastern United States: Survey Findings and Implications', *The College Student Journal* 31, 3 (1997): 272–381.

non-smokers began to smoke (ibid.). As Figure 3.6 shows, the decline in teenage smoking is the mirror image of the increase in tax levels.

Women smoke for the same reasons that men do, and for some additional reasons as well. Among the reasons are (1) because of addiction, (2) to enhance social acceptability, (3) to improve self-esteem and relieve stress, and (4) to control

weight (Cunningham, 1996: 165–73). Prevalence of smoking also declines as people age, because of both quitting and because of the relatively earlier deaths of those who do smoke. The decline in smoking has been associated with public health campaigns, warnings on cigarette packages, banning of cigarette advertising, and increased tax levels. In some jurisdictions there have been con-

Table 3.5   Alcohol Consumption by Sex and Age Group, 1998–1999 (Regular Drinkers)

	Total	12–14	15–17	18–19	20–4	25–34	35–44	45–54	55–64	65–74	75+
					%						
Males	65	x	38	71	76	71	75	69	66	53	42
Females	45	x	33	58	61	49	53	52	44	36	22

Source: Statistics Canada, Catalogue no. 82M0009XCB: <http://www.statcan.ca/english/Pgdb/People/Health/health05a.htm>.

Table 3.6	Regular Drinkers and Level of Education
Less than high school	45%
High school	57%
College diploma	57%
University diploma	63%

Source: Statistics Canada, Catalogue no. 82M0009XCB: <http://www.statcan.ca/english/Pgdb/People/Health/health05a.htm>.

Table 3.7	Smokers Aged 15–19 and Other Unhealthy Behaviours	
	Current smoker	Never smoked
	%	
Heavy infrequent drinker[1]	19	7
Heavy frequent drinker[2]	23	6
Used marijuana or hash in the last year	49	12
Used marijuana or hash at least once during the last month	28	4

[1]Drinks less often then once a week, usually five or more drinks when alcohol is used.
[2]Drinks once a week or more frequently, usually five or more drinks when alcohol is used.

Source: W. Clark (1996).

certed efforts to charge store owners who sell cigarettes to underage people. On the other hand, the increase in smoking among adolescent women is difficult to understand and explain.

Very few adults begin smoking. New smokers usually begin in their youth. In the homes of adult smokers, children typically 'try smoking' as early as five years old, and most have tried by seven or eight years old. The tobacco industry's advertising is directed towards a young market. Tobacco manufacturers regularly do surveys and hold focus groups for the youth market. That they recognize the importance of this youth market is illustrated in an Imperial Tobacco document:

> If the last ten years have taught us anything, it is that *the industry is dominated by the companies who respond most effectively to the needs of younger smokers.* Our efforts on these brands will remain on maintaining their relevance to smokers in these younger groups in spite of the share performance they may develop among older smokers. (Cunningham, 1996: 170; emphasis in original)

To be sure, smoking has harmful effects on health. Males who are regular smokers have a greater risk of many health problems. There is a time-lagged parallel between the rise of lung cancer deaths and tobacco consumption. Second-hand smoke also poses a significant health

Figure 3.6	The Relationship between the Prices of Cigarettes and the Rate of Teen Smoking

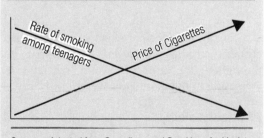

Sources: Adapted from *Canadians and Smoking: An Update* (Ottawa: Health and Welfare Canada, 1991).

problem. In 1995, 7.5 million non-smoking Canadians aged 15 and over, about 46 per cent of all non-smokers, were exposed to second-hand smoke. This exposure puts them at risk for heart disease, lung cancer, bronchitis, and pneumonia, asthma, and breast cancer (Clark, 1998; *Canada Year Book*, 2001).

Box 3.11   Occupational Mortality among Bartenders and Waiters

Dimich-Ward et al. (1988) studied death registrations in British Columbia to determine the strength of the association between exposure of waiters and bartenders to smoking and alcohol consumption, and their risk of death from lung cancer and cirrhosis of the liver. Records on 254,920 males and 165,912 females, representative of deaths in British Columbia between 1950 and 1978, were selected through the Division of Vital Statistics. Of these deaths, 1,280 men and 436 women had their occupation recorded as bartender or waiter.

It was found that alcohol- and tobacco-related causes of death were predominant among male bartenders and waiters. Measured in terms of proportional mortality ratios (PMR), their death rates from cancer of the mouth, esophagus, larynx, and lung, and from bronchitis and emphysema, cirrhosis, accidental poisoning due to drugs or alcohol, and homicides were higher than average. Elevated risks for female bartenders or waitresses included esophageal cancer, lung cancer, cirrhosis, and accidental death.

There are many potential explanations for these rates. A survey of smoking habits of US workers found that bartenders and waiters are among the highest percentages of cigarette smokers. It is, however, not only active smoking that is a contributing factor. Pollutants in the air of bars include carbon monoxide, nicotine, particulates, and aromatic hydrocarbons.

If 400 cigarettes are smoked per hour within a poorly ventilated tavern, the benzo(a)pyrene content would be the equivalent of 36 cigarettes smoked in an eight-hour period. Cooking fumes also contribute to benzo(a)pyrene levels. Benzo(a)pyrene has carcinogenic properties and is therefore likely to be involved in the etiology of respiratory cancers. It is said that ease of access to alcoholic beverages contributes to the elevated rates of cirrhosis for those whose occupation is bartender or waiter. These findings are important in identifying ways to cut the risks involved in such occupations.

Finally, it is worth noting that as the rates of cigarette smoking are declining in Canada and throughout the developed world, the rates are increasing in the developing world.

Physical Activity

Canadians of all ages have increased their levels of physical activity recently. In 1991, 32 per cent of Canadians over 15 years of age were 'physically very active' as compared to 27 per cent in 1985. Physical activity rates are highest among the younger age groups of Canadians. In 1991, 55 per cent of Canadians 15–24 years old and 36 per cent in the 24–44 age group were physically active; 21 per cent of men and 12 per cent of women over 65 were physically active. Men are more likely to be physically active than women,

although the rates of activity are increasing for both men and women (Millar, 1992). Still, it is estimated that 63 per cent of Canadians do not get enough exercise to provide health benefits.

The Impact of Weight, Body Image, and Eating Disorders

In spite of the increased levels of physical activity, the number of overweight Canadians has increased. Thirty-four per cent are now overweight (Gilmore, 1999). Overweight is more common among older Canadians. Men are more likely to be overweight than women, but women are more likely to be underweight. Despite women's tendency to underweight (especially when young) a sizable proportion of Canadian women with normal weights believe that they weigh too much.

Box 3.12   Why Do Young People Smoke?

Do you smoke cigarettes? If so, do you remember how and why you started? Have you ever tried to quit smoking? Smoking among young people is affected by a number of different factors. We will discuss just a few here. Consider for yourself some of the reasons not included in the following discussion.

(1) Smoking among young people is affected by school policy and by teaching in the schools.

(2) Students who attend schools that ban cigarette smoking entirely on school property are less likely to smoke than students at schools that offer restricted areas for smoking (13 per cent of those whose schools had banned smoking as compared to 20 per cent of those whose schools had simply restricted smoking areas smoked).

(3) Smoking rates are also related to the levels of academic achievement in young people. 8% of those who report that their academic achievement is above average smoke as compared with 15% of those who say their

achievement is average and 25% of those who say their achievement is below average. More than half of those (53%) of those who have quit school smoke.

(4) Having a smoker in the home is also associated with smoking in young people: 50 per cent of those in homes where both parents smoked, 33 per cent of those in homes where one parent, smoked and only 10 per cent of those in homes where no one smoked took up the habit. Prices also affect levels of smoking.

(5) When the government decreased the tax on cigarettes in 1994 in response to the high rates of smuggling of cigarettes across the US border there was an immediate increase in smoking among 5 per cent of smokers 15–19 years old. Moreover, 19 per cent of those in this age group began smoking.

(6) There is also a relationship between smoking cigarettes, drinking alcohol, and using soft drugs (Clark, 1996).

Source: Warren Clark, 'Youth Smoking', *Canadian Social Trends* (Winter 1996): 2–7.

The incidence of overweight and obesity is growing in spite of the proliferation of a wide range of products and services designed to help people lose weight. Fat-free, low-fat, and sugar-free products now control major market shares of every conceivable foodstuff and beverage category; personal exercise machine ownership continues to accelerate and health and fitness clubs have become routine locations for social interaction. This is not only an issue that relates to the aesthetics of gender or the related experience of self-esteem. Obesity is an excess of body fat frequently resulting in threats to health. People who are 20 per cent above their ideal body weight are considered obese (www.weight.com). Now considered

an epidemic, obesity is a significant risk factor for a variety of diseases, including cardiovascular disease, non-insulin-dependent diabetes mellitus (NIDDM), cancer of the breast, colon, and prostate, musculoskeletal problems, and gall bladder disease (Katzmarzyk, 2002). Obesity also leads to declines in the quality of life. There is a direct relationship between excess body weight and higher mortality. Approximately 35 per cent of men and 27 per cent of women are obese today.

Think for a minute about the causes of eating and of food choice. When do you eat? Are you always hungry when you eat? When you are hungry, how often do you stop to make a fresh salad or to eat a piece of fruit? How often do you stop at a fast-food outlet? What do you know about nutrients in various foods? What social changes do you think have led to the 'obesity epidemic'?

Sexuality and AIDS

Consideration of the health of Canadians would not be complete without a brief discussion of sexuality and some of its health consequences. In 1996, 25.3 per cent of males and 16.5 per cent of females in Canada between the ages of 15–29 had at least two different sexual partners. The numbers were much fewer for those 30–59: 6.9 per cent for men and 3.5 per cent for women. Among those who had sex with two (or more) partners, 39.7 per cent of the men and 3.6 per cent of the women over 20 used a condom with their regular partner and 53.9 per cent and 50.6 per cent of the men and women, respectively, used a condom for a casual partner (http://www.whobarcelona.info/AIDS2002/Canada_En.pdf). These figures reflect a need for continuing concern about AIDS and other sexually transmitted diseases among Canadians.

AIDS IS an infectious and contagious disease. Discovered in the late 1970s in the US, its presence was not officially noted until 1981. The first case recorded in Canada was in 1982 (Frank, 1996). It is estimated that by 1991 some 50,000 Canadians were infected with the HIV virus, which is believed to be the precursor of AIDS, and by 1995, 9,133 Canadians had died due to AIDS-related conditions (ibid.). In 2001, 55,000 Canadians have been diagnosed with HIV and are still alive and there have been 62,247 cases of HIV/AIDS as of 2001 (Ghosh, 2002). The rate of heterosexually transmitted HIV is growing while that of homosexually transmitted HIV is decreasing. Of cases reported by 30 September 1995, risk categories for men and women can be broken down as follows: 76 per cent are men who have sex with men; 9 per cent are the result of heterosexual contact; 4 per cent are men who have sex with men and inject drugs; 4 per cent are recipi-

ents of contaminated blood products; and 3 per cent are from injection drug use. Now the percentages are 11 per cent heterosexually transmitted, 69.1 per cent homosexually transmitted, 10.7 per cent transmitted via injected drug use, 3.4 per cent by blood, 0.9 per cent perinatally, and 4.9 per cent through an unknown route of transmission (http://www.whobarcelona.info/AIDS2002/canada_En.pdf). Table 3.8 shows the numerical distribution of sources of transmission.

It is estimated that over 35 million cases of AIDS have occurred around the world since the late 1970s. A significant majority of these cases have occurred in sub-Saharan Africa, South Asia, and the Americas. The disease is much more common in the US than in Canada. There were 1,542 cases per million people in the US and 380 cases per million in Canada. By comparison, there were 7 cases per million in Japan, 578 cases per million in France, 426 cases per million in Italy, 302 cases per million in Australia, and 173 cases per million in the UK (World Health Organization, *Weekly Epidemiological Record*, cited ibid.). Figure 3.7 indicates the global nature of the HIV/AIDS epidemic.

The incidence of HIV/AIDS among women is increasing rapidly in Canada. In 1986, 2 per cent of the HIV-positive population was female; by 1993, 15 per cent of the cases were female; and by 2001 25 per cent of newly reported cases were female (Ghosh, 2002). Globally, too, women make up the fastest-growing group infected with HIV. The modal age range of those diagnosed with HIV is 15–30 and the mean age is 30. Nearly half are under 34. The average age for HIV infection is declining. This has important implications for targeting information and education programs (ibid.).

Summary

(1) Over the past 150 years there have been dramatic changes in life expectancy rates in Canada and other developed nations. Many explanations have been suggested for this,

Table 3.8   AIDS in Canada by Mode of Transmission

Sex	Transmission Group	<1997	1997	1998	1999	2000	Total	%
All	All	15,628	688	599	416	260	17,591	100.0
	Hetero	1,592	116	113	81	38	1,940	11.0
	Homo/Bi	11,237	352	274	165	124	12,152	69.1
	IDU	1,444	137	143	103	60	1,887	10.7
	Blood	561	14	10	5	3	593	3.4
	Perinatal	138	11	4	4	2	159	0.9
	NS	656	58	55	58	33	860	4.9
Male	All	14,400	577	501	345	231	16,054	100.0
	Hetero	928	69	74	52	24	1,147	7.1
	Homo/Bi	11,237	352	274	165	124	12,152	75.7
	IDU	1,255	103	103	82	51	1,594	9.9
	Blood	409	11	7	3	3	433	2.7
	Perinatal	0	0	0	0	0	0	0.0
	NS	572	42	43	44	29	730	4.5
Female	All	1,049	97	94	64	26	1,330	100.0
	Hetero	664	47	39	29	14	793	59.6
	IDU	189	33	40	21	9	292	22.0
	Blood	121	3	3	2	0	129	9.7
	Perinatal	0	0	0	0	0	0	0.0
	NS	75	14	12	12	3	116	8.7

Hetero: Heterosexual contacts.
Homo/Bi: Homosexual contacts between men.
IDU: Injecting drug use—this category also includes cases in which other high-risk behaviours were reported in addition to injection of drugs.
Blood: Blood and blood products.
Perinatal Vertical transmission during pregnancy, birth, or breast-feeding.
NS: Not specified/unknown.

Source: Adapted from UNAIDS/WHO epidemiological fact sheet: <http://www.whobarcelona.info/AIDS2002/canada_En.pdf.>.

such as improvements in public health, improved nutrition, improvements in hygiene, and improvements in birth control. Immunization is also important for the health of a population.

(2) The chief causes of disease and death in Canada today are heart disease, cancer, and accidents. These can be referred to as diseases of civilization and affluence and are typical of developed nations. Causes of death

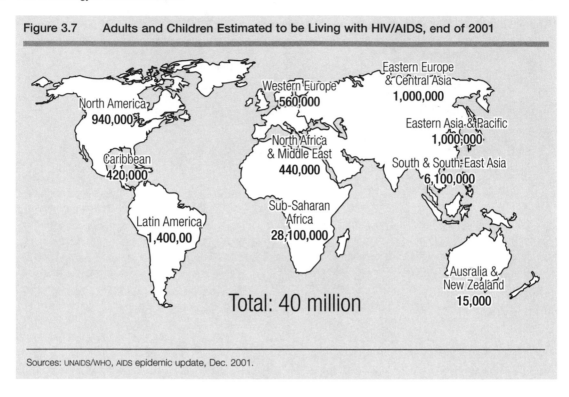

Figure 3.7   Adults and Children Estimated to be Living with HIV/AIDS, end of 2001

North America 940,000

Western Europe 560,000

Eastern Europe & Central Asia 1,000,000

Eastern Asia & Pacific 1,000,000

Caribbean 420,000

North Africa & Middle East 440,000

South & South-East Asia 6,100,000

Latin America 1,400,00

Sub-Saharan Africa 28,100,000

Ausralia & New Zealand 15,000

Total: 40 million

Sources: UNAIDS/WHO, AIDS epidemic update, Dec. 2001.

are related to lifestyle, environmental, and work-related factors. Self-imposed contributions to mortality include: smoking, drug abuse, excessive alcohol consumption, nutritional inadequacies, lack of exercise or recreation, overwork, reckless driving, and sexual carelessness. The diseases that result from smoking and alcohol consumption and the social characteristics of their users are discussed.

(3) Physical activity and obesity levels are related to the health of Canadians.

(4) AIDS is an important new disease with both spreading and devastating effects in populations around the world. Today the greatest incidence is in sub-Saharan Africa.

Questions for Study and Discussion

1. What is the relevance of medical treatment to the overall extension of life expectancy in Canada today? Consider the work of McKeown and McKinlay and McKinlay in your answer.

2. Why do women tend to live longer lives than men?

3. What are the major social interventions neces-sary to reduce global disparities in health and death rates?

4. Why is the position of women central to social and economic development in a worldwide context?

5. Compare and contrast the morbidity and mortality rates in Cuba and the Dominican

Republic and explain the differences.

6. What are the most important interventions today to increase the life expectancy of people in the developing world?

7. Explain the changing gender ratio with respect to HIV/AIDS.

Suggested Readings

Canada Year Book. Various years. Ottawa: Statistics Canada. A source of summary information on Canadian health, the labour force, demography, and so on.

Epp, Jake. 1986. *Achieving Health for All: A Framework for Health Promotion*. Ottawa: Minister of National Health and Welfare. Health policy today in Canada is influenced by the reports of Lalonde and Epp.

Lalonde, Marc. 1974. *A New Perspective on the Health of Canadians*. Ottawa: Information Canada. A government document of historical importance both in Canada and in an international context.

McKeown, T. 1976. *The Role of Medicine: Dream, Mirage or Nemesis*. London: Neufeld Provincial Hospitals Trust. An interesting work providing an important analysis of reasons for the decline in mortality over the last few hundred years.

World Health Organization. Various years. <www.who.org> This Web site has a great deal of information on health conditions around the world.

Chapter 4 | *Environmental and Occupational Health and Illness*

Learning Objectives

- Water, air, and land are the three fundamental parts of the environment upon which we depend for health.
- Environmental threats to all three are ubiquitous and increasing.
- Five important environmental threats are carbon dioxide and climate change, acid rain, the depletion of the ozone layer, insufficiently restricted introduction of new chemicals, and the disposal of hazardous wastes.
- Medical wastes and second-hand smoke are two other new and growing environmental threats.
- Occupational health and safety are significant causes of morbidity and mortality in Canada and around the world.
- There are important gender differences in occupational health and safety.
- Traffic, sports, and other accidents are also important challenges to health.

The Major Environmental Issues

Have you heard of the twentieth-century disease? Do you know anyone diagnosed with allergies or asthma? Is housework safer than factory work? Are occupational hazards greater for men or for women? Is environmental degradation a threat to health? What are the specific relationships between environments, occupations, and health? What is the significance, for health, of Chernobyl, Bhopal, Love Canal, the PCBs in the Great Lakes, the depletion of the Newfoundland fisheries, Walkerton, or the Westray Mine disaster? The purpose of this chapter is to provide an overview of some of the major environmental and occupational health hazards, their effects on health, and the potential sociological explanations.

There are three fundamental components of the environment: air, water, and land. They affect our health both directly (e.g., through the air we breathe and water we drink) and indirectly (e.g., through the food we eat). Environmental hazards in air, water, and land have increased tremendously in the twentieth century. It has been estimated, amid great controversy, that from 60 to 90 per cent of all cancers are environmentally caused.

Moreover, environmental hazards may affect our health in ways that are unseen in the short term and only evident in the long term in the health of future generations. Many diseases of major organ systems such as the lungs, heart, liver, and kidneys, as well as reproductive problems, birth defects, and behavioural disorders, seem to be associated with environmental factors. There are between 50,000 and 70,000 chemical substances in commercial use in farming, manufacturing, and forestry industries. Every year about 1,000 new chemicals are introduced in North America and about 2,000 worldwide (World Health Organization, 1997: 12), the majority of which have not been tested for potential ill effects. Radioactive waste with a half-life of 250 centuries, uranium mine tailings, and low-level radiation leakage from routinely functioning nuclear power plants and weapons facilities are taken for granted as an inevitable part of the environment by most Canadians. Nuclear accidents are almost 'normal' events. Yet they have the ongoing potential for massive death and destruction.

Environmental risks are now ubiquitous—and growing. The whole world is a united ecosystem. Changes in one nation-state's environmental policies and procedures, in the amounts of allowable air, water, and land pollution, for example, have the capacity to affect aspects of the ecology of the rest of the world. Even the snows of the remote, virtually uninhabited Antarctic contain residues of PCBs, DDT, and lead, which have emanated most directly from industries in North America and the former Soviet Union. Water, air, and soil have all been infiltrated with various types and degrees of toxic chemicals. Like other health threats, environmental hazards are unequally distributed. Poorer people in both the developed and developing worlds are less likely to be able to move away from a toxic waste dump, to drink bottled water, to buy organically grown foodstuffs, and so on. A study in the US noted that visible minorities (particularly Aboriginal, black, and Hispanic peoples) are more likely to live near

uncontrolled waste sites (Lee, 1987). A recent Canadian study expresses this relationship as follows: 'the victims, of course, are not a random group. There is an undeniable correlation between employment in lower-status, lower social class jobs and an increased risk of developing a work-related cancer. . . . it is precisely this group that is likely to be most affected by a company's environmental pollution when they leave the workplace' (Firth et al., 1997: xi). Socio-economic status has been shown to influence the likelihood that people live near noxious facilities (Been, 1994). In addition, decisions about locating noxious facilities discriminate against the poor and racial minorities (Hamilton, 1995).

The poorer, less-developed countries, too, are unequally subject to the destructive effects of environmental degradation when they, for instance, cut down precious rain forests to provide timber for furniture, housing, or other purposes for the developed world. Moreover, cash-strapped economies of the developing world, lacking alternatives, are more likely to allow the dumping of wastes within their borders in return for cash payments. Thus, there are ways that the environment of the underdeveloped South, in spite of a relative lack of industrialization, is more vulnerable than that of the developed North.

A number of environmental issues threaten the everyday health and safety of all people on the planet. Among the most critical environmental issues arguably are: (1) *carbon dioxide and climate change* (the greenhouse effect); (2) *acid precipitation*; (3) *the depletion of the ozone layer*; (4) *chemicals*; and (5) *the disposal of hazardous wastes* (*Economic and Ecological Interdependence*, 1982), (6) *industrial pollution of air, water, and land*, and (7) *medical wastes*.

Carbon dioxide is produced by the burning of fossil fuels used to provide heat for residential purposes and power for industry. Fossil fuels are one of the causes of increasing amounts of carbon dioxide in our atmosphere. Carbon dioxide reflects additional quantities of the sun's radiant

Box 4.1   Bhopal

One example of the effects of the political economy on the health of peoples in the developing world brings to light a number of issues. In 1984, in one of the worst industrial disasters ever, an explosion in a Union Carbide plant in Bhopal, India, spewed more than 40 tons of lethal methyl isocyanate gas into the slums immediately surrounding the plant. Over 6,000 people were killed. Many thousands of others were blinded, disabled, and diseased as a result of the 'accident'.

The 'accident' was absolutely avoidable; that it happened is the result of a number of important factors common in industries imported from the West to the developing world. First, the Union Carbide plant in Bhopal was relatively unprofitable as compared to other divisions of Union Carbide elsewhere in the world. At the time of the accident, the Bhopal plant was for sale. It lacked top-level interest or support. A number of divisions within the plant had been closed down. Personnel had been let go and not replaced.

Thus, it was operating with only a partial complement of workers and with equipment that was in poor repair. It was also, however, involved in the manufacture of dangerous chemicals such as methyl isocyanate. In spite of the objections of the municipal authorities, the central and state governments allowed it to continue operating without adequate safety precautions and regulations. There were no adequate plans for dealing with a major accident and the company personnel did not really understand the potentially lethal effects of the chemical they were producing (methyl isocyanate gas). The external regulation was extremely weak. In the interest of fostering the importation and investment of capital to their countries, governments in developing countries frequently ignore or are unaware of even minimal health and safety standards. The 'accident' at Bhopal is just one example of the potential for widespread industrial-based devastation in the developing world.

---

energy back to earth, causing a warming trend that affects, among other things, the growing of crops and the probability of flooding from the melting of glaciers. The depletion of the ozone layer, which is already happening rapidly as the result of the use of aerosol spray containers, among other things, has increased this warming trend and has led to and will continue to cause an increased incidence of skin cancer and extensive damage to animal and plant life.

The primary agents in the production of acid precipitation are sulphur and nitrogen. They are released as gases from ore smelters, coal-fired generating stations, automobile exhausts, and ore and gas refineries. Sulphur and nitrogen combine with water vapour in the air to form acidic solutions—primarily sulphur dioxide and several nitrous oxides. These acids then fall as precipitation and enter the soil and surface water, ulti-

mately affecting plant and animal life. There is evidence that acid precipitation can lead to gastroenteritis and respiratory damage (Weller, 1986). Air pollution may result from the more than 70,000 chemicals on the commercial market, many of which are released into the environment; little or nothing is known of their potential long-range effects. Finally, the problems of disposing of hazardous wastes particularly threaten those less economically able to resist dumping in their own backyards.

Pollutants pose significant threats to health. Polluted water and air affect rates of dysentery, typhoid, various bacterial and infectious diseases, lung disease, including cancer, various respiratory problems, and cardiovascular diseases. Pesticides such as DDT are known to kill or induce disease in fish and wildlife. They may also have an adverse effect on people when they enter

Box 4.2   Environmental Illness

An increasing number of North Americans are suffering from what they claim to be the results of low-level exposures to synthetic chemicals (Ashford and Miller, 1991) and what has been called by a variety of names, including 'multiple chemical sensitivity', 'chemically induced hyper-susceptibility', 'immune system dysregulation', 'environmental illness' or EI, and 'twentieth-century disease'. These are similar to other new diseases such as AIDS (see Sontag, 1988: 104) in which the sufferer is subject to a whole range and variety of signs and symptoms, of varying severity, some of which change considerably from day to day. Among the various symptoms often reported are the following: headaches, rashes, depression, shortness of breath, muscle and joint inflammation, fatigue, nausea, and other gastrointestinal and nervous system disorders. Those with EI are often sensitive to a wide range of synthetic environmental contaminants. Equally troubling, because of its delegitimizing character, is the fact that symptoms often cannot be detected by standard methods. One consequence of the lack of reliable diagnostic markers is that most allopathically trained medical doctors do not recognize this as a real disease. In 1965 a small group of physicians, scientists, and health professionals founded the Society for Clinical Ecology to address the issues being brought forward by sufferers. Renamed the American Academy of Environmental Medicine in 1984, it now has about 600 physician members (Oberg, 1990: 6).

In 1987 the Environmental Research Foundation and the National Academy of Scientists in the United States suggested that between 15 and 20 per cent of the US population may have allergic sensitivity to chemicals in the environment. The Environmental Protection Agency has also stated that health problems result, for some people, at levels of exposure considered below regulatory concern. People with environmental sensitivities have to be careful about where they live, where they go to school and play, what they eat, drink, and smell. Their whole lives may be affected by their sensitivities. Some have even established a protected community, in Wimberly, Texas, an area with little industry or farming (Belkin, 1990).

the food chain. Solid wastes (such as plastics, rubber, glass, and metals) that do not break down except over a very long period of time pollute the environment and take up space that could be used by living things. Noise pollution may lead to loss of hearing, accidents, stress, cardiovascular disease, and disturbed sleep. Critical environmental issues threaten the quality of the air, the water, and the land. Some specific contemporary concerns with respect to air, water, and land will be examined in turn.

Air Pollution and Human Health

Both indoor and outdoor air contribute at least low levels of pollutants, including ozone, sulphur oxides, nitrogen oxides, carbon monoxide, and other particulates that may irritate eyes and inflame the respiratory tract. There is evidence that long-term exposure may have a negative effect on the immune system and be implicated in long-term respiratory problems such as emphysema and chronic bronchitis, cancer, asthma, cardiovascular disease, chronic obstructive pulmonary disease, and various respiratory infections (Raven et al., 1993: 435).

Air pollution is already known to kill men and women in Canadian cities. Burnett, Cakmak, and Brook (1998) examined daily deaths in 11 Canadian cities from 1980 to 1991 and evaluated the association of these deaths to concentrations of ambient gaseous air pollutants. They found that nitrogen dioxide had the largest effect on mortality, a 14.1 per cent increased risk, followed by ozone (1.8 per cent), sulphur dioxide (1.4 per cent), and carbon monoxide (0.9 per cent). The five cities that were able to reduce sulphur content in gas to 30 ppm were able to show a risk reduction (Montreal, Toronto, Winnipeg, Edmonton, Vancouver). A number of adverse health effects are also associated with ambient air pollution, including respiratory symptoms, lost school and work time, restricted activity, asthma attacks, emergency room visits, hospital admissions, and deaths. An extreme case of indoor pollution is the 'sick building syndrome' in which the presence of air pollution inside tightly sealed buildings can lead to a whole variety of illnesses. As well, total environmental sensitivity, in which a person is allergic to myriad components in the modern environment, has forced some people to live in a totally sterile environment.

The most seriously harmful indoor pollutant may be radon, a tasteless, odourless gas that forms naturally during the radioactive decay of uranium in the earth's crust. Radon seeps through the earth and through basements. It greatly increases the deleterious effects of smoking on the lungs. Another indoor pollutant with serious health costs is asbestos. Often used as insulation because it does not conduct heat or electricity, asbestos also can break down into almost invisible fibres that can be inhaled. When inhaled it irritates the lungs and is known to be related to lung cancer and mesothelioma, a rare and almost always fatal cancer. Many millions of workers in Canada and around the world have been exposed to asbestos in mining, textile industries, and construction industries (Firth et al., 1997). In the last several decades various levels of government have acknowledged the dangers of asbestos that have been known since the 1920s and have introduced laws to remove asbestos insulation from public buildings such as schools and offices and eliminate its use in new buildings. Unfortunately, some research has shown that removing asbestos

can release fibres that would otherwise remain stable and thus it is sometimes safer to seal asbestos in place.

Apart from yet related to harmful pollutants in the air, temperature alone can be a contributing factor to mortality rates, as extreme cold and extreme heat result in higher mortality rates

Second-hand Smoke

Second-hand smoke is both an environmental and occupational health issue. It is an environmental issue because smoking may affect others in homes, on the streets, in public buildings, on public transportation, and in restaurants and stores. It is a workplace issue because workers may be involuntarily exposed to the second-hand smoke of their colleagues.

Not only is smoking a direct cause of lung cancer but so is breathing in the second-hand smoke of others, and here young non-smokers are most likely to be exposed to second-hand smoke (Figure 4.2). Researchers at Canada's Laboratory Centre for Disease Control have estimated that as many as 330 non-smoking Canadians may die yearly from lung cancer due to regular exposure to second-hand smoke (Canadian Cancer Society, 1994). There are two sources of second-hand smoke: sidestream smoke (given off by the burning tip of a cigarette, pipe, or cigar) and exhaled smoke (puffed out by the smoker). Among the toxic chemicals released into the air in these ways are nicotine, tar, carbon monoxide, formaldehyde, hydrogen cyanide, ammonia, and nitrogen oxide. Among the health effects are lung cancer, bronchitis, emphysema, asthma, hay fever, cystic fibrosis, headaches, coughs, throat irritation, heart and circulatory diseases, pregnancy complications, and low-birth-weight babies, among others. Table 4.1 lists the major air pollutants, their sources, and their health consequences.

Automobiles and other motor vehicles continue to be a major source of air pollution (Goodall, 1992), although emissions have been

Figure 4.1   A Model of the Relationship between Temperature and Deaths from Heart Disease and Stroke

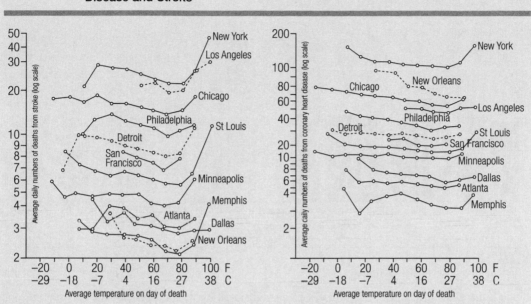

Source: Adapted from A. Haines, 'The Implications for Health', in S. Leggett, ed., *Global Warming: The Greenpeace Report* (New York: Oxford University Press, 1990).

Box 4.3   Last Gasp

Asthma is often seen as an elusive disease. Although it tends to run in families, it also develops in those who have no history of asthma among their kin. This disease may strike at any age, but children, with their small breathing tubes, are particularly vulnerable.

Several millions of Canadians suffer from asthma, the sometimes lethal inflammation of the airways to the lungs. In asthma sufferers, the bronchial tubes or airways are extremely sensitive to a variety of triggers unique to each patient. These triggers include those in modern office buildings, such as the more than 900 chemical and biological agents in the air, including chromium dust, acrylates, and epoxy resins. In factories and shops, there are more

unseen dangers like fluorocarbon propellants breathed in by beauticians, sulphur dioxide fumes inhaled by brewery workers, and chlorine gas encountered by petrochemical workers.

There are other triggers in homes. Central heating and wall-to-wall carpeting are breeding grounds for dust mites, microscopic animals that produce a potent allergen in their dung. Common household products like vapours from cleaning solvents and paint thinners and the fumes from such personal products as spray deodorants and scented cosmetics can also set off an attack. Some individuals display fewer symptoms while others face life-threatening attacks. Some physicians confuse this disease with respiratory infections, especially in children.

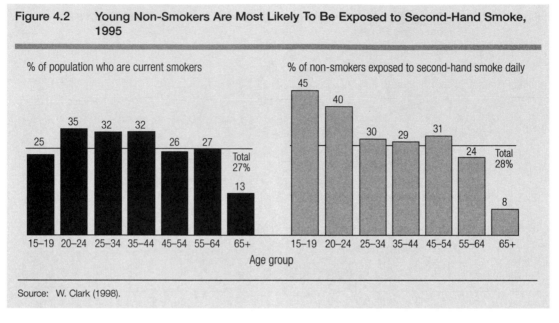

Figure 4.2   Young Non-Smokers Are Most Likely To Be Exposed to Second-Hand Smoke, 1995

Source: W. Clark (1998).

reduced since the Clean Air Act of 1971. The number of vehicles has grown and the total number of kilometres driven has increased over that time. Four common air contaminants from automobiles (although to a lesser extent, they arise from other sources as well) are carbon monoxide, nitrogen oxides, hydrocarbon, and ground-level ozone. In high concentrations, these substances can affect pulmonary function, suppress the immune system, and result in toxic and carcinogenic effects. They also contribute to acid rain, depletion of the ozone layer, and global warming.

Greenhouse Effect

The greenhouse effect, which has received considerable media attention in recent years, can be thought of as a rise in the earth's average temperature due to increasing concentrations of carbon dioxide (and other similar gases) in the environment. This global warming has both direct and indirect effects on human health. The indirect effects operate through the many changes in the physical environment, such as

drought on the Prairies, decline of water supplies in southern Canada, soil degradation, erosion, and flooding of coastal regions (*Canada's Green Plan*, 1994: 99). These changes result in changes in quality and availability of primary requisites for human life—food and water. Temperature increases may also directly cause certain health problems, especially affecting the cardiovascular, cerebrovascular, and respiratory systems. For instance, one US study noted increased rates of death and stroke at about 25°C (Chivian et al., 1993). As the concentration of carbon dioxide increases the number of deaths can be expected to increase. For example, during summer heat waves in Los Angeles, when temperatures averaged about 41°C, the peak mortality was between 172 per cent and 445 per cent higher than would have been expected (at all ages). Among people over 85 the peak mortality was considerably higher. It ranged from 257 per cent to 810 per cent more than the expected mortality levels. Figure 4.1 illustrates the striking correlation between temperature and stroke in 12 American cities.

Table 4.1   Principal Air Pollutants, Their Sources, and Their Respiratory Effects

Pollutant	Sources	Health effects
Sulphur oxides, particulates	Coal and oil plants Oil refineries, smelters Kerosene stoves	Bronchoconstriction Chronic bronchitis Chronic obstructive lung disease
Carbon monoxide	Motor vehicle emissions	Asphyxia leading to heart and nervous system damage, death
Oxides of nitrogen (NO_x)	Motor vehicle emissions Fossil fuel power plants Oil refineries	Airway injury Pulmonary edema Impaired lung defences
Ozone (O_3)	Motor vehicle emissions Ozone generators Aircraft cabins	Same as NO_x
Polycyclic aromatic hydrocarbons	Diesel exhaust Cigarette smoke Stove smoke	Lung cancer
Radon	Natural	Lung cancer
Asbestos	Asbestos mines and mills Insulation Building materials	Mesothelioma Lung cancer Asbestosis
Arsenic	Copper smelters Cigarette smoke	Lung cancer
Allergens	Pollen Animal dander House dust	Asthma, rhinitis

Source: From H.A. Boushey and D. Sheppard, 'Air pollution', in J.F. Murray and J.A. Nadel, eds, *Textbook of Respiratory Medicine* (Toronto: Saunders, 1988).

Medical Pollution

Burning medical wastes is another serious, yet relatively unknown source of air pollution, particularly in urban areas. On average, each hospitalized patient contributes 13 pounds of waste on a daily basis. The wastes emitted include soiled bandages and bedding, replaceable syringes and other surgical/medical tools, contaminated plastics, and pathogenic remains, such as blood and body parts. The problem is compounded by the fact that most medical incinerators do not meet adequate standards of waste disposal. Waste is burned incompletely, thereby emitting acidic gases, heavy metals, toxic organics, and dioxins that can be from 10 to 100 times higher than waste from municipal incinerators (Rabe, 1992).

Water Pollution and Human Health

The Great Lakes comprise one-fifth of the world's fresh surface water. Their destruction is a Canadian and an international disaster. The Great Lakes are both a source of drinking water for about 40 million people on both sides of the

Box 4.4   Global Warming: Is It So Bad?

Stephen Strauss, a science writer for the *Globe and Mail*, finally said it, that a hotter climate has many benefits. Accompanied by a cartoon featuring a 'Welcome to Whitchorse' sign surrounded by palm trees, the article playfully suggests that Canadians are not likely to be opposed to shorter winters. Among the advantages of a shorter winter would be fewer traffic accidents. Between 1988 and 1997 there were over 4,500 fatal traffic accidents and over one-quarter of a million people hurt on snowy, ice-packed, slippery, and slushy winter roads. Not only are traffic accidents more frequent in the winter, but apparently people are more likely to die. Mortality rates are 10 to 25 per cent higher in the winter than in the summer. However, deaths are not the only rates that could go down in a warmer Canada. Taxes could as well. Snow removal currently costs Canadians about $1 billion a year. Icebreakers for ferry crossings on the east coast, which cost about $75 million, might not be needed. Individually owned snow-blowers apparently consume millions of Canadian consumer dollars. On average, Canadians pay about $1,000 a year to heat their homes. This, too, could diminish, as could the cost of winter boots, coats, hats, and mitts. These are just a few of the benefits of global warming put forth by Strauss. Have some fun thinking about what some of the others might be.

Source: Stephen Strauss, 'Global Warming May Not Be So Bad', *Globe and Mail*, 18 May 2002, F7.

Box 4.5   Just Some 'Facts' from a World Health Organization Fact Sheet on Air Pollution

Inside and outside air pollution is a major environmental problem around the globe. Every year millions of people die or suffer serious health effects from it, including, most directly, respiratory diseases, asthma, chronic obstructive pulmonary disease, cardiovascular disease, and lung cancer. The elderly, the very young, and those who are otherwise compromised with respect to health are among the most vulnerable.

- About 3 million people die every year from air pollution (this comprises about 5 per cent of annual deaths).
- Around 30–40 per cent of asthma may be linked to air pollution.
- Adult cigarette smokers raise their chance of dying from lung cancer between 20 per cen-

tand 30 per cent if they work or live in an atmosphere where others also smoke.
- Indoor exposure to air pollution (from indoor fires, for example) is directly linked to mortality and acute respiratory infections and is a prime cause of child and infant mortality in the developing world.
- Air pollution is responsible for about one-third of all occupational illnesses around the globe.
- Traffic and industry are major causes of outdoor pollution.
- Indoor cooking and heating produces many pollutants and a pollutant released indoors is 1,000 times more threatening to the respiratory system than the same fumes would be outdoors.

Source: <http://www.who.int/inf-fs/en/fact187.html>.

Canada-US border and a garbage dump for industrial and domestic waste. Already, over 1,000 chemical and metal pollutants have been observed in the Great Lakes (Harding, 1994: 653). In the Golden Horseshoe between Oshawa and St Catharines in southern Ontario there are more than 50 sources of industrial pollution and more than 30 sources of municipal sewage. Moreover, for many years, untreated industrial and human wastes have been dumped directly into the lake from both Canada and the US (ibid.).

The overuse of water is another environmental threat. Canada already has one of the highest per capita consumption rates of any country. Ninety per cent of water is used for industrial and agricultural consumption. Free trade agreements and the pressure from the US to divert some of Canada's water to its southern neighbour potentially comprise a great threat to Canadian health via the decreased availability of clean water for Canadian consumption.

More recently, overfishing and bottom dredging by foreign and Canadian ships have contributed to the exhaustion of the cod stocks off Newfoundland. In response the Canadian government declared a moratorium on cod-fishing. This is a disaster for the province as cod has long been the staple basis for the vulnerable economy of the island.

Land Pollution and Human Health

One of the most contested of contemporary issues is what to do with solid waste—domestic, manufacturing, hospital, radioactive, or from any other source. Debates about waste disposal have even spawned a new acronym, NIMBY (not in my backyard). Without doubt, this environmental problem concerns the effect on humankind of the thousands of by-products and wastes of our industrial society, ranging from slightly annoying products to deadly toxins and chemicals.

Increasingly, literature on hazardous waste disposal in Canada and the United States points to

a growing problem with seemingly fewer and fewer solutions (Rabe, 1992). Many facilities, unable to meet tightening regulatory standards, have closed. Others have been planned but have been prevented from opening because of local opposition. Deciding the location for the hundreds of millions of metric tons of hazardous wastes is one of the most important political and policy issues of the day. Alberta, Manitoba, and Quebec appear to be among the most effective jurisdictions involved in providing sites in North America. Success in these jurisdictions has taken place via a procedure that has rejected top-down planning in favour of extensive public participation, creative types of community compensation, and solid partnerships among public and private organizations and local and provincial governments (ibid.).

As the deleterious effects of hazardous waste disposal become more widely known, dumping wastes becomes a complicated legal and political issue. Chapter Sixteen discusses drug dumping in the less-developed world. Hazardous waste dumping in countries of the South is a similar problem. When some industries in the richer developed world have needed to get rid of hazardous wastes they have shipped them to countries in the developing world. Some nations around the world have tentatively committed to some controls on international shipments of wastes, such as those from hospitals and pharmaceutical companies, PCBs, mercury, lead, and other chemicals that are known to be harmful. Such commitments are almost impossible to monitor effectively.

Biodiversity

All of these threats to the air, water, and land have another profound implication for the future of life on the planet—the decline in biodiversity. For instance, although the rain forests comprise only 7 per cent of the earth's surface, they are home to almost half of the living species of the planet. While it is impossible to know exactly how many

Box 4.6   Why Is It Difficult To Demonstrate Effects of the Environment on Health?

For a number of reasons it is difficult to assess the effect of the environment on health. Among these reasons are the following:

- The environment is complex: differentiating among different parts of the environment and their independent effects is practically impossible.
- Since new chemicals are released into the environment almost daily, noting and then measuring the particular amount of the chemical in the changing environment is exceedingly difficult.
- The ratio of the potential contaminant to the environment is usually so extremely small that instruments capable of measuring such minuscule amounts are not readily available.
- Double-blind studies with human subjects are considered unethical, yet the amount of the contaminant necessary to account for the time lag and for the low weight of the typical laboratory mammal (rat) is relatively enormous.
- Synergistic relationships are inevitable in the environment, yet because all of the elements in the synergistic relationship are not known the effects cannot be duplicated.
- There is a variable latency period between exposure and the onset of disease. Both this variability in latency and its length make identifying causal connections between toxic substance and illness difficult.

- Few physicians are trained in environmental and occupational health.
- A definite cause-effect link demonstration is required as proof.

Consequently, only a small number of environmentally based illnesses have yet been noted and a fraction of occupationally caused illnesses compensated (one out of 17 occupationally induced cancers is estimated to be compensated by Workers' Compensation in Ontario) (Makdessian, 1987). The ideological/financial issues include the following:

- Frequently, sponsors of research are pharmaceutical and medical device companies with a vested interest in research that involves their products.
- When research is funded by interest groups, independent research is difficult at best.
- Medical journals, the major legitimate purveyors of new scientific findings, are also often funded by major pharmaceutical companies.
- Certain types of basic research have dominated to date and because of the peer review system (a good old boys' network, some would say) basic research has a greater likelihood of support than other types of research.

species there are at present, some scientific estimates suggest that the total number of species is in the range of 30 million. In fact, researchers have identified more than one thousand species of ant (Wilson, 1991, in Macionis, 1995). The impact of the decline in biodiversity on the health of human populations is not entirely known. However, given the enormous interdependence in this complex ecosystem, the extinction of some species may very well indirectly lead to the extinction of others and ultimately may lead to the destruction of species that serve to protect human life.

Occupational Health and Safety

Worldwide, 200,000 people are killed and 120 million injured annually in reported work-related incidents (World Health Organization, 1997).

Table 4.2   Claims by Year of Accident, Ontario, Selected Years

	1988		1991		1994		1997	
Allowed lost-time	208,499	43%	155,475	39%	125,644	34%	101,806	30%
Allowed no lost-time	226,850	47%	195,204	48%	177,022	48%	168,463	50%
Not allowed	43,703	9%	48,645	12%	62,482	17%	64,737	19%
Abandoned	33,974		39,149		50,416		53,768	
Denied	9,729		9,496		12,066		10,969	
Pending	8,602	2%	3,680	1%	4,002	1%	4,470	1%
Total	487,654	100%	403,004	100%	369,150	100%	339,476	100%

Source: Ontario Workers' Compensation Board, *Annual Report* (1997), 3.

Table 4.3   Lost-Time Claims by Gender, Ontario, Selected Years

Gender	1988		1991		1994		1997	
Male	155,546	74.6%	110,859	71.3%	88,395	70.4%	71,160	69.9%
Female	52,244	25.1%	44,063	28.3%	37,098	29.5%	30,571	30.0%
Not available	709	0.3%	553	0.4%	151	0.1%	75	0.1%
Total	208,499	100%	155,475	100%	125,644	100%	101,806	100%

Source: Ontario Workers' Compensation Board, *Annual Report* (1997), 7.

Canadians face a relatively high degree of danger when they go to work. Statistics on workplace accidents and work-related injuries likely underestimate the number of injuries that occur because many people do not receive or request compensation. Others may be transferred to lighter jobs during the time of recuperation so that compensation is unnecessary. Nonetheless, there has been a significant decrease in the rate of job-related accidents. In 1988 there were 487,654 registered occupational accidents in just one province, Ontario. By 1997, the number for Ontario had dropped to 339,476 registered accidents (see Table 4.2). This dramatic shift certainly reflects the change in the economy as globalization and North American free trade have sent primary and secondary manufacturing jobs out of Canada and the tertiary service sector has grown. The downward shift also may reflect an increased unwillingness to report accidents due to the fear of job loss or the lack of faith that the claimant is likely to receive compensation. As Table 4.3 indicates, there has been an increase in disallowed claims, from 9 per cent in 1988 to 19 per cent in 1997. Reflecting the differences in male and female occupations and their changes over time, Table 4.3 shows that while women make fewer claims as a result of on-the-job accidents, the proportion of claims made by women has increased from 25.1 per cent in 1988 to 30.0 per cent in 1997.

In addition to workplace accidents, workers

Box 4.7   Problems with Pesticides

Fifty million people in the world are estimated to work on plantations and to experience direct contact with pesticides. Another 500 million people are exposed through seasonal agricultural work. Even the 'non-exposed' population is exposed through water and food contaminated with pesticides. Chronic poisoning with heavy metals, such as lead, can result in many other serious health problems. This risk is growing in urban areas as reliance on automobiles increases. The incidence of thyroid cancer is growing already among those children who live near Chernobyl, Ukraine. In the years 1980–5 there were three cases. In the 1986–95 period there were 420 reported cases of thyroid cancer in children under 15. About 3 million deaths each year are estimated to be the result of air pollution around the world (World Health Organization, 1997: 12).

The use of pesticides, chemical fertilizers, and insecticides on the land has been found to be associated with a variety of human cancers. The hormone-disrupting capabilities of organochlorides have been observed repeatedly. Coburn et al. (1998) trace their use to the decline in mating and nesting behaviour in bald eagles between 1947 and 1952. The best explanation was that the birds had become sterile. In 1970, herring gulls on Near Island in Lake Ontario were observed to have a chick death rate of 80 per cent. The dead chicks exhibited 'grotesque deformities', including 'adult feathers instead of down, club feet, missing eyes, twisted bills' (ibid., 4). Despite the links of fertilizer use to morbidity and mortality for animals and humans, its use continues to rise. Three countries alone, the United States, China, and India, account for half of the world's fertilizer use.

face a number of hazards on the job. These can be classified as physical (e.g., noise, heat or cold, postural, radiation), chemical (e.g., solvents, heavy metals, pesticides, pharmaceuticals), biological (e.g., HIV, hepatitis B and C), and psychological (e.g., stress and violence). Workplace hazards, too, are likely to increase under globalization and free trade. To attract multinational companies to use their labour and resources, poor countries will compete with one another. One way (in the short run) to compete effectively is to lower labour costs. Lower labour costs involve, among other things, fewer health and safety precautions for workers as well as an absence of workers' compensation.

The US government has estimated that as many as 40 per cent of all cancers may be caused by the work environment. Others have estimated that up to 90 per cent of cancers are related, in part, to the working environment (Epstein, 1998; Firth et al., 1997). Exposure to the following substances has been found to increase the risk of cancer by the amount indicated in brackets: arsenic (2 to 8 times for lung cancer); benzene (2 to 3 times for leukemia); coal, tar, pitch, and coke oven emissions (2 to 6 times for cancer of the lung, larynx, skin, and scrotum); vinyl chloride (200, 4, and 1.9 respectively for cancer of the lining of the heart, brain, and lung); chromium (3 to 40 for cancers of the sinus, lung, and larynx) (Tataryn, 1979: 157–8). High exposure to levels and consequent risks are more prevalent among the working classes and those with lower incomes (ibid., 158). Firth et al. (1997) have documented the extensive occupationally induced health problems from asbestos in Thetford Mines, Quebec, and at Bendix Automotive in Windsor; radiation exposure in Elliot Lake; and arsenic exposure in drinking water.

Occupational health and safety are major concerns for all working women, both those who work in the paid labour force and those who do not. Less publicized than the hazards associated with blue-collar work, the places where most

Box 4.8   Occupational Health and Safety

Paradoxically, workers' compensation boards work, on the one hand, to provide benefits to certain workers who have suffered ill health as the result of work, and on the other hand, to reinforce the notion that health is commodifiable—that it has a certain monetary value. Doran (1988: 460) argues that in spite of the evident advantages from workers' compensation legislation, an equally important loss has been suffered: workers have to battle to preserve their health at the expense of industrial production. The commodification of health has been characterized by an increasingly narrow definition of health that largely denies the experience of the sufferer/worker while valorizing the medical and legal definitions. Thus, illness is not defined by the sufferer but by the medical/legal authorities who label a narrow set of experiences as, first, medically relevant and, second, occupationally induced. One primary modality through which this is accomplished is the bureaucratic necessity of a workers' compensation form that includes some categories of symptoms as relevant and, by exclusion, deems other symptoms irrelevant. Moreover, accidents are prioritized over long-term chronic conditions as more likely to be worker-related (ibid).

Canadian women work, including 'offices, banks, stores, restaurants, hospitals, medical laboratories, schools, child care centres and hairdressing establishments' (CACSW, 1987: 85–6), have their own peculiar health risks.

Clerical workers may be subject to poor lighting and ventilation, excessive noise, and toxic substances such as emissions from computer terminals. Often they spend long hours sitting on uncomfortable furniture, which may lead to back pain, and working at relatively monotonous jobs, which may lead to stress. Retail and service workers may be vulnerable to health hazards from bending, lifting, and carrying; varicose veins and foot and back problems are often experienced. Hairdressers, who usually stand all day, suffer back and foot problems along with the dangers of exposure to toxic chemicals such as hair permanents, dyes, and aerosol sprays. Respiratory difficulties and skin reactions are frequent results. Teachers and child-care workers are continually exposed to a variety of contagious and infectious diseases. Health-care workers may be exposed to radiation, toxic chemicals, and contagious diseases, and may have to cope as well with lifting, bending, and standing. Women who work at home may be subject to dangers from all sorts of household cleaning substances such as abrasives, astringents, soaps, and detergents (ibid., 85–8).

Occupational stress has recently been recognized as a significant problem associated with a number of health problems, such as alcoholism (see Figure 4.3). 'Symptoms of persistent stress include physiological, psychological, and behavioral changes that result in depression, job dissatisfaction, increased blood pressure, increased blood serum cholesterol, increased risk of coronary disease, migraine headaches, and increased drug and alcohol consumption' (Geran, 1992: 14). Among the sources of stress listed in the General Social Survey of 1990 were (a) unreasonable deadlines (27 per cent), (b) conflicts with people at work (23 per cent), (c) lack of feedback (23 per cent), (d) unclear duties (22 per cent), and (e) not enough influence over the job (22 per cent). Some people have suffered psychiatric illness as a result of workplace stress and have been able to prove this link to the satisfaction of workers' compensation boards and commissions across Canada (ibid., 17). The physical environment was also noted as a source of stress, including poor air

Box 4.9   Occupational Diseases of Hairdressers

There are 66,855 hairdressers in Canada, representing 0.6 per cent of the workforce. The most frequent occupational diseases among hairdressers are skin diseases, followed by respiratory disease, certain cancers, and other miscellaneous diseases.

Hairdressers are in daily contact with cosmetic preparations and metallic instruments for shampooing, drying, bleaching, tinting, and permanently waving; these preparations can lead to dermatitis and eczema of the fingers and hands and occasionally the forearms. 'Cosmetologists perform other beauty services such as massaging the face and neck with creams and oils, colouring eyebrows and eyelashes, manicuring fingernails and toenails, and carrying out depilatory techniques' (Heacock and Rivers, 1986: 109). Other skin diseases include hair implantation granulomas as a result of hair cuttings becoming embedded in the skin, infection and inflammation from cuts, abrasions, and burns, and allergic contact dermatitis of the upper eyelids from nail polish and other manicure products.

Respiratory disorders are also common among hairdressers. A 1976 study showed female cosmetologists to have an increased prevalence of chronic respiratory symptoms, small airway obstruction, and atypical sputum cytology. These increases were found to be related to duration of occupational exposure. Exposure to large amounts of hairspray appears to be a factor in these disorders. It has also been found that asthma could be a result of occupational exposure to henna dyes.

Certain types of hair dyes are mutagenic and, in laboratory testing, one type produced liver cancer in rats. The results of exposure to hair dyes for humans are less conclusive; no appreciable risk of breast cancer among female hairdressers was found in a 1977 study. However, a 1984 study found that female hairdressers have increased risk of death from multiple myeloma and ovarian cancer.

Miscellaneous risks associated with professional hairdressing include varicose veins from prolonged standing, nervous fatigue from working long, irregular hours in sometimes adverse conditions, and occupational cramps from moving muscles constantly the same way.

Recommendations for hairdressers' health and safety, as suggested by Heacock and Rivers, include: better room ventilation, proper lighting, clean floors, freshly laundered working clothes, towels, and aprons, sitting or reclining breaks at regular intervals, and regular hours of work with limited overtime.

Beauticians should be warned of potential hazards associated with hairdressing products, and protective gloves should be worn to prevent contact with irritating chemicals or solutions. Hands should be washed with non-irritating or neutral Ph soap, and hand moisturizers should be readily available at sinks. More research should be done to identify real health threats to hairdressers, including lifestyle factors. Chemical constituents of hairdressing products in Canada should appear on product labels.

quality (16 per cent), dust and fibres in the air (15 per cent), loud noise (11 per cent), exposure to computer screens (7 per cent), and exposure to dangerous chemicals or fumes (9 per cent). Figure 4.3 presents a model of occupational stress.

Many women work in female-dominated job ghettos at jobs that are different from the jobs men do. Many jobs done by women are positions with lower pay, less power, and often with little independence, autonomy, or control. Yet there is a lack of research and intervention related to occupational health for women (Messing, 1994). Women tend to be poorly paid—just over 70 cents for every dollar made by men. Women are often the

Box 4.10   Rotational Shift Work: What Are the Adverse Effects?

Shift work affects about one-quarter of the population in North America. It is common in industrial work, mining, hospitals, transportation, and food service work. A great deal of evidence suggests that shift work can disrupt the family and personal life, and can lead to a myriad of health problems. Among the negative consequences are the following:

1. Persistent fatigue is common.
2. Gastrointestinal and digestive problems are frequent.
3. Shift workers are more vulnerable to heart disease and heart attacks. In general, shift workers have lifestyles associated with ill health, including smoking, obesity, little recreation or regular exercise, and poor diets.
4. Medication may affect the person on shift work in an unpredictable way.
5. Shift work has negative effects on family activities and relationships. This can lead to depression, isolation, and loneliness. The lack of daycare associated with most shift work may mean that children are sometimes left unattended. Participation in 'normal' parent-child, husband-wife, and family socializing is severely restricted because of the unpredictability of the schedule.
6. There is some evidence that there are more accidents at work among shift workers.
7. Working conditions can be poorer (lighting, ventilation, cafeteria services, and opportunities for socializing may be restricted).

last hired and the first fired. To the extent that women's jobs are considered less important than men's jobs, then women have less ability to demand safe, clean, and healthy working standards. Women's occupational health and safety issues are thus both different and potentially more problematic than those of men. Even if the risks women face tend not to be as dramatic and acute—that is, they are not as likely to result in immediate or almost immediate death—the long-term chronic health problems that result are serious. Women workers are exposed to a broad range of occupationally related health hazards. In clerical work, which continues to be dominated by women, the types of problems are wide-ranging. In addition, the work life of women is problematic because of their multiple roles. Observations made about the relative poverty and lack of control in the female-dominated parts of the labour force are exacerbated among women of minority status who may be likely to work in even more marginalized settings such as domestic

work, agriculture, cottage industries, and prostitution. Women with disabilities are also more likely to be underemployed and unemployed.

Moreover, women's problems at work may have serious consequences for the next generation. So may those of men. Damage to the reproductive organs, to developing fetuses, and to sperm quality and quantity, as well as the potential for sterility, miscarriage, or genetic problems in offspring, is among the most devastating effects of occupational health and safety inadequacies. Unfortunately, concern over potential reproductive hazards has focused almost exclusively on women, so that women have been banned from some jobs entirely and from others during their child-bearing years or during pregnancy. Such legislation both discriminates against women and simultaneously ignores the real danger to the reproductive health of men. Instances of such stereotyping and discrimination have been frequent enough that the Canadian Advisory Council on the Status of Women has recom-

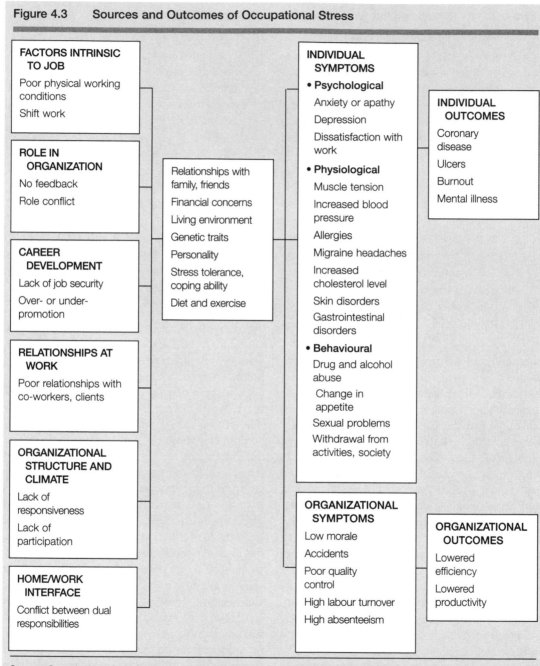

Figure 4.3   Sources and Outcomes of Occupational Stress

FACTORS INTRINSIC
TO JOB
Poor physical working
conditions
Shift work

ROLE IN
ORGANIZATION
No feedback
Role conflict

CAREER
DEVELOPMENT
Lack of job security
Over- or under-
promotion

RELATIONSHIPS AT
WORK
Poor relationships with
co-workers, clients

ORGANIZATIONAL
STRUCTURE AND
CLIMATE
Lack of
responsiveness
Lack of
participation

HOME/WORK
INTERFACE
Conflict between dual
responsibilities

Relationships with
family, friends
Financial concerns
Living environment
Genetic traits
Personality
Stress tolerance,
coping ability
Diet and exercise

INDIVIDUAL
SYMPTOMS
• **Psychological**
Anxiety or apathy
Depression
Dissatisfaction with
work
• **Physiological**
Muscle tension
Increased blood
pressure
Allergies
Migraine headaches
Increased
cholesterol level
Skin disorders
Gastrointestinal
disorders
• **Behavioural**
Drug and alcohol
abuse
Change in
appetite
Sexual problems
Withdrawal from
activities, society

ORGANIZATIONAL
SYMPTOMS
Low morale
Accidents
Poor quality
control
High labour turnover
High absenteeism

INDIVIDUAL
OUTCOMES
Coronary
disease
Ulcers
Burnout
Mental illness

ORGANIZATIONAL
OUTCOMES
Lowered
efficiency
Lowered
productivity

Source: Geran (1992: 15); adapted from C.L. Cooper, 'The Six Major Causes of Stress at Work', in *Health Promotion in the Working World* (1989).

mended that the federal government amend the Canadian Human Rights Act and the Canada Labour Code to prevent discrimination in hiring, job replacement, promotion, and other conditions of employment based on factors related to reproductive physiology, such as reproductive capacity, pregnancy, or childbirth; that exclusionary policies and practices arising from such issues be prohibited by law; and that the legislation be monitored and enforced on a continuing basis (CACSW, 1987: A14.3).

Estimating the actual prevalence of occupationally related disease is problematic for a number of reasons (Dickinson and Stobbe, 1988). First, there may be a long period of latency between exposure to the damaging substance or activity and the resultant disease. Second, there is a lack of information and indeed a great deal of misinformation about which chemicals are being used, and about which chemicals or activities have damaging long-term effects. Even when information is available about the negative consequences of a substance, the information may be withheld. Moreover, the effects may be difficult to monitor. One additional set of problems has to do with the fact that physicians are often poorly trained in recognizing occupationally related diseases.

The average Canadian in 1991 lost 6.2 days per year on average as the result of perceived exposure to workplace hazards. The most important cause of missing work was the risk of accident or injury. This was more important for male than for female workers: 18.5 days as compared to 10.7 days annually. Women were more likely than men to lose days of work as the result of excessive job demands, poor interpersonal relations, and other physical hazards, chemicals, noise, or dust or fibres in the air.

Time-Loss Work Injuries in the Health-Care Industry

There may be some irony in the fact that the health-care industry is itself a source of accidents, illness, and death. In fact, for one province,

British Columbia in 1995, where the figures are available, the health-care industry was associated with a higher injury rate than the provincial average for all industries combined. Moreover, 71 per cent of all claims were from within the health-care industry. The most frequent claims were made by those lowest in the hospital hierarchy— the practical nurses, nurse's aides, and orderlies, followed by registered nurses, cleaners, and housekeepers (Tan et al., 1996: 23). Compared to the other occupations, that of the registered nurse is one of the most vulnerable to acts of force or violence (Figure 4.4).

Injury and illness among health-care workers is a significant cost to the health-care system (CIHI, 2002: 88). According to the National Population Health Survey, 5.6 per cent of Canadians working in health-care occupations reported work-related injuries in the year prior to the survey. This is substantially higher than the 3.6 per cent of Canadians working in all other industries.

A recent survey of 9,000 nurses in Alberta and British Columbia found a significant number of nurses reported verbal and physical violence in their workplaces in the previous five shifts they had worked. Among the most common problems were hurtful attitudes or remarks (38 per cent of nurses had experienced these). Seventeen per cent of the nurses in Alberta and 21 per cent of those in British Columbia reported that they had been spit at, bitten, hit, or otherwise physically assaulted. Eight per cent reported sexual harassment of a verbal nature. While most of this was from patients, approximately one-quarter was from other health-care providers (about half from fellow nurses and half from physicians). Another study noted that compensation claims related to violence had increased over 10 times in British Columbia (ibid., 91).

Agricultural Work

Agriculture has long been associated with a pastoral, idyllic, and healthy style of life. In fact, after mining and construction, agricultural work is the

Figure 4.4   Serious Claims from Acts of Force or Violence to Nursing Professionals Compared to Other Occupations, 1991–1995

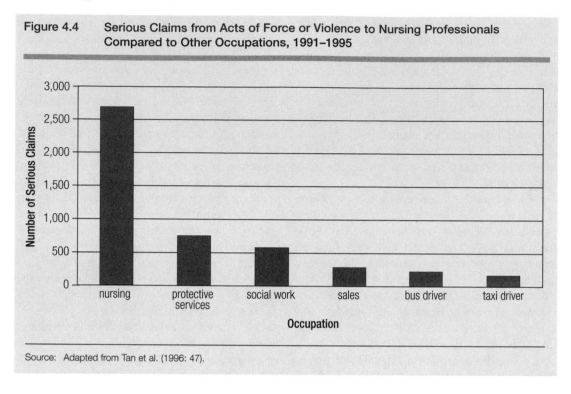

Source: Adapted from Tan et al. (1996: 47).

most health-threatening occupation (Bolaria, 1994: 684). Not only do agricultural workers suffer a high rate of accidents and associated fatalities, but also the working conditions, including working with and repairing farm machinery, the intensification of the farm labour process, poor housing, and sanitation, as well as low wages and long hours of hard labour, can be a heavy burden. As the ozone layer thins the rate of skin cancer is bound to increase among farm labourers.

Pesticides are another major threat to human health, as a result of both direct ingestion via pesticide-coated fruits and vegetables and indirect ingestion because of long-term accumulation in soil, water, and air. Pesticides also are known to have a tendency to break down or to combine with other compounds over time, which may be even more dangerous to human health. Short-term effects of mild pesticide poisoning include nausea, vomiting, and headaches, as well as more

serious permanent damage to the nervous system, miscarriage, birth defects, sterility, and reproductive disorders. Long-term pesticide exposure has been found to be associated with various cancers of the lungs, brain, and testicles (the herbicide 2,4-D, for example, has been found to be associated with a type of lymphoma). It has been suggested that pesticide (whether insecticide, herbicide, fungicide, or rodenticide) use constitutes a potentially catastrophic experiment with human life (Raven et al., 1993).

Compounding the problems resulting from agricultural work itself is the fact that much of the hired labour force is composed of migrant (temporary), immigrant, illegal, or undocumented workers (Bolaria and Bolaria, 1994: 440). The tenuous nature of a permanent stay in Canada for such immigrants and refugees has meant that many have had to take whatever job was offered and to accept its working conditions without

---

Box 4.11   Drought in Africa

What has caused the repeated droughts in Africa? Many theories have been proposed over the years. Perhaps it was the fact that the borders of the African countries were so frequently redrawn because of wars. Perhaps it was a simple consequence of the large mass of desert in the centre of the continent. Maybe it was simply an accident of geography and nature. Recent research suggests that the drought suffered by the corridor of land and peoples from Senegal to Ethiopia, which resulted in massive famine and death by starvation of 1.2 million people, was actually, in part, the result of pollution originating in North America, Europe, and Asia. A group of Canadian and Australian scientists has recently suggested that it may have been the result of tiny particles of sulphur dioxide emitted from factories and power plants. These particles work by altering the physics of cloud formation and reduce rainfall a continent away by as much as 50 per cent. Over the years the disastrous lack of rainfall has been blamed on everything from El Niño to overgrazing. One important clue to the link is the fact that when the industrialized West banned aerosols in the 1990s the rain returned to Africa.

Source: Joseph B. Verrengia, 'Pollution Blamed for African Drought', *Toronto Star*, 22 July 2002, A3.

---

complaint. Racism, a lack of language facility, and, in some instances, a lack of skills or training render these people particularly vulnerable. 'In summary, immigration laws, contractual obligations, lack of protection by labour legislation, lack of alternative job opportunities, poverty and unemployment in the country of emigration and the absence of union organization place many foreign workers in a vulnerable position and render them powerless vis-à-vis the employer' (ibid., 442).

Other Accidents and Violence

Accidents and violent deaths are the major causes of potential years of life lost among Canadians 1–75 years of age. To some extent accidents result from human error—driving under the influence of alcohol and drugs and driving at excessive speed. Many traffic fatalities and deaths from accidental falls and fires result from alcohol-related impairments. A new type of traffic accident is associated with the use of a car phone (Min and Redelmeier, 1998). Some countries have laws that prevent the use of a cellular phone while driving. However, a recent study in Toronto found that over the period 1984–93 locations with the largest increases in collision rates tended to have the smallest increases in estimated cellular telephone use (ibid.).

Sports-related accidents comprise 23 per cent of all accidents. Most of these (65 per cent) occurred to men, and in 1990 such accidents resulted in almost as many outpatient hospital visits (535,000) as did work-related accidents (591,000). Clearly, sports injuries are an important public health problem that needs to be more clearly defined. This problem is particularly serious because its incidence is related to age. The 15–24 age group is considerably more likely to experience sports injuries than those in any other age group. Among people 15–24, sports injuries were responsible for approximately 42 per cent of all injuries. Approximately 8.7 million activity-loss days and 1.5 million bed-disability days in 1987 resulted from sports injuries. The most dangerous sports in order were: ice hockey, cycling, skiing, and baseball (Statistics Canada, 1991). Of every 1,000 ice hockey injuries, 106 were serious, involving, for example, spinal or neurological damage. Figure 4.5 portrays the age

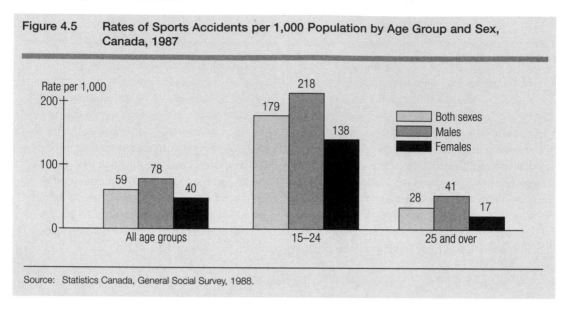

Figure 4.5   Rates of Sports Accidents per 1,000 Population by Age Group and Sex, Canada, 1987

Source: Statistics Canada, General Social Survey, 1988.

and sex incidence of sports-related accidents.

Violence against women and children is an important factor in ill health and death, a factor that has long been under-reported. In 1993, Statistics Canada conducted the Violence Against Women (VAW) survey (Strike, 1995). Four per cent of women over 18 in a total of 431,000 women reported that they had been sexually or physically assaulted in the previous year by a stranger, while 7 per cent reported that they had been assaulted by someone they knew. The numbers were much higher when women were asked whether they had ever been assaulted—19 per cent said they had been sexually assaulted and 8 per cent said that they had been physically assaulted. The health consequences are not entirely clear, but some evidence suggests that they are serious and last a long time. Aside from long-term health consequences, women who have been assaulted are more likely to be afraid in various situations, such as taking public transportation, entering or leaving a car alone, or staying alone in a home.

In the same survey, 29 per cent of women who had ever been married or lived common law had been physically or sexually assaulted by their partner (Rogers, 1994). Although many men used weapons and physically injured their wives, few victims reported the incidents to the police or used support services. Among the reasons given for not involving the police are the following: too minor (52 per cent); wanted to keep the incident private (10 per cent); didn't want or need help (10 per cent); didn't want to get involved with the police or courts (9 per cent); fear of partner (8 per cent); didn't think police could do anything (7 per cent); shame/embarrassment (5 per cent); and didn't want partner arrested (3 per cent) (ibid., 6). Violence reflects prevalent socialization patterns and culturally based value systems. It is extolled as glamorous and exciting. It is featured in popular television shows and films and young boys are given toy guns and military equipment to play with, while macho superheroes are provided as role models. The several cases of mass shootings at Canadian and US schools in recent years are not entirely shocking when we consider, among other things, the prevalence of the culture of 'macho' violence and the availability of guns.

Violence is sometimes used to control

women and children—to keep them in their place. Long subservient, first to their parents and then to their husbands, women are logically the victims of the greater strength and power of their 'keepers'. In a society that gives men the dominant roles in economics, politics, law enforcement, and religion, it is no wonder that men frequently dominate women and children physically as well. Nor is violence restricted to the home. Women and children are vulnerable to sexual harassment, rape, and physical abuse on the streets and in the homes of friends, neighbours, and other family members.

Summary

(1) There are three fundamental parts of the environment—air, water, and land. All affect our health both directly and indirectly.

(2) The major environmental issues facing Canadians today include: carbon dioxide production and climate change, acid precipitation, the depletion of the ozone layer, industrial pollution of air, water, and land, and the disposal of hazardous wastes and medical wastes.

(3) Other significant environmental issues related to air quality include air pollution and second-hand smoke.

(4) Water pollution in the Great Lakes continues to be a serious concern.

(5) With respect to land, the issue of waste disposal is critical.

(6) Occupational health and safety issues are a major concern, even in today's post-technological era. It has been estimated that a significant proportion of all cancers are related to working and the environment.

(7) The health and safety issues of working women in female job ghettos, while less dramatic (and less studied) than those of predominantly male occupations, are nevertheless myriad and consequential.

(8) Particular health and safety issues are related to agricultural work, which is among the most dangerous kinds of work in Canada.

(9) Sports accidents are a significant cause of morbidity and mortality, especially among young people.

(10) Accidents and violence have a considerable impact on the morbidity and mortality rates of Canadians.

Questions for Study and Discussion

1. Why is it difficult to demonstrate the effects of the environment on human health? Scientifically? Politically?

2. Could the industrial accident in Bhopal have been prevented? How? Are there lessons to be learned from Bhopal regarding the rest of the developing world?

3. Is the world's sustainability under threat? Explain.

4. Why is prevention not a more important part of the message that Canadians receive from the Canadian cancer establishment?

5. What problems do pesticides cause? Should they be banned?

Suggested Readings

Burnett, Richard T., Sabit Cakmak, and Jeffrey R. Brook. 1998. 'The Effect of the Urban Ambient Air Pollution Mix on Daily Mortality Rates in 11 Canadian Cities', *Canadian Journal of Public Health* 89, 3: 152–5. This is a tidy research-based report on the relationship between mortality and air pollution.

Epstein, Samuel S. 1998. *The Politics of Cancer Revisited*. Fremont Centre, NY: East Ridge Press. A book that brings together research on environmental and occupational causes of cancer.

Harding, Jim. 1994. 'Environmental Degradation and Rising Cancer Rates: Exploring the Links in Cancer', in Bolaria and Dickinson (1994: 649–67). A description of the fate of the world's largest non-saltwater basin—the Great Lakes.

Messing, K. 1998. *One-Eyed Science: Occupational Health and Women Workers*. Philadelphia: Temple University Press. Messing is a well-known Canadian researcher in the area of women's occupational health. This book is an excellent example of a critical approach to the subject.

O'Connor, Dennis R. 2002. *Report of the Walkerton Inquiry*. Toronto: Queen's Printer for Ontario. The O'Connor Inquiry followed the Walkerton water crisis in Ontario that resulted in at least seven deaths and thousands of illnesses in the town of Walkerton.

Chapter 5

Social Inequity, Disease, and Death: Age and Gender

Learning Objectives

- Health, illness, and death are not randomly distributed across society.
- Morbidity and mortality rates differ in different parts of the social structure and in different subcultures.
- The age structure of society can be shown through an age pyramid. This demographic portrayal can be useful in developing health and social policy.
- The most significant change in life expectancy over the last century and a half has been in the infant and child mortality rates.
- Infant mortality rates are one of the best indicators of the overall health profile of a people or society.
- At every age, women are more likely to be counted in morbidity rates and men in mortality rates.
- Explanations for differential morbidity by age include differences in lifestyle, psychosocial aspects of symptoms and care, and differential access to health-giving resources.
- Explanations for differential morbidity and mortality in men and women include biological factors, attentiveness to bodily sensations, ability to remember and describe health, and ability to engage in preventive behaviours.

Introduction

The next two chapters will describe and examine the ways that the social structure and associated subcultures correspond to different rates of death and disease among Canadians. Social structure refers to location in society. You and I are in different locations. Right now I am in Ontario, at a summer cottage, looking out over Lake Huron.

When you read this book I will undoubtedly be somewhere else. However, you and I will still be in different places. We will not be occupying the same space. Geographic or spatial location is one aspect of the social structure. People who live in different places have different life chances and different opportunities for and challenges to health. Many of these are related to environmental issues because water, air, and land, the bedrock of health, differ in different locations. Major cities and their environs tend to be more vulnerable to smog. Forested rural areas are more likely to succumb to forest fires and the smoke generated by these fires.

The examples provided so far suggest the structure could be horizontal. Spatial structure is also hierarchical. Hierarchy or vertical placement can be observed along a number of different dimensions. It can be seen in economic, educational, and social status variations. For example, it is possible to consider that society is structured so that those with more money are at the top and those with less money are at the bottom. It is also structured so that those with more education, or those who hold more prestige because of their families or jobs, for example, can be seen as being located at or near the top of an invisible hierarchy. This hierarchy can also be thought of as reflecting inequality or inequity. From the perspective of conflict theory or of social justice, hierarchical structure is indicative of inequity. Inequity is most obviously notable in economic disparity from one level to another. It is also evident, and often correlated with economic position, in the different places in the structure held by people of different ages, ethnicity, and gender. Inequity can also be seen in the distinctions between people with respect to rural/urban location, religion, region, province, and so on. Indeed, often such systems of inequality are linked together so that, for example, the elderly are more likely to be female, and elderly women are more likely to be poor. Such linked socio-demographic characteristics can be called an axis of inequality.

How does inequity relate to health and illness? The research is clear and becoming clearer. There is a consistent and positive relationship between good health and location further up the social structural hierarchy. This means that in a society such as Canada people who have more wealth tend also to have more health and people who have less wealth tend to have poorer health.

Thus the individual level of well-being tends to correspond to the location of the individual in the social structure. In addition, the overall degree of equity or inequity within society affects the well-being of everyone within the society. Societies that are more equal, where the hierarchy is less extensive, tend to have better overall health among the population than those that are more differentiated. As the degree of overall inequality declines or increases, so, too, can we expect that the level of health will vary (see Figures 5.1 and 5.2).

How do these processes work? First, why would economic inequality be associated with health? There are a number of different types of answers. The most obvious one is *material and social class* differences. Human health depends fundamentally on available, accessible, and good quality food, water, transportation, and housing. Without these health is compromised and challenged. Two aspects of income are relevant: income sufficiency or adequacy for such things as the purchase of food, affording the rent or mortgage, buying a car or paying for public transportation; income stability so that the money is available consistently and predictably, from month to month and from year to year. At minimum some material goods are absolutely necessary for the health of the individual and the individual family. Moreover, there are ways that income inequity perpetuates itself. One of the most important of these is through class-associated premarital or teenage pregnancy. Teenage and unmarried women tend not to take good care of themselves when they are pregnant. Compared to those whose pregnancies are planned, they are less likely to eat sufficient and well-balanced diets and less likely to engage in prenatal care. They may, in trying to hide the pregnancy, not gain adequate weight. Low-birth-weight babies are more likely to be born to women in these circumstances. Low birth weight is a significant problem that tends to result in all manner of difficulties for the child, including a greater likelihood of death, disability, and disease.

Figure 5.1   A Hypothetical Model of the Relationship between Socio-Economic Status and Health for an Indivudual

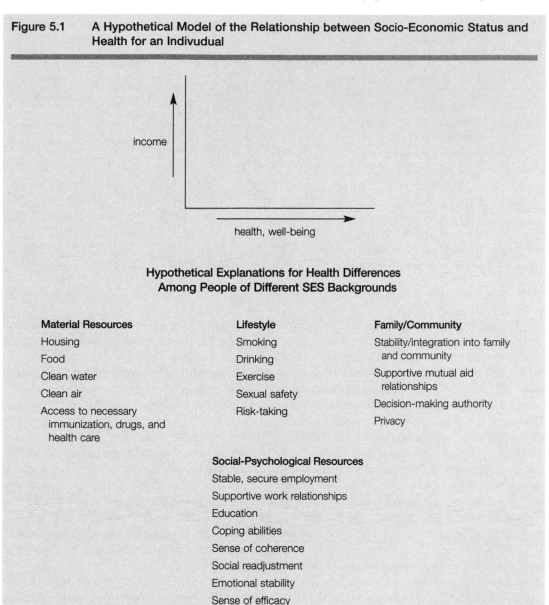

income

health, well-being

**Hypothetical Explanations for Health Differences
Among People of Different SES Backgrounds**

Material Resources

Housing

Food

Clean water

Clean air

Access to necessary
immunization, drugs, and
health care

Lifestyle

Smoking

Drinking

Exercise

Sexual safety

Risk-taking

Family/Community

Stability/integration into family
and community

Supportive mutual aid
relationships

Decision-making authority

Privacy

Social-Psychological Resources

Stable, secure employment

Supportive work relationships

Education

Coping abilities

Sense of coherence

Social readjustment

Emotional stability

Sense of efficacy

Low-birth-weight babies, as they become of school age, tend to be poorer students and to have learning difficulties and various chronic illnesses. Thus the results of this one behaviour associated with income may lead to complex and extensive health-and income-related threats to the newborn and to the growing child. There is evidence, too, that perception of social class location is related to socio-psychological issues such as self-esteem.

**Figure 5.2   A Hypothetical Model of the Contributions of Equity to the Health of a
Population**

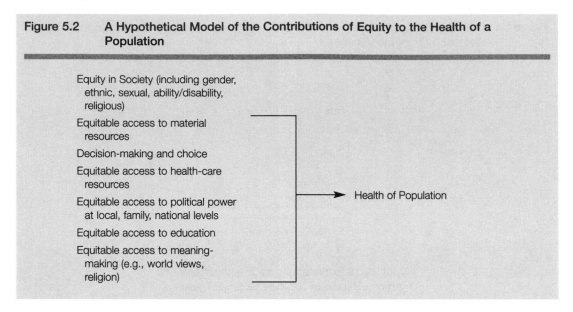

Gender is an important basis for inequality. This is both the result of the fact that women working full-time earn a fraction of what men who work full-time earn and because women have different bodies, social experiences, and some would even argue different social worlds. With respect to income, the arguments made above regarding material deprivation and its relationship to ill health tend to relate more often to the circumstances in which women find themselves. Women have different health profiles from men for other reasons as well, and these relate to their different roles in pregnancy and childbirth and their different roles and responsibilities in the family. Age, too, is relevant to health both because it is correlated with income and because people's worlds and bodies change over the life cycle. Women tend to live longer lives and to live these lives in the context of chronic illnesses and disabilities.

Education is related to employment as well as to health-related behaviours and to awareness and access to health information. People with more formal education are more likely to work in jobs in which they have control and autonomy.

Jobs requiring more education also are more likely to be the jobs that are predictable and have higher social status and prestige. These, too, are associated with self-esteem, respect, and health and well-being.

Ethnicity is another important hierarchical and cultural component of the Canadian social structure. People of different ethnic groups can be ranked according to income. They can also be differentiated with regard to their views and attitudes towards health and treatment. Racism is a reality that many people in visible minority ethnic groups have to deal with on a daily basis. Racism can independently cause assaults to self-concept and self-esteem and lead to illness and illness coping behaviours.

These 'variables' are described separately in the text. However, the next two chapters examine some of the inequities in morbidity and mortality as they relate to social structural positions reflected in age, gender, socio-economic status, and ethnicity. Consider, for example, the following questions.

Are women more often sick than men? Do men and women suffer from different illnesses?

Table 5.1   A Model for Analysis of Morbidity and Mortality Rates at the Societal Level

Culture	Political-Economic System	Ecological System	Social Structure	Social Psychology	Micro Meaning
the degree of medicalization	capitalism socialism communism	environmental quality and condition (water, air) quality of agricultural land and foodstuffs transportation and communication systems	gender age ethnicity education religious affiliation working limitations employment and unemployment rates	stress type A behaviour* sense of coherence* perceived social support	the definition and meaning of health, disease, and death

*These will be defined fully in Chapter Seven.

Does sexism enter into medical treatment? Does old age bring increasing infirmity and illness? Are the elderly overprescribed medicines by their doctors? Do the elderly themselves rely too heavily on doctors? Do the elderly feel that their health is poor? These are some of the questions that this chapter addresses.

Health, illness, and death are not randomly distributed in a society. Rather, their incidence and prevalence are inextricably linked to the social organization of the society. One aspect of this social organization, as we have noted above, is the extent of inequity in the social structure. Inequity causes different life chances and experiences, as well as unequal access to fundamental social resources such as food, recreation, satisfying work, and adequate shelter. Because of unequal access, people who differ in age, sex, income, class, occupation, race, ethnicity, marital status, rural or urban background, and religiosity differ in their rates of sickness and death. This chapter will examine how illness and death rates vary depending on age and sex. It will then discuss some of the possible explanations for the observed variations. As a first step to this analysis, however, it is essential to put the relationship between illness and death and the social structure into a broad, com-

prehensive context. Table 5.1 is a model of the major social variables and their possible connection with rates of illness and death.

On the broadest level, cultural differences between societies manifest themselves through such things as varying definitions of health and illness and varying views regarding appropriate types of medical treatment, for example, the degree to which a society is 'medicalized'—that is, influenced by medical explanations and treatments for social problems, such as hyperactivity, which used to be regarded as naughtiness but is now treated with a drug. This concept will be developed in greater depth in later chapters. A historical illustration will suffice here. The handling of 'problem drinking' is a good example of the process of medicalization.

At the beginning of the twentieth century and earlier, when Canadian society was less medicalized, when religious concepts were more prominent, problem drinking was considered to be a sign of weakness or a sin. Moral responsibility and societal opprobrium were advocated to control drinking. Today, in a more medicalized society, 'alcoholism' is considered not a sin but a sickness. Alcoholism is treated medically, and addictive behaviour is explained in terms of bio-

Figure 5.3   Population Projections for Canada, Percentage of the Population Aged 60 and
Over, 2001–2051

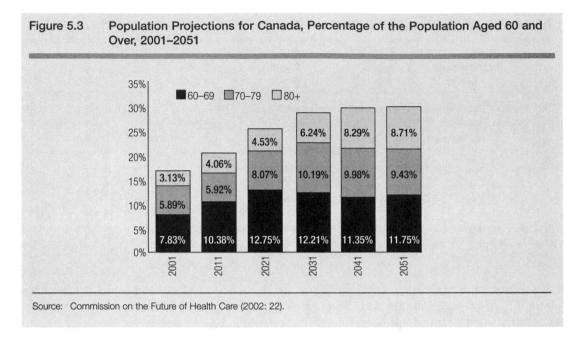

Source: Commission on the Future of Health Care (2002: 22).

chemistry, or psychiatrically, as the result of continuing psychological dependence.

Differences in mortality and morbidity are
related to political-economic systems as well as to
cultural differences. The level and distribution of
numerous resources such as food, shelter, access
to meaningful work, environmental quality, and
satisfying social relations vary within societies. If
the political-economic system causes differences
in people's access to resources, there will be structured inequities in rates of death and illness
(Stronk and van de Mheen, 1996).

Age and Mortality

Age is associated with morbidity and mortality
rates in both predictable and surprising ways.
The most obvious projected change in the population over time, as shown in Figure 5.3, is the
overall aging of the population and the corresponding decrease in the younger proportion of
the population. It is also evident that population
aging is expected to continue to increase signifi-

cantly until at least 2036, as is the decline in the
proportion of the population under 20.

The *population pyramid* is the most basic
method used to describe the age distribution of a
population. Figure 5.4, which includes population pyramids for Canada from 1925 to 2050,
clearly illustrates the demographic shift in the
population over more than a century. The rapid
growth of the older population is especially evident among women (the right-hand side of the
pyramids).

A number of explanations have been offered
for this complex phenomenon. The most important factor in population aging is the overall
decline in the birth rate. As people have fewer
babies, there are correspondingly fewer young
people. With fewer young people in the population there is necessarily a greater proportion of
elderly. A second and somewhat less important
factor is the increase in life expectancy over the
past century and a half in Canada.

Life expectancy increases are the result of a
number of changes. As we discussed in Chapter

Figure 5.4   Population Pyramids for Canada, 1925–2050

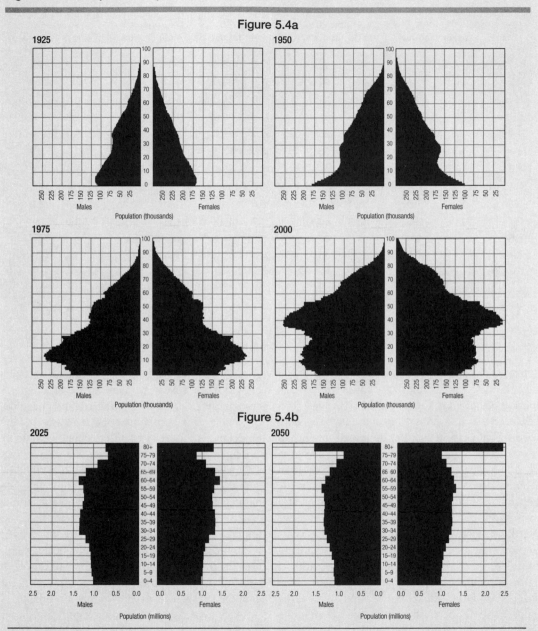

Figure 5.4a

Figure 5.4b

Sources: For 1925–2000: Statistics Canada, 'Age Pyramid of Population of Canada, July 1, 1901–2001', at: <www12.statcan/english/cencus01>; for 2025–2050: US Census Bureau, International Data Base, 'Population Pyramid Survey for Canada', at: <www.census.gov/cgi-bin/ipc/idbpyrs.pl?cty=CA&out=s&ymax=25>.

Table 5.2   Expected Years of Life Remaining, 1921–1991

	At birth		At age 20		At age 40		At age 60		At age 80	
	male	female	male	female	male	female	male	female	male	female
1921*	n.a	n.a.	49.1	49.2	32.2	33.0	16.6	17.1	6.0	6.1
1931	60.0	62.1	49.1	49.8	32.0	33.0	16.3	17.2	5.6	5.9
1941	63.0	66.3	49.6	51.8	31.9	34.0	16.1	17.6	5.5	6.0
1951	66.3	70.8	50.8	54.4	32.5	35.6	16.5	18.6	5.8	6.4
1956	67.6	72.9	51.2	55.8	32.7	36.7	16.5	19.3	5.9	6.8
1961	68.4	74.2	51.5	56.7	33.0	37.5	16.7	19.9	6.1	6.9
1966	68.8	75.2	51.5	57.4	33.0	38.2	16.8	20.6	6.4	7.3
1971	69.3	76.4	51.7	58.2	33.2	39.0	17.0	21.4	6.4	7.9
1976	70.2	77.5	52.1	59.0	33.6	39.7	17.2	22.0	6.4	8.2
1981	71.9	79.0	53.4	60.1	34.7	40.7	18.0	22.9	6.9	8.8
1986	73.0	79.7	54.3	60.7	35.5	41.2	18.4	23.2	6.9	8.9
1991	74.6	81.0	55.7	61.7	36.9	42.3	19.4	24.1	7.4	9.5

*Excludes Quebec.

Source: Statistics Canada, *Report on the Demographic Situation in Canada 1994*, Catalogue no. 91–209E (Ottawa: Minister of Industry, Science and Technology, 1994), Table A6, 106.

Three, first and most important is the rapid decline in the infant mortality rate. The average life expectancy for Canadians over the last 160 years or so has grown substantially. As well, women's life expectancy has increased more than that of men. Significantly, while men, in all of the years recorded, have lived shorter lives than women, the difference between the average life expectancies of men and women has been greater in the past 25 years than at any point in history.

Life expectancy figures from the last 50 years demonstrate another feature of the changing causes of death. If we compare life expectancy at birth with life expectancy at age 60 (see Table 5.2), an important fact comes to light. Most of the gains, for both men and women, have been in the ages below 60 years. The rapid decline in the infant and child mortality rates has been the major cause of increased life expectancy rates. The data in Table 5.2 provide one answer to the question of the differences in life expectancy between the sexes: women have gained more years of life than men both at birth and at age 60.

Table 5.3 explains this increase in life expectancy by portraying the decline in mortality among infants and those 85 years of age and older. The most significant decline for both sexes is clearly in the early years of life. Women's mortality rate has declined so that it is almost half the earlier rate (1921). The drop is not so dramatic for men. An important part of women's increasing longevity is improved nutrition and other public health measures for pregnant women, as well as advances in neonatal medical procedures that are associated with the subsequent decline in infant mortality.

Life expectancy has grown significantly over the last century and a half. Some obvious questions are: How much more is it likely to grow? Will new diseases and new epidemics threaten the health of the population as in the past? Will

Table 5.3   Death Rates by Sex and Age, Canada, 1921–1990

	Overall mortality rate		Infant mortality rate		85+ mortality rate	
	Male	Female	Male	Female	Male	Female
1921	10.9	10.2	98.2	77.4	228.2	224.9
1931	10.5	9.6	94.4	74.4	228.1	212.6
1941	10.8	9.1	67.0	51.9	241.9	229.3
1951	10.1	7.8	42.7	34.0	235.1	212.0
1961	9.0	6.5	30.5	23.7	208.9	192.2
1971	8.5	6.1	19.9	15.1	198.6	163.3
1981	8.0	6.0	11.0	8.5	188.5	141.6
1990	7.9	6.5	7.5	6.1	182.8	139.5

Notes: (1) Deaths per 1,000 (male and female) population.
(2) Data not available for Newfoundland prior to 1949, Quebec (1921–5), the Yukon and Northwest Territories prior to 1950.
(3) Infant mortality: number of deaths per 1,000 live births.

Source: *Selected Mortality Statistics, Canada 1921–1990* (Ottawa: Statistics Canada, Mar. 1994).

the advances of the past continue on into the future? And if these advances do continue, can we expect that these additional years will be lived in a state of disability (see Figures 5.5 and 5.6) or, as some have speculated, will people live an increasingly lengthier and healthier life, becoming ill only in the few months before death? (Fries, 1980).

Interestingly, none of these causes of the dramatic decline in mortality are explicitly sex-specific, with the exception of the relatively unimportant (numerically speaking) matter of birth control. Moreover, the early and more rapid increases in life expectancy for women as compared to men have diminished since about 1978 or so (Nault, 1997: 36). The difference between the life expectancies of males and females is due partly to the changing sex-specific incidence of certain diseases. For instance, while the rate of disease has declined for both men and women, the absolute decline has been faster among men than women. The gap between men and women in regard to chronic obstructive pulmonary dis-

eases and lung cancer has diminished because of an increase in mortality rates among women. The mortality rate decline for accidents has been larger for men. In addition, death rates in such male-dominated industries as mining, construction, transportation, and storage have fallen since the mid-1970s. Still, men are more likely to die from a variety of causes and this has been true over a period of time.

Sex differences in two major risk factors for serious disease, smoking and obesity, have also decreased over the relevant time period. The smoking rate declined for both males and females from 1977 to 1994–5, but for males the decline was greater, at 11 per cent, than for females, at 4 per cent. In 1985, 22 per cent of men and 14 per cent of women were overweight. In 1995, 25 per cent of men and 21 per cent of women were overweight (ibid., 39). This trend has continued to the present, as discussed in Chapter Three.

The question must then be raised, why is it that men today live shorter lives than women? Several lines of inquiry might be followed to

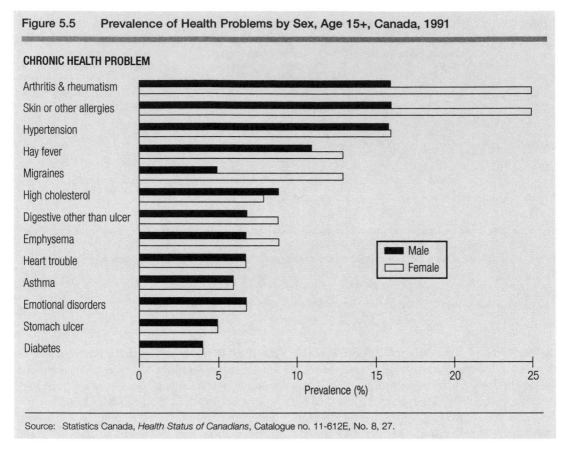

Figure 5.5   Prevalence of Health Problems by Sex, Age 15+, Canada, 1991

CHRONIC HEALTH PROBLEM

Source: Statistics Canada, *Health Status of Canadians*, Catalogue no. 11-612E, No. 8, 27.

answer the question. First, the genetic superiority of women is an aspect of the explanation. More males are conceived and yet more male fetuses die (Waldron, 1981). Males, in a number of different species, have higher death rates than females (although this is not universal). However, even if genetics does play a significant part in the sex-mortality differential, it cannot be the only factor. For one thing, as Rutherford (1975) points out, the increase in the sex-mortality differential over the past 50 years could not be due entirely to genetics because genetic structures do not change that quickly. Furthermore, men are less likely to be ill. If the cause of the mortality differential were genetic, surely it would be paralleled in differences in morbidity rates for men and women.

Second, to explain this anomaly—that men are more likely to die, even while women are more likely to get sick—we must look at the causes of mortality by sex. One important distinction between male and female causes of mortality occurs in early to middle adulthood as the result of external causes such as motor vehicle and other accidents and suicide (Wilkins, 1996: 12). Men and women die from essentially the same causes, although at different rates and ages: cardiovascular disease and diseases of the heart, cancer in general and lung cancer in particular, accidents and adverse effects associated with motor vehicle accidents, and chronic obstructive pulmonary disease (Nault, 1997: 38). However, the differences between the sexes in 1995 were

Figure 5.6   Life Expectancy and Health, by Sex

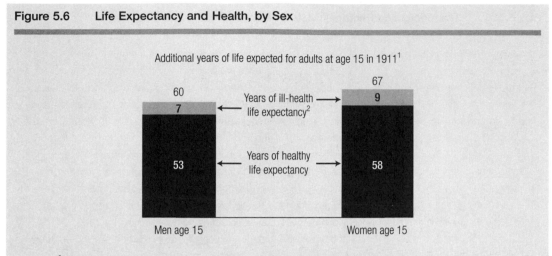

Additional years of life expected for adults at age 15 in 1911[1]

60   Years of ill-health ——→   67
7   ←—— life expectancy[2]   9

Years of healthy
53   ←—— life expectancy ——→   58

Men age 15   Women age 15

[1] Life expectancy figures were adjusted with HSI to produce an estimate of Health-adjusted Life Expectancy.
[2] The difference between total life expectancy and Health-adjusted Life Expectancy represents the duration of all episodes of ill health.

Source: *Canadian Social Trends* (Summer 1995), which used Statistics Canada, Health Status Index (HSI) using the 1991 *General Social Survey*,

much smaller than they were in 1979.

In the context of health policy one very useful set of calculations is PYLL, potential years of life lost. This essentially refers to premature mortality and takes into account the age at which people die from different causes. The younger the average age of death for a given cause of mortality, the greater the PYLL (see Table 3.4).

The most important contributions to higher male mortality can be argued to be related to the following causes. The higher rate of cigarette smoking among men has a significant impact on the sex differential for lung cancer, cardiovascular disease, and respiratory diseases (Waldron, 1981), although the sex differential for lung cancer is narrowing. Significantly, the rate of cigarette smoking among women is also increasing. Another important contribution to the respiratory and lung cancer differential is likely linked to the higher risks occurring at men's employment venues, as discussed in Chapter Four. Men are

more prevalent in the workforces of industries that work with carcinogenic substances. (It is worth noting, however, that some cleaning products used primarily by women in the home have been found to be carcinogenic and of significant risk to women's health. More research needs to be done on the safety of products used to clean and maintain homes.)

Risk factors for heart disease include smoking, high-fat diet, and stress (particularly type A behaviour). These risk factors are more prevalent among men than women (ibid.). Higher alcohol consumption among men is implicated in several causes of mortality—but chiefly accidents and suicide (see Tables 5.4 and 5.5).

Men drive more than women and less safely (Waldron and Johnston, 1981: 19). They consume more alcohol than women. At least half of all fatal motor vehicle traffic accidents involve alcohol. The probability of other accidents and suicides is also increased by alcohol consumption.

Box 5.1   The Social and Personal Costs of Alzheimer's Disease

Have you ever forgotten the name of a word for a thing or a person? I have, and in fact I find such forgetfulness is happening more frequently today than it did a few years ago. Among the most troubling and important of the disorders facing elderly Canadians are the various types of dementia, and memory loss is one of the most noticeable symptoms of dementia, a condition that increases sharply as people age.

Alzheimer's disease is the most common form of dementia, which is characterized by a progressive deterioration and destruction of cells in the brain and leads to increasingly severe declines in memory, thinking, and reasoning. People suffering from Alzheimer's often begin with an inability to remember information, words, or names. Over unpredictable periods of time, these memory difficulties result in greater and greater problems with reasoning, judgement, and emotional and personality stability—and denial by the Alzheimer's patient that anything is wrong can be one of the most difficult aspects of the disease, both for the patient and for the caregiver. Eventually people with the disease become unable either to care for their own basic needs or to engage in the activities of daily living on their own. Alzheimer's is eventually fatal.

It is still impossible to diagnose Alzheimer's with certainty until biopsy but, according to the Alzheimer Society (www.alz.org/AboutUs/faq.htm), widely accepted practice criteria, including such diagnostic tests as the 'mini mental inventory', have led to a diagnosis accuracy rate of about 90 per cent. Numerous different hypotheses regarding disease causation have been examined but there are still no definitive conclusions. While no medical treatments are available for the cure of the disease, several drugs now work to delay and moderate temporarily the worsening of symptoms. Between 30 and 40 experimental treatments and preventative strategies are being developed and tested in various places around the world.

In the context of both an aging population and lack of clear or certain methods of prevention, the disease is likely to grow in the next 30 years or so as the approximately 10 million baby boomers turn 65. In the absence of effective treatments, knowledge about prevention, or adequate financing and support for home or institutional care, the burden of this disease for the sufferers and their friends and families is bound to increase (Burke et al., 1997). Today, one in 13 people over 65 is estimated to have Alzheimer's or another related dementia. By 2031 approximately three-quarters of a million Canadians likely will be affected. There were approximately 83,200 new cases of dementia in 2001. Of these, 50,500 were female and 32,700 were male (www.alzheimer.ca/english/disease/articles-boomers.htm).

About one-half of those diagnosed with dementia live in institutions such as nursing homes, homes for the aged, and retirement homes. Others typically live at home, i.e., the residence of the caregivers, and are cared for by family members— spouses, daughters, daughters-in-law, sons, grandchildren—with only a small amount of voluntary or paid assistance. Indeed, a mere 3.4 per cent of caregivers apparently use respite care (designed to give caregivers a brief break). Partly because of inadequate levels of home care and support services for people with dementia and their caregivers, not to mention the financial cost of respite care, informal caregivers seem to have more chronic health problems than others in their cohort. Forty per cent of those caring for a person with severe dementia and 16 per cent of those caring for someone with moderate dementia report symptoms of depression. Depression is twice as prevalent among caregivers of Alzheimer's patients as it is among other caregivers (www.alzheimer.ca/english/disease/stats-caregiving.htm).

One of the challenges facing the health-care system of the future, in the absence of discoveries leading to prevention, is that of providing programs and supports for caregivers and sufferers of Alzheimer's to enable both to cope as well as possible in difficult circumstances. A great deal of research has been carried out on the biomedical aspects of the disease. There needs to be significant additional study of the related social, sociological, and personal issues.

Thus, while there may be gender-based genetic differences, it is clear that the male lifestyle, including cigarette smoking, industrial employment, excess alcohol consumption, and high-fat diet, contributes to male mortality. In addition, the male tendency to engage in violent, aggressive, and high-risk activities cannot be overlooked in gender-specific mortality rates. Such gendered characteristics are also implicated in the much higher suicide rate among men. Women are more likely to attempt suicide but men, in part because they tend to choose more violent means, are more likely to succeed at dying by suicide.

Age and Morbidity

Health problems affecting the elderly are of growing concern as the population ages. The elderly go to the doctor more frequently than young people and they are more likely to be hospitalized and to use prescribed medications (Jennett et al., 1991). In addition, evidence indicates that the elderly are more likely to be given prescriptions inappropriately (Ferguson, 1990; Shorr et al., 1990; Brook et al., 1989) and that as many as 19 per cent of hospital admissions may result from inadequate or inappropriate drug prescriptions (Grymonpre, 1988). In addition to over-prescribing by doctors, some of the problems associated with medicine use among the elderly result from metabolic changes due to aging that affect the absorption rates of drugs, side effects from multi-drug use associated with the simulta-neous treatment of several problems, and drug-taking mistakes made by the elderly themselves as the result of problems with their visual, motor, or memory abilities (Tamblyn et al., 1994).

Eight per cent of Canadians over 64 suffer dementia of various kinds, including vascular dementia and Alzheimer's disease. More common in women than men, dementia is expected to grow in incidence over the next decades (Burke et al., 1997). Dementia, characterized by severe cognitive and emotional deficits, increases over the life course. The 1991 Canadian Study of Health and Aging (CSHA) found the following prevalence of dementia: 8 per cent of those over 64, 2.4 per cent of those who were 65–74; 11 per cent of those 75–84; and 35 per cent of those over 84.

Women are more likely than men to be diagnosed with dementia (ibid., 25). Alzheimer's disease (a primary degenerative disease of the brain involving progressive memory loss up to, at times, extreme disability resulting in the need for round-the-clock care) is the most common type of dementia, accounting for 64 per cent of all cases. As the population continues to age, this disease is expected to grow in significance so that the number of Canadian seniors with dementia is likely to triple by 2031 (Figure 5.7). Women are also more likely to try to commit suicide, although they are less likely than men to be successful (Figure 5.8). This is partly because of the different means to suicide used by men and women. The one exception is elderly men, who are more likely than elderly women to attempt to kill themselves.

Table 5.4   Mortality Rates*, by Causes, 1994–1997

	1994			1995			1996			1997		
	Both Sexes	Male	Female	Both Sexes	Male	Female	Both Sexes	Male	Female	Both Sexes	Male	Female
All Causes	685	886	536	680	881	532	671	864	529	661	848	524
Malignant neoplasms	191	243	156	188	240	152	188	238	156	182	231	149
Intestine, except rectum	20	26	16	21	26	17	20	25	16	19	24	16
Lung	51	76	32	49	74	32	50	73	34	48	70	33
Breast	—	—	30	—	—	29	—	—	29	—	—	28
All other malignant neoplasms	120	141	77	118	141	76	118	140	77	115	137	74
Diabetes	17	20	15	18	21	15	17	21	14	17	21	15
Diseases of the heart	187	250	140	184	246	138	181	241	135	173	232	130
Ischaemic heart diseases	145	200	104	141	195	101	137	190	98	132	182	94
All other heart diseases	42	49	36	43	51	37	43	51	38	42	50	36
Cerebrovascular diseases	50	55	46	49	55	45	48	53	44	48	53	44
Atherosclerosis	6	7	6	5	6	4	4	5	4	4	5	4
Respiratory diseases	60	88	43	60	87	44	60	86	44	60	86	45
Pneumonia & influenza	24	31	19	23	31	19	23	31	18	24	32	19
Bronchitis, emphysema, & asthma	7	10	5	6	9	5	6	9	5	6	8	5
Chronic liver diseases & cirrhosis	30	47	19	31	47	21	30	46	21	31	47	21
Congenital anomalies	4	4	4	4	4	4	4	4	4	4	4	4
Perinatal mortality excluding stillbirths	4	4	4	4	4	3	4	4	3	4	4	3
Injuries and poisonings	45	66	25	46	66	26	44	64	26	42	61	24
Motor vehicle accidents	11	16	6	11	16	7	10	15	6	10	15	6
Suicide	13	21	5	14	22	5	13	21	6	12	20	5
Homicide	2	2	1	2	2	1	2	2	1	2	2	1
All other injuries & poisonings	19	27	12	19	26	13	19	26	13	18	25	12
Other causes	114	138	94	116	141	96	114	138	95	120	143	102

*Rates are age-standardized using the 1991 populations for Canada.

Source: Statistics Canada, Catalogue no. 82F0075XCB, at: <www.statcan.ca/english/Pgdb/People/Health01.htm>.

Table 5.5   Suicide Rates per 100,000 Population, by Age and Sex, 1997

	All ages	1–14	15–19	20–4	25–44	45–64	65+
Males	19.6	1.4	19.9	24.9	25.0	25.5	23.0
Females	5.1	0.4	5.5	3.6	6.6	7.6	4.5

Source: Adapted from Statistics Canada, Catalogue no. 82F0075XCB, at: <www.statca.ca/english/Pgdb/health01.htm>.

Box 5.2   Population Aging

You have probably heard the concern voiced that as the population ages in the next several decades in Canada as a result of the increase in age among the baby boom generation that the costs to health care will skyrocket. In fact, people over 65 are more likely to be ill than adults at other ages. Moreover, they are also more likely to use the health-care system when they are ill. Recent research from the Canadian Health Services Research Foundation demonstrates that the increasing use by seniors is not the result of their increasing numbers in the population but rather their relatively higher rates of use. There is evidence that it is not the sick seniors who are responsible for the increase in costs but rather healthy seniors. In Manitoba, for example, the rate of doctor visits among the well between the 1970s and 1983 increased 57.5 per cent for specialists and 32 per cent for general practitioners. The rates for unhealthy seniors increased less than 10 per cent. It appears that the elderly routinely receive more care than they formerly did. The cost of health-care increases due to the simple aging of the population is estimated to be only 1 per cent of the total health-care costs. The significant impact of population aging then appears to be the result of increased treatment of the elderly, including such interventions as flu shots, hip replacement, and cataract surgery (CHSRF, 2001).

Box 5.3   Alzheimer's Is Expensive

Alzheimer's is already proving to be an expensive disease for corporations and will be increasingly so as the population ages in the next part of this century. The cost is estimated to be about $9 billion in Canada annually. This figure is the result of absenteeism, losses in productivity, and replacement and insurance costs for workers. One part of this is due to the losses resulting for the person with the disease; the other is due to the lack of social and health support services that necessitate that family members take time from and are sometimes unable to concentrate at work because of worries about the diagnosed person. In a recent study, caregivers of people with Alzheimer's reported that they spent an average of 46 hours per week over and above their hours at work in caregiving. Today the estimates are that approximately 238,000 Canadians have the disease. The numbers are expected to increase.

Source: Andre Picard, 'Alzheimer's taking huge economic toll, study says', *Globe and Mail*, 25 July 2002, A6.

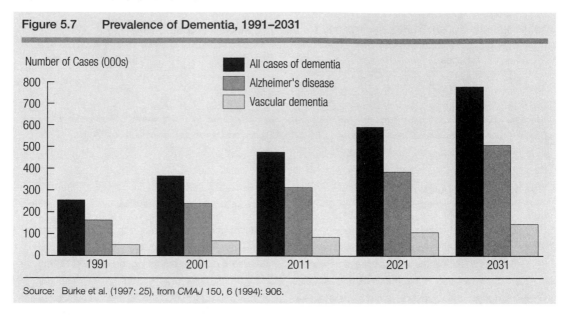

Figure 5.7   Prevalence of Dementia, 1991–2031

Source: Burke et al. (1997: 25), from *CMAJ* 150, 6 (1994): 906.

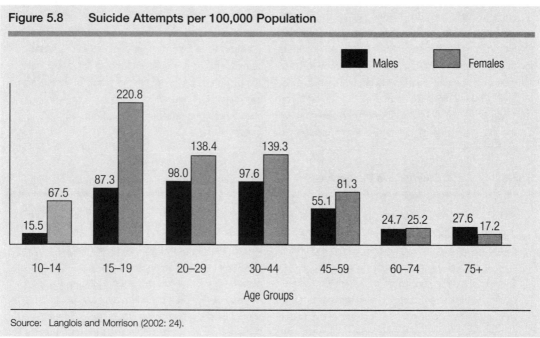

Figure 5.8   Suicide Attempts per 100,000 Population

Source: Langlois and Morrison (2002: 24).

The elderly have more chronic conditions, are more likely to be hospitalized and medicated, and yet they are still likely to self-report excellent or good health and health satisfaction (Table 5.7). This may be because they see and evaluate themselves in relative terms in comparison with others of the same age. This finding is also true of those over 85. In a recent national study of Canadians over 65 a separate analysis for those over 85 was calculated (Ebley et al., 1996). Most Canadians over 85 years of age rated their health as either pretty good or very good. Furthermore, recent research has shown how psychosocial factors such as a sense of purpose in life, a sense of control, social participation, and life satisfaction (Anstey et al., 2001; Pinquart, 2001; Ranzijin, 2001), as well as socio-economic factors (Martin, 2001), are positively related to quality of life and appear to be implicated in longevity. The figures in Table 5.7 show differences in men and women and in people of different age groups with regard to one psychosocial illness—depression.

When we think about a link between age and health, we tend first to associate aging and health decline. Newborns are another age group whose health is of great significance to the overall health of the population. The weight of newborn babies is a 'key predictor of their survival chances' (Millar et al., 1993: 26). Low birth weight, said to be less than 2,500 grams or about five and a half pounds, is associated with physical and mental disabilities and infant death. Despite various types of preventive strategies, such as prenatal programs for pregnant women at high risk, the rate of low-birth- weight babies has declined only slightly, to about 5 per cent of live births in Canada. Mothers either younger than 20 or older than 35 are more likely than those in other age groups to have low-birth-weight babies. Also, mothers who smoke during pregnancy are more likely to have low-birth-weight babies. First-born female and pre-term babies are more likely to fit into this category (ibid.). Income, too, makes a difference. Poorer women are more likely to have low-birth-weight babies. The first three years of life are also significant to subsequent health. During this time children's brains and nervous systems are growing and developing, and they are acquiring language and other essential skills.

Table 5.6   Self-Reported Health and Happiness Status of Canadians Ages 55 and Over, 1990

	Men	Women
HEALTH STATUS		
Excellent	32%	27%
Good	46	48
Fair	17	19
Poor	4	6
Not stated	1	1
HAPPINESS STATUS		
Very happy	56	49
Somewhat happy	39	43
Somewhat unhappy	2	5
Very unhappy	1	1
No opinion, not stated	3	2

Source: *Canadian Social Trends* (Summer 1992): 26.

Table 5.7   Depression Rates (Self-Perceived) by Age and Sex

	Male (000s)	Female (000s)
All ages (over 12)	480	834
12–14	9	18
15–17	26	60
18–19	22	48
20–4	42	80
25–34	110	184
35–44	134	210
45–54	78	122
55–64	29	66
65–74	18	30
75+	12	16

Source: Statistics Canada, *National Population Health Survey, 1996–1997.*

Box 5.4   Women in the Labour Force and Increasing Life Expectancy

There are numerous health risks associated with employment. They include chemical toxins, air pollution, hazardous materials and equipment, shift work, and stress. Still, a new study from the European Commission says that a major factor in health outcomes is the economy. Further, this study notes that the increased number of women in the labour force is an important source of declining mortality rates. Often the benefits of women's involvement in the labour force seem to appear very quickly. In some countries drops in mortality occurred in the same year as the increase of women in the labour force. The effects remain for at least 10 years. The opposite is also true: the lower the employment of women in a given year the higher the mortality rate over the next decade.

To what would you attribute the health benefits? Is it the fact that women have more money? Is it related to their greater sense of belonging when at work? Is it because they are too busy to get sick? Outline a few hypotheses that might help us to understand this interesting link between working among women and mortality rates.

Source: Rory Watson. 'More women in the workforce reduces mortality', *British Medical Journal* 324 (8 June 2002): 1352. Available at: <http:bmj.com/cgi/content/full/324/7350/1352/b>.

Gender and Mortality

Throughout the nineteenth and twentieth centuries, where records are available for industrializing and industrialized societies, they show that males have often experienced greater mortality rates than females. This difference begins even before birth, for more male than female babies are stillborn (Lewis and Lewis, 1977). In fact, there are significant differences between men and women in both mortality and morbidity rates. Morbidity rates are higher for women. While men are more likely, at every age during their life cycle, to die, women are more likely to be ill. However, this has not always been the case. Before industrial capitalism, the mortality rates for men and women were approximately the same (Eyer, 1984). At times, the female rate was higher than the male rate. The higher rate for women was often associated with the high rate of maternal mortality because of women's limited access to important health-giving resources such as adequate nutrition, foodstuffs, and birth control. Over the past century, improvements in nutrition, the spread of more effective contraception, and the overall improvement in the status of women have had a dramatic effect on their life expectancy.

A comparison of the overall life expectancy with the overall disability-free life expectancy reinforces the point made earlier: men are more likely to die, women to get sick. The rank ordering of overall causes of death is the same for both men and women. The most important cause of death is circulatory system disease. The second is cancer or all malignant neoplasms. Within this category, lung, bronchial, and tracheal cancers are the largest causes of male death, while breast and lung cancer are competing as the largest cause of female death. These are followed closely by bronchial and tracheal cancer for women. Moreover, these two cancer rates are growing for women, and as women continue to take up smoking their lung cancer rate will continue to increase while the male rate will continue to decrease. Another interesting difference is that the death rate by accident is more than twice as high among men as among women. This figure includes automobile accidents as well as all other accidents and suicide and homicide.

Box 5.5   Women and AIDS

The first wave of the spread of AIDS was largely among men. Most often the transmission was either the result of homosexual relations or, later, injection drug use. In more recent years there has been a growing incidence of HIV resulting from heterosexual relations and an increased number of infected women. Up to 31 December 2000, 7.7 per cent of all AIDS cases in Canada were among women. However, in 2000 women comprised 24 per cent of the positive HIV tests. Of all of the cases of AIDS among women so far recorded, 66.9 per cent are due to heterosexual contact, 22.8 per cent are the result of injection drug use, and 10.1 per cent are the result of the transfusion of blood and blood products. There has been consistent growth in the proportion of injection drug use as a cause of AIDS in women. Thirty-four per cent of women who received a positive test for AIDS in 2002 were infected by injection drug use.

Women are particularly vulnerable to AIDS for a number of social-structural, cultural, and biological reasons, including women's relative poverty, their cultural devaluation, and the thinness and greater extent of vaginal skin, which makes it more vulnerable to rips and tears and thus infection. In fact, women are about four times more vulnerable to sexually transmitted diseases than men and the area of women's genitalia exposed to sexual fluids is four times that of men. In addition, men's semen carries greater amounts of the virus than vaginal fluids. Moreover, because they can pass the virus on to the fetus during pregnancy, AIDS among women can be an even more devastating disease than AIDS among men.

Sources: <http://www.hc.sg.ca/pphb-dgspsp/publicat/epiu-depi/index.html>; 'The female condom and AIDS: UNAIDS point of view', Geneva: UNAIDS, 1997.

Gender and Morbidity

Women can expect to live longer than men, yet a higher percentage of their years alive involve the experience of some disability. Expected years of life free of severe disability represent 97 per cent of total male life expectancy and 94 per cent of female life expectancy (*Canada Year Book*, 1994). Women's greater life expectancy is clearly at a cost of more years of disability. Women are more likely than men to be ill, no matter how the illness rate is determined: by self-report, clinical records, physiological testing, days of disability, doctor visits, or hospitalization. In short, the incidence of illness among females is higher than it is among males. A small part of this difference is accounted for by the fact that pregnant women are expected to visit the doctor for regular prenatal checkups and to give birth in hospital. In addition, childbirth is followed by routine medical checkups for both mother and baby (medical care for pregnancy and childbirth is included as illness in the statistics). The sex difference for acute illnesses is between 20 and 30 per cent greater for women (Verbrugge, 1985), including childbirth-related illness. It is only slightly lower when childbirth-related illnesses are excluded (ibid).

Most non-fatal chronic illnesses are also generally more prevalent among women. Figure 5.5 shows some of these health differences between the sexes. There is a remarkably higher incidence of reports of certain problems among women than among men: for instance, migraine, arthritis and rheumatism, and skin and other allergies. It is notable that the health problems reported more often by men are more often causes of fatality, e.g.,

---

BOX 5.6   Men, Steroids, Sports, and Health

Anabolic steroids are synthetic testosterone. They are often used by athletes to build mass and muscle in order to improve their competitive status. Used by professional and amateur athletes in national and international competitions and in local gyms, their deleterious effects are numerous. Steroid use is associated with a number of different changes. The increased amount of testosterone is, for instance, related to increased violence, sexual interest, and prowess. One researcher in fact has suggested that the use of steroids is a factor in the overall increase in violence—violent rapes, murders, and violence towards gays in the US (Taylor, 1991: 69). Steroid use is also related to megorexia—the opposite of anorexia. Megorexia involves a distorted body image and a voracious, even insatiable appetite. The steroid user then would have an unattainable desire to acquire, not thinness as in the case of anorexia, but mass. A constant preoccupation with appearance can sustain dependency on steroid use. Steroids are also addictive and may cause serious psychological symptoms upon withdrawal. Moreover, when the user stops the body returns to the pre-steroid strength and shape. The dramatic physiological change can have devastating physical and psychological consequences. There are, too, a number of physical health conditions associated with steroid use, including liver and cardiovascular diseases, hypertension, acne, fluid retention, and sleep disturbance. Because steroid use is often not made public, its association with other health conditions may be invisible but widespread. Finally, in the age of HIV and AIDS, the needles used for injecting steroids may become infected and passed from athlete to athlete in a particular gym or a particular team.

Sources: Taylor (1985, 1991).

---

high cholesterol as associated with heart disease.

When the leading types of illness for men and women are ranked, they are largely comparable. In effect, men and women generally suffer from the same sorts of illness and disability, but men tend to experience them more severely. Furthermore, men's illnesses proceed more quickly to death. In summarizing a decade of research based on morbidity and mortality data from a variety of sources in the US, Verbrugge (1985: 668) concludes as follows: 'Women have more frequent illness and disability, but the problems are typically not serious (life-threatening) ones. In contrast, men suffer more from life-threatening diseases, and more permanent disability and earlier death from them.'

The morbidity rates for men and women are potentially inaccurate for three known reasons. In the first place, male rates are likely under-reported. Household surveys tend to rely on the answers of available subjects, and these have tended to be women. Interview subjects are known to under-report the morbidity of the absent person (Nathanson, 1977: 20). In the second place, health statistics probably minimize reports of women's illness because such statistics focus on the most publicly visible health problems rather than relatively minor, private complaints. Yet women are more likely to suffer any number of minor yet uncomfortable sensations associated with non-fatal chronic or acute conditions (Verbrugge, 1985). The American National Health Interview Survey has shown that women report more minor health problems such as headaches, insomnia, palpitations, and tremors than men. Such problems may or may not lead to preventive health actions such as visits to a doctor, which then get counted in morbidity statistics.

Box 5.7	Premenstrual Syndrome

Recently, PMS, premenstrual syndrome, has gained credibility as a term that may provide medical and even legal legitimacy. Some women have expressed relief at having their cyclical and bodily experiences medicalized and their discomfort or unhappiness legitimized as due to a medically recognized syndrome. Other women regret the medicalization of what they consider to be a largely normal occurrence. Women who take this perspective ask questions such as how to distinguish real PMS from a normal menstrual cycle. PMS was used as a legal defence by two women accused of murder in Britain in the 1980s. In both cases evidence as to the woman's cyclical irrationality and aggressive impulsivity just prior to menstruation was accepted as a defence. One woman received probation and the other was acquitted.

The dubious advantages of the diagnosis of PMS—late luteal phase dysphoric disorder (LLPD)—are hotly debated among feminists and physicians. The symptoms are all quite subjectively defined and include: (1) marked mood lability; (2) persistent and marked anger or irritability; (3) marked anxiety or tension; (4) marked depressed mood or thoughts; (5) decreased interest in usual activities, work, friends, hobbies; (6) fatigue or marked lack of energy; (7) difficulty concentrating; (8) marked change in appetite; (9) hypersomnia or insomnia; and finally (10) a variety of other physical symptoms such as breast tenderness, bloating, headaches, etc.

Source: Stoppard (1992: 123).

Box 5.8	Viagra

Women's health has been and continues to be an important issue for both social science and medical understanding. However, the peculiar discrimination that men experience with respect to health should not be ignored. The near-epidemic of desire unleashed with the marketing of Viagra, a drug designed to produce an erection in a male with erectile dysfunction, is one indication of how little is known about the ways that men suffer in their bodily functions. Until Viagra was introduced into the market, few knew of the extent of erectile dysfunction among men. Perhaps they weren't talking about it with their doctors and were thus not getting counted in morbidity figures. The recent politicalization of prostate cancer is an example of men organizing for health advocacy for other men. Some researchers, concerned about the high incidence of prostate cancer and the reluctance of men to be tested for the disease, have suggested that the cultural construction of masculinity is a threat to men's health.

Third, preventive or early stage medical care is also more frequent for women because of visits to the doctor for pregnancy, childbirth, and their children's health care. But should preventive action be considered morbidity?

The conclusion that must be drawn, still, is that women are more likely to suffer from a variety of illnesses than men and that men are more likely to die at every age than women. Which is the better measure of parity? To live (and be ill longer) or to die earlier? What will the future bring? Are women actually 'dying to be equal', as evidenced by their growing rates of cigarette smoking, alcohol consumption, and increased

Table 5.8   Summary of Explanations of Inequalities in Morbidity and Mortality

Four Factors in the Social Structure that Are Linked to Health

Age	Gender	Class	Ethnicity
Older people more likely to use medical facilities and experience chronic illness, but less likely to perceive themselves as ill	High incidence of minor illness in females High incidence of serious illness in males	The lower the social class, the greater mortality and morbidity	Native people have high incidence of morbidity and mortality from contagious and infectious diseases and from alcohol and violence

Hypothesized Causal Links

Age	Gender	Class	Ethnicity
1. Biological differences 2. Differences in lifestyle 3. Psychosocial aspects of symptoms and care-taking behaviours 4. Material inequities	1. Biological differences 2. Acquired (lifestyle) differences 3. Psychosocial aspects of acknowledgement of symptoms 4. Willingness to talk about health and illness 5. Frequent use by women of medical care system because of childbirth procedures as well as illness 6. Differing responses by doctors to male and female patients	1. Biases in measuring and recording processes 2. Illness causes downward mobility 3. Class-based cultural and behavioural differences 4. Class-based material inequities	1. Racism 2. Lifestyle differences 3. Class-based material differences leading up to inequities 4. Biological differences 5. Environmental hazards

involvement in non-traditional, high-risk, and high-stress careers? These questions will be addressed in the last section of this chapter.

Explanations for Differences in Disease and Death

Before attempting to discuss the reasons for age, gender, class, race, and ethnic differences in morbidity and mortality, it is important to understand the causes of illness and death. *A New Perspective on the Health of Canadians* (Lalonde, 1974) distin-

guishes among four components of health: human biology, environment, lifestyle, and health-care organization. Human biology covers all aspects of the mental and physical health of the body, including genetic inheritance, the processes of maturation and aging, and the many complex internal systems in the body. Environment covers all factors external to the body that affect health: clean drinking water, clean air, adequate food-stuffs, garbage and sewage disposal, and also the social environment—gender, social class, ethnic and cultural differences. Lifestyle refers to the

Box 5.9   *Shape* versus *Men's Fitness*

Shape and *Men's Fitness* are two popular fitness magazines; the first is directed towards females, the second towards males. Published by the same publisher, the circulation figures of *Shape* and *Men's Fitness* are 781,000 and 240,000, respectively. A comparative analysis of the two magazines over 1992 indicated a contrast of stereotypical images of the health and fitness of males and females. Some examples of stereotypical differences follow. (1) Cover models in *Men's Fitness* tend to be action-oriented males observed biking, running, hiking, weight-lifting, walking, and skiing. In contrast, the models on the cover of *Shape* tend to be in inactive poses such as sitting by the pool or standing on the beach. (2) The attire of the male models in *Men's Fitness* appears to be appropriate to the particular sports in which they are involved. However, the female models often wear costumes that would often be banned, as too revealing, in a typical fitness club.

(3) Each month, the magazines present 'success' stories submitted by readers. Although the ostensible purpose of the magazine is the promotion of health and fitness, the success stories for women tended to describe weight-loss achievements. By contrast, the success stories of males tended to describe weight gain. (4) An analysis of the portrayal of holidays noted that Valentine's Day was an important issue for females (*Shape*) in that two articles were dedicated to it. On the other hand, there were no articles in *Men's Fitness* on Valentine's Day. This seems to reflect a continuing focus on men as instrumental and woman as socio-emotional specialists.

This is a very brief overview of a report that compared two gender-specific health and fitness magazines in the 1990s (Johnstone and Robinson, 1995). It is not to be generalized but to be read as a series of observations you might test as you observe your own selection of mass media.

aggregate of individual health habits such as exercise, diet, smoking, alcohol use, seat-belt use, promiscuity and sexual carelessness. Finally, health-care organization covers the technologies, facilities, personnel, and organizations devoted to medical care.

The question then becomes, what is the link between inequities in the social structure and the components of health? Table 5.8 simplifies and summarizes some of the explanations for health inequities for age, gender, class, and ethnicity.

Age

It is a biological fact that people age and their bodies undergo some degeneration. Many kinds of chronic diseases seem to be largely associated with old age, such as cancer, arthritis, stroke, and heart disease. Certainly, biological factors are part of the explanation for age differences in mortality

and morbidity. But there are social and economic causes as well. These are listed in Table 5.8 and described below.

Differences in lifestyle. People of different age groups or generations have lived through different historical and political-economic circumstances. Such events as war and economic depression have significant and long-term consequences for the health and disability levels of each age group.

Psychosocial aspects of symptoms and care. Different historical periods have different cultures and social norms regarding the recognition of symptoms and signs and the action to be taken to respond to them (e.g., whether to 'doctor' oneself, do yoga, or go to the doctor). Any and all of these things may result in different health outcomes.

Differential access to health-giving resources. Significant political and economic differences certainly exist between different age groups. It is also clear that poverty accompanies aging, particularly for women. Income disparities lead to differences in nutrition, stress levels, density in living quarters, access to transportation, and the like. Such resources affect health status.

Gender

Verbrugge (1985, 1989) and Verbrugge and Wingard (1987) have made a major contribution to understanding gender differences in morbidity and mortality. After a thorough examination of the research literature available on the effects of differences in biology, lifestyle, preventive measures, the use of medical facilities, and treatment, Verbrugge (1985) reached the following conclusions.

(1) Because of both biological factors and lifestyle, women have more illness of a mild, transitory type and men of a more serious type. Mild illness accumulates over time, so that women suffer more bed-days and disability days and are more likely to see themselves as ill than men are. When men get sick, however, it is more likely with a serious or fatal condition.

(2) Women are more attentive to bodily sensations and more willing to talk about them. They tend to take more care for each episode of illness. When the illness is serious (e.g., cancer) men and women are equally likely to take action.

(3) While the sexes have similar levels of ability to remember major health problems, women are better 'describers' of mild problems because they are willing to talk about them. Women are more likely to include their feelings in their descriptions of their health.

(4) Women's greater attention to minor signs and symptoms and their greater willingness to take preventive and healing actions (i.e., bed rest, diet) mean that their health problems tend not to become as severe as those of men of the same age. This greater carefulness regarding their health helps women extend their lives.

Summary

(1) Illness and death rates vary depending on social-structural conditions: cultural differences, the political-economic system, the socio-demographic structure, social psychology, and existential phenomenology.

(2) One socio-economic characteristic that affects morbidity and mortality rates is age. Typical of most of the industrialized world is the aging of the population, which occurs with an overall decline in fertility rate and an increase in life expectancy, among other factors.

(3) Life expectancy increases are the result of many changes, including a rapid decline in the infant mortality rate and medical advances and their impact on the later stages of the life cycle. Both men and women have undergone great increases in life expectancy in the past 160 years, yet the excess of male mortality over female mortality has been greater in the last 25 years.

(4) Potential years of life lost (PYLL) is a useful figure because it calls attention to causes of death among the younger population. From this statistic, we can see that males are more than twice as likely as females to die prematurely from causes such as motor vehicle accidents, ischemic heart disease, accidents, and suicide.

(5) As people age they are more likely to be ill, yet older people are more likely to perceive themselves as 'healthy for my age' and to be fairly satisfied with their health.

(6) At every stage in their life cycles, men are more likely to die and women are more likely to be ill. This disparity seems to be related to industrialism and capitalism.

(7) Table 5.9 offers explanations of the health differences by age, gender, class, and ethnicity.

Questions for Study and Discussion

1. How can we explain the different life expectancies of men and women?
2. What is the relevance of the decline in the birth rate?
3. Compare a magazine that is written for a male audience and one that is written for a female audience with respect to the description of body and health issues.
4. Contrast the medicalization process involved in the construction of premenstrual syndrome as compared to male sexual inadequacy or impotence.
5. Why is there a new emphasis on research on women's health? What is your assessment of this initiative?
6. Should there be a new emphasis on men's health? Why or why not?

Suggested Readings

Clarke, Juanne N. 1983. 'Sexism, Feminism and Medicalism: A Decade Review of the Literature on Gender and Illness', *Sociology of Health and Illness* 5 (Mar.): 62–82. A useful critique of research on the relationships of gender, morbidity, and mortality.

MacPherson, Barry. 1983. *Aging as a Social Process.* Toronto: Butterworths. An excellent overview of issues relating to aging Canadians.

Verbrugge, Lois M. 1985. 'Gender and Health: An Update on Hypothesis and Evidence', *Journal of Health and Social Behavior* 26: 156–82. Another important reference for examining gender differences in health.

Waldron, Ingrid. 1981. 'Why Do Women Live Longer than Men?', *Journal of Human Stress* 2: 19–30. This study provides a good overview of issues regarding gender differences in morbidity and mortality that continue to be important.

Walters, Vivienne. 1992. 'Women's Views of Their Main Health Problem', *Canadian Journal of Public Health* 83, 5: 371–4. This is an important document because it signals a turn in health-related and gender-based research to the experience of the woman whose health is under examination.

Chapter 6 | *Social Inequity, Disease, and Death in Canada: Class, Race, and Ethnicity*

Learning Objectives

- Inequity in a society impacts on health at the level of both the individual and the population as a whole.
- Individual health and population health are both significant factors in the health status of people around the globe.
- Income and illness rates are negatively related.
- Income and death rates are negatively related.
- Education is an important resource for health.
- Ethnic status, because of income inequalities, discrimination, and racism, is associated with poorer health.
- Aboriginal Canadians have dramatically different life chances (in respect to morbidity and mortality) than non-Aboriginal Canadians.
- Political power seems to be associated with health status.
- Visible minority status is also relevant to health and illness rates.

Introduction

What sorts of relationships exist between inequity, perceived inequity, and health? Of what relevance for illness is the overall degree of inequity in a society as compared to individual poverty? Do morbidity and mortality rates differ in different regions of the country? What does the level of education have to do with health, illness, and death? Do poor people live shorter lives? Are the poor more often sick than their wealthier counterparts? These are some of the questions

that this chapter addresses. Health, illness, and death are linked to the social and economic structures of the society. One crucial aspect of this socio-economic structure is the extent of inequity, which is associated with different life chances and unequal access to resources such as food, recreation, satisfying work, and adequate shelter. People who differ in age, sex, income, class, occupation, ethnicity, marital status, rural or urban background, and religiosity differ in their rates of sickness and death. People who live in societies that are relatively unequal experience

---

Box 6.1   Income Distribution within a Society and Its Effect on Health

---

In developed countries, death rates are lowest when the degree of egalitarianism between classes is highest. 'Income distribution is now probably the single, best predictor of longevity among developed nations' (Wilkinson, 1990: 391). Moreover, there is a tendency for diseases for which nations have unusually high rates to be those that show the greatest socio-economic differences internally. This pertains to cirrhosis of the liver in France, respiratory disease in England, and homicide in the United States.

The absolute GNP or the average income of the people within the country is less important than the relative equality of wealth of people in a given society. In the developing world, health is a function of the physical effects of living circumstances as well as the meaning of the social conditions. Moreover, the social tensions exacerbated by inequality impact on the poor and the wealthy alike. 'It looks as if it may damage social relations among people at all levels of society, and lead, where relative deprivation is greatest, to a complete breakdown of the social fabric' (ibid., 409). Those countries where the poorest 70 per cent of the population have the most tend to have the highest rates of life expectancy.

Source: Wilkinson (1990), from Luxembourg Income Study, Working Paper 26, World Bank, World tables.

---

greater morbidity and higher death rates than people who live in societies characterized by greater equality.

This chapter will examine how illness and death rates in Canada vary depending on specific social conditions: income, education, and ethnicity. It will then discuss some of the possible explanations for the observed variations.

Social Class

One of the most consistent of epidemiological findings supported by a wide variety of evidence is that there is an inverse relationship between social class and mortality. Low socio-economic status has repeatedly been associated with a high incidence of infectious and parasitic diseases and high rates of infant mortality. Antonovsky (1967) noted that the high mortality of the lower classes from all causes of disease has been recorded since the twelfth century. The data highlighted in the following section show how this general finding has particular relevance for Canada. In spite of a national health insurance system of about 30 years' duration in this country, a significant and

consistent class gradient in health outcomes remains. Figures 6.1 and 6.2, based on 1986 data, portray the differences in life expectancy at birth for males and females of different neighbourhood income levels in Canada. Figure 6.3, using 1996–7 data, shows the consistency of the relationship between household income and health for children under 12.

As these figures indicate, average neighbourhood income and household income are directly related to life expectancy and health. This is true for both males and females, although the class gradient is steeper for men than women. A more sensitive indicator is health-adjusted life expectancy. This considers more than whether people live or die. It is an indication of the health-related quality of life. This measure corroborates the previous findings. Table 6.1 shows a relationship between both life expectancy overall and health-adjusted life expectancy. In both instances, people with more education fare better than people with less. Moreover, within every neighbourhood 'type', women live longer than men: those of the highest social class can expect to live the longest.

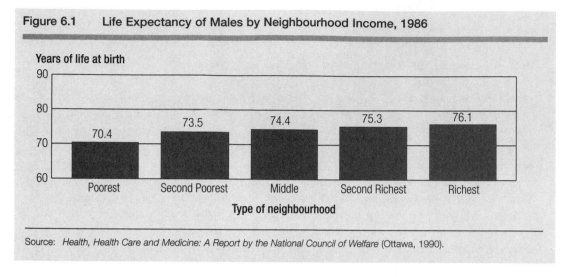

Figure 6.1   Life Expectancy of Males by Neighbourhood Income, 1986

Source: *Health, Health Care and Medicine: A Report by the National Council of Welfare* (Ottawa, 1990).

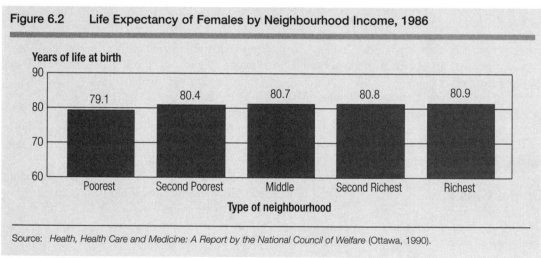

Figure 6.2   Life Expectancy of Females by Neighbourhood Income, 1986

Source: *Health, Health Care and Medicine: A Report by the National Council of Welfare* (Ottawa, 1990).

The life expectancy range for men from highest to lowest educational attainment is 3.2 years; for women, 2.2 years. The difference between men in the lowest quartile and those in the highest quartile, at 37.5 and 42.8 years of health-adjusted life expectancy, is even greater than the straightforward life expectancy. The same pattern is true for women. As Table 6.2 indicates, income adequacy is directly related to activity limitation, disability in the two weeks prior to the survey,

and satisfaction with health. Again, the poorest suffer more disability and are least satisfied with their health.

Class or income differences are also evident in the prevalence of illness. Table 6.3 illustrates the relationship between income adequacy and selected health problems for men and women. Overall, for both sexes, 73 per cent of those in the lowest income bracket have health problems, while 61 per cent in the highest income bracket have health

Figure 6.3   Percentage of Children under Age 12 Reported to Have Excellent or Very Good Health, by Household Income Group, Canada (excluding Territories), 1996–1997

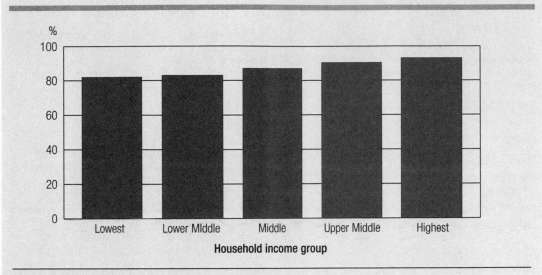

Source: National Population Health Survey, Cross-sectional file, 1996–7.

Table 6.1   Life Expectancy and Health-Adjusted Life Expectancy at Age 30, by Sex and Educational Attainment, Canada, 1990–1992

Educational attainment	Life expectancy Years	Health-adjusted life expectancy Years	Difference Years	%
Men				
Lowest quartile	44.5	37.5	7.0	16
Second quartile	45.2	39.5	5.7	13
Third quartile	47.6	41.8	5.8	12
Highest quartile	47.7	42.8	4.9	10
Women				
Lowest quartile	51.0	41.0	10.0	20
Second quartile	52.0	44.1	7.9	15
Third quartile	52.2	44.5	7.7	15
Highest quartile	53.2	46.3	6.9	13

Source: Wolfson (1996: 44).

Table 6.2   Prevalence of Three Health Status Indicators by Income Adequacy, Age 15+, Canada, 1991

	HEALTH STATUS INDICATOR		
Income adequacy	Activity limitation (%)	Two-week disability (mean no. of days)	Very satisfied with health (%)
Total	11	0.64	55
Lowest	25	1.34	37
Lower middle	19	0.96	47
Middle	13	0.70	54
Upper middle	9	0.53	57
Highest	7	0.48	65
Not stated	10	0.56	55

Source: Statistics Canada, *Health Status of Canadians*, 1991, Cat. no. 11–612E, no. 8, 46.

problems. When this is specified by sex, the overall class difference is the result of differences among women, not men (i.e., 79 per cent of women in the lowest income category report health problems while only 60 per cent of those in the highest income category report health problems). This pattern is reversed among men: those in the highest income category report more problems than those in the lowest (62 per cent as opposed to 61 per cent). However, when particular conditions are considered, income adequacy appears very important for both men and women. Canadians with the lowest income adequacy are more than three times as likely to experience arthritis and almost nine times as likely to experience emotional difficulties as those in the highest income categories. By comparison, hay fever tends to be slightly more common among those with higher income. One of the most sensitive indicators of class differences in health is the health of children. Figure 6.4 portrays this relationship.

Class correlates not only with death and specific diagnoses, but also with self-reported health. Yet, not all diseases and causes of death are related in the predicted way to social position; some

diseases, such as breast and prostate cancer, increase as social class increases (Gorey et al., 1998). And while a majority of adult Canadians feel that their health is excellent or very good, those in the highest social classes are considerably more likely to claim very good or excellent health than those in the lowest income groups (Figure 6.5).

Repeated studies have demonstrated a relationship between income and mortality. Most of these studies have been cross-sectional, which means that they have implicitly assumed stability of income over time in a person's life. But income may vary across a lifetime and sometimes the change in income is quite dramatic, as after a job loss. Recent American research has examined the relationship between the stability of income and mortality, showing that people who experienced an income loss of more than 50 per cent over a period of five years were 30 per cent more likely to die (McDonough, 1997: 3). Income loss has an impact on mortality regardless of actual dollar income, but it appears to affect the mortality rate of those who had lower incomes more than those with higher incomes.

Table 6.3   Prevalence of Selected Health Problems by Sex and Income Adequacy, Age 15+, Canada, 1991

Sex and income adequacy	Total population 15+ (000s)	Any health problem	Hyper-tension	Heart trouble	Diabetes	Arthritis/ rheuma-tism	Asthma	Emphy-sema, etc.	Hay fever	Skin or other allergies	Stomach ulcer	Other digestive problems	Recurring migraines	High blood cholesterol	Any emotional disorders
BOTH SEXES															
Total	20,981	63%	16%	7%	4%	21%	6%	8%	12%	21%	5%	8%	9%	8%	5%
Lowest	799	73	22	15	4	37	8	19	14	24	9	12	16	9	17
Lower middle	1,633	71	22	12	7	31	8	15	9	21	7	11	12	12	9
Middle	4,766	63	17	8	3	23	5	9	9	19	6	10	10	8	6
Upper middle	5,743	60	14	5	3	16	5	6	13	22	4	7	9	8	4
Highest	2,171	61	14	4	3	12	6	4	16	18	2	6	7	9	2
MALE															
Total	10,266	59%	16%	7%	4%	16%	6%	7%	11%	16%	4%	7%	5%	9%	4%
Lowest	261	61	19	1C	–	31	–	15	17	17	10	10	–	–	10
Lower middle	686	70	19	13	9	29	10	17	9	17	8	11	6	13	6
Middle	2,264	59	16	8	4	21	4	8	9	14	6	9	6	8	5
Upper middle	3,067	56	16	5	3	13	6	5	12	16	3	6	4	9	3
Highest	1,340	62	18	4	3	10	6	3	16	14	–	6	5	10	–
FEMALE															
Total	10,715	66%	16%	7%	4%	25%	6%	9%	13%	25%	5%	9%	13%	8%	7%
Lowest	538	79	23	17	5	40	9	20	12	27	8	13	19	11	20
Lower middle	947	72	24	12	6	33	6	13	9	24	7	10	15	10	11
Middle	2,503	66	17	3	3	25	5	9	10	23	5	12	14	8	7
Upper middle	2,676	64	13	5	3	20	4	6	15	23	5	8	14	7	5
Highest	831	60	9	3	–	16	7	4	15	25	–	4	10	7	–

Source: Statistics Canada, *Health Status of Canadians*, Mar. 1994, Cat. no. 11–612E, no. 8.

Figure 6.4   Children with Lower Functional Health

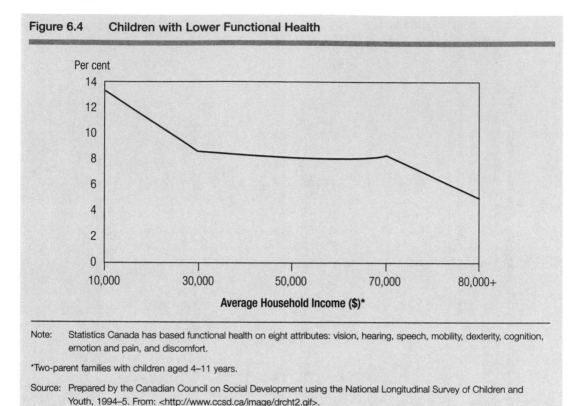

Note: Statistics Canada has based functional health on eight attributes: vision, hearing, speech, mobility, dexterity, cognition, emotion and pain, and discomfort.

*Two-parent families with children aged 4–11 years.

Source: Prepared by the Canadian Council on Social Development using the National Longitudinal Survey of Children and Youth, 1994–5. From: <http://www.ccsd.ca/image/drcht2.gif>.

Power, like income, is often considered a component of social class. The relationship between power and illness was raised by the findings of the British-based Whitehall Study, which compared the health of more than 10,000 British civil servants over nearly two decades. None were impoverished. None were deprived. All were white-collar workers in office jobs. Nevertheless, there was a direct decrease in mortality associated with higher status and more power in the organization. A similar finding was noted in a larger Swedish study—heart disease was more prevalent among those whose work was psychologically demanding and lacking in decision-making power. Researchers noted that while the level of stress was as high for those in the more powerful positions, it declined dramatically when

they left work and went home. They seemed much more able to turn off the stress response (Taylor, 1993).

Education

Education is also an important resource in Canadian society. It opens doors to certain (and often safer) occupations; it increases the chances of promotion to a more satisfying occupation. It may also have a direct effect on health. Figure 6.6 indicates that education is related to health status and activity level. As the level of education rises, fewer Canadian adults report poor or fair health or activity limitation. Important indicators of health are prevention and health promotion activities. Mammograms are advised for all

Figure 6.5   Self-Reported Health Status and Income

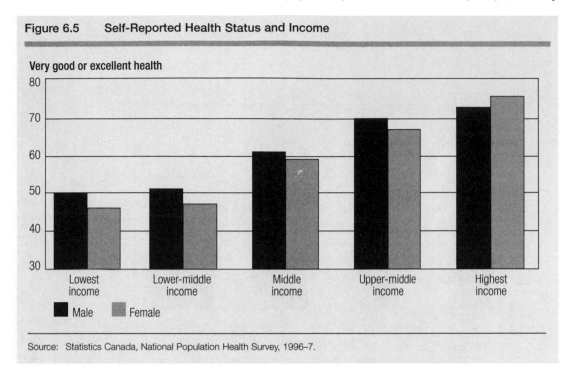

Source: Statistics Canada, National Population Health Survey, 1996–7.

women ages 50–69 for early detection of breast cancer. The likelihood of having a mammogram varied considerably according to a number of socio-demographic factors. Women who were single, who had relatively little education, who were not in the paid labour force, who had not recently visited a physician, and who were immigrants from South or Central America, the Caribbean, Africa, and Asia were less likely than other women to have had a mammogram (Gentleman and Lee, 1997: 23).

'Race', Ethnicity, and Minority Status

'Race', ethnicity, and minority status are also important factors affecting health in Canadian society and around the world. They should be defined and distinguished. 'Race' is a social and political construct that has been used to distinguish among people on the basis of physical

characteristics such as skin colour, bone density, blood types, and facial structure. Historically, there have been thought to be three broad categories of race: Caucasians, Mongoloids, and Negroids. In fact, there are no pure races and the concept is an outdated one. However, the effects of the beliefs in race continue and can be considered to be racism. 'Ethnicity' is a term that refers to a common cultural background. 'Minority status' refers to the numerical distribution of different ethnic categories of people.

There is a close and persistent relationship between ethnicity and class. A significant amount of economic inequality can be attributed to differences in ethnic background (Reitz, 1980). Inequality has significant implications for social relations between people and among those of differing backgrounds. Furthermore, how others view an individual has important consequences for the individual's self-esteem. To the extent that ethnicity is related to occupational status,

Figure 6.6   Canadians Age 15+ Reporting Fair or Poor Health Status and Activity
Limitations, by Education Level

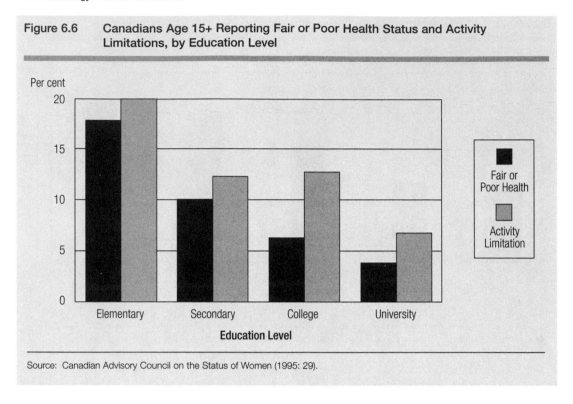

Source: Canadian Advisory Council on the Status of Women (1995: 29).

income, and education, then people of different ethnic groups will differ in their morbidity and mortality rates. There is a wide variation in adjusted income by education in various ethnic groups in Canada. Little research has been done on the relationship between ethnicity and health status in Canada. However, it is reasonable to assume that as ethnicity and class are correlated and class and health are correlated, then ethnicity and health will be correlated.

One way to consider the issue of the health of ethnic groups is to examine the relative health of immigrants through a comparison of their subjective reports with those of other Canadians (Table 6.4). Immigrants report that they perceive themselves to be healthy to a greater extent than do other Canadians regardless of various socioeconomic and demographic characteristics when they arrive. However, the longer they remain in

Canada the closer their self-reported health status becomes to the rest of the population. The life expectancy of immigrants to Canada is also greater than that of the Canadian-born (D'Arcy, 1998: 80).

The one ethnic 'group' for which some data are available is Canadian Aboriginals: First Nations, Inuit, and Métis. The variety of terms, including the older terms 'Indians' and 'Eskimos', reflects the struggle to find a name that best reflects the history and identity of peoples whose cultures were colonized by the European immigrants over the past 500 years. There is some debate about whether Aboriginal Canadians ought to be considered an ethnic group or not. Those who favour the ethnic group designation argue that there are cultural similarities among all 55 or more sovereign Aboriginal peoples, and all are colonized peoples, so that together they con-

Box 6.2   The Native Peoples of Grassy Narrows

The experience of the Ojibwa of the Grassy Narrows Reserve provides a poignant and trenchant critique of the disastrous impact the Canadian state and Canadian industry can have on a people and their way of life. Until 1963, the Grassy Narrows Ojibwa lived a settled, traditional life, hunting and fishing on and around the English-Wabigoon River in northern Ontario. Then, in 1963, they were relocated by the Department of Indian Affairs, so the reserve would be nearer to a road and thus nearer to a number of services and amenities in modern life, such as schools, various social services, and electricity. Uprooting and moving the people had a tumultuous impact on their health and lifestyle. Before the Ojibwa had time to adjust to this crisis, another hit. This time it was the discovery that the English-Wabigoon River system, which had been their main source of livelihood for many years, was poisoned by methyl mercury.

Before 1963, over 90 per cent of all deaths among the Ojibwa were attributed to natural causes. By the mid-1970s, only 24 per cent of the deaths resulted from natural causes. By 1978, 75 per cent of

the deaths were due to alcohol-induced violence directed against the self and others. Homicide, suicide, and accidental death rates soared. Child neglect and abuse grew rapidly, and numerous children were taken into the care of the Children's Aid Society and placed in foster homes. As Shkilnyk (1985: 3) says: 'Today the bonds of the Indian family have been shattered. The deterioration in family life has taken place with extraordinary swiftness.' Despite the good intentions of the Canadian government in relocating the people, their socio-economic conditions deteriorated. 'All the indications of material poverty were there—substandard housing, the absence of running water and sewage connections, poor health, mass unemployment, low income, and welfare dependency' (ibid.).

The Grassy Narrows Ojibwa experienced too much change, too quickly. Their autonomy and cultural traditions were destroyed. Because of mercury pollution, they were robbed of their means of livelihood. There are many lessons to be drawn from this situation. Still, the solutions remain complex.

Box 6.3   'Race', Political Power, and Health

Political empowerment may become an important consideration in efforts to understand the crisis of morbidity and mortality. In a recent study, LaVeist (1992) examined all US central cities with a population of more than 50,000 residents and with blacks comprising at least 10 per cent of the population. The selection process resulted in 176 cities in 32 states. The two crucial variables were the absolute and relative degree of African-American political power and the post-neonatal mortality rate (deaths occurring between the second and twelfth months of life). African-American political power was measured as the proportion of African-American representatives on the city council divided by

the proportion of African-Americans in the voting age population. The sum measure is an indication of absolute black political empowerment—i.e., the percentage of city council members who are African-American. The results underscore the importance of relative political power to mortality rate. Where African-Americans were well represented on city councils, the African-American post-neonatal mortality rate was relatively low. LaVeist discusses some of the processes that could be implicated in the correlation, including the most obvious explanation that black people's needs (water, welfare, hospitals, protective services, etc.) would receive some priority.

Table 6.4   Age-adjusted Prevalence of Any Chronic Condition and Specific Chronic Conditions, by Immigrant Status, Duration of Residence, Sex, Income, and Education, Canada, 1994–1995

	Total[†]	Canadian-born	All immigrants[‡]	European immigrants Years in Canada			Non-European immigrants Years in Canada		
				Total[§]	0–10	11+	Total[§]	0–10	11+
Age-adjusted %									
Any chronic condition	55.5	56.8	50.3*	55.3	46.7	57.7	44.7*	37.2*	51.2
Sex									
Men	51.7	53.0	46.6*	51.1	39.8	54.7	40.8*	33.8*	46.7
Women	59.2	60.5	53.8*	59.3	52.3	60.5	48.1*	40.1*	55.6
Annual household income									
Less than $30,000	57.6	59.7	51.3*	57.4	46.3	59.5	45.8*	37.4	55.5
$30,000 or more	53.9	54.7	49.8*	54.0	46.4	56.8	44.6*	39.0*	48.7
Education									
Less than secondary graduation	55.5	56.3	52.5	57.7	55.2	58.8	45.7	37.0*	58.3
Secondary graduation or more	54.9	56.2	49.6*	54.4	45.8	57.0	44.6*	35.8*	50.1

Notes: Household population aged 18 and over.
†Includes unknown immigrant status.
‡Includes unknown country of birth.
§Includes unknown years in Canada.
*Difference compared with Canadian-born significant at 95% confidence level.

Source: *Health Reports* 7, 4 (Spring 1996).

stitute an ethnic group. Others, however, argue that because the cultural diversity of the Aboriginal peoples at colonization has been seriously compromised by the dominance of the state, they cannot be considered one cultural or ethnic group. Regardless of which side of this complex controversy one takes, the evidence remains clear that Aboriginal peoples have experienced different life chances and different life expectancy rates than non-Aboriginal Canadians.

The Aboriginal Peoples' Survey, conducted in conjunction with the 1991 census, enumerated just over a million people of Aboriginal origin, including 49,255 Inuit and 212,650 Métis, or 3.7 per cent of the Canadian population (Dickason, 1997: 410–11). This total figure, however, is low, because some bands refused enumeration, because of the difficulty in enumerating off-reserve status and non-status Indians, and due to inevitable under-reporting on the part of Métis. 'Everywhere in Canada they are struggling to overcome the effects of colonialism and its associated assimilationist practices. Such effects include, but are not limited to, cultural loss, discrimination, unemployment, and poverty' (McCormick et al., 1997). Colonialism also has had broad health effects, with epidemics of smallpox, measles, and tuberculosis devastating large

Box 6.4   Medical Care and Mortality: Racial Differences in Preventable Deaths

Blacks suffer higher rates of sickness and death than whites. This is particularly evident in regard to essentially preventable health problems. A study based in Alameda County in California (Woolhandler et al., 1985) provided a number of details that help explain this racially based inequity.

1. Blacks are less likely than whites to have private health insurance.
2. A greater proportion of blacks have never been to a physician for a checkup.
3. Blacks are four times as likely as whites to rely on public sector care.
4. More than twice as many blacks as whites have not received immunizations.
5. Fewer black women receive pap smears.
6. Fewer black than white people with hypertension are under treatment.

7. When admitted to hospital, blacks are more likely admitted through an emergency room.
8. Blacks are more likely to be transferred to a public emergency room.

These disparities in health care are an important part of the explanation for the morbidity and mortality differential between blacks and others. While this study is based in California, where universal health care is absent, a similar study is not available to compare Canadians of different racial background. Nevertheless, it is possible to put forth the hypothesis that although the morbidity and mortality inequities may not be as strong in the Canadian situation, because of differences in both racism and economic inequalities, it is likely that black Canadians have higher age-adjusted rates of morbidity and mortality than Euro-Canadians.

numbers of people. The residential school system, reserve life, and extensive racism have also played a part and resulted in high poverty rates (54 per cent, as compared to 35 per cent of the Canadian population over 15 years old, report an income of less than $10,000 per year). Not surprisingly, these differences in levels of poverty are mirrored in morbidity and mortality differences. The continuing differences in income, education, employment, and housing are a fundamental contribution to the poorer health of Aboriginal Canadians.

Box 6.5   Karoshi

Overwork itself is an insured cause of mortality in Japan. 'Karoshi' is the Japanese term that means death from overwork. The Japanese Labour Ministry has resisted the organizing and lobbying efforts made by spouses and family members of victims of Karoshi through the Association of Families of Karoshi Victims. The government, until now, has refused to keep statistics. But the United Nations Human Rights Commission has recognized Karoshi

sufficiently to organize a hearing and to accept testimony. This action may lead to formal human rights investigations. The Japanese Ministry of Labour has been forced to respond. It now offers compensation to the families of overwork victims only if certain conditions demonstrating excessive overtime are met. These include the following: the victim must have worked for 24 hours preceding death or seven days straight with more than four hours' overtime a day.

Figure 6.7   Infant Death Rates for Selected Causes: Aboriginals, 1989–1991, and Canada, 1990

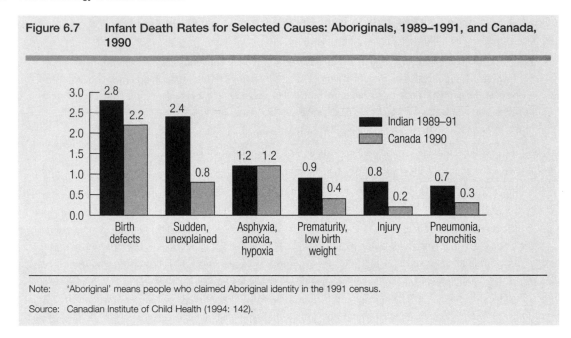

Note: 'Aboriginal' means people who claimed Aboriginal identity in the 1991 census.

Source: Canadian Institute of Child Health (1994: 142).

The life expectancy of Aboriginal males at birth is 64 years while the life expectancy of the overall Canadian male population is 73 years. Aboriginal females can expect to live 71 years while the Canadian female average at birth is close to 80 years. The infant mortality rate (Figure 6.7) is a significant part of the explanation (Newbold, 1998: 61), as are high rates of alcohol and substance abuse, suicide, and violence among the young. Both the birth and the infant mortality rates are higher for registered Indians than for other Canadians (Bolaria and Bolaria, 1994: 249), although the discrepancy appears to be diminishing over time. The rate of sudden, unexplained infant death is three times as high among Aboriginals. Low birth weight and premature birth are twice as frequent causes of death among Aboriginal infants. In addition, Aboriginal young people are more likely to die as the result of injuries. The injury death rate is five times greater for preschoolers, four times greater for infants, and three times greater for teenagers (Figure 6.8). The suicide rate among Aboriginal young people is also much higher than among young Canadians as a whole (Figure 6.9).

Another examination of the health of Aboriginal peoples has looked at their own self-described health status as well as the incidence of particular diagnoses. Interestingly, Aboriginal peoples are comparable to other Canadians with regard to this subjective measure (Newbold, 1998: 65).

The health of Aboriginal peoples is related to gender, class, age, and area of residence (Wotherspoon, 1994). That being said, a number of dramatic differences in disease type/incidence exist between Aboriginals and other Canadians. The rate of diabetes (Figure 6.10) is 10 times the Canadian rate (Anderson, 1994: 317). Aboriginal men are twice as likely and Aboriginal women are five times as likely to be obese than their non-Aboriginal counterparts (Barsh, 1994: 21). In some Native communities more than 40 per cent of the population has some form of 'disability' (Demas, 1993: 53). Overall, 31 per cent of adult Aboriginals, as compared to 13 per cent of non-Aboriginals, are 'disabled' (Ng, 1996). AIDS is

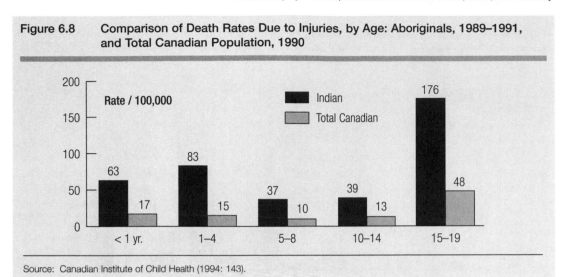

Figure 6.8   Comparison of Death Rates Due to Injuries, by Age: Aboriginals, 1989–1991, and Total Canadian Population, 1990

Source: Canadian Institute of Child Health (1994: 143).

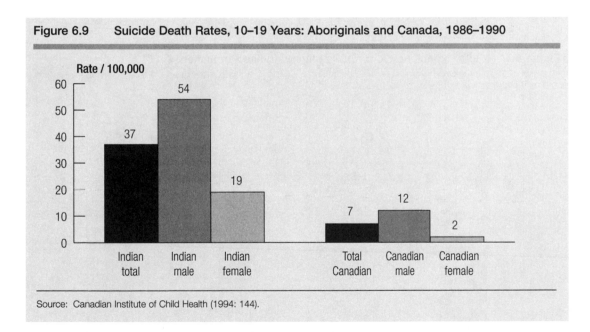

Figure 6.9   Suicide Death Rates, 10–19 Years: Aboriginals and Canada, 1986–1990

Source: Canadian Institute of Child Health (1994: 144).

expected to be a leading cause of death for Aboriginals in the years to come (Frideres, 1994: 279), and Aboriginal women are especially susceptible because of other higher rates of sexually transmitted disease and inequitable gender rela-

tions. As Figure 6.11 indicates, the life expectancy at birth for both male and female registered Indians is significantly lower than for the total Canadian population. In 2002 the gap in life expectancy between First Nations people and

Figure 6.10   Incidence of Diabetes among First Nations and Canada, by Age Group, 1991

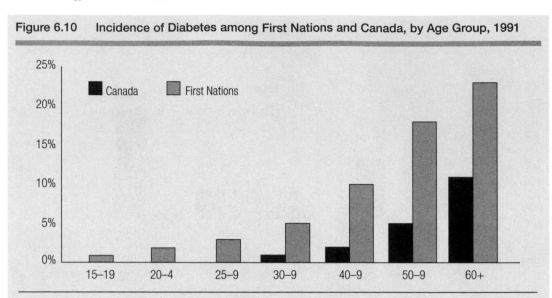

Source: Commission on the Future of Health Care (2002: 220).

Figure 6.11   Life Expectancy at Birth, Registered Indian Population, 2000

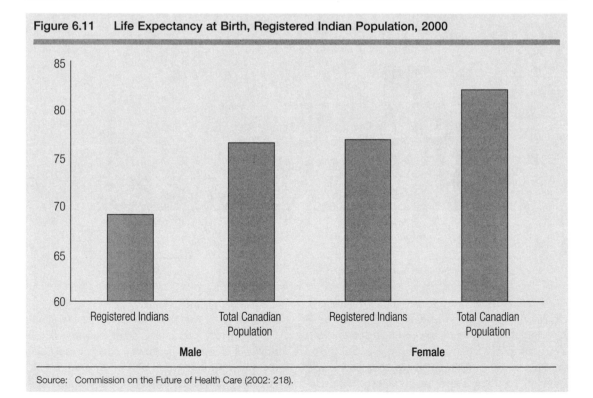

Source: Commission on the Future of Health Care (2002: 218).

Figure 6.12   Life Expectancy at Birth, Aboriginal Peoples and Canadian Population, 1991

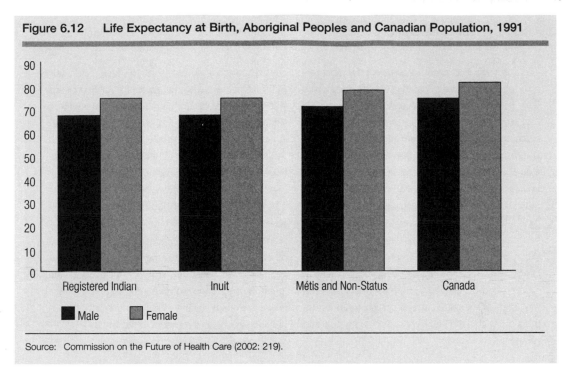

Source: Commission on the Future of Health Care (2002: 219).

other Canadians was 7.4 years for men and 5.2 years for women (Romanow Report, 2002: 218). Figure 6.12 shows an estimate of the disparities in life expectancy between the Canadian population as a whole and Aboriginal groups (ibid., 218–19). (This is just an estimate because good statistics on the health of First Nations and other Aboriginal groups have not been kept.)

In 1993, one Innu community, Davis Inlet (Utshimassits), Labrador, made front-page news and headlines when 'six children were pulled from an abandoned shed, high on gasoline fumes, shrieking that they wanted to die' (www.southam.com/NewsMedia/SI/sdavis/davsection/./.html). These children, in some ways, represented the results of a loss of culture. The people were one of the last groups of nomadic hunters in North America. Until about 30 years ago they lived in tents. Then they were resettled on an island 275 kilometres north of Goose Bay, where they have struggled with alcoholism, glue-

sniffing, physical and sexual abuse, and suicide. More recently, millions of dollars have been spent to build a new village, Natuashish (Sango Bay), on the mainland for the people of Davis Inlet, but this anticipated move may prove to be too little and too late. Their former way of life was destroyed. Their future is uncertain, as the research presented by British medical sociologist Colin Samson in his aptly titled book, *A Way of Life That Does Not Exist: Canada and the Extinguishment of the Innu*, clearly attests. Indeed, a recent British study led by Samson found that the Innu of northern Quebec and Labrador have the highest suicide rate in the world—a rate 13 times higher than for anyone else in Canada (McAndrew, 1999: A1; Samson et al., 1999; Samson, 2003: 227–9). As the National Chief of the Assembly of First Nations, Matthew Coon Come, explained, 'It took an investigation by the Assembly of First Nations, which led to a stinging human rights report by the Canadian Human

Box 6.6   The Great Dying

The numbers have been debated, but the most reliable recent estimate is that the New World peoples likely numbered between 90 and 112 million before they were devastated. Not only were the Amerindians numerous, they also enjoyed good health. In fact, before contact they were apparently in better health than Europeans. They did not have measles, smallpox, leprosy, influenza, malaria, or yellow fever. For most, staying healthy and living well were essential to their religion. In an age before Europeans' hygiene included regular bathing, the peoples of the New World kept clean and the Europeans could not help noticing the 'good smells' emanating from the healthy, robust people. Apparently, they especially admired their even, white teeth and clear complexions, 'something most pockmarked Spaniards, Portuguese and French had lost at an early age' (Nikiforuk, 1991: 80). At this time, the average life expectancy of Europeans was about 20 years less than that of the Amerindians. It is suggested that the good health was the continuing result of the origins of these people, who had had to cross the frozen Bering Strait to the New World. Because of the harsh cold, the diseased immigrants and their germs were killed.

Into this context of good health the new disease smallpox entered—an unknown yet voracious predator that spread, as an epidemic, until it and other strong killers such as the plague and tuberculosis killed probably 100 million people. This, the 'great dying', occurred over about one century. Some historians rank this as the greatest demographic disaster in the history of the world.

Rights Commission, to force the federal Crown to begin to take steps to return the Innu of Davis to their traditional lands.'

The problems continue today, not only in Davis Inlet but in reserves across the country as traditional land is taken away and people are resettled. There are many attempts to solve the 'behavioural problems' such as those described above regarding the people of Davis Inlet. Many would argue, however, that prevention of the problems through First Nations self-government is the only real possible direction for lasting social change.

Explanations for the Health Effects of Inequalities

The Black Report (1982), an evaluation of Britain's National Health Service and its impact on the health of the population, highlighted four different types of explanation for class differences in health. These differences have persisted for the past 50 years, since the introduction of the National Health Service, which was designed to equalize health status in Britain. These four explanations are: measurement artifact, natural or social selection, cultural/behavioural differences, and materialism. The authors of the Black Report prefer the materialist explanation, which sees health as the result of political-economic differences or differences in the way members of different social classes are constrained to lead their lives. The alternative explanations offered by the Black Report follow.

Measurement artifact. The findings of class-related health differences are merely the result of the biases involved in the measurement and recording processes. Certainly measures both of class and of health are of imperfect validity. The argument is that the association itself is false because it is due to a measurement bias that affects the measurement of class and health simultaneously (see Blane, 1985, for a discussion of some of the finer points of this explanation).

Natural or social selection. An explanation

Box 6.7   How Does Racism Work?

A great deal of research documents the many ways that discrimination hurts adults. It has been shown to cause psychological distress, experiences of depression, low self-esteem, anxiety, and declines in physical health. Are these effects the same in adolescents and children? What are the consequences of growing up as a person who is a member of a stigmatized and stereotyped ethnic minority? It makes sense to suggest that the impact of racism is even greater on children than on adults because young people are at the stage of developing their identities and understandings of what it means to be a member of an ethnic group. Perceived discrimination may interfere with the ongoing internalization processes because of the difficulties of identifying with a group one sees being rejected and hated.

Whitbeck and his colleagues (2001) studied 195 American 'Indian' children in grades 5–8 in three different reservations in the upper Midwest of the United States. Although this study is based in the US there is no compelling reason to believe that the processes are different in Canada. They found that the experience of prejudice and discrimination had significant consequences for the development of American 'Indian' adolescents. The experience of the lack of being the same as others and of being rejected by the majority groups during early adolescence may lead to self-hatred, anger, delinquency, and substance abuse. Beginning substance abuse behaviours early compounds the difficulties associated with them and may seriously challenge later life chances. Children who use substances are more likely to drop out of or fail at school and to have problems getting along with other people, including peers and family members. These are among the adaptations to discrimination that can accumulate and severely limit opportunities in later life.

What can be done? Do you have any experiences with discrimination and prejudice? Have you felt critical or disparaging of people because of their ethnicity or visible minority status? Can you remember where and how that feeling started? What maintains your feelings of ethnic superiority or inferiority?

Source: Les B. Whitbeck, Dan R. Hoyt, Barbara J. McMorris, Xiaojin Chen, and Jerry D. Stubben, 'Perceived Discrimination and Early Substance Abuse among American Indian Children', *Journal of Health and Social Behavior* 42 (Dec. 2001): 405–24.

based on cause and effect is questionable. It is argued here that perhaps class differences result from human biological differences rather than that the human biological differences result from the class inequities. One view is that resources unequally available to people in different social classes cause changes in human biology so that the poorer classes, lacking adequate nutrients, clean drinking water, safe working conditions, and the like are more likely to become ill. The competing view is that people suffer from ill health first and then drop down in the social class hierarchy. Illness itself, because of resultant dis-

ability, unemployment, or demotion, according to this argument, causes the decline in social class. A number of studies have suggested that this explanation has some validity and that illness certainly may cause a drop in class level for some. Overall, however, the impact of ill health on downward mobility is very slight and tends to be limited to certain sexes and age groups, namely, men in their later middle age.

Cultural/behavioural. Class (and here minority racial and ethnic status groups are also relevant) does cause illness; the explanation stipulates that the mechanism through which this occurs is class

Box 6.8   Poverty

Women are poorer than men. This finding varies from the 9.1 per cent difference between men and women who are unattached to the 33.8 per cent difference among single parents. In 1999 men's incomes were $4,882 higher among unattached individuals and $18,258 among single parents. The child poverty rate in Canada in 1999 was 18.7 per cent. Children under six were the most likely to have lived in poverty from 1993 to 1998. Between 1993 and 1998 visible minority immigrants comprised 6 per cent of the Canadian population. About 42.5 per cent of these people lived in poverty for at least one of these years. The comparable figure for the total population was 29.5 per cent. In addition, 15.6 per cent of the visible minority immigrant population as compared to 5 per cent of the total population lived in poverty for all of these years.

Between 1993 and 1999, Aboriginal people who did not live on the reserve made up 0.9 per cent of the total Canadian population. Almost half (49.4 per cent) lived in poverty at least one year, while 12.6 per cent lived in poverty throughout this period.

Also, the risk of poverty is inversely related to the level of education achieved. As well, 31.9 per cent of senior unattached men and women lived in poverty. The poverty rate among senior couples is much lower.

Source: National Council of Welfare, *Poverty Profile* (Ottawa: National Council of Welfare, Summer 2002).

differences in lifestyle preferences and behaviours, including such things as the consumption of harmful commodities (refined foods, tobacco, alcohol), leisure-time exercise, and the use of preventive health measures such as contraception, 'safe sex', prenatal monitoring, and vaccination. This explanation implies that lifestyle behaviours are the result of a number of individual, free-choice decisions. The suggestion is that because of the culture of poverty, those in the poorer classes choose to live for today, to ignore preventive health guidelines, and to indulge themselves in smoking and eating fatty, rich foods, all the while lying around on the couch and neglecting to exercise. The problem with this notion is that individual decision-making must always be seen in the context of the social structure and of the constraints that impede the behaviours of the people placed in different locations in the social structure. Furthermore, there is no evidence that the lower classes or minorities tend uniformly to fail to practise good health habits. To take just one example, class is inversely related to alcohol consumption and alcoholism.

Materialist. Illness is the result of lifestyle. In this case, however, the lifestyle and class differences result from conditions of work, adequate supply of money to provide for nutritious foods, amount of leisure time, availability of transportation, housing quality, air pollution, and clean drinking water. Cigarette smoking, which is higher in the lower classes, is expensive. Thus the materialist cannot be the only explanation. In the materialist explanation, lifestyle differences are not thought of as based on individual choice, as they are above. Blane (1985) reviews a number of studies documenting the materialist argument and concludes that the materialist explanation appears the most promising and yet has been largely neglected.

More recently, research on global and national inequalities and health has noted the importance of the overall level of equality or equity in a society as predictive of the average life expectancy in the society. This perspective is sometimes called the population health perspective. There is evidence in this research tradition that those who are financially better off but live in a more inequitable society will have poorer health than those who are less well off in material terms but live in a more equitable society. This suggests the importance of the *perception of fairness* and of *social capital* or *cohesion* in a more complete understanding of the link between health and equality.

Ethnicity

The final question is, why are there ethnic differences in morbidity and mortality rates? The explanations offered are similar to those for the previous three variables, particularly class. The most important additional explanation is racism, which through prejudice and discrimination may have an additional impact on the health of Canadian Aboriginal peoples, African Canadians, and other visible minorities. Ethnicity is largely explained as a subset of class.

Racism leads to bias in how people are treated in all aspects of their lives. It limits their job, educational, religious, recreational, marital, and family choices and chances. One of the effects of racism is the environmental destruction of the lands of First Nations peoples. As Table 6.5 shows, the threats to the environment include a wide variety of such things, including flooding as the result of the construction of dams and hydroelectric projects, water contamination, and depletion of fisheries.

Canadian Indians on reserves suffer from isolation, remoteness, and limited power in the control of their own housing, location, education, and occupation. Furthermore, there are numerous examples of the pollution of Native waterways and the destruction of what had been their staple foodstuffs.

Economics and Health

Why are there pervasive correlations between death, disability, and disease and age, gender, class, and ethnicity? What do these social-structural characteristics have in common? Is the relationship between the social-structural variables and health variables the result of one overriding mechanism? Or are there different relationships between each pair of variables?

Marxist analysis attempts to integrate all discrete and superficially unique explanations into a unified explanation. A substantial body of scholarship documents the relationship between the economy and health status. Beginning with the work of Friedrich Engels in *The Condition of the Working Class in England*, analysis has focused on the state and the economy as they affect health outcomes. Engels noted the contradictions between the workers' need, in the earliest industrialist economies, to sell their labour power and the capitalist factory owners' need for profit. Because industrial profit was necessary to maintain factory-based production, the wages of workers were kept low and their working conditions poor. Shelter for the poor was frequently inadequate, crowded, unheated, and unsanitary. Poor hygiene and inadequate nutrition resulted in widespread contagious diseases such as tuberculosis and typhoid.

The first principle of capitalism is that business requires profit. Profit, as the colloquial saying puts it, is the bottom line. According to Marxist analysis, all capitalist states are arranged in such a way as to maximize profits. Furthermore, competition forces capitalists to maximize outputs while minimizing the costs of production. The growth of profits results in the accumulation of capital. Excess capital is invested in new or more efficient production units. New and greater profits are then realized. Increased production invokes a need to find and create new markets. When domestic markets are saturated, new foreign markets must be opened up. Profits from these markets are reinvested, and the cycle of profit, competition, accumulation of capital, investment, and expanded markets repeats itself.

When the state is based on capitalism, state decisions are guided by the necessity of supporting the most successful profit-making initiatives. Usually when a choice between profitability and

Table 6.5   Selected Contaminants and Their Impact on First Nations Health Conditions

Source and contaminant	Areas of major concern (number of projects or developments)
Impact: Destruction of wildlife; restrictions on hunting and fishing rights; contamination of food, air, and water	
Flooding of First Nations lands through dams and hydroelectric developments	Atlantic (8) Northern Quebec (11) Ontario (17) Manitoba (4) Saskatchewan (2) British Columbia (9)
Acid rain and toxic chemicals from smelters, coal-fired electricity, transportation, and industrial processes	Quebec and Ontario (43% of lakes contaminated) Ontario (Serpent River, Big Trout Lake, Weagamow, Wawa-Sudbury, 65% of headwaters in Muskoka-Haliburton area) Arctic and Northern Canada (lakes and coastal regions contaminated) Canada (40% of forest affected, a dozen rivers no longer support trout or salmon)
High water temperature from large-scale forest harvesting	British Columbia (Meares Island, Lyell Island, Moresby Islands, Stein watershed)
Aquaculture and fish farming in marine water	Bays traditionally harvested by First Nations in maritime waters
Oil and gas exploration, drilling, pipelines, refineries, and potential for spills	West coast offshore High and eastern Arctic (Beaufort Sea, Mackenzie Delta) Northern Alberta
Noise from military	Northern Canada
Impact: Water contamination and destruction of fisheries	
Mercury and other heavy metals from mining, smelters, and acid rain	Northwest Territories (lakes and rivers) Ontario English-Wabigoon River system, St Clair River, Sarnia
Toxic chemicals, including PCBs, DDT, dioxin, and endusulfin	Great Lakes (1,000 chemicals) Ontario (Niagara River) Quebec (St Lawrence River system) Northern Canada
Impact: Social and economic disruption	
Dislocation of whole communities, disruption of industries, depletion of resources	All regions noted above

Source: Bolaria and Bolaria (1994: 263).

human need is confronted, profitability must, in the final analysis, come first. The argument is that the good of the whole, not the good of individuals, is advanced when economic productivity and profitability prevail. Consequently, when the need for profit is the determining principle, the health needs of the population assume secondary importance. The worth of individuals in a capitalist economy is measured by their relationship to the means of production. Because of upturns and downturns in the economy, a reserve labour force is required. The reserve labour force is made up of people who are peripheral to the paid labour force and can be brought into it or dismissed from it depending on market demands.

The more marginal the worker is in the capitalist economy, the more easily he or she can be replaced. Occupational health and safety precautions are expenses to the capitalist owner. To the extent that the cost of such precautions threatens the level of profit, and in the absence of state legislative requirements, health and safety standards will be minimal. Accidents, job-related sickness, and alienation will be most prevalent in the workers who are most marginal and most replaceable. One overriding reason for income, gender, age, and ethnic differences in health is the variation in access to safe, satisfying, adequately remunerated work. Marxist analysis provides an important explanation for inequities in health outcomes.

To conclude: health is the outcome of access to fundamental resources. Poverty, poor nutrition, inadequate housing and transportation, and the lack of effective birth control all contribute in known ways to ill health. In a capitalist economy there are significant differences in access to these life-giving resources in respect to differences in age, gender, income, and ethnic group.

Commodification

One other contribution of Marxist analysis to understanding inequities in death, disease, and disability is through the concept of commodities or commodification. Commodities are objects or activities having an 'exchange value'. They can be bought and sold in the marketplace and can be used to acquire other things. Their value is determined by market factors such as supply and demand. Health can be seen as a commodity. It is no longer simply the individual experience of well-being but, in a capitalist economy, is subject to supply and demand. The buying and selling of organs for transplantation into unhealthy bodies is perhaps the most blatant example of commodification. Health is purchasable for those with the money. There is also a way in which health itself is an object that reflects value and worth back on the individual. In this case, health is used to indicate the productive value of the person to the society. Healthy people are thought to be good people. Health is believed to embody a certain level of conspicuous consumption and a degree of much valued self-control (Crawford, 1984).

Whenever a government or a corporation decides to allow the continuance of a practice that is destructive to the health of a population in the interests of financial benefits such as taxes or profits, health is being commodified. Cigarette smoking is a case in point. There is absolutely no doubt that cigarette smoking is a significant cause of disability and death in Canadian society. Yet neither the cigarette industry nor the government has been willing to pull cigarettes from the market or to limit their production to low-tar cigarettes. Cigarettes are a fundamental and crucial aspect of contemporary economies. According to Doyal (1979), the state made a deliberate decision to allow the tobacco industry to continue. The British Department of Health showed that a reduction in cigarette smoking would be costly to the state. Not only would the tax on cigarettes be lost, but also there would be the additional financial costs of caring for people longer into their old age, which would be the inevitable result of increased life expectancy.

Recent research has delved more deeply into the reasons that socio-economic inequality is associated with health inequality. Clearly, the variation in physical resources, such as a clean, adequately sized living space and sufficient, nutritious foods and beverages, is an important reason for the link. Lifestyle differences in smoking and alcohol consumption play a part. Occupational hazards are influential. However, according to new studies, there may be a paradigm shift in approaching the correlation between health and inequality. Including social stress, self-efficacy, emotional well-being, and social cohesion into the equation (between health and material inequality) provides a meaningful, deeper context for understanding (Elstad, 1998). Health differences are a function of materialist constraints, some of which are translated into behavioural differences. The next chapter continues with an examination of this paradigm.

The Link between Social Class and Cigarette Smoking

Cigarette smoking is the major cause of premature mortality in the developed world today (Pampel, 2002). This is despite the fact that the rate of cigarette smoking, except among the young, has declined dramatically over the past 30 years or so. Thus the excess mortality presently being experienced should abate somewhat in a few years until the consequences of the high rate of smoking among teenagers begins to have the devastating effects that can be expected in the absence of a change in this behaviour.

Given the strong link between cigarette smoking and social class and given its significance as a cause of both high levels of premature morbidity and mortality, it is important to understand how and why poorer people are drawn to it. Deaths from diseases such as bronchitis and emphysema, lung cancer, cardiovascular disease, and all cancers combined increase by factors of 12.1, 11.8, 1.6, and 1.7 in the presence of cigarette smoking. In addition, people who smoke have lower rates of self-rated health and higher rates of death from crime, violence, accidents, and alcohol abuse.

What is the link between smoking and social class? The *materialist* explanation is not appropriate here. Cigarettes are expensive and their cost is significant in the overall budget of the relatively lower income groups. For example, an average of 15 per cent of the disposable income of the smoking poor in Britain is expended in maintaining the cigarette habit.

Socio-psychological explanations would suggest that the reason might be the sense of relative deprivation felt by the poorer people in a society. This experience, the argument goes, causes emotional, social, and psychological stress and smoking is taken up and continued as a 'cheap' form of therapy and stress reduction. Poorer people usually cannot afford warm vacations in the cold winter months, cottages in the north, ski trips, or even psychotherapy, massage therapy, or other individual therapeutic interventions chosen by those with higher income levels.

Alternatively, people of lower status may tend to have generally higher levels of *fatalism and anomie* because they realize the almost impermeable borders between their own life chances and circumstances and those of people further up the socio-economic hierarchy. They may not know how or believe that it is possible to change their own socio-economic position. Feeling blocked and expecting to live shorter and sicker lives, they may just tend to think that smoking cessation does not really matter in their situation. They may not, after years of negative experiences, feel that they have the self-efficacy to change their lives or those of their families.

Social capital is another possible explanation of the negative relationship between smoking and social status. There is evidence that those lower in status have less social capital in terms of, for instance, friendship, neighbourhood, and acquaintance networks that provide the basis for the development and maintenance of experiences of social cohesion via networks of trust, shared values, and common goals and obligations. Lacking strong networks of relationships, poorer people are less likely to have alternative coping strategies modelled, social control mechanisms offered, and social support.

These explanations suggest that the lower the education, occupational prestige, status, and income the greater the likelihood of smoking within a society; they may also be used to help to explain the adoption of smoking around the world by poorer, developing countries at a higher rate overall than in the developed countries.

Another explanation comes from *diffusion* theory. Here it has been shown that innovations are generally picked up first by the wealthier and more highly placed individuals in a society. Only later are innovations picked up by those lower on the social hierarchy. This is also the case with cigarette smoking. Thus the correlation between high rates of cigarette smoking and lower social class are related to the fact that cigarettes have more recently been picked up by the lower-status groups as those higher on the social ladder have rejected them. Pampel's extensive research, which included data from 15 European nations, demonstrated that diffusion theory rather than social inequality is the better explanation of status-based smoking patterns.

The Growth of Inequality

The growth of inequality over the globe is paralleled by an increase in inequity in Canada as well as in other developed nations such as the United Kingdom, the United States, Australia, New Zealand, and Sweden. This is a concomitant to the changing economic policies favouring the dominance of market principles for governing over principles of justice and equity. Rather than policies that focus on a balance between the protection of the weak, poor, and vulnerable in society and economic prosperity and growth, current policies increasingly support free markets first and foremost. There has been growing evidence of declines in government involvement in the provision of adequate and universal health and

social services, coupled with decreasing taxes for the corporations and the richest members of society (Moss, 2002; Raphael, 2002; Hurtig, 2001). Societies with greater inequality tend to have higher morbidity and mortality rates. Countries with more internal equity tend to have higher levels of life expectancy. As well as the overall degree of relative societal equality and inequality, the socio-economic status of individuals within societies is negatively correlated with both morbidity and mortality. Those lower in the socio-economic hierarchy tend to have higher levels of sickness and death. Those higher in a societal socio-economic hierarchy tend to have lower levels of morbidity and mortality. If the availability of material goods and services were the entire explanation for health disparities between people located at different places in the social structure, then overall inequity in a society would not affect life expectancy or other health outcomes. However, it does. Do people feel unhappy and stressed when they live in a society where there is a great deal of disparity? Are people happier and less stressed when they feel that there is a generally high level of similar life circumstances and life chances among most other people in their country? If so, how does this work to affect their health and well-being? There are a number of explanations for the fact that poorer people and more inequitable societies tend to have higher rates of disease and death.

The most obvious explanation is simply materialist. Poorer people are less able to buy healthy foods, to afford stable, clean, and otherwise adequate housing, to have access to efficient transportation, to live and work in environmentally 'friendly' places, and to have all of the basic requirements of living. This problem is compounded when the 'people' of whom we are talking are children. Not only are their immediate life circumstances constrained through poverty, but their life chances are compromised because they are more likely to have been born at low birth weight, are less likely to have food provided to them that is adequate for their health and growth. Such early deprivation multiplies. The effects of poverty on children born to such situations increase as they grow, and is exacerbated as they have less access to quality education and health care and experience a myriad of other social circumstances associated with high morbidity and mortality. Thus, simple material deprivation is one important cause of ill health.

Another possible explanation is lifestyle 'choice'. Here lifestyle factors such as choice of healthy foodstuffs (e.g., fresh vegetables vs bags of chips), smoking, alcohol consumption, illicit drug consumption, and risky behaviours such as speeding, fighting, and unprotected sex can be considered relevant. In addition, the utilization of early detection strategies such as the Pap smear, mammography, PSA testing for prostate cancer, and the like might be noted. However, there is no consistent relationship between all of these factors and socio-economic status. Each has to be investigated separately. For example, alcohol consumption is positively associated with social class and cigarette smoking negatively. That is, despite relative material deprivation poorer people are more likely to smoke cigarettes and thus it is reasonable to assume that their families are also more likely to be exposed to second-hand smoke.

Socio-psychological factors such as the experience of relative deprivation, high stress (perhaps from unemployment, seasonal employment, or otherwise insecure, poorly paid, or problematic employment situations), and family and relationship insecurity may affect health. Social capital or social cohesion has recently been investigated as an important characteristic of social life with significant health consequences. Social capital is found in integration into friendship, neighbourhood, and acquaintance networks that provide the basis for developing shared values and feelings of belonging, trust, and social cohesion (Pampel, 2002; Kawachi et al., 1997; Kawachi et al., 1999; Wilkinson, 1997). Here,

too, poorer people tend to inhabit social worlds that provide less stability for the development of strong friendships, shared norms and values, and access to community-level decision-making and service-providing structures that would provide the mechanisms and strategies to enable the development of social cohesion.

Summary

(1) Illness and death rates vary depending on social-structural conditions: cultural differences, the political-economic system, the socio-demographic structure, social psychology, and existential phenomenology.

(2) As social class increases, life expectancy increases. Class is also related to the length of life that is lived with a disability. Low-income earners do not have poorer health habits overall yet they are less likely to engage in some preventive health measures. They are also more likely to be exposed to occupational health hazards.

(3) Race and ethnicity affect mortality and morbidity rates. For example, the life expectancy rate is lower and the PYLL is higher among Canadian Native people when compared with non-Native people. The causes of death also differ: Aboriginals tend to die from illnesses related to poverty, inadequate nutrition, lack of potable water, crowding, and social stress; non-Aboriginals tend to die from 'diseases of affluence', such as diseases of the circulatory system.

(4) Biological risks are part of the explanation for inequities in mortality and morbidity. Historical differences in lifestyle, differences in culture and cultural norms, and differential access to health-giving resources are also factors.

(5) Other factors that contribute to different rates of morbidity and mortality are class, ethnicity, lifestyle, environmental contaminants, and social capital or social cohesion.

Questions for Study and Discussion

1. How does income affect the health of the individual?
2. How does the overall degree of inequity in society affect the health of the population?
3. Why and how is education level related to morbidity and mortality?
4. How and why do prevention-related behaviours relate to socio-economic status?
5. What are the major challenges to the health of the Aboriginal peoples? What social and health policies do you advocate with respect to this issue?

Suggested Readings

Antonovsky, A. 1967. 'Social Class, Life Expectancy and Overall Mortality', *Milbank Memorial Fund Quarterly* 45: 31–73. Antonovsky's work on the sense of coherence deserves to be read and reread.

Gorey, Kevin M., Eric J. Holowaty, Gordon Fehringer, Ethan Lauckkanen, and Nancy L. Richter. 1998. 'The association of socio-economic status with cancer incidence in Toronto, Ontario: Possible confounding of cancer mortality by incidence and survivorship', *Cancer Prevention and Control* 2: 237–48. A classic epidemiological study of the relationship between cancer and social class.

McDonough, Peggy. 1997. 'Income Dynamics and Mortality', *Institute for Social Research Newsletter* 12, 3: 1–3. This brief report presents an interesting analysis of social class and mortality.

Raphael, Dennis. 2001. *Inequality Is Bad for Our Hearts: Why Low Income and Social Exclusion Are Major Causes of Heart Disease in Canada*. North York, Ont.: North York Health Network. Available at: <http://www.yorku.ca/wellness/heart.pdf>. This report demonstrates a link between heart disease and inequality.

Wilkinson, Richard G. 1990. 'Income Distribution and Mortality: A "Natural" Experiment', *Sociology of Health and Illness* 12, 4: 391–412. Wilkinson examines the link between mortality rates and inequality in different national situations.

Chapter 7

Some Social-Psychological Explanations for Illness

Learning Objectives

- Socio-psychological factors are related to morbidity and mortality.
- Stress, social support, coronary-prone behaviour, sense of coherence, prayer, and religiosity are related to wellness, sickness, and death.
- Psychoneuroimmunology is a new field of study that looks at mind/body interactions.
- Stress was first defined and studied by Canon and Selye.
- There are a variety of new ways to measure stress, including the frequently used and critiqued Social Readjustment Rating Scale (SRRS).
- The health consequences of stress appear to be highly diverse.
- Social support appears to be supportive of health.
- Coronary-prone or Type A behaviour has been found to be related to heart disease.
- Sense of coherence and spirituality have associations with health.
- People go to the doctor for a variety of social and economic reasons.

Introduction

What is the role of interpersonal relationships in illness? Is it true that people can die of a broken heart? Does the repression of feelings, particularly anger, cause cancer? Can a person choose to live or die? What is stress? Is stress good or bad? Does prayer help when a person is sick? Is religion of any benefit to well-being? Why do people go to the doctor? When do people choose to visit a physician rather than 'carry on' or go to bed with an aspirin? The symptoms of a head cold, backache, digestive difficulties, or influenza will send one person to bed, another to the doctor, and others to the drugstore, acupuncturist, nurse practitioner, or neighbour. What determines the actions that people take when they are feeling ill?

On any day, for every person at the doctor's office, there are many more people not at the doctor's office who are suffering from the same or similar symptoms. The least common response for ill people is to seek medical care. The enormous expenditures on over-the-counter medications bear testimony to the frequency of this type of self-help care. So does the prevalence of folk remedies such as 'feed a cold and starve a fever'.

Yet doctors' offices are often filled with people with conditions that cure themselves or conditions for which the doctor cannot provide medical assistance.

Many people visit doctors for psychosocial reasons such as stress, emotional distress, social isolation, and information rather than for strictly medical reasons (Barsky, 1981). Some studies, for instance, show that 50 to 70 per cent of patient visits to primary-care providers include psychosocial complaints (Ashworth et al., 1984; Good et al., 1987). Most patients who go to physicians do not have serious physical disorders (Weiss and Lonnquist, 1992).

This chapter is divided into two parts. The first part will deal with just a few of the many socio-psychological factors found to be associated with illness, including stress, coronary-prone behaviour, social support, sense of coherence, religion, and prayer. The second part will discuss the processes through which people come to define themselves as ill and as needing care, and the actions they take in regard to their health when deciding to seek help from an allopathic practitioner.

Stress

Stress occurs when an organism must deal with demands much greater than or much less than the usual level of activity. As such, stress is ubiquitous. All of us are stressed to some degree or we would not be alive. The presence of at least some stress in life is beneficial. Stressful experiences can be healthy and can fit us for positive and flexible adaptations to stress later on. Or stress can be so overwhelming that it leads to serious illness or death. Too much change, in too short a time, can overtax the resources of the body.

Two major writers, Cannon (1932) and Selye (1956), were involved in the early articulation and measurement of stress. Cannon suggested that health is ultimately defined not by the absence of disease but rather as the ability of the human being to function satisfactorily in the particular environment in which he or she is operating. People must constantly adapt to changes and assaults—to changes in weather, conflicts at work, failure in school, great success on the hockey team, promotion, flu germs, and so on. The body adapts to such changes by maintaining a relatively constant condition. For example, when the body becomes overheated, it will evaporate moisture to help keep it cool; when confronted with bacteria, it will produce antibodies. The process of maintaining a desirable bodily state (the constant condition) is called homeostasis. The body is thus prepared to meet threats by adapting in ways that will return it to the desired state.

Cannon described the typical bodily reaction to stress as 'fright or flight', and detailed the accompanying physiological changes. Somewhat later, Selye defined stress as a state that included all the specific changes induced within the biological system of the organism. It is a general reaction that occurs in response to any number of different stimuli. Both positive and negative events can cause stress. It does not matter whether the event is the happy decision to become engaged to be married or the disappointing failure in a course in university—each requires adaptation.

Building on several decades of research on the pituitary-cortical axis, Selye proposed the General Adaptation Syndrome (GAS) as the body's reaction to all stressful events. The 'syndrome' has three stages: (1) an *alarm reaction*, (2) *resistance or adaption*, and (3) *exhaustion*. During the first stage, the body recognizes the stressor and the pituitary-adrenal cortical system responds by producing the arousal hormones necessary for either flight or fright. Increased activity by the heart and lungs, elevated blood sugar levels, increased perspiration, dilated pupils, and a slowing of the rate of digestion are among the physiological responses to this initial stage of the syndrome. During the adaptive stage the body begins to repair the damage caused by arousal and most of the initial stress symptoms

Table 7.1   Stress Self-Assessment Checklist

Use the following scale for each symptom and circle the number that best applies to you.

1. Never
2. Occasionally
3. Frequently
4. Constantly

In the last month I have experienced the following

1. Tension headaches	1	2	3	4
2. Difficulty in falling or staying asleep	1	2	3	4
3. Fatigue	1	2	3	4
4. Overeating	1	2	3	4
5. Constipation	1	2	3	4
6. Lower back pain	1	2	3	4
7. Allergy problems	1	2	3	4
8. Feelings of nervousness	1	2	3	4
9. Nightmares	1	2	3	4
10. High blood pressure	1	2	3	4
11. Hives	1	2	3	4
12. Alcohol/non-prescription drug consumption	1	2	3	4
13. Minor infections	1	2	3	4
14. Stomach indigestion	1	2	3	4
15. Hyperventilation or rapid breathing	1	2	3	4
16. Worrisome thoughts	1	2	3	4
17. Skin rashes	1	2	3	4
18. Menstrual distress	1	2	3	4
19. Nausea or vomiting	1	2	3	4
20. Irritability with others	1	2	3	4
21. Migraine headaches	1	2	3	4
22. Early morning awakening	1	2	3	4
23. Loss of appetite	1	2	3	4
24. Diarrhea	1	2	3	4
25. Aching neck and shoulder muscles	1	2	3	4
26. Asthma attack	1	2	3	4
27. Colitis attack	1	2	3	4
28. Periods of depression	1	2	3	4
29. Arthritis	1	2	3	4

Table 7.1 (continued)

30. Common flu or cold	1	2	3	4
31. Minor accidents	1	2	3	4
32. Prescription drug use	1	2	3	4
33. Peptic ulcer	1	2	3	4
34. Cold hands or feet	1	2	3	4
35. Heart palpitations	1	2	3	4
36. Sexual problems	1	2	3	4
37. Angry feelings	1	2	3	4
38. Difficulty communicating with others	1	2	3	4
39. Inability to concentrate	1	2	3	4
40. Difficulty making decisions	1	2	3	4
41. Feelings of low self-worth	1	2	3	4
42. Feelings of depression	1	2	3	4
TOTAL SCORE				

Source: Neidhardt et al. (1985). © 1985, 1990 International Self-Counsel Press Ltd. Reprinted by permission.

diminish or vanish. But if the stress continues, adaptation to it is lost as the body tries to maintain its defences. Eventually the body runs out of energy with which to respond to the stress and exhaustion sets in. During this final stage, bodily functions are slowed down abnormally or stopped altogether.

Continued exposure to stress during the exhaustion stage can lead to what Selye calls the 'diseases of adaptation'. These include various emotional disturbances, schizophrenia, migraine headaches, certain types of asthma, cardiovascular and renal diseases, ulcers, hypertension, lowered resistance to viruses, and immune deficiency. Table 7.1 provides a stress self-assessment checklist. People are not always aware that they are living under stressful circumstances. Sometimes bodily and emotional symptoms are the first sign that something is amiss. Table 7.1 lists many of the warning signs or symptoms of stress that may result in subsequent health problems. A typical person will have a score of between 42 and 75 in any given month. The higher the score, the greater the likelihood of illness. The evidence is strongest for the relationship between stress and cardiovascular disease, infectious disease, and pregnancy complications (Adler and Mathews, 1994: 232).

As well as the symptoms and diseases listed, stress can also lead to death. To study such effects of stress Engel collected 170 reports of sudden death. He discovered that the deaths usually occurred within an hour of hearing emotionally intense information, which could be either positive or negative. Of the sudden deaths, 21 per cent occurred on the collapse or death of a close friend, 20 per cent during a period of intense grief, 9 per cent at the threat of the loss of a close person, 3 per cent at the mourning or anniversary of the death of a close person, 6 per cent following a loss of status or self-esteem, 27 per cent when in personal danger or threat of injury (whether real or symbolic), 7 per cent after the danger was over, and, finally, 6 per cent at a reunion, triumph, or happy ending (Engel, 1971).

Stress can be short-term, medium-term, or long-term. Briefly, the short-term stressors arise from small inconveniences, for example, traffic jams, lost keys, or waiting for the doctor. Such things usually result in a temporary sense of anxiety. These have been called daily hassles (Lazarus and Delongis, 1983). Medium-term stressors develop from such things as long, cold, dark winters, a layoff from work, stress at work, or an acute sickness in the family. Long-term stressors result from such incidents as the loss of a spouse or the loss of a job. Holmes and Rahe (1967) have systematized the stress value attached to a list of life events in a scale called the Social Readjustment Rating Scale (SRRS). Using extensive interviews with 394 people of varying ages and socio-economic statuses, Holmes and Rahe were able to develop average scale values representing the relative risks of a number of specific life events. Marriage was assigned an arbitrary value of 50. The adjustment value of other items was estimated in comparison to marriage. The resulting scale itemizes 43 changes and quantifies their hypothetical impact (see Table 7.2). In general, the higher the score, the greater is the likelihood of illness. It is important to note that, while some of the events are considered negative or undesirable and others might be considered positive or desirable, they all require psychosocial adjustment and are, thus, potentially stressful.

As the scale and other related research indicate, stressors can be the result of changes in any area of life and at a variety of levels, such as: (1) the individual level (e.g., bacterial infections); (2) interpersonal situations (e.g., loss of a spouse); (3) social-structural positions (e.g., unemployment, promotion at work); (4) cultural systems (e.g., immigration); (5) ecological systems (e.g., earthquake); or (6) political/state systems (e.g., wars). The greater the number of stressors, and we might hypothesize the greater the number of levels of stressors, the more vulnerable a person is to the possibility of disease and emotional and bodily dysfunction.

It should be emphasized that stressors are not to be thought of as objective things that affect an unthinking organism in a monolithic way. A person's evaluation of the stressful situation, the strategies available for coping, the degree of control felt, and the amount of social support experienced all mediate the impact that the stressor ultimately has on that person. As Viktor Frankl (1965) has pointed out, some people, even in the most atrocious of circumstances such as a concentration camp, have been able to use their experiences in a manner that was meaningful to them, and thus these people ultimately became stronger and healthier as a result of this most extreme of stress-filled situations. Frankl's work has, by the way, been used to develop a school of psychotherapy called logotherapy.

The SRRS has been used among a wide variety of different people in North America. It has also been used in a number of cross-cultural studies that have included Swiss, Belgian, and Dutch peoples (Bieliauskas, 1982). Overall, researchers have found significant similarities among different cultural groups in their evaluation of the impact of various events. Such studies have shown the SRRS to be a remarkably stable or reliable instrument. It has also been used to 'predict' illness and symptoms of distress. Holmes and Masuda's 1974 study concluded 'that life-change events . . . lower bodily resistance and enhance the probability of disease occurrence.' Several researchers have correlated high SRRS scores with symptoms and with illness, including major illnesses such as heart disease (Theorell and Rahe, 1971; Rahe and Paasikivi, 1971). High SRRS scores have also been found to be associated with psychological distress in a number of studies (Bieliauskas, 1982). Several researchers have used SRRS successfully to predict the onset of illness. One interesting example of this research is the study that examined the SRRS of 2,600 navy personnel prior to their departure on voyages of 6–8 months; the researchers found significant correlations between the levels of stress before

Table 7.2   The Stress of Adjusting to Change

Events	Scale of impact	Events	Scale of impact
Death of spouse	100	Son or daughter leaving home	29
Divorce	73	Trouble with in-laws	29
Marital separation	65	Outstanding personal achievement	28
Jail term	63	Wife begins or stops work	26
Death of close family member	63	Begin or end school	26
Personal injury or illness	53	Change in living conditions	25
Marriage	50	Revision of personal habits	24
Fired at work	47	Trouble with boss	23
Marital reconciliation	45	Change in work hours or conditions	20
Retirement	45	Change in residence	20
Change in health of family member	44	Change in schools	20
Pregnancy	40	Change in recreation	19
Sex difficulties	39	Change in church activities	19
Gain of new family member	39	Change in social activities	18
Business readjustment	39	Mortgage or loan less than $10,000	17
Change in financial state	38	Change in sleeping habits	16
Death of close friend	37	Change in number of family get-togethers	15
Change to different line of work	36	Change in eating habits	15
Change in number of arguments with spouse	35	Vacation	13
Mortgage over $10,000	31	Christmas	12
Foreclosure of mortgage or loan	30	Minor violations of the law	11
Change in responsibilities at work	29		

Source: Holmes and Rahe (1967: 214).

the start of the voyage and the subsequent levels of disease during the voyages (Rahe et al., 1970).

The SRRS has also met its share of criticism for the following reasons.

(1) It ignores differences in the meaning people place on the various events. There is evidence that the impact of the death of a spouse, for instance, varies depending on whether or not the death was sudden or occurred after a protracted period of illness.

(2) Some of the events listed may be signs of illness or the results of illness, such as changes in eating habits, sleeping habits, personal habits, or sex difficulties. Thus the scale is, in part, tautological and its ability to predict illness is questionable because some items on the scale are symptomatic of illness.

(3) Some research has found that distinguishing between the desirable and undesirable events enhances the predictive value of the scale. Marriage is generally taken as a reason for celebration, death as an occasion for mourning. It has been argued

Box 7.1   Moderate Wine Drinking Is Good for You

It's good for you! No it's not! Yes it is! There has been a lot of debate over the last number of years about the benefits of moderate drinking. Another new study, which has tracked 4,500 graduates of the University of North Carolina since 1964, has found that wine consumption seems to be associated with good health. This time it is not thought to be primarily because of the biochemistry of wine but rather because of the lifestyles associated with those who drink wine. Apparently, according to this recent study, those who drink wine also tend to eat less saturated fat and cholesterol, eat more fibre, smoke less, and exercise more frequently. They tend to be less likely to be overweight than those who drink beer or spirits. They tend to drink alcohol in moderation as compared to those who regularly choose other types of alcohol. As compared to abstainers they tend to eat less red meat, more fruit and vegetables, and to be less likely to smoke. These findings are consistent across social status categories. Thus wine drinkers from lower-income backgrounds had good health outcomes, while high-income abstainers had poorer health outcomes.

Source: Andre Picard, 'Wine lifestyle touted as promoting health', *Globe and Mail*, 25 July 2002, A3.

that the stress-related effects of death are therefore more pronounced than those of marriage.

(4) The ability to control events has been shown, in a number of studies, to be an important factor in determining the degree of stress experienced.

(5) Whether stress affects the incidence of disease or merely behaviour during illness has been questioned. It may be that life events affect the likelihood of people reporting illness rather than affecting the disease process.

(6) The SRRS asks about events that have occurred during a specified period of time. Some research has shown that the association between stress and subsequent illness or disease cannot be studied separately from the previous stress level and the history of past illnesses. Thus experiences of the years before the time period referred to in the SRRS may also have a powerful effect on the level of stress experienced. A car accident followed by the loss of a driver's licence and a household move in the years before the designated SRRS time period might exacerbate whatever level of stress is experienced during the year of the srrs measurements.

There have been a series of critiques of and improvements on the SRRS in the 1980s and 1990s. Turner and Avison (1992) refer to 16 different reviews and critiques that have altered how life events are measured. Zimmerman (1983) describes 16 alternative inventories designed to measure life stress through life events. These critiques and improvements address some of the problems and issues of the SRRS. Two such refinements will be briefly described here.

Turner and Avison (1992) note that crisis situations (life events) can pose opportunities as well as problems. When life events are managed well and resolved, the researchers hypothesize, they may not contribute negatively to stress for the individual. Using large samples of both physically impaired and community-based comparison groups, Turner and Avison found support for the idea that resolution of a life event generally eliminates or minimizes its stress impact. Thoits (1994) continued and replicated the findings of the elaboration of the relationship between resolved and unresolved life events and health outcomes. She emphasizes that men and women must be actively involved in managing stress,

Table 7.3	Some Examples of Indicators of Excess Stress	
Physical	**Psychological**	**Behavioural**
Rapid pulse	Inability to concentrate	Smoking
Increased perspiration	Difficulty making decisions	Medication use
Pounding heart	Loss of self-confidence	Nervous tics
Tightened stomach	Cravings	Absent-mindedness
Tense arm, leg muscles	Worry or anxiety	Accident-proneness
Shortness of breath	Irrational fear or panic	Hair-pulling, nail-biting, foot tapping
Tensed teeth and jaw	Feelings of sadness	Sleep disturbance
Inability to sit still	Frustration	Increased use of alcohol
Sore back and shoulders		Addictive eating

Source: Adapted from Neidhardt et al. (1985: 5–6).

more and less successfully. Moreover, she notes that people with the personality characteristics of mastery and self-esteem manage stress more successfully.

Conger et al. (1993) compared the reports of exposure and vulnerability to specific types of life events made by men and women. Their findings were consistent both with the social-structural positions of men and women (primarily with respect to labour force participation and other daily role responsibilities) (Aneshensel et al., 1987) and with their identity perspectives (primarily with respect to the self-concepts and identities of men and women) (Thoits, 1983, 1991). Men were more likely than women to report exposure to and be distressed by work and financial events. Women, by contrast, were more likely to be upset by exposure to negative events within their families. Further, men and women responded differently to negative events. Men were more likely to become hostile whereas women's somatic complaints increased. Table 7.3 lists physical, psychological, and behavioural indications of stress.

Stress research has continued to dominate the field of the sociology of health and illness, especially in the United States. In fact, in an analysis of the relative ranking of the 'top' journals in the field of sociology, the *Journal of Health and Social Behavior* was ranked as the second most important journal for sociologists on the basis of the 'objective' measure of citation impact. Johnson and Wolinsky (1990) compared this journal with *Social Forces*, the *American Journal of Sociology*, and the *American Sociological Review* over an 11-year period beginning in 1977 and found that the *JHSB* always outranked *SF*, outranked *AJS* 7 of 11 years, and outranked *ASR* 4 out of 11 years. They argue that this ranking is largely attributable to the widely cited work on stress, coping, mental health, and social support and to the reputations of the editors over this period of time as superb stress researchers. While the claim made by Johnson and Wolinsky is passionately debated in a series of articles in the same volume of the journal, the point that stress has been among the most central areas of research in the field remains plausible.

The idea that stress is both a predictor of ill health and a particular sort of suffering is now so legitimated and widespread beyond sociology journals that it is routinely studied by Statistics Canada. In Statistic Canada's General Social Survey of 1992, a number of stress-related questions were

Table 7.4   Canadians' Responses to Stress-related Questions

	Total*	Men*	Women*
1. I plan to slow down in the coming year.	21	19	22
2. I consider myself a workaholic.	25	26	25
3. When I need more time, I tend to cut back on my sleep.	44	45	43
4. At the end of the day, I often feel that I have not accomplished what I had set out to do.	46	44	48
5. I worry that I don't spend enough time with my family and friends.	32	33	32
6. I feel that I'm constantly under stress trying to accomplish more than I can handle.	33	31	35
7. I feel trapped in a daily routine.	34	32	37
8. I feel that I just don't have time for fun any more.	28	25	31
9. I often feel under stress when I don't have enough time.	45	41	48
10. I would like to spend more time alone.	22	19	26

*Per cent of Canadians 15 and over who agree with each statement.

Source: Statistics Canada, General Social Survey, 1992.

asked of Canadians (Table 7.4). Those most stressed had the greatest number of role responsibilities. For instance, mothers of infants reported feeling stressed 72 per cent of the time. Workers with compressed workweeks and with on-call work were highly likely to be stressed continually.

The theory that ties the mind and body together in modern biological science is called psychoneuroimmunology (PNI). It is the study of the interrelations between the central nervous system and the immune system. The immune system is chiefly located in the bone marrow, thy-

mus, lymph nodes, spleen, tonsils, appendix, and Peyre's patches (clumps of immune tissue in the small intestine). Because so little is presently known about this interacting system, the present-day study is primarily of 'circulating peripheral blood' (Cohen and Herbert, 1996: 115).

A number of studies have shown how stress affects the immune system, including the suppression of cellular immune functioning leading to viral reaction and suppression of antibody responses. 'Through well-developed research methodologies, the emerging field of PNI is pro-

Box 7.2   Spiritual Beliefs and Bereavement

One hundred thirty-five relatives and close friends of terminally ill patients were studied for their reactions to bereavement. Those who had spiritual beliefs were more able to resolve their grief. People without spiritual beliefs had a more difficult time and often were not able to resolve their grief even after 14 months.

Source: Kiri Walsh, Michael King, Louise Jones, Adrian Tookman, and Robert Blizard, 'Spiritual beliefs may affect outcome of bereavement: prospective study', British Medical Journal 324 (29 June 2002): 1551.

viding scientific evidence to support the mind/body connection' (Caudell, 1996: 494).

In addition to understanding more of the mind/body connection and its relationship to illness, researchers have also begun to investigate the effects of behavioural interventions on increasing immune system functioning. Interventions such as relaxation training, meditation, guided imaging, and therapeutic touch have been found to improve aspects of the immune system (ibid.). Many people are also using yoga, biofeedback, tai chi, and pranic healing, for example, because of their belief in the mind/body connection.

Social Support

Almost all people think they understand social support, on an intuitive if not on a cognitive level. If you were to ask your friends whether they knew the meaning of social support, you would probably find unanimous affirmation. If you were then to ask each to define its meaning, you would likely hear as many definitions as there are people giving them. For some, social support would be defined as 'a feeling that you have or don't have'. For others, it would be defined as friends with whom to party. Another would define it as someone with whom to do things. Still another might see social support as having someone on side in case of an argument. Material and practical aid might be necessary components of social support for others.

When sociologists attempt to measure social support, the varieties and idiosyncrasies of meaning become apparent. An early and often used definition of social support comes from the work of Cobb (1976), who thought of social support as information that would lead a person to believe (1) that he or she is cared for and loved, (2) that he or she is esteemed and valued, and (3) that he or she belongs to a network of communication and mutual obligation. A group of researchers used this definition as the basis for a scale that

was later revised and subjected to a number of uses (see Turner et al., 1983). The scale asks people to describe themselves in comparison to others with respect to the amount of social support they feel they have. It is, in essence, a subjective measure based on each person assessing his or her felt degree of social support. It includes both social support in the sense of a person's feeling of being loved and esteemed by others, and social support as an experience of being part of a 'network' of people.

This definition of social support emphasizes the subjective perception of the respondent. Others have considered social support as something that can be objectively measured—social support exists to the extent that a person can count on others to offer specific services such as cooking, cleaning, snow shovelling, or transportation when the need arises (Thoits, 1982). In this case, the degree of social support is reflected in the reliability and extensiveness of the actual aid supplied rather than in the subjective feeling of the individual. In a further refinement, others have pointed out that different kinds of 'support' are desired and expected from different 'kinds' of others. That is, people may expect different things from their friends than from their kin. Whether or not the network is made up of people who know each other or not may also affect the experience of social support.

A number of studies have examined the impact of social support on health outcomes. From 1978 to 1999 the *Journal of Health and Social Behavior* published numerous articles concerning social support in a variety of situations. There were articles on all of the following: the health consequences of being unemployed, self-assessments of the elderly, occupational stress, mental health, psychological well-being, primary deviance among mental patients, life stress, psychotropic drug use, psychological distress and self-rejection in young adults, adolescent cigarette smoking, health in widowhood in later life, teenage pregnancy, social support among men

Box 7.3   Uncertain Identities and Health Risk

We have discussed the frequency of smoking in society today. We have talked about the ways that schools, cigarettes taxes, and families contribute to smoking rates. We have also, again, only briefly, talked about some of the serious health consequences of smoking. Taking another tack, Martyn Denscombe (2001) has used the symbolic interactionist perspective to understand the meanings of smoking to young people who do smoke. While the rates of smoking among adults have been declining over the last 30 years or so, the rates among young people have been increasing despite aggressive government anti-smoking campaigns. This is particularly true among young women. In this battle the government campaigns are clearly less effective than tobacco industry advertising campaigns. A number of researchers have studied the enigma of the increase in smoking among young people. Among the explanations that have been investigated are peer pressure, feelings of immortality, stresses of adolescence, an addiction to smoking based on just 'trying it', susceptibility to advertising, influence of parents and older siblings, low self-esteem, and fun.

The explanation Denscombe investigates is uncertain identities among young people. He argues that uncertainty is particularly endemic and problematic for a number of reasons in a postmodern society. As a result of interviewing and conducting focus groups with young people he described the ways in which cigarette smoking is used to develop and maintain a desired identity. The following is a list of identity-related motives given by young people about why they smoke:

- to look grown up
- to look cool
- to look hard
- (among girls) for girl power
- to be in control.

Denscombe concludes that smoking can be seen as a way to enhance self-image, self-empowerment, and self-affirmation. What about you? Do you smoke? If so, do any of these explanations fit for you and your experience?

Source: Martyn Denscombe, 'Uncertain identities and health-risking behaviour: the case of young people and smoking in late modernity', *British Journal of Sociology* 52, 1 (2001): 157–77.

with AIDS, and depressed patients. This list gives some idea of the range of situations in which social support has been shown to act. It is also worth emphasizing that offering social support as well as receiving social support has health benefits. Note the frequencies of the positive effects that offering care to others is perceived to have in Table 7.5.

Some researchers have emphasized that social support has a direct relationship to health so that the person who has support is less likely to become ill; others have noted that adequate social support can minimize the harmful effects of stress on a person's mental or physical health. These two notions are compatible with one another: social support may have both direct and indirect effects on health (see Turner et al., 1983).

In 1973, Gove analyzed causes of mortality and noted that married people tended to live longer. Analyses of the dates of death of famous people (Phillips and Feldman, 1973) showed that death rates declined just before a significant occasion, such as a birthday, wedding, or Christmas celebration—an occasion on which these people would have the opportunity to reaffirm social ties with the group of significant others. A very large

Table 7.5   Caregivers Generally Feel Positive about Their Activities

	Never	Rarely/ Sometimes	Nearly always	Don't know/ Not stated	Total
How often do you feel . . .					
you don't have enough time for yourself, because of the time you spend helping people?					
Women	55	31	12	–	100
Men	65	25	9	–	100
Total	59	29	11	1	100
others help you more often than you help them?					
Women	64	26	9	–	100
Men	63	28	6	–	100
Total	63	27	8	2	100
stressed between helping others and trying to meet other responsibilities for family or work?					
Women	41	40	18	–	100
Men	55	32	12	–	100
Total	46	36	15	2	100
by helping others, you simply give back what you have received from them?					
Women	21	27	50	3	100
Men	25	27	45	–	100
Total	22	27	48	3	100
angry when you are around the person(s) you are helping?					
Women	75	19	3	2	100
Men	82	14	–	–	100
Total	78	17	3	2	100
by helping people, you simply give back some of what life has given you?					
Women	15	22	60	3	100
Men	15	26	56	3	100
Total	15	24	58	3	100

– Sample too small to be released

Source: Cranswick (1997: 4).

study (Beckman, 1977) charted the lives of 7,000 people over a period of some nine years; during that period 682 of the 7,000 people died. After controlling for a variety of socio-demographic and risk factors, the data revealed that those who died tended to lack social ties (family, church, informal and formal group associations). Beckman concluded that isolation and the lack of

Box 7.4   Some Hypothetical Explanations of Health Differences among People of
                 Different Socio-economic Status Backgrounds

Material Resources   **Lifestyle**

Housing   Smoking

Food   Drinking

Clean water   Exercise

Clean air   Sexual safety

Access to necessary immunization, drugs, and medical care   Risk-taking

Family/Community

Stability/integration into family and community

Supportive mutual-aid relationships

Decision-making authority

Privacy

Social-Psychological Resources

Stable, secure employment

Supportive work relationships

Education

Coping abilities, emotional stability

Sense of coherence, sense of efficacy

social and community networks likely increases vulnerability to disease in general.

One study that made an effort to move beyond the correlational connections between social support and health outcomes is based on interviews with teenage mothers during pregnancy and then after childbirth. The purpose of this study was to investigate the impact of social support (Turner et al., 1992). These researchers examined the impact of social support on what has been argued to be a very important indicator of the health of a population—infant birth weight. Consistent with their hypothesis, the researchers noted that pregnant teenagers who received more support from family, friends, and partners had higher-birth-weight babies. Not only did the level of social support positively affect birth weight but also the psychological health of the new mother. This research also

found that socio-economic background influenced the relationship between social support and the health outcomes of mothers and their infants. Social support was especially helpful to young women with lower-class backgrounds, although it was not unimportant for those from higher socio-economic backgrounds.

The relationship between social support and specific diseases such as cancer and heart disease has also been examined. A number of studies have reiterated the relationship between cancer and the loss of a marriage partner (LeShan, 1978). Relationships have also been discovered between the incidence of cancer and other indicators of social connections. For example, the greater the religious cohesion, e.g., among Mormons, the lower the incidence of cancers (although it is important to note here that there are many differences in lifestyle and diet exhibit-

Box 7.5   Types of Social Support

Emotional Support
(offering affection, acceptance)

Informational Support
(providing desired/requested information)

Instrumental Support
(washing dishes, cutting grass, bringing a meal)

Cognitive Support
(reframing and recontextualizing)

ed by Mormons). While the studies neither establish a causal connection nor explain all of the variance, there seem to be sufficient grounds to pursue further research on the potential association between social connections and cancer.

Professor David Spiegel, a psychiatrist and researcher at Stanford University Medical School, set out to refute the notion that the mind could be used to affect the outcome of disease. He observed 86 women with breast cancer for 10 years. To his surprise, he found that women who took part in group therapy and who had been taught self-hypnosis lived twice as long as those who had not (Spiegel et al., 1989). Subsequent research has repeated this finding, although not consistently. The promise of such research has proven to be so great that a new field, psycho-oncology, examines the psychological aspects of getting and surviving cancer and includes a now classic text, *Handbook of Psycho-oncology* (Lerner, 1994: 139). According to the author of this book; 'Social support is, as we shall see, one of the most important and interesting categories which psycho-oncologists address' (ibid., 14).

What are the mechanisms through which support operates? How does social support affect health? Does support influence the interpretation of stressful life events? Are people who feel supported likely to feel that they can manage to cope with the sudden death of a spouse because they believe that others will listen and continue to care? Does social support have different meanings among people of different social categories, such as the elderly, minority populations, or the poor?

Can stress lead to the destruction of potentially supportive relationships at times? Do those lower on the social ladder, lacking relative power, also experience a daily lack of social support in their interactions with mainstream and powerful social institutions such as churches, schools, and health clinics? The mechanisms through which social support affects health need to be further studied and clarified.

From a slightly different perspective, a growing body of research demonstrates the positive effects of social support, longevity, and enhanced quality of life once a person has been diagnosed with a serious disease (ibid.). In addition, evidence indicates that both stress and low social support negatively impact on health-injurious behaviour such as smoking and excess alcohol consumption, direct correlates of coronary heart disease (CHD) (Adler and Mathews, 1994). Still, the costs to health of living alone are growing and are particularly high among elderly women. Figure 7.1 shows that there has been an increase in the percentage of the population over 15 who live alone and Table 7.6 shows that as of 2001 the elderly are more likely to be living alone than those of other age groups. This is especially true for women.

Coronary-Prone or Type A Behaviour and Heart Disease

Scientific interest in the socio-psychological causes of heart disease can be traced to the beginning of this century. Sir William Osler, a renowned

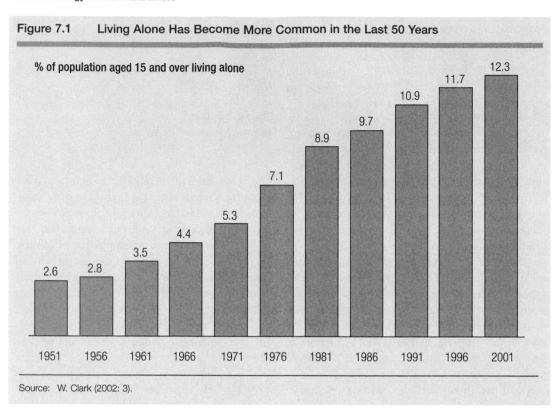

Figure 7.1   Living Alone Has Become More Common in the Last 50 Years

% of population aged 15 and over living alone

Year	%
1951	2.6
1956	2.8
1961	3.5
1966	4.4
1971	5.3
1976	7.1
1981	8.9
1986	9.7
1991	10.9
1996	11.7
2001	12.3

Source: W. Clark (2002: 3).

Table 7.6   Living Alone, by Age and Sex

Age	Both sexes 000s	Both Sexes	Men	Women
		% of population living alone in private households		
15 and over	3,030	12	12	13
15–24	140	3	4	3
25–44	980	10	14	7
45–54	450	10	11	9
55–64	400	14	11	16
65 and over	1,060	29	17	38

Source: W. Clark (2002: 4).

physician, made the following observation about people who had heart disease in his famous lecture on angina pectoris at Oxford in 1910: 'In a group of 20 men [with angina], every one of whom I know personally, the outstanding feature was the incessant treadmill of practice' (Osler,

1910: 698). Osler thus commented on his own casual observation of the particular 'speeded-up' character of those with angina.

Researchers have continued to study the possible relationship between CHD or myocardial infarction and what has come to be called type A behaviour, in which individuals who are competitive, achievement-oriented, easily annoyed, and time-urgent are compared to their easy-going counterparts, type B individuals. Recent research has found the link to be inconclusive. However, an association continues to be found for a relationship between type A behaviour and general poor health, including chest pains, general health problems, and injuries (Adler and Mathews, 1994). Several particular components of the type A construct, including hostility, anger, and the expression of anger, appear to be correlated with CHD (see Smith, 1992). Evidence suggests that 'workaholism' is associated positively with income and that it is a significant problem among Canadians. Figure 7.2 shows the relationship between income and self-reported workaholism. The link between workaholism and Type A behaviour needs further research.

There is continuing research on the effects of depression, distress, exhaustion, and negative affect as well as optimism and self-esteem on health outcomes. Measurement has proven to be difficult and the findings are inconclusive, but research on the relationship between health and specific moods and attitudes continues to show promise.

Sense of Coherence

Still on the socio-psychological level, Antonovsky reversed the usual questions about what sorts of things cause illness. Instead he asked: How do people stay healthy? Rather than look at the deleterious effects of such things as the lack of social support and the consequences of stress, Antonovsky focused on the positive and beneficial. Citing evidence from many studies, he argued that a 'sense of coherence' or a belief that

things are under control and will work out in the long run is a crucial component of the state of mind that leads to health. People who have good or excellent health are, all things being equal, likely to have a strong sense of coherence, which is defined as follows:

> . . . A global orientation that expresses the extent to which one has a pervasive, enduring though dynamic feeling of confidence that (1) the stimuli deriving from one's internal and external environments in the course of living are structured, predictable, and explicable; (2) the resources are available to one to meet the demands posed by these stimuli; and (3) these demands are challenges, worthy of investment and engagement. (Antonovsky, 1979: 19)

The 'sense of coherence' concept draws attention to the fact that the extent to which a person feels that he or she can manage whatever life has in store is an important factor in health. It is important to note that this socio-psychological factor is also associated with social class.

There are three components to this concept. The first is *comprehensibility*—the basic belief that the world is fundamentally understandable and predictable. Such a belief in the comprehensibility of the self and of human relationships is absolutely essential for coping. People with a high sense of coherence feel that the information they receive from the internal and external environment is orderly, consistent, and clear. People with a lower sense of coherence tend to feel that the world is chaotic, random, and inexplicable. A person with a high sense of coherence feels that his or her actions in the past have had the expected consequences, and they will continue to do so in the future. The student who knows how hard to study or how many drafts of a paper to do in order to get the desired A or B (or, heaven forbid, C) grade is someone with a high sense of comprehensibility.

Susan provides an example of someone with a strong belief in comprehensibility. Susan was

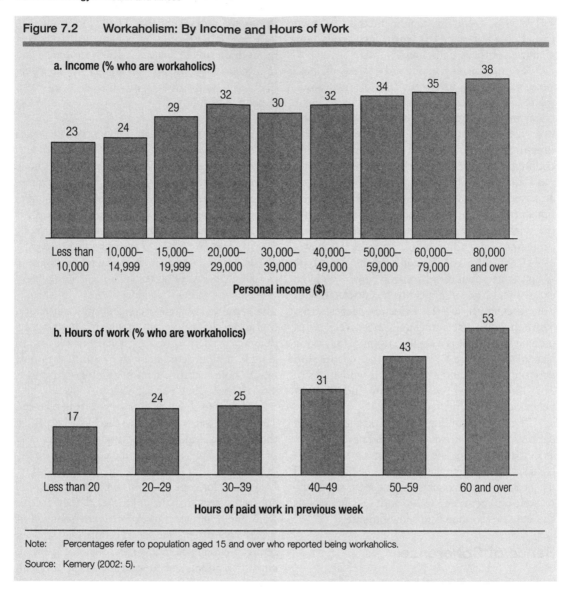

Figure 7.2   Workaholism: By Income and Hours of Work

a. Income (% who are workaholics)

Personal income ($)

b. Hours of work (% who are workaholics)

Hours of paid work in previous week

Note: Percentages refer to population aged 15 and over who reported being workaholics.

Source: Kemery (2002: 5).

interviewed during a study of women who had received a diagnosis of cancer.

> Oh sure, I'm very sick, I've lost both breasts and I'm scheduled for eighteen months of chemotherapy, but it'll be okay. My mother and sister had breast cancer. They were caught early enough. I have been having regular checkups for the past 10 years, and so when the doctor first noticed that something wasn't right he immediately booked me for a mammography and then exploratory surgery, and finally, almost as a preventative thing, he took off both breasts, but he believes that I will be fine now, and I guess I do too. (Clarke, 1995)

During the same study Rose was also interviewed; she could be characterized as having a low sense of comprehensibility.

> I don't know why everything always happens to me. I go to church regularly. I am a good wife and mother. I keep the house clean, and as a grade three teacher, I've certainly done my share for the neighbourhood, the PTA, and the church. It's not fair that I am the one to get this colon cancer. I've even watched our diets—fibre, protein, low cholesterol, and so on. It just doesn't make sense. (Ibid.)

The second component of the sense of coherence is *being able to cope*. The person with a sense of coherence understands what the world expects and feels that he or she has the ability and the resources necessary to meet whatever is demanded. Not only does the student know what is necessary to get an A, B, or C grade, he or she feels able to obtain the desired grade.

Data from people with multiple sclerosis provide some sense of the meaning of this component. At 20, Josh played baseball and hockey for his college teams. He did reasonably well in school, held a part-time job, and had an active social life. At 21 he was lethargic, felt weak, and was often discouraged about his future. After numerous tests and false diagnoses, Josh was told that he had multiple sclerosis. He didn't think he could cope with his life. Before, he had been absolutely tied up in activity and doing, doing, doing. That was all he knew and all he wanted from life. The multiple sclerosis limited his strength, mobility, and energy. He felt that there were few alternatives to his previous lifestyle, and besides, he didn't want any of them.

Jan, at 23, had recently been diagnosed as having multiple sclerosis. Jan, too, had been socially very active. A cheerleader and an avid tennis player, she had done reasonably well in high school, had graduated as a nurse, and was working at her local hospital when she was diagnosed. She quickly realized that she would prob-

ably have a difficult time working in this career because of the physical strength and energy required for such work. She began taking courses to prepare herself to work in nursing administration. A desk job on a nine-to-five basis would be much more manageable, she felt. She cut back on her sports activity but stayed active by walking to work. By making sure she had at least 10 hours of sleep at night, Jan felt that she could manage whatever the future had in store for her.

The third component of a sense of coherence—*meaningfulness*—refers to the motivation to achieve a desired outcome. This component depends on the extent to which life makes sense, has a purpose, and is worth the effort. The student values learning, and the grade achieved is important because grades and education have a purpose to play in life's satisfactions and goals.

Laura was the mother of Alex, a mentally challenged eight-year-old boy who also had cerebral palsy. Apparently he hadn't received enough oxygen at birth. Laura was naturally shocked and even devastated when she was first told about his disabilities. Over time, though, she organized her life around Alex's difference and used this to give her life particular meaning. She started a local self-help group for parents of disabled children, was active on the local board of a community organization designed to provide volunteer social activities for people with special needs, and worked with the school board and the teachers in developing special programs to integrate such children in the schools.

Joan, on the other hand, provides an example of a parent who could not find meaning in the severe mental challenges of her daughter. Again, the disability was the result of an accident at birth. From the time of Amanda's birth Joan had been furious. She was furious with the doctors, the nurses, the hospital, and, it seemed, with most everyone. Her fury turned inside and she became depressed. She isolated herself and continued to bewail her fate and that of her daughter. She tried one new kind of treatment after another—diet, vitamins, acupuncture, hypnosis, patterning, and prescription drugs. She tried them all, but nothing worked and nothing made sense to her. She was without hope or meaning.

The student with a high sense of coherence, when confronted with an unexpected (and seemingly undeserved) failure, does not give up in bitterness and disgust but rises to the challenge: he or she questions the mark, takes the course again, or takes a different course. In other words, the student with a high sense of coherence would be able to explain the failure to himself or herself, and willing and able to take action to improve the grade, believing that such action would have the desired outcome and that the whole process of learning and being examined is meaningful. Not surprisingly, an aspect of the sense of coherence—perceived control—is associated with socio-demographic variables. In an analysis of the 1994–5 National Population Health Survey, based on a national probability sample, Segall and his colleagues found that people of higher socio-economic status had a greater sense of perceived control over their lives than those of lower status (Segall et al., 1997).

All of these aforementioned socio-psychological issues—stress, social support, type A behaviour, and sense of coherence—appear to operate on the body through the immune system. For an extensive overview of the research in psychoneuroimmunology that is accessible to social scientific understanding, see Kaplan (1991) and Lerner (1994).

Religion and Health: Theoretical Views

Religion and religiosity are associated with both physical and mental health. Durkheim's studies of suicide were the first to investigate aspects of this relationship. His concern was with the degree of integration into a social group as well as the regulation of behaviour provided by religious affiliation. Today, to a significant extent, building on Durkheim, researchers have investigated a variety of components of religious affiliation in relationship to various aspects of health. According to Ellison's (1991) review there are four means through which religion has been theorized to enhance well-being: (1) social integration and support; (2) personal relationship with a divine other; (3) provision of systems of meaning; (4) promotion of specific patterns of religious organization and personal lifestyle. First, religion may increase social integration through friendship and social ties entered into on a voluntary basis. It can provide a social support network available in a crisis, regular community celebration of ritual events, normative social control regarding behaviour associated with good health (such as dietary and drinking norms), and interpersonal and business ethics and norms. Second, a personal relationship with a divine other may involve frequent prayer and meditation, as well as identification with a supreme being or with various benevolent figures from religious texts. Third, the personal system of meaning is an explanatory framework through which believers can understand themselves, their personal relationships, their work, and personal crises, tragedies, and joys, indeed, the whole 'round of life', including death and life after death. The fourth component refers to ways in which church membership may provide direction and support for patterns of behaviour such as church attendance and family mores, as well as other patterns having to do with such health-related activities as dietary restrictions.

In *Le Suicide*, Durkheim explained the protective and destructive effects of various forms of integration and regulation with respect to the suicide rate. In particular, he examined the results of too little integration or too much integration into the social group of which the individual was a part and the corresponding rates of egoistic and altruistic suicide. He also examined too little regulation and too much (normative) regulation and the corresponding tendency for anomic or fatalistic suicide. In *Elementary Forms of Religious Life*, Durkheim moved beyond the focus on the integrative and regulative functions of society and religion and examined such other topics as the division of time and space into the sacred and the profane and the impacts of ritual and group worship on the collectivity.

Religion and Health: Empirical Study

It has been nearly 150 years since Benjamin Travers remarked that he had never seen a case of cancer of the penis of the Jew, and almost that long since Regoni-Stern first observed that Catholic nuns in Verona, Italy, were at significant risk for breast cancer yet significantly protected against uterine cancer (Levin and Schiller, 1987: 9). The history of the empirical study of the relationship between religion and health is a long, circuitous, and complex one. Yet the refinement of the concepts of religion and health and the pathways between the two variables are still poorly understood. Religion and religiosity have a wide variety of components, such as denominational adherence and interaction with the divine. Health outcomes, too, have been investigated in a variety of ways, such as the increase or decrease in specific diagnosis (e.g., heart attack), overall morbidity and mortality, and health risk factors such as smoking. Among the control and intervening variables considered are ethnicity, class, and religious density in a specified geographical area. But what aspect of religion contributes to health? What pathways relate these two to one another? Levin has reviewed over 250 studies (1993: 5). Regardless of the definitions of the independent variables (various religious factors) or the dependent variables (e.g., specific diagnoses or overall morbidity and mortality), the results across all of the studies find that the greater the intensity or degree of religious involvement of the individual, the better the health. Levin's review of this literature concluded that nine hypotheses have been investigated.

1. *Behaviour.* The relationship between religion and health results from the health-relevant behavioural prescriptions, including such things as alcohol consumption, dietary patterns, and smoking.

2. *Heredity.* The genetic pools of different religious groups, particularly the most conservative and the smallest, tend to be concentrated. This may lead to greater or lesser health. For instance, Tay-Sachs disease seems to be more frequent among Eastern European Jews. Sickle-cell anemia is more prevalent among members of the predominately black National Baptist Convention than among those of the predominantly white Southern Baptist Convention. (This religious difference is likely confounded by the racial composition of the two groups.)

3. *Psychosocial effects.* Here, involvement in a congregation of religious adherents provides a sense of belonging, and receiving and giving social support promote better health. This type of investigation corresponds to the tradition of research that has independently demonstrated the benefits of good and supportive social relationships, perhaps through buffering the negative effects of stress and anger through psychoneuroimmunological pathways.

4. *Psychodynamics of belief.* The beliefs of adherents to particular denominations may engender a sense of hope, purpose, peace, and self-confidence, on the one hand, or guilt and self-doubt, on the other. Such beliefs may be associated with health benefits or decrements. For example, the 'Protestant ethic' could provide the epistemological and theological foundation for type A behaviour and the internal locus of control.

5. *Psychodynamics of religious rites.* The very practice of regular, recurrent public and private rituals, such as church attendance, daily scripture reading, and prayer, may serve to moderate anxiety, dread, and loneliness and

establish a sense of being loved and accepted.

6. *Psychodynamics of faith.* It is possible that belief in a God and an ordered universe may operate as a placebo. For example, 'various scriptures promise victory or survival to the faithful. The physiological effects of expectancy beliefs such as these are now being documented by mind-body researchers' (ibid., 10).

7. *Multifactorial explanations.* It is likely that the relationship between religion and health is due to a combination of the factors listed and hypotheses that have not yet been considered.

8. *Super-empirical explanations.* The preceding hypotheses are social, psychological, and biological. It may be that the best hypothesis is one for which concepts and measurement tools are not yet available. Consider, for example, the beliefs of ancient religious traditions in a universal life force or 'energy'. To date, this is largely a mysterious idea to the Western researcher. In the future, empirical observations may be available to further understanding of this 'energy' or life force.

9. *Supernatural influence.* Another possible explanation is supernatural, 'in other words, a transcendent being who exists fully or partly outside of nature chooses when and why to endow and bless individuals with health or healing, presumably on the basis of their faithfulness' (ibid., 11). Such a hypothesis, by definition, cannot be studied.

At an ecological rather than individual level the degree of concentration or density of a religious group is another component of the religious influence on health that has been examined. Areas with a higher concentration of religious groups have been shown to have different morbidity and mortality rates than areas that are similar in all regards but lack religious density. For example, Fuchs (1974) compared the mortality rates of two similar western states, Utah, where there is a very high concentration of Mormons, a religion that, among other things, prohibits cigarette smoking, alcohol, and caffeine, and Nevada, a more secular state, which at the time had high rates of alcohol and cigarette smoking. There were also important differences in marital, family, and geographical stability in these two states. The death rates for cirrhosis and for cancer of the respiratory system were higher in Nevada. At the county level, the impact of religious concentration and denominational affiliation on cancer mortality rates has also been examined, controlling for demographic, environmental, and regional factors known to affect cancer mortality. The findings noted the cancer-protective effects for all inhabitants of living in a densely religious area, perhaps the result of diminished exposure and increased social disapproval of cancer-causing behaviours.

Prayer and Health

Prayer for health is as ancient as civilization. Lately, under the modern positivistic scientific paradigm, a number of studies have been published establishing that prayer affects changes in human beings as well as a number of other bodily systems, including cells, fungi, yeast, bacteria, plants, single-celled organisms, and animals (Targ, 1997). It doesn't matter whether the prayer includes the laying on of hands or if the 'prayer' and 'prayee' are geographically separated even by a wide distance, with or without intervening barriers. How does this work? Scientists cannot investigate whether or not God heals through prayer because, by definition, God is outside (some would say inside, too) and greater than human senses. God is infinite and perfect. Human powers of observation and measurement are flawed and finite. Thus, we cannot 'study' God empirically. But is there some empirical force, energy, or information whose effects, emanating from prayer, can be studied? Prayer is believed to be communication with the deity, the Creator who, once asked, answers the petitioner. Healing in this context is the supernatural response of God to the desires of people.

Prayer has also been investigated as a natural phenomenon with some interesting results. Levin and Vanderpool (1989) have reviewed empirical studies and found a link between religion and health. These ideas can also be related to prayer. For instance, (1) to prepare to pray some will make behavioural adjustments, such as dietary restrictions (the best known of these may be fasting); (2) knowing that one is being prayed for may, in and of itself, lead to a feeling of being supported; (3) knowing that one is being prayed for and praying for oneself and others may be comforting and result in changes in the immune system through psychoneuroimmunologic mechanisms and pathways; and finally (4) a belief in prayer may, through psychoneuroimmunologic pathways, lead to well-being.

The most often cited study of prayer and healing was done by Randolph Byrd at the San Francisco General Medical Center in 1982–3 (Lerner, 1994: 128). A devoutly religious yet scientifically trained medical doctor, Byrd set out to investigate the effects of prayer on healing by looking at the health effects of being prayed for among 393 cardiac patients. He randomly assigned the patients to two groups and assigned people from nearby evangelical and Catholic prayer groups to pray for a total of 192 patients in the experimental group. The control group consisted of 201 patients who were alike in all respects at the beginning of the study as a result of the random assignment. After the prayers, six conditions differentiated the control and experimental groups. The experimental group was healthier in the following ways: (1) the need to be ventilated or intubated; (2) the need for antibiotics; (3) the frequency of cardio-pulmonary arrest; (4) the frequency of congestive heart failure; (5) the frequency of pneumonia; and (6) the need for diuretics. In this double-blind situation,

prayer by distant and unknown others worked.

Another study, with parallels to Byrd's, a double-blind clinical investigation of post-operative patients, documented psychological and physical improvements. In this study, 53 males who underwent hernia surgery were divided into three groups. The first group received a pre-recorded tape with suggestions for a speedy recovery. The second group experienced distant healing during the surgery by a healer who was concentrating on the individual and sending him/her healing thoughts, and the third group was a control. The group receiving distant healing was more significantly associated with recovery than either of the other two groups (Targ, 1997: 75). Other studies have noted the effectiveness of distant healing for various physiological measures, such as electro-dermal activity, heart rate, blood volume, and relaxation (ibid.).

The Illness Iceberg

The distribution of illness in a population has been described using the simile of an iceberg (Last, 1963; Verbrugge, 1986). The simile implies that most symptoms of disease go largely unnoticed by the people who have the symptoms, by health-care practitioners, and by epidemiologists interested in measuring the incidence and prevalence of disease. There are a number of reasons why a great deal of illness goes undetected. In the first place, people often explain away or rationalize physical changes in their bodies in ways that seem to make sense and therefore do not require a medical explanation. Sudden or extensive weight loss and a long-standing cough that doesn't seem to get better can both be signs of very serious illness. They are both, however, easily explainable in lay terms: 'I've been too busy to eat' or 'if it would only stop raining my cough would go away.' In the second place, some signs of latent illness develop slowly over a long period, so that the patient is not alerted to them. High blood pressure and cholesterol buildup in the arteries are two examples. Some of these diseases can only be detected by clinical tests such as X-rays, CAT scans, and blood and urine tests.

Practitioners, too, are limited in what illness they can detect. Some diseases that are not observable through any specific clinical measures can be diagnosed only by a myriad of complex tests, plus symptoms described by the patient, and some element of luck or art. Also, practitioners are often limited in their ability to detect illness because their patients do not provide sufficient information. Epidemiologists face all of the obstacles described above. In addition, epidemiologists frequently rely on a wide range of data collection strategies (as discussed in Chapter Two), all of which are subject to various limitations of validity, reliability, recall, response rate, truth-telling, and the like.

In the face of such ambiguity and variability in the recognition and acknowledgement of signs and symptoms of illness, what are the processes that lead some people to decide to do something about them and others to ignore them?

Why People Seek Help

What makes you decide to go to the doctor? Do you go when pain becomes severe? Is it when your symptoms interfere with your responsibilities at home, school, or work? Do you go for reassurance that a symptom is not a reflection of anything serious? Do you try to avoid going to the doctor? When you feel cold or flu symptoms do you generally just go to bed early or take a day or two off work? Do you tend to begin a course of vitamins? Do you go to the local drugstore to buy something from the shelf? Or do you go to a naturopath, chiropractor, nutritionist, allopathic physician, acupuncturist, or other therapist? The processes by which people come to notice signs they think may be symptomatic of illness, the kinds of attention they pay to these signs, and the action they decide to take are all a part of the study of illness behaviour. Whether someone seeks help and what kind

of help is sought are the result of complex social and psychological determinants.

The first stage of illness is the acknowledgement or notice of symptoms or signs. Sometimes symptoms are noticeable as little more than a minor behavioural change, such as tiredness or lack of appetite. Some common symptoms, such as a cough, cause only a mild discomfort; others may cause a searing pain. Sometimes symptoms are noticeable as measurable physical anomalies such as a heightened temperature or an excessive blood-sugar reading. At times, illness is not experienced until it is diagnosed after a routine medical examination.

People with similar symptoms may respond very differently to them. One may go straight to the doctor; another may 'let nature take its course', even with severe symptoms. Although early responses may be quite variable, they will make sense within the context of the social, cultural, economic, and psychological conditions of each person.

An early study, 'Pathways to the Doctor' (Zola, 1973), was based on interviews with more than 200 people at three clinics. For each person it was the first visit for that particular problem. According to Zola's analysis, the decision to seek treatment was based on a great deal more than the mere presence of symptoms. Rather, this decision was associated with one or more of the following: (1) occurrence of an interpersonal crisis; (2) perceived interference with social or personal relations; (3) sanctioning by others; (4) perceived interference with vocational or physical activity; and (5) a kind of 'temporalizing' of symptoms.

Each of the five motivations to seek medical care will be illustrated by a description of a case. John's case exemplifies action on the basis of an interpersonal crisis. John had been feeling tired for the last six months; he had explained it to himself as overwork. As he said:

I knew that as soon as I finished the presentation, I'd feel better. This was the big one. We'd been working on preparing this series of ads for a major soft drink company for just about two years. My promotion, my future was tied up in it. I didn't want to let down.

Then in the final week, Mac [his co-worker] was really upset one day and quit. He said it was my entire fault, that I had been impossible to work with, that I didn't co-operate, and that I was too busy. That night I decided I had to go to the doctor to get this thing diagnosed and fixed. (Clarke, 1996)

Perceived interference with social or personal relations can be illustrated by the case of Mary Beth, who had a cough that seemed to be hanging on amid increasing tiredness. Walking the stairs to her second-floor flat seemed to be more and more of an ordeal. She managed to get to work regularly and stay through what seemed like very long days. When a skiing vacation with a group of friends came up and she realized that she wouldn't be able to go, she decided that she had had enough and made an appointment with the doctor. In both of these cases, the symptoms had continued for a long period. The point of decision was not marked by new symptoms or symptoms that suddenly become more severe, but rather by changes in the social environment.

Sanctioning occurs when someone insists or ensures that the person with symptoms goes to the doctor. Men visit physicians less often than women, and it appears that a large percentage of their visits result from the urging of women (wives, sisters, mothers, or female friends). Charles's situation is illustrative. Charles had been experiencing chest pains for some weeks. He had been telling his wife Carol about them but insisted, since they seemed to occur only after meals, that they must be caused by heartburn and were not serious. Carol, however, thought otherwise, and made an appointment with their doctor. Faced with an appointment and a worried wife, Charles went to the doctor.

The fourth impetus to seeking medical aid is rooted in the Protestant work ethic. Sometimes the only changes that merit medical attention are those that interfere with work. Zola (1973) gives the example of a man with multiple sclerosis who, despite losing his balance and falling in a number of different locations, did nothing until he fell at work. Then he decided to seek medical advice.

The final impetus noted by Zola is 'temporalizing'. Sometimes symptoms only become problematic when they seem to have continued 'too long' or to have developed 'suddenly' and 'unexpectedly'. For example, at least three times over the winter Larry had had a cold with a very dry cough that lasted for a few weeks. He bore with it. When the first weekend of warm, sunny weather arrived at Easter, he noticed that he had the cough again. This time he decided that he had had it too long, that spring was here and the cough needed 'looking after'. Susan's situation shows that sometimes it is the suddenness rather than the duration of the symptom that causes a person to seek help. Susan described herself as 'healthy as a horse'. When she woke up one day with a very bad headache, she decided quickly that 'something was wrong' and went to the doctor.

Mechanic (1978) proposed that seeking help depends on 10 determinants: (1) visibility and recognition of the symptoms; (2) the extent to which symptoms are perceived as dangerous; (3) the extent to which symptoms disrupt family, work, and other social activities; (4) the frequency and persistence of symptoms; (5) amount of tolerance for the symptoms; (6) available information, knowledge, and cultural assumptions; (7) basic needs that lead to denial; (8) other needs competing with the symptoms; (9) competing interpretations that can be given to the symptoms once they are recognized; and (10) availability of treatment resources, physical proximity, and psychological and financial costs of taking action.

Mechanic and Zola do not contradict one another. Each takes a somewhat different point of view and focuses on some aspects of the reasons for seeking help while ignoring others. In particular, Mechanic acknowledges the relevance of the symptoms themselves—their severity, perceived seriousness, visibility, frequency, and persistence—and the knowledge, information, and associated cultural assumptions people use in determining whether or not to take action because of the symptoms. In Zola's 1973 model, 'symptoms' per se are not discussed except with regard to how long they continue or how suddenly they emerge. Zola's point of departure, given certain symptoms, is what action will likely be taken. Aside from this major difference, both models accentuate the importance of the disruption in family, work, and recreation and other competing goals in determining when an individual will to go the doctor. Zola stresses the necessary role that others sometimes play in determining health actions. Mechanic notes the real constraints that may exist with regard to the access to medical resources.

Summary

(1) Stress is a process that occurs in response to demands that are either much greater than or much less than the usual levels of activity. Historically, the bodily reaction to stress has been termed 'fright or flight' by Cannon. Later, Selye suggested that the General Adaptation Syndrome (GAS) is the body's reaction to all stressful events. It has three stages: an alarm reaction, resistance, and exhaustion. Exposure to stress in the third stage can lead to 'diseases of adaptation'.

(2) Some researchers have developed scales to measure degrees of stress.

(3) Several factors affect the amount of stress experienced. One important one is social support, which has been seen to be a buffer against the degree of stress experienced.

(4) Coronary-prone behaviour has been defined as that which is compulsive, dominating, and aggressive. People with these characteristics have type A personalities. Type A behaviour may include impatience and a wish to do things quickly, job involvement, and hard-driving conscientiousness. The type A person may be more likely to suffer premature cardiac disease.

(5) People are more likely to stay healthy when they have a feeling of comprehensibility, manageability, and meaningfulness in their lives and are able to develop a sense of coherence and a belief that things are under control.

(6) Religion and prayer have been associated with healing both historically and, more recently, empirically.

(7) The first stage of illness is the acknowledgement or notice of symptoms or signs. What people do about the illness, how illness is experienced and handled or treated, is called illness behaviour. Illness behaviour varies according to the individual's social circumstances. Factors that lead an individual to seek treatment include the occurrence of an interpersonal crisis, the perceived interference with social or personal relations, sanctioning by others, the perceived interference with vocational or physical activity, 'temporalizing' of symptoms that have continued 'too long' or develop 'suddenly' and 'unexpectedly', and the availability of treatment resources, physical proximity, and psychological and financial costs of taking action.

Questions for Study and Discussion

1. Assess yourself with regard to all of the socio-psychological variables that seem to be related to health status. What changes can you make now to improve your health?
2. Design a study to measure the sense of coherence of students at your university.
3. Critically evaluate the studies examining the relationship between prayer and health.
4. What do you estimate to be the proportion of the contribution of each of the various factors said to be associated with going to the doctor as Mechanic and Zola outline them?
5. Define, describe, and critically analyze ideas associated with the illness iceberg.

Suggested Readings

Frankl, V. 1965. *Man's Search for Meaning*, trans. I. Lasch. Boston: Beacon Press. A positive interpretation of the concentration camp experience.

Holmes, T.H., and R.H. Rahe. 1967. 'The Social Readjustment Rating Scale', *Journal of Psychosomatic Research* 11: 213–18. A useful discussion of the development and uses of the scale.

Journal of Health and Social Behaviour. Various years. Examine library copies over the past decade or so to see how they have portrayed the issues of social support and health.

Lerner, Michael. 1994. *Choices in Healing*. Cambridge, Mass.: MIT Press. This is a new classic on complementary treatments and practices for people dealing with cancer and other serious illnesses.

Levin, J.S. 1993. 'Esoteric vs. Exoteric Explanations for Findings Linking Spirituality and Health', *Advances* 9, 4: 54–6. Any of Levin's work on the relationship between religion and health is well worth reading.

Segall, Alexander, Michael J. Mahon, Judith G. Chipperfield, and Daniel S. Bailis. 1997. *Understanding the Relationship between Perceived Control, Personal Health Practices, and Health Status*. Final Report. Winnipeg: University of Manitoba, Max Bell Centre. A Canadian research report on some of the socio-psychological issues that relate to health behaviours and outcomes.

Zola, Irving. 1973. 'Pathways to the Doctor: From Person to Patient', *Social Science and Medicine* 7, 9: 677–89. Try to read at least one piece of Zola's useful and exciting approach to the sociology of medicine.

Chapter 8   *The Experience of Being Ill*

Learning Objectives

- Illness is experienced in subjective and personal terms.
- Illness experience is reflexively constructed by social meanings as well as personal stories.
- Illness, disease, and sickness need to be understood as distinct from one another.
- Among the variety of popular conceptions of illness are the following: illness as choice, as despair, as secondary gain, as a message of the body, as communication, as metaphor, as statistical infrequency, and as sexual politics.
- The insider's view of living with illness over time (chronic illness) describes it as involving a great deal of work and management of, among other things, treatments, symptoms, disease, and health-care providers.
- Illness affects self and identity.

Introduction

What is it like to acknowledge for the first time symptoms of a potentially serious illness? For instance, how do women feel and how do they talk to themselves and to others upon first noticing a lump in a breast? How do men or women manage to cope with a diagnosis of myocardial infarction? How do people who feel awful but cannot get a diagnosis, such as some people with chronic fatigue syndrome, fibromyalgia, or environmental sensitivities, manage? What is it like to be told that your child has epilepsy, Tay-Sachs disease, or Down's syndrome? What is it like for the doctors, the nurses, the siblings, and signifi-

cant others? How do people talk to themselves when they come to realize that they have cancer, diabetes, or AIDS? How do people manage the uncertainty surrounding the diagnosis and the possible or probable future prognosis of illness? How do people tell their significant others once they have received a diagnosis from the doctor? And how, then, do family members and significant others manage the news? How are such mild and self-limiting diseases as the flu or a cold understood in the whole context of the lives of people? These are the sorts of questions that might be asked about the experience of illness.

The purpose of this chapter is to describe and explain something of the experience of being ill in Canadian society. Most published sociological research to date assumes that the object of sociology is the observation of the institutions and structures of society that constrain people's thoughts, feelings, beliefs, and actions. This view prevails in most of the articles published in all the major North American journals of sociology.

Chapters Four through Seven have been written in this positivist tradition, using quantitative and 'objective' data about social phenomena to provide causal explanations. These four chapters do not examine the processes whereby these external 'objective' forces come to be integrated into the social actions (thoughts, feelings, beliefs, and behaviour) of human beings. Nor do they offer an explanation of the meanings and interpretations that people give to these factors.

Chapter Eight is written in the symbolic interactionist tradition: it draws attention to the meanings, interpretations, and world views of human beings in relation to illness, sickness, disease, and death. The chapter examines the subjective reality, the consciousness of people making and finding meaning in interactive and social context. The analysis in this chapter is at the individual level. However, it must be emphasized that a person's views are affected by a particular society and by a particular place at a unique point in time in that society. Meanings are constructed out of social interactions in specific social, political, economic, and historical contexts. Meanings reflect a person's position in the social structure and that person's personal relationships and experience. Cultural attitudes to illness vary. The meaning of illness to people varies.

Illness, Sickness, and Disease

Sociologists generally distinguish among disease, illness, and sickness. Disease is that which is diagnosed by a physician; it is usually believed to be located in specific organs or systems in the body and curable through specific biomedical treatments. Illness, by contrast, is the personal

experience of the person who acknowledges that he or she does not feel well. Sickness refers to the social actions taken by a person as a result of illness or disease, such as taking medication, visiting the doctor, resting in bed, or staying away from work. Patients feel illness and act sickness; physicians diagnose and treat disease.

Sickness, disease, and illness may, in some ways, be independent of one another. The fact that people can feel ill and act sick and yet not visit a physician confirms this, as in the case of a mild condition such as a cold. People can act sick without either feeling ill or having a medical diagnosis, as when a student complains of having flu in order to get an extension for an essay or an exemption from an examination. A physician may tell people that they are not ill and ought not to be acting sick. This may happen when a person is experiencing sleeplessness from the stress of final exams, and thus feels ill, but does not have a medical condition. Finally, a person may have an illness diagnosed as a disease by a physician. Such a diagnosis legitimizes sick-role behaviour. In this case sickness, illness, and disease may occur together. Figure 8.1 is meant to clarify the relationships among illness, sickness, and disease. Illness, sickness, and disease are integrally related because they are all socially constructed experiences. People do not experience or talk about their illnesses in a social or cultural vacuum. Everything that people feel, say, think, and do about their illness is culturally and socially mediated. For example, a sore back conjures up one set of meanings, ideas, and actions when it happens to a person with bone cancer. A sore back conjures up a different set of meanings, ideas, and actions when it happens to a world-class skier just before the Olympics. In fact, noticing that a part of the body, such as the back, is sore is only possible within a particular social-cultural context and its resultant language categories.

Sickness behaviour is also socially mediated. Social-structural and cultural factors influence whether a person visits a chiropractor, natur-

Figure 8.1   A Model of the Relationships among Illness, Sickness, and Disease

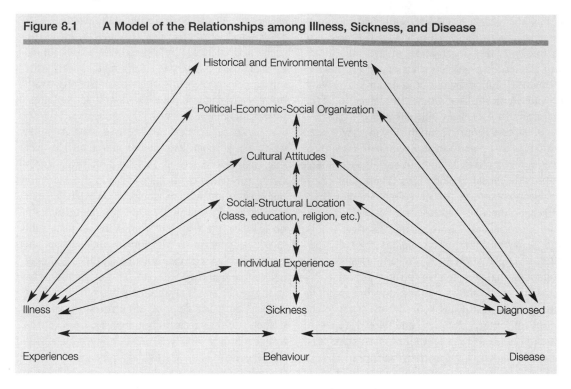

opath, masseuse, or the health food store. Whether a woman goes to the hospital at the first sign of labour or does not go until she is ready to deliver depends in part on cultural influences. Old-order Mennonite women, according to the nurses in the obstetrics department of a local hospital, often have their babies on the way to the delivery room because they tend to wait through several stages of labour before travelling in buggies to the hospital. According to the same source, women from some other ethnic backgrounds usually enter the hospital at the first sign of contractions, and once there they are likely to engage in long, protracted, painful, and 'noisy' labour.

Disease, too, is a socially mediated event. Doctors make their diagnoses from a complex mix of socio-cultural, historical, economic, medical, scientific, technological, and clinical data, and in the context of their own age, specialty, class, gender, and ethnicity. That death, too, is

socially mediated was described first by Sudnow (1967) and later by Timmermans (1998), as described in Box 8.1.

Outrageous Acts and Everyday Rebellions is the title of a witty satire by Gloria Steinem (1983) illustrating how illness, sickness, and disease may be sociological or, in this case, gendered determinations. Steinem suggests, for example, that beliefs about menstruation are socially determined: if men menstruated rather than women, menstruation would have very different meanings and consequences. First of all, if men menstruated, it would be a laudable, dramatic event, symbolic of strength and manhood. Men would compete with one another about how large their 'flow' was, how long it lasted, and whose blood was the brightest. Menstruation would be celebrated as a recurring, ritual reminder of the power of masculinity. To prevent problems such as cramps and premenstrual syndrome (PMS), bil-

Box 8.1   Social Value of the Patient and Death

David Sudnow (1967), in what has by now become a classic text, described in great detail, as the result of lengthy participant-observation at two US hospitals, how the 'presumed social value of a patient' affected the type of death-care the patient received. For example, poorer people, less 'functioning' people, and people who were less 'valuable' because of 'race'/ethnicity or age were given less aggressive treatments. Timmermans (1998) has recently reinvestigated the question of whether or not and how a patient's social worth continues to be a factor in the type and quality of treatment received. In particular, Timmermans examined how the use of resuscitation

technologies may have altered this finding. How do health-care practitioners 'make sense of engaging in a practice with the small chance of saving lives and the potential to severely disable patients'? (ibid., 469). Apparently, in the face of controversial options, the health-care practitioners continue to distinguish between people on the basis of their 'social viability' and on the basis of attempting 'to avoid a lawsuit'. In sum, 'in the liminal space between lives worth living and proper deaths, resuscitative efforts in the emergency department crystallize submerged subtle attitudes of the wider society' (ibid., 471).

lions of dollars in research money would be spent. Doctors specializing in menstruation would be thought to hold the most prestigious specialty; the most highly paid and desired medical position. Sanitary napkins and tampons would be free. Epidemiological research would demonstrate how men performed better and won more Olympic medals during their periods. Menstruation would be considered proof that only men could serve God and country in war, in politics, or in religion (ibid., 338).

Variations in the Experience of Being Ill

In all societies people experience illness, pain, disability, and disfigurement. Sorcery, the breaking of a taboo, the intrusion of a disease-causing spirit into the body, the intrusion of a disease-causing object into the body, and the loss of the soul are all seen as possible causes of disease (Clements, 1932). All these explanations, except for the intrusion into the body of a disease-causing object, involve the supernatural or magic in an attempt to understand illness. Westerners tend to see illness as empirically caused and

mechanically or chemically treatable. To a large extent, since Descartes, we have separated the mind, the body, and the spirit. But in most of the non-Western world, non-empirical explanations and cures for disease seem to dominate: illness is seen as a combination of spiritual, mental, and physical phenomena.

The experience of pain varies from one ethnic group and culture to another. For instance, Zborowski (1952) found that patients in New York City from Jewish and Italian backgrounds responded emotionally to suffering and tended to dwell on their painful experience. He also noted a difference in the attitudes of each of these groups to discomfort. Italians saw pain as something to be rid of and were happy once a way to relieve their pain was found. Jews were mainly concerned with the meaning of their pain and the consequences of their pain for their future health. 'Old Americans' and the Irish, by contrast, reacted stoically.

What is viewed as disease or health varies from society to society. Disfigurement or illness may or may not be seen as normal. 'Afflictions common enough in a group to be endemic, though they be clinical deformities, may often be accepted as part of man's natural condition' (Hughes, 1967: 88).

Disagreement is widespread over which states of physical being are desirable and which are not. Among some people, the obese woman is an object of desire; others define obesity as repugnant or even as a symptom of emotional or physical illness. People with epilepsy are some-times the object of ridicule and fear, but some people think they possess supernatural powers. There are many examples to illustrate how health and illness evaluations depend on value judge-ments (Clements, 1932; Hughes, 1967; Fitzpatrick et al., 1984; Turner, 1987).

It is clear that for many people health and religion, the natural and the supernatural, are often closely related. This is true of people's con-ceptions of the causes of disease and accident, and of their cures. As Freidson (1970: 211) has said, 'human and therefore social evaluation of what is normal, proper, or desirable is as inherent in the notion of illness as it is in notions of morality.'

Popular Conceptions of Health, Illness, and Disease

Medical anthropologists and sociologists who have examined beliefs about illness in modern Western communities have found that beliefs vary depending on the cultural background. Non-medical people hold immensely strong beliefs about illness, its causes, and its appropri-ate treatments (Cornwell, 1984). Cornwell distin-guished between medicalization-from-above and medicalization-from-below. The first refers to def-initions of the reality that are the result of devel-opments in scientific medicine. The second refers to the acceptance and the rejection of such defi-nitions on the part of lay people. It is particular-ly important to note that medical and lay ideas may be similar but are often quite different and even, at times, contradictory. The following sec-tions describe a number of popular conceptions of health and illness.

Illness as Choice

Illness is a choice. We choose when we want to be ill, what type of illness we'll have, how severe it will be, and how long the illness will last. Because the body and mind are connected, illness is a result of thinking and feeling as well as of bodily processes. We give ourselves illnesses to take a break from the busy obligations of everyday life. We choose to be ill to allow for 'time out' from our routines: to rest, to take stock, to escape, and to withdraw. A host of research in fields such as psychoneuroimmunology and psychosomatic medicine attests to the prevalence of this belief, on both theoretical and empirical levels. A great deal of work has been done on the mind-body interaction in the case of cancer, in particular. Several physician writers have addressed mind-body relationships in various ways. For an overview of several of the most popular, consider the work of Chopra (1987, 1989) and Dossey (1982, 1991).

Oncologist Carl O. Simonton and his col-leagues were the earliest contemporary 'popular-izers' of the role of the mind in both sickening and healing the body. They argued that cancer is a disease that arises from a sort of emotional despair. Simonton's book, *Getting Well Again*, is full of examples of people who come to recog-nize, with the help of the psychotherapeutic skills of Simonton's staff, that their cancer has been, in a sense, a personal choice. Once a patient comes to understand the reason for the choice of cancer as a way of coping with a personal problem, he or she can confront the problem on a conscious level and seek solutions (Simonton et al., 1978).

Simonton's method includes a number of techniques. One of the best known is the system-atic use of imaging—conjuring up mental pic-tures of cells. People are directed to imagine their cancer cells as, for example, black ants and their healthy cells as knights in shining armour, for example. The hypothesis is that the more power-ful the imaging of the anti-cancer forces, the more likely it is to be effective. Effective imaging usually results in one of the following outcomes: increased longevity; moderation of symptoms, including pain; increased sense of well-being, autonomy, and control; improved quality of life; and even, at times, remission of the disease.

Imaging may be the most dramatic of the techniques used to combat cancer 'psychologically'; but numerous other methods are being used around the world by psycho-oncologists. Alastair Cunningham, a psychologist and immunologist at Princess Margaret Hospital in Toronto, has for a number of years been running groups for people with cancer. Included in Cunningham's program for coping with cancer and minimizing its impact are stress-management techniques such as writing a journal or diary and meditating. Dr Cunningham has written a workbook called *Helping Yourself* that is accompanied by two audiotapes, one for deep muscle relaxation and the other on imagery for healing. These were sponsored by and are widely available through the Canadian Cancer Society. The effects of all of these on quality of life, longevity, and the disease itself are under investigation. The point to be made here is that within this model of health/illness an important part of healing (along with medical interventions) and of improving the quality of life is taking responsibility for one's state of health and choosing to try to do something about it.

Illness as Despair

Closely related to the idea that illness reflects choice is the idea that illness reflects and results from a sort of despair. Many social commentators, psychologists, and medical researchers have thought of illness as a sort of emotional despair. Lawrence LeShan (1978), a psychotherapist who counselled and then studied cancer patients, came to the conclusion that a common type of emotional experience among the majority of cancer patients predated the development of the disease. Examples of these emotional experiences include long-standing, unresolved grief over the loss of someone close, such as the death of a mother or father in childhood, childhood loneliness or isolation and the loss of someone close in adulthood, and the loss of a job. For LeShan's patients, understanding their grief and expressing feelings of sadness and anger became pathways towards being healed.

Norman Cousins's work, which formed the basis for his book, *Anatomy of an Illness as Perceived by the Patient*, is the foundation of another similar and newly popular approach to illness, health, and healing. This book, a long-time best-seller, translated into at least 13 different languages and 'must' reading in a number of medical schools throughout the world, tells the story of Norman Cousins's reaction to and healing from a severe and potentially fatal case of ankylosing spondylitis, a degenerative disease of the connective tissues in the spine.

Cousins's story of his 'miraculous' recovery focused on three aspects of his 'systematic pursuit of salutary emotions' (1979: 35). The first was his partnership with his doctor. Cousins asked his doctor to engage in a collaborative partnership. The physician had the traditional armaments to offer. Cousins had done some reading about how healing could be affected by the power of positive thinking and by massive doses of vitamin C. Because he found the hospital forbidding, noisy, and thoroughly unhealthy, Cousins asked his doctor to treat him in a nearby motel. The second important component of his recovery was that his doctor agreed to his request for massive intravenous doses of vitamin C, in which Cousins, having done considerable research on his own, believed. The third aspect of his rehabilitation strategy, and the most important for our purposes in this chapter, was laughter. Cousins had books of jokes and cartoons, tapes, and old movies brought to his room for his enjoyment. Laughing deeply relieved his pain and generally made him feel better. As he says, 'It worked. I made the joyous discovery that ten minutes of genuine belly laughter had an anesthetic effect and would give me at least two hours of pain-free sleep. When the pain-killing effect of the laughter wore off, we would switch on the motion-picture projector again, and, not infrequently, it would lead to another pain-free sleep interval' (ibid., 39). As he was interested in demonstrating the credibility of his experience, Cousins instituted some small experiments. He found that each episode of laughter decreased the level of inflammation in his connective tissues.

Five years after recovering from this disease, and having achieved some renown in the area of holistic health (he was appointed senior lecturer at the School of Medicine, University of California at Los Angeles, and consulting editor of *Man and Medicine*), Cousins suffered a serious heart attack. Rehabilitation resulted in another book, *The Healing Heart* (1983), in which he further developed his arguments regarding the importance of positive emotions in maintaining and achieving health that he had first elaborated in *Anatomy of an Illness*. Cousins's work is based on the idea that the mind and body are a single entity; positive change in one, for example in the body by the use of pharmaceuticals such as vitamin C, or in the mind by mood elevation through, for instance, laughter, can lead to healing.

Illness as Secondary Gain

Sometimes illness has definite benefits. Remember the last time you were conveniently sick on the day of a big test for which you had not had time to prepare. Small children quickly learn to complain of sore tummies when they do not really feel like going to church, to school, or to grandma's house. Illness may provide an opportunity or permit someone to behave in ways he or she would like to but otherwise would feel constrained from doing.

Or illness may allow someone to meet needs that would otherwise go unmet. The benefits of illness are as varied as people's illnesses. A case example will illustrate. Brett was a high school guidance counsellor and history teacher; he had also taken on the job of basketball coach and was supervising set-building for the school play. Brett was married and had two preschool children in daycare while he and his wife Lucy worked. Lucy was required to do a great deal of travelling in her job as a buyer for a large department store. Brett was often responsible for driving the kids to and from daycare, as well as for feeding and bathing them. He hadn't expected so much responsibility: he had been raised to assume that his wife would handle the children, the house, the cooking, and most of their domestic life.

He felt trapped. On the one hand, he supported and applauded Lucy's success and realized that if she was really going to 'make it' in her business of choice she would have to continue at her present pace for three or four years. On the other hand, he frequently felt overwhelmed by his responsibilities. The day his doctor diagnosed mononucleosis, Brett was secretly relieved. At least now he had a way out.

The question of secondary gains has been explained in a more systematic way in research on welfare mothers (Cole and Lejeune, 1972). In this case the focus was on whether and in what situations mothers on welfare would be likely to claim that they were ill. The researchers hypothesized that illness could be seen as a legitimation, or acceptable explanation, for failure. Being on welfare is thought by a substantial number of welfare recipients to be the result of and also a continual reminder of a personal failure. This being the case, then women on welfare would be likely to look for a rationalization and legitimation for their situation. Indeed, the researchers found that women on welfare who felt that they had little hope of changing their status were more likely to use illness as their explanation for being on welfare than women who hoped or expected to move off welfare. The point here is that sometimes claiming illness seems to be a better choice and to provide a greater level of reward than the other available options. In such a case illness can be thought of as providing secondary gains.

Box 8.2   It Can Happen to Anyone—It Happened to Me

. . . In the spring of 1995 . . . I developed a bronchial infection and was sick for two weeks. My doctor prescribed some easy, quick-acting antibiotics to cure me. . . . What followed . . . were three months of me feeling more tired than usual. Nothing happened that, in and of itself, would cause alarm, but eventually things built up to reveal a larger problem.

I was a French camp counsellor that summer. We did a lot of different activities: singing in French, making slime out of corn starch and water, playing soccer, and other things of that nature. I found that after the first five minutes or so of chasing children I was exhausted. I blamed it on the sun, not having eaten enough breakfast, anything that could have been true once or twice, but not repeatedly. What ended up happening was that my partner would take the outdoor activities as primary counsellor and I would do the indoor. This eliminated the 'problem', or so I thought.

Later that same summer I went on a hike with my family. My 'hike' consisted of finding the start of the trail, looking at the map, and deciding that I was too tired to walk it. I ended up sitting, in the shade, for the hour and a half that the rest of my family walked. Even when they came back, my stroll over to the concession stand to get pop for my sister was exhausting. This was definitely not the way a healthy 17-year-old was supposed to be feeling.

Continually, throughout this period, I needed to sit down while taking showers. After about three minutes I would need to turn off the water and sit until I felt strong enough to stand up and rinse off. Again, this was not normal, but at the time I made excuses.

Summer ended, and I went back to school. There, I needed to rest after climbing from my first-floor English class to my locker on the second floor. There, I was told by a science teacher in front of the class that I looked green. I shrugged this off, thinking that the teacher was impolite, but not incorrect. Later that week a different teacher said that I looked pale. I was (and am again) a vegetarian, so I thought that my paleness was due to anemia, caused by my diet.

Eventually, I noticed an enlarged lymph node on my neck. My mom and I went to a walk-in clinic. We were quickly and efficiently (as those clinics are) dealt with and sent forth as healthy into the healthy world. The doctor told us to come back if it didn't go away on its own. It wont away in a few days.

Three weeks later, after further incidents of flashing lights and perpetually needing to sit down to clear my head, I woke up thinking that something was wrong. Placed together like this on a page it is so blatant, so apparent that my conclusion was correct.

However, during that time, everything could be (and was) explained away. The flu, my vegetarianism, waking up too early and staying too late at school: all of this could add up to what was happening to me on a daily basis. But not for three months. I decided that I couldn't go to school that day. This was after attempting to shower, and needing to sit down as soon as I put the water on, after about five seconds. My mom decided to take me back to the walk-in clinic (we were in between doctors at the time, ours being newly retired). . . .

Less than three hours after I had gone to get my blood taken, the doctor was calling. This seemed a little strange. Now, I am so thankful for that doctor's action; he helped get the ball rolling for my (future) cure. My mom answered the phone and the doctor said: 'I think there might be something serious here.'

As we know, he was quite right.

Source: Clarke, with Clarke (1999: 5–7), from *Imprint* (University of Waterloo), 10 Oct. 1997.

Illness as a Message of the Body

Within the homeopathic perspective, illness is an expression of a unique person at a particular point in time and engaged in a special set of circumstances. Illness is also the expression of a whole person—body, mind, and soul. Illness and health are not polar opposites: both exist in a person continuously in a state of dynamic equilibrium. From this perspective symptoms are not signs of illness but indications that the person is responding to a challenge and is engaging in what is called a healing crisis. The healing crisis (or the symptom) is a manifestation of what has been happening for a time but has been repressed and therefore unnoticed. Fever, rash, inflammation, coughing, crying, sleeplessness, and tension are revelations of a deep disturbance of the whole person. Symptoms are valuable and useful because they allow the person to acknowledge the crisis and to seek help. The role of the healer is to support the person emotionally and to enhance the natural recuperative powers of the physical body through the administration of minuscule amounts of natural medications that are known to create the symptoms the individual 'patient' is presenting (see Chapter Fifteen for a more complete discussion of homeopathic medicine).

Illness as Communication

People communicate through words and by signs or body language. People also send messages through the way their bodies are functioning. Illness sends a message that one part of the body is alienated from the 'self'. The body expresses the soul. One may even say that illness expresses the soul more impressively than health, in the same way that a good caricature expresses essential aspects of a personality more clearly than photographs taken in a characteristic situation (Siirla, 1981: 3).

Through particular sets of symptoms or particular kinds of illnesses, people convey messages about themselves. A woman with breast cancer may be saying that her need and desire to nurture have been frustrated. Since the breast is important in mothering, feeding, and soothing, it becomes the most appropriate symbol for communication about frustrated nurturing. Thus a person's needs may be expressed through illness. 'If these [needs] cannot be expressed in a realistic, "healthy" form, symbolic organ language takes over' (ibid., 8).

In this view, different diseases express different frustrations. Rheumatism, a disability that affects the muscles and the joints, may express the frustration of a person who once liked to be very active but who had to limit his or her activities. Cold symptoms such as runny nose and sneezing may result from a frustrated desire to cry. All illnesses can be examined as attempts by the body for expression that otherwise cannot be expressed or are frustrated or repressed.

Illness as Metaphor

Related to the suggestion that illness is communication is the idea advanced by Susan Sontag that illness is metaphor. Illness communicates by conveying a particular message for a person at a special point in his or her life. Illness as metaphor suggests that cultures bestow meanings on various illnesses. In Sontag's view, however, metaphors are most likely to be related to illnesses that have no clear or obvious cause or treatment. The two examples that she examines in some depth in *Illness as Metaphor* (1978) are cancer in the twentieth century and tuberculosis in the nineteenth century. In 1988 she examined the metaphoric meanings of AIDS. Her basic argument is that the metaphors attached to diseases are often destructive and harmful. They frequently have punitive effects on the patient because they exaggerate, simplify, and stereotype the patient's experience. Metaphors may function as stigma. They may serve to isolate the person with the disease from the community. Metaphors often imply adverse moral and psychological judgements about the ill person. They have perpetrated the view, for example, that cancer is a form of self-judgement or self-betrayal.

Table 8.1   Images of Cancer, Heart Disease and AIDS

CANCER	HEART DISEASE	AIDS
Cancer is described as an evil, immoral predator.	Heart disease is described as a strong, active, painful attack.	Little is said about the nature of the disease other than it debilitates the immune system. Much is said about the moral worth of the victims of the disease.
Euphemisms such as the Big C are used rather than the word 'cancer'.	Heart disease, stroke, coronary/arterial occlusion, and all the various circulatory system diseases are usually called the Heart Attack.	Acquired immune deficiency syndrome is called AIDS. The opportunistic diseases that attack the weakened immune system are often not mentioned.
Cancer is viewed as an enemy. Military imagery and tactics are associated with it.	The heart attack is described as a mechanical failure, treatable with available new technology and preventable with diet and other lifestyle changes.	AIDS is viewed as an overpowering enemy, as epidemic and scourge.
The whole self, particularly the emotional attitude of the person and the disease, is subject to discussion. Because the disease spreads and because the spread is often unnoticed through symptoms or medical checks, the body itself becomes potentially suspect.	It occurs in a particular organ that is indeed interchangeable with other organs.	It is described as affecting the immune system and resulting mostly from immoral behaviour— connotes 'shameful sexual' acts and drug abuse.
Cancer is associated with hopelessness, fear, and death.	There is a degree of optimism about the preventability and the treatability of the disease.	It is associated with fear, panic, and hysteria because it is contagious through body fluids, primarily blood and semen.
Prevention through early medical testing is advised.	The heart attack is described as very preventable. Suggestions for lifestyles that will prevent it are frequently publicized.	Prevention through monogamous sexual behaviour or abstinence, and avoidance of unsterilized needles and drug abuse.
There are innumerable potential causes listed. They range from sperm to foodstuffs to the sun.	There is a specific and limited list of putative causes offered again and again.	Initially the causes for AIDS were very general: being homosexual, a drug user, or a Haitian.
There is little consideration of the socio-political or environmental causes, e.g., legislation that limits smoking.	There is little mention of socio-political causes.	There is little mention of socio-political causes.
There is uncertainty about cause.	There is certainty about cause.	There is uncertainty about cause.

Media Images of Cancer, Heart Disease, and AIDS

One recent study of the way cancer, heart disease, and AIDS have been portrayed in the mass print media illustrates how diseases come to have unique meanings and metaphors associated with them. Disease is seen as much more than a mechanical failure, a physiological pathology (Clarke, 1992a). Table 8.1 portrays the findings.

The moral worth of the person with cancer is attacked by the invasion of an evil predator so fearsome it is not even to be named, but fought as a powerful alien intruder that spreads secretly through the body. The person with cancer is not offered much hope of recovery. By and large, the media portray cancer as associated with horrid symptoms, mutilations, excruciating suffering, and finally death. To some extent the person with cancer is held to be blameworthy because the cancer could have been detected through early medical checkups or prevented through practising positive emotions. There is a great deal of uncertainty about the cause of cancer. There are numerous putative causes. They are usually described as the result of individual lifestyle decisions. Again, then, it is the individual who is ultimately culpable.

The media description is radically different when the disease is a heart attack. The heart attack is presented as an objective, morally neutral event that happens at a specific time and place and causes a great deal of pain. Heart disease is portrayed in optimistic terms. Not only are there very clear and precise steps to be taken to prevent it, but also when it occurs it can be treated in a variety of mechanical ways, including using technology to replace a malfunctioning heart. Heart disease does not affect the whole person or the moral being of the person. It 'attacks' one part only. Heart disease is an 'outsider' that can be repelled through quick, decisive action and the use of medical marvels. The person with heart disease may experience acute fear and pain, but the period of recovery is likely to be dominated by optimism about a cure and a resolve to change the lifestyle habits that led to the disease in the first place.

The person with AIDS is portrayed as a diseased person and as somewhat morally repugnant. He (usually a 'he' in the developed world although equally male and female in the developing world) is described as hopelessly doomed and isolated from potentially significant sources of emotional support such as lovers and family members. The disease itself is described in mechanical and biomedical terms. The media do not dwell on the painful or debilitating symptoms of the disease. They do not focus on the inevitable terminal stages of the disease, on death itself, or on the mortality rate. Rather, they focus on the fear of contagion and the uncertainty about the causes of contagion. The person afflicted with AIDS is stigmatized because of the connection with a deviant lifestyle, and is isolated because people are afraid of the contagion that might result from being close. This fear of being close affects not only the close friends and significant others of the person with AIDS, but also more distant others such as medical personnel.

It must be emphasized that these are images of cancer, heart disease, and AIDS drawn from selected Canadian and American magazines—*Newsweek*, *Time*, *Maclean's*, *Good Housekeeping*, *Ladies' Home Journal*, and *Reader's Digest*—over a 20-year period. Think about whether this analysis fits your understanding of the mass print media stories that you have read on disease. These magazines are the highest circulating magazines in North America. However, they are not the only magazines with a mass circulation available in North America. They may or may not be the most widely read. Little research has been done on the impact of such media depictions on people in society.

Illness as Statistical Infrequency

From this point of view illness is essentially an infrequent state of mental or physical malfunctioning. When a condition, no matter how uncomfortable, is prevalent among a group of people, it is usually not considered pathological. Illnesses such as the common cold and flu are so prevalent as to be considered largely unimportant (it is clear that they are not taken seriously because few research dollars are allocated to investigating them).

Illness as Sexual Politics

Many feminist thinkers have analyzed the ways in which disease can be seen as sexual politics. Reissman (1987) has done a theoretical/empirical review of the medicalization of women's bodies and lives with a focus on childbirth, reproduction and contraception, premenstrual syndrome, 'beauty', and mental health and illness. Currie and Raoul (1992) discuss 'women's struggle for the body' in the face of culturally and historically entrenched bodily constraints and restrictions. From the feminist perspective the constraints and limitations of gender roles are associated with the conceptualization and the subsequent diagnosis of various diseases. For example, Ehrenreich and English (1978) document how the 'mysterious epidemic' experienced by nineteenth-century middle- and upper-class women was the outgrowth of the conditions that characterized their lives. The journals and diaries of women of the time give hundreds of examples of women who wasted away into lives of invalidism. The symptoms included headache, muscular aches, weakness, depression, menstrual difficulties, and indigestion. The diagnoses were many: 'neurasthenia', 'nervous prostration', 'cardiac inadequacy', 'dyspepsia', 'rheumatism', and 'hysteria'. The diseases were not fatal. They were usually chronic, however, and lasted throughout a woman's life until her death.

The feminist analysis explains that these diseases provided an appropriate role for women in the middle and upper classes. These women were utterly dependent on their husbands, and their sole purpose in life was the provision of heirs. Household tasks were left to domestic servants. Hired help cared for children. The wife's job was to do precisely nothing—and thus to stand as a symbol to the world of her husband's great financial success. Medical ideology buttressed this view of the appropriate role of middle- and upper-class women with the theory of the conservation of energy. This was the belief that human beings had only a certain amount of energy. Since the primary functions of women of these classes were procreation and decoration it behooved them to save all their vitality for childbearing and not to waste any in studying or in doing good works. Such activities would drain energy away from the uterus, where it was needed, into the brains and limbs, where it served no good purpose. This issue, from the point of view of medicalizing women's emotions, is further discussed in Chapter Thirteen.

Contemporary feminists have suggested that the eating disorders bulimia and anorexia nervosa are logical expressions of women's role today (Currie, 1988). Eating disorders can best be understood, in this perspective, as the internalization of conflicts that result from the prevailing contradictory images of women. Anorexia is almost exclusively a disease of adolescent women, particularly those from middle- and upper-middle-class backgrounds, and occurs primarily in modern Western capitalist societies. Some have applied traditional Freudian psychoanalysis to these disorders and have attributed their causes to a fear of sexuality and an attempt to avoid femininity. Others have explained them, from a family systems perspective, as a result of mothers who overprotect and overidentify with their daughters. Daughters differentiate from mothers and become separate individuals, in this perspective, by rebelling and refusing to eat. Several feminist authors have argued that eating disorders constitute a protest by women against the contradictory images of women as independent, competent wage-earners and as sexual objects who earn only a portion of male salaries in work that is devalued because it is done by women (ibid.; Wolfe, 1990).

During two discrete periods in the twentieth century anorexia was a notable problem—the 1920s and the final two or three decades of the century. Both of these periods were times when equality of opportunity for men and women was being stressed. These were times of expanded educational and employment options for women. They were also times of contradictions. In theory, choices for women were expanding; in practice, they still earned only a fraction of men's incomes. Furthermore, women were and continue to be notoriously underrepresented at all levels of the political process—municipally, provincially, and federally. Nor have their domestic responsibilities declined. Inadequate public, subsidized child care and excessive domestic responsibilities mean that women who work outside the home also have full-time jobs inside the home. Yet a woman's identity is still tied up with her appearance. In these circumstances eating disorders, as Orbach (1986) claimed, can be seen as a women's 'hunger strike'.

The next section of this chapter moves from a consideration of models of illness in contemporary society to some empirical analyses of the experience of illness from the perspective of the subject.

The Insider's View: How Illness Is Experienced

Most sociological analyses of illness have treated it as an objective phenomenon measured by questionnaires and by biophysical or clinical tests. From this perspective the varieties of personal experiences are irrelevant. What matters is the explanation of the incidence and prevalence of various types of disease. However, in keeping with the arguments and traditions noted in the work of people such as Weber, Husserl, Schutz, Blumer, Mead, Cooley, Simmel, Garfinkel, and Goffman, some researchers have turned their attention to the symbolic meanings and the social constructions of illness in the context of people's everyday experiences. These researchers focus on analysis at the individual level. It must be emphasized, however, that individual attitudes must always be set in a social context at a particular place and at a particular point in time.

Analyzing illness at the individual level has a long and noteworthy tradition in the sociology of medicine and the sociology of health and illness. One of the first published studies, mentioned earlier, was that of Mark Zborowski (1952, 1969), who compared the understandings and meanings of pain among Jewish, Italian, and 'Old

American' ethnic groups in New York City. Erving Goffman's *Asylums* (1961) described the experience of hospitalization from the perspectives of the patients or inmates and from that of the staff. Later, Goffman (1963) examined stigmas associated with illnesses and other 'unusual or abnormal' conditions.

Roth (1963) described his own experience of hospitalization for tuberculosis. Myra Bluebond-Langer (1978) described the world of children dying of leukemia and the experiences of their parents, their nurses, and their doctors. Her work is particularly instructive in illustrating the control and spread of information. Bluebond-Langer documented the children's extensive detailed knowledge of their conditions, the next stages in their diseases, the probable side effects of various medications, and which medications they were likely to be given, even when parents and hospital staff would attempt to shield them from this information.

Speedling (1982) expanded the description of the experience of illness from the point of view of the person with the disease to that of the family when one of its members suffers a heart attack. His research looks at the impact of a person's hospitalization on the family, on how the family defines heart attack, on the person who has had the heart attack, and on his or her later ability to cope with the changes brought about by the disease. Stewart and Sullivan (1982) have examined the processes through which multiple sclerosis came to be diagnosed, the various phases and stages and uncertainties associated with its history, its emotional impact, and the changes it brings in interpersonal relationships.

In her study of a community, Cornwell (1984) examines common-sense ideas about health, illness, and health services held by families and households in East London. Their ideas are described within the context of the life of the respondents. Thomas's (1982) work focuses on the experiences of people with impairment, disability, and handicaps. Thomas distinguishes among impairment, which is physical or psychological pathology, disability, which is the limitation on everyday activities such as eating, dressing, and walking, and handicap, a socially derived concept that labels a person pejoratively. As Thomas says, these three are not necessarily inextricably linked to one another.

Thomas pays particular attention to the self-identities of the various people involved, the 'disabled' person, societal attitudes towards 'disability', and the attitudes of parents and professional caregivers. Like most books in this genre, his work is filled with lengthy quotations drawn from accounts given by the people involved. Schneider and Conrad's (1983) study of epilepsy examines living with epilepsy—its diagnosis, living with uncertainty, managing the symptoms, concealing the disorder, strategies of relating to others, the views of parents and family members, coping with the stigma, and handling medical regimens.

More recently, sociologists have turned to narrative description of illness experience, including emotional experiences. Marianne Paget, a sociologist whose work was the study of medical error, was coincidently the subject of medical errors. The series of errors made by different physicians were ultimately responsible for her death. Before she died, however, she wrote of her experience in *A Complex Sorrow*, which includes a play text. As she says:

> It was while attending the first trial [for medical negligence/malpractice] in late 1987 that I began to experience back pain. Eight months later, I learned I had cancer. Almost simultaneously, I learned that the errors made in my diagnosis had jeopardized my life. I was told that my condition was incurable. (Paget, 1993: 5–6)

Such symbolic interactionist and phenomenological writing is becoming more frequent in a postmodern sociology of the body, emotion, and health and illness, but it represents a significant and reflexive move from studying others' meanings to studying one's own.

Strauss and Glaser (1975) studied the impact of a number of different chronic illnesses and noted that people with such illnesses and their family members had to face a variety of common concerns. Strauss and Glaser distinguished all of the following issues: (1) preventing and managing medical crises; (2) managing medical regimens (taking medications, administering needles, physiotherapeutic exercises); (3) controlling symptoms and preventing symptom eruption; (4) organizing and scheduling time (including necessary rests and treatments) efficiently; (5) preventing or coping with social isolation; (6) dealing with uncertainty and adjusting to changes during the course of the disease; (7) normalizing social and interpersonal relationships; (8) managing stigma; and (9) managing knowledge and information. Each of these will be discussed in turn.

Crisis management requires constant vigilance on the part of the ill person and those who are taking care of him or her. A diabetic, for instance, must continually monitor blood-sugar levels and weigh and measure food intake and insulin levels. Such monitoring may not be completely accurate, nor are the results entirely predictable. A reaction to an imbalance may be infrequent, but it is a constant possibility. People with colitis or other bowel disorders have to be prepared all the time for an unexpected and potentially embarrassing and even humiliating bowel evacuation. People caring for those with Alzheimer's in their own homes are well aware that the patient is constantly at risk. Newspapers often carry stories of Alzheimer's patients who have left home and become lost, often without adequate clothing for protection from the elements.

Managing medical regimens is often a complex matter. The physician tells the patient to take a certain number of pills or to have injections at certain intervals. The patient often adapts and adjusts the quantity or frequency to a level at which he or she feels comfortable. Most medications have side effects. The patient must learn to balance the need for the medication with the need to be free of side effects. Cancer patients may have to cope with chemotherapy, radiation, and surgery. Each of these treatments has negative psychological and physical side effects. People with cancer who are scheduled for chemotherapy on a regular basis by doctors may decide to take a week or more off because they cannot bear the side effects, need or want a holiday, have a party or other special event to attend, or have any of a number of other social and personal priorities. For the person with diabetes, managing the medical regimen is not as simple as just obeying the doctor's orders. Diabetics must make complicated calculations about the quantity of insulin they require. The amount of insulin necessary will vary with the amount of rest or stress the diabetic is experiencing. The patient has to learn to manage the medication in order to be comfortable and yet to avert a coma. Diabetics may also experience restrictions on their social lives—they may not be able to go to eat with friends. People with ulcerative colitis and with a colostomy or ileostomy must devote considerable time to managing their diet, monitoring their liquid intake, and being prepared to cope with a loss of control.

The control of symptoms is a related issue. This involves managing the medical regimen daily, hourly, or even more frequently so that a crisis does not erupt. It also involves taking enough medication to prevent a crisis but not enough to cause uncomfortable side effects. Minor symptoms may lead to changing some habits; major symptoms may require redesigning the patient's house and lifestyle. Someone with colitis may be severely restricted in mobility by the necessity always to be near a toilet. A person with arthritis might have to move to a one-storey house without steps up to the door.

Organizing and scheduling time can be important in many chronic diseases because available time is almost always limited. Time is needed to manage the required medications, to visit doctors

and hospital, to change clothes or apparatus, to cope with restrictions, to be able to move about, and so on. Often the symptoms, too, such as headaches and backaches, require that the ill person drop the daily routine in order to go to bed to cope with the pain. Tiredness and fatigue are almost inevitable accompaniments to most chronic illnesses.

Preventing or coping with isolation and trying to maintain social relationships when the person can no longer do what 'normal' people do is another never-ending struggle. Sometimes people restrict their friendships to others who have the same problem and therefore understand. The ubiquity of self-help groups for most chronic diseases attests to the importance of social relationships with similarly disabled people, and perhaps, also, to the isolation felt by these people. Those with cancer and their families have repeatedly stated in interviews that they are almost glad they have had the disease because through it they have met so many wonderful people. People have also said that they can talk to others who have a similar disability in a way that they have never been able to talk to anyone else before the diagnosis.

Another underlying experience that seems to be common among people with a variety of chronic illnesses is *uncertainty* (see Conrad, 1987; Strauss and Glaser, 1975), which affects every stage of illness, beginning with the diagnosis and ending with cure, confirmation that an illness is chronic, or death. Most chronic illnesses have variable and unpredictable prognoses. Cancer is perhaps the archetypal disease of uncertainty. Its very cure is measured by the diminishing probability of recurrence one, two, three, or more years after the initial diagnosis and treatment.

Diseases such as epilepsy, multiple sclerosis, and Alzheimer's are characterized by uncertainty. In all three the uncertainty is endemic to the whole diagnostic process. They are each very difficult to diagnose and require the results of a number of different tests before a reasonably confident diagnosis can be reached. But uncertainty also prevails during the stages of treatment, of spread of the disease, and of resurgence and remission. Under such circumstances, it is difficult to *normalize social relationships*—to make plans for the future, to be considered and consider oneself a reliable friend, companion, spouse, parent, or worker when faced with a disease with an unknown prognosis.

People who have once experienced a heart attack may distrust their bodies for a long time. They may avoid work and exercise and radically alter their lifestyle. They may feel unable to count on being alive in six months or a year. Because a heart attack frequently occurs without warning, those who have had a heart attack may lose the ability to take their bodies for granted. Yet this ability is often the prerequisite for life satisfaction.

Managing stigma is another issue the chronically ill must face. The sociological use of the term 'stigma' originated with the work of Goffman (1963), who examined varieties of social interactions that were impaired by people's identity problems. Goffman designated a stigma as an attribution that discredits the value of a person. Goffman distinguished between the effects of stigma that are known only to the person involved and those that are known to others, and analyzed various strategies designed to handle the stigma in each case. The discredited person, whose deviant stigma is known to others, is challenged to 'manage impressions' when interacting with others in order to maintain acceptable relationships. The discreditable person whose stigma is not known has another problem to contend with: he or she must manage information to hide the stigma and prevent others from discovering it. Many chronic illnesses carry stigma that can radically affect both the sense of self-identity and interpersonal relationships, for as Cooley has said, the way that we see ourselves is related to (1) our imagined idea of how we appear to others, (2) our imagined understanding of how others view us, and (3) our resultant feelings of pride or mortification. Even cities can experience disease-based stigma, as with the recent SARS outbreak in Toronto. For a period of time people were warned by the World Health Organization to avoid the city. Chinese restaurants lost customers and money as Torontonians and visitors stayed away, fearing transmission of the virus because of its high incidence in China, and Toronto lost millions in tourist dollars.

Cancer has been experienced as one of the most stigmatized of diseases. Among the denigrating beliefs are the following: (1) cancer is fatal; (2) cancer means mutilation; (3) cancer implies a wretched death; (4) it is traitorous; (5) it is unclean; (6) it is contagious; and (7) it is caused by emotional repression (Peters-Golden, 1982). Susan Sontag claims that the stigma associated with cancer is often more painful than the disease itself. As she says, 'Since getting cancer can be a scandal that jeopardizes one's love life, one's chances of promotion, even one's job, patients who know what they have tend to be extremely prudish, if not down-right secretive about their diseases' (Sontag, 1978: 7).

Dunkel-Schetter and Wortman (1982), researchers who have reviewed substantial amounts of literature on the subject and worked as clinicians with cancer patients, confirm that one of the most painful aspects of the disease may be its stigma. An incisive illustration of this point is found in Orville Kelly's book on the subject of coping with cancer. He describes a situation in which a woman approached him after he had given a public lecture and told him that the doctors had once thought that her husband had cancer. The following conversation then ensued:

'Thank God it wasn't cancer!' she exclaimed.
'What was it?' I asked curiously.
'Heart disease,' she replied.
'How is he doing?' I asked.
'Oh, he died later of a heart attack,' she said.
(Kelly, 1979: 5)

Box 8.3   Living With Cancer

What were you doing on 12 October 1995? It was the Thursday just after Thanksgiving of that year. Maybe you were handing in papers to professors or teachers. Maybe you had a cold and were lying in your residence, trying to down the orange juice your roommate had so graciously picked up for you at Brubaker's. Maybe you have no recollection of that day. I do.

That was the day I sat on a hospital bed surrounded by my family at a large teaching hospital. At noon that day I heard for the first time why I had been tired and lacking in strength and energy that summer and the first month of grade twelve. This was also when I learned a little about what would consume the next two years of my life.

My doctors told me that I had been diagnosed, after blood tests and a bone marrow test, with acute lymphoblastic leukemia: cancer of the blood. My doctors were quick to inform me that the disease had been caught early. It was the 'easiest' leukemia to deal with and it had a higher than 80 per cent survival rate. These were great signs. All in all, things couldn't have been better under the circumstances.

I received my first massive chemotherapy dose the next morning. What started so abruptly is a process that I am still living through. Now, almost a tenth of my life has been spent in treatment. I receive steroids and other drugs that, while poisoning and killing my good, healthy powerful cells, are also saving me.

It is amazing to me that so much of my life has been so 'normal' the past two years and yet this shadow, this elephant, has been consistently walking beside me, and at times, nudging me from my path to go off and graze.

Cancer is not a disease that newborns, children, or young adults are supposed to get. Neither is cancer an illness that adults and seniors should have to deal with. It kills, maims, and hurts the millions who receive the diagnosis.

It also has an enormous impact on these individuals' support networks. My family has been walking this path with me, sometimes in more fear and pain than I. Some of my friends have not known what to do or say, and some have pulled through in ways that still keep me warm. . . .

Source: Clarke, with Clarke (1999: 23–4), from *Imprint* (University of Waterloo), 26 Sept. 1997.

Recent research, however, has found that women with breast cancer no longer report feeling stigmatization (Bloom and Kessler, 1994). Indeed, women with breast cancer perceive themselves to have more, not less, social support following the diagnosis. Moreover, women with breast cancer report experiencing more social support following surgery than those with gall bladder disease or benign breast disease.

Schneider and Conrad (1983) emphasize the importance of the stigma of another disease—epilepsy. Epilepsy may imply disgrace and shame. Borrowing a term originally used by the homo-sexual subculture, people with epilepsy are living 'in the closet'. This means that, like gays and lesbians, those with epilepsy have frequently tried to manage their perceptions of being different by isolation and concealment. 'Coming out of the closet', for gays and lesbians, is a political move designed to end the shame and isolation, and to empower and instill pride in people who formerly have felt stigmatized. People with epilepsy and their families have evolved a number of techniques designed to manage information about epilepsy and thus to come out of the closet. Rather than being entirely closet-bound, people with epilepsy go in and out through a 'revolving door' (ibid., 115). Some people can be told, others not. Some can be told at one time but not at another. People with epilepsy have been denied driver's licences, jobs, and even housing. Some people with the disease have therefore learned to hide their diagnosis when filling out application forms or applying for jobs, or when first meeting new people. Managing the anxiety that surrounds the concern about when and whom to tell is an ongoing problem.

People with epilepsy have also developed ways of telling—as therapy and as prevention. Sometimes telling others from whom the epilepsy has been kept secret has therapeutic consequences. It can be cathartic, for example, when a person has kept up a close friendship over a period of time, all the while keeping the truth of epilepsy secret. Telling can also serve preventive purposes. Sometimes this occurs when epileptics believe it likely that others will witness their seizures. It may be hoped that the knowledge that the seizure is due to a defined medical problem and that there are clear ways to deal with it will prevent other people from being frightened.

People with epilepsy have frequently said that these negative social attributions were often more difficult to manage than the disease itself. A superlative account of the processes through which mutual denial of a stigmatized disease is maintained on a verbal level is found in the work of Bluebond-Langer (1978) on children with terminal leukemia. She devotes considerable detail to documenting how doctors, nurses, and parents practised mutual 'pretence' to provide the 'morale' for the continuation of hope through often painful and debilitating treatments. Although they all knew the children were dying, they all agreed not to acknowledge this fact. Meanwhile, the children knew in astonishing detail how long they were likely to live.

There are times when the lack of evidence that a disease exists elicits negative attributions. People with psychosomatic illness may be viewed as malingerers. Because the symptoms of multiple sclerosis can grow and then regress, people with this disease may not seem ill, and friends and acquaintances may complain that they are poor sports or 'just psychosomatically' ill: 'Knowing that I did have the disease was a great relief, but despite this I could not really believe it for some years to come. Other people could see nothing wrong with me and I feared that they regarded me as a malingerer' (Burnfield, 1977: 435).

Managing knowledge and information about the disease and its probable course and effects is crucial in the successful adaptation to chronic illness. Full knowledge can benefit both the person with the disease and the key others who are involved with the person. Knowledge aids not only in the treatment of the disease as a physical entity, but also as an emotional and social challenge to the person with the disease. In *Having Epilepsy*, Schneider and Conrad document the ways in which knowledge is a scarce and valuable resource in coping with epilepsy. Frequently, children with a diagnosis of epilepsy are kept in the dark about the name of the disease, about its duration, and about how to manage it. Often, parents are 'shocked, embarrassed, fearful, and ashamed' that their children have epilepsy, or they are afraid that their child will be ostracized when the diagnosis is made known. Hiding it from the child, according to Schneider and Conrad's findings, is often a source of resentment in the child and leads to greater disability and dependence in the future. As one woman said, talking of her parents, 'I mean, they, the fact that they had never told me and couldn't cope with me, I felt was a total rejection of a child by that parent' (Schneider and Conrad, 1983: 86–8).

Two newer trends in the work on the experience of chronic illness need to be highlighted. The first is the work of Corbin and Strauss (1987) on the BBC chain and the second is the work of Charmaz (1982, 1987) on the struggle for the self. Each brings to the literature a fresh focus on understanding the experiences of chronic illness.

Table 8.2	Identity Preferences
Supernormal Identity	Persons seeking this identity try to do everything even better than those who are 'normal'.
Restored Self	Persons seeking this identity try to be like they were before the illness.
Contingent Personal Identity	Persons in this category try to achieve the above two identities at times but also recognize ongoing rules.
Salvaged Self	Persons seeking this identity try to attain some parts of their previously healthy selves.

Source: Adapted from Charmaz (1987).

Corbin and Strauss consider that the essential social components of this experience involve what they call the BBC chain—*biography, body, and self-conception*. By this, they point out that all who suffer from chronic illness are confronted, through their bodies (and their illness-related constraints, pains, freedoms, change, and so on), with challenges to both self-concepts and personal biography (i.e., the detailed story that the individual tells oneself about his or her life). The point here is that as the body is changed, so, too, are integral parts of the person—the self and the self-story in historical and future context.

Charmaz focuses on one aspect of the chain: *the self*. She argues that when individuals live with the ambiguities of chronic illness they develop preferred identities that 'symbolize assumptions, hopes, desires and plans for the future now unrealized' (1987: 284). Moreover, coping with or managing chronic illness requires a balancing of identities and abilities through what Charmaz thinks of as a hierarchy of preferences. In her studies of people with various types of chronic illness she observed a tendency for people to have a hierarchy of preferences (or levels) for identity. In particular, she suggested a hierarchy beginning with, as a first choice, a supernormal identity and ending with, as last choice, a salvaged identity. Table 8.2 portrays the hierarchically arranged preferred identities of the chronically ill and describes their meaning.

This new focus on the self has also been described by Arthur Frank (1993), based on his analysis of published, book-length illness narratives. His research uncovered three typical change narratives: (1) the rediscovery of the self who has always been; (2) the radical new self who is in the process of becoming; and (3) the no-new-self assertion. Frank, a sociologist who survived two very serious illnesses in his late thirties, a heart attack and then cancer, has written an insightful book about his illness experiences (1991). He has done so as a sociologist and the book is a wealth of sociological theorizing based on bodily and health-related experience.

Case Study: Women and Cancer

The symbolic interaction approach focuses on people's actual experiences and the meaning made of them. To provide an understanding of such research, one case study will be given in detail. It was described in the book *It's Cancer: The Personal Experiences of Women Who Have Received a Cancer Diagnosis* (Clarke, 1985). The research was based on a series of long, unstructured interviews with women who had received a cancer diagnosis at some time in their lives. For some women, the diagnosis was relatively recent; for others it had been made in the distant past. Subjects ranged in age from 17 to 85; some lived in small towns; others in large metropolitan

---

Box 8.4   Becoming Ill

One day my body broke down, forcing me to ask, in fear and frustration, what's happening to me? Becoming ill is asking that question. The problem is that as soon as the body forces the question upon the mind, the medical profession answers by naming a disease. This answer is useful enough for practising medicine, but medicine has its limits.

Medicine has done well with my body, and I am grateful. But doing with the body is only part of what needs to be done for the person.

What happens when my body breaks down happens not just to that body but also to my life, which is lived in that body. When the body breaks down, so does the life. Even when medicine can fix the body, that doesn't always put the life back together again. Medicine can diagnose and treat the breakdown, but sometimes so much fear and frustration have been aroused in the ill person that fixing the breakdown does not quiet them. At those times the experience of illness goes beyond the limits of medicine.

Source: Frank (1991: 8).

---

areas; some worked outside their homes for pay, others worked inside their homes without financial remuneration. These women also varied in religious affiliation and in their degree of religiosity. While most were married, some were single and several were divorced or widowed at the time of the interviews. They had, however, a number of things in common. One was that once they were asked to talk about the impact of cancer on their lives they all had a great deal to say. This was in spite of the fact that many of the women had said to the researcher beforehand that they would not know what to talk about and would need a series of precise questions asked of them.

Subjects were selected because of the commonality of the cancer experience. However, the research focuses not on the disease or on its treatment. Rather, it is concerned with the social world, the family relationships, the concept of the self, and other issues relating to the whole context of the lives of the particular women studied. Being a patient represents a crucial but nevertheless small part of the daily round during a chronic or terminal disease. For most of the women interviewed, the greater part of their lives had no connection with the medical community. Among the questions asked were the following: What is it like when symptoms that are known to be associated with cancer are first noticed—a lump, a persistent cough, or any other the 'warning signs'? How is the time at which the diagnosis was received remembered, thought of, and talked of in the whole context of life? In our cancerphobic society, how does the diagnosis affect the self-concept of the person who is ill? Is there a sense of stigma associated with cancer, as some social commentators have suggested? How do women with cancer feel friends, family, and acquaintances treat them? How do they talk and think about their treatment by medical care personnel?

A number of experiential themes can be drawn from the analysis. Many are useful in attempting to place the experience of cancer in the context of the experience of chronic illness in modern society. The analysis highlights the major issues faced by women as they come to assimilate the diagnosis. The first stage is frequently shock: the person questions realities that were taken for granted, the continuity of the body, the image of the self as a healthy and functioning person. At this stage, women often asked questions such as: Why me? And why here in this organ?

The sense of time changes after a shock. The

assumptions that time is sequential and that activities occur in a managed way are radically altered. Time was experienced by some as external and chaotic. Women said such things as, 'I just didn't know what to do, how to handle it. Should I tell John? Should I call the doctor? Should I eat lunch? Should I go to the grocery store and finish shopping? I just didn't know what to do' (Clarke, 1985: 19). While carrying out routine actions, women were preoccupied with themselves and were isolated in the midst of continuing activity. They were confused about what to do, when and how to do it, and who, when, and what to tell.

Most of us, most of the time, believe we exercise a certain degree of control over our internal and external worlds. Women who had just received a diagnosis of cancer felt they had lost their belief that the world made sense and that most things were, after all, meaningful and controllable. For some, 'magical thinking' seemed to dominate. Women reported thinking that perhaps if they tried to forget about it, it would go away, or perhaps if they didn't tell anyone, if no one else knew, then it would lose its reality. The body, long taken for granted as the house of the self and the source of action, was suddenly untrustworthy. Family heritage, too, sometimes became the subject of new scrutiny.

Once the diagnosis was assimilated, women talked of changed images of themselves— changed self-identities. A number of women talked of how cancer was considered a taboo subject. It was something that was not talked about except in euphemisms such as 'the Big C'. This sense of having been touched by the untouchable led a number of women at this early stage of the disease to see themselves as outcasts and marginal to society. The self-image of a healthy person with nothing to hide quite abruptly changed to a sense of shame and secrecy. Women talked of how at this time they felt themselves to be undesirable as women, sometimes because of the loss of a breast, at other times because of the loss of

other body organs and the necessity of attaching appliances to the body, to control elimination, for example. But even if the diagnosis did not mean surgery and physical alteration of the body, the brush with mortality that cancer seemed to imply for many people was the source of a radical revision in self-concept.

A diagnosis of cancer may lead a woman to re-examine her whole life and its meaning. Existential questioning such as 'Why me?' is an example. Women asked themselves how they could make sense of their cancer diagnosis. By such questions they were expressing an interest in much more than the medical understanding of the causes of their disease. Rather, they asked themselves how it could have been predicted from their past lives and how it could be said to make sense and to be meaningful in the whole context of life. This process is similar to what has been called the legitimation of biography (Marshall, 1980). Marshall describes this as an inevitable process in aging people who, as their lives are drawing to a close, want their story to be a good one, not necessarily a story of success, happiness, fame, and wealth, but a story that 'makes sense', that is meaningful (ibid., 114).

Such a review of life involves criticizing and editing past experiences and decisions so that they make good sense in the whole context of life. For some, cancer was a message from God to return to the fold. For some, it was a message from the fates to eliminate stress or to change life's priorities. Cancer was considered a threat to the continuity of life. Women usually attempted to understand it as a message of symbolic importance and to gain from it a sense of new direction for the future.

This process can also be seen as an aspect of the search for control and mastery that all human beings require. Thus, whether or not they were cognizant of the biomedical analyses of the causes of their disease, women seemed to explain it in their own ways and within the context of their own lives. Women who saw themselves as busy and productive contributors at work and in their family might, for example, explain the anomaly of cancer as a result of the stress they had been feeling. They could then try to reduce that stress. Women for whom religion provided an important sense of identity and social connectedness tended to see their illness in the context of a loss of faithfulness to God or to the church. They could then return to involvement with religion and the church. Those whose primary focus had been the needs of others often decided to put themselves first. Those who were medically more sophisticated, or who had medical doctors or scientists in the immediate family, might tend to attribute the disease to external factors such as pollution or to lifestyle factors such as diet. These things, too, they could attempt to alter. Not only did women understand the meaning or cause of their illness within the context of their whole life story, but they also attempted to change the direction of the life story on the basis of what they had learned from the disease.

A diagnosis of cancer may generate profound self-doubt and renewed self-analysis. It is often accompanied by changed attitudes in friends, family members, acquaintances, and even medical personnel. People may relate to the person with cancer as if she or he has been changed not only physically but morally as well. People often said that other people didn't seem to know how to talk to them or what to talk about. It is as if the whole person has changed. This disease is not seen as just a malfunctioning in one part of the body, but often as a symbol of an inadequate and questionable half-person. The person in many ways becomes, as a result of cancer, marginal to the mainstream of social affairs.

Unlike normal social interaction, interaction with a person with cancer can become confusing and problematic. Cancer is such a feared disease. In fact, according to a survey by James and Lieberman (1975), it may be the most feared disease. As an illustration, one woman talked of meeting a new person and going out to lunch to become better acquainted. She was startled when her 'new friend-to-be' said that she was sorry, that she would really like to become her friend but was not willing to invest in someone who wouldn't be around much longer. Another woman spoke of walking down her street just after she arrived home from the hospital and seeing a neighbour hide behind a curtain rather than wave or walk outside for a chat, as would have been normal before the diagnosis. Fear of future loss or unpredictable disruption in the relationship may be one of the threats faced by people in contact with a person who has received a diagnosis of cancer.

Summary

(1) Disease is an abnormality, diagnosed by a doctor, in the structure and function of body organs and systems. Illness is the personal experience of one who has been diagnosed by a doctor or who does not feel well; it involves changes in states of being and in social function. Sickness is the social actions or roles taken up by individuals who experience illness or are diagnosed with a disease.

(2) Illness, sickness, and disease are all socially and culturally mediated experiences.

(3) In the Western world, illness is thought to be empirically caused and mechanically or chemically treatable. In non-Western cultures, illness and cure have a non-empirical basis. The experience of pain differs from culture to culture and, at times, so does what is viewed as illness and as health.

(4) Western industrialized society has become increasingly medicalized. The medical profession understands illness through a biomedical model, three perspectives of which are the germ theory, the mechanistic concept, and the cellular concept.

(5) Life experiences of individuals as they encounter illness, such as cancer, are of concern to sociologists. People with cancer tend

to experience shock and to find social interaction confusing and problematic. This could be a result of the stigma placed on cancer, which, at times, can be more painful for the patient than the disease itself. This is common to all stigmatized diseases, for example, epilepsy and AIDS.

(6) Uncertainty is another common reaction among those with chronic illnesses. It affects the individual's self-image and also his/her interpersonal relationships. Uncertainty prevails at all stages of illness, including diagnosis, treatment, spread and resurgence, and remission. It is difficult to make plans for the future.

(7) How to manage medical regimens is another issue for those who are chronically ill.

Lifestyle changes and learning how to manage medication and treatment serve to add to the problems of one who faces chronic illness.

(8) Knowledge and information about the disease and its probable course and effects help the individual and significant others to adapt to chronic illness. Information that the public has about the disease is also important to the individual when dealing with normal social interaction. A significant source of information in modern society is the mass media.

(9) The media can associate certain meanings with diseases. From these meanings that we get from the media, we may create images of people who have certain diseases.

Questions for Study and Discussion

1. Describe a situation in which you experienced illness, sickness, and/or disease and consider the tensions among these three aspects of the experience.

2. Provide examples of five of the several popular conceptions of illness.

3. Examine a popular magazine for discussions of illness, disease, and sickness. What images of disease are evident?

4. Look for 10 Web sites on a disease of interest to you. What meanings are assumed and portrayed?

5. Do you think the images of heart disease, cancer, and AIDS described in the research discussed in the chapter are still relevant today? What might be the relevance of the portrayal of disease, illness, or sickness for the individual and family experience of the disease?

6. Do you suffer from or do you know anyone who has a chronic illness? Do the challenges articulated in this chapter reflect your understanding of the experiences that you or this other person have?

Suggested Readings

Cousins, Norman. 1983. *The Healing Heart*. New York: Norton. Cousins's work was part of the revolution in health care pointing to a new focus on the relationship between the mind and body.

Currie, Dawn. 1988. 'Starvation Amidst Abundance: Female Adolescence and Anorexia', in Bolaria and Dickinson (1988: 198–216). One of the best

overviews of the sociological perspective on eating disorders.

Dossey, Larry. 1991. *Meaning and Medicine*. New York: Bantam Books. Dossey is a popular writer in the area of mind/body relationships and health.

Freidson, Eliot. 1970. *Professional Dominance: The Social Structure of Medical Care*. New York: Atherton

Press. A theoretical examination of power and medical practice.

Paget, Marianne A. 1993. *A Complex Sorrow: Reflections on Cancer and an Abbreviated Life*, ed. Marjorie L. Devault. Philadelphia: Temple University Press. Both emotionally moving and intellectually challenging, this book tells the story of a medical sociologist whose own misdiagnosis led to an early death.

Simonton, Carl O., Stephanie Matthews Simonton, and James L. Creighton. 1978. *Getting Well Again.*

Toronto: Bantam Books. Mostly of historical interest, but immensely valuable as one of the first popular studies of the influence of the mind on cancer.

Weitz, Rose. 1999. 'Watching Brian Die: The Rhetoric and Reality of Informed Consent', *Health* 3, 2: 209–27. Weitz's work exemplifies a new type of sociological method called autoethnography. In this paper she discusses her personal reactions to a serious accident of a family member.

Part III Sociology of Medicine

The next eight chapters of the book discuss issues in the sociology of medicine. Rather than investigating and discussing the causes of death and disease, how they vary across different parts of the social structure, or the experience of sickness, illness, and disease, this component of the book will examine the ways that medical practitioners and scientists define illness and sickness as disease and the implications of this social construction.

Chapter Nine focuses on the sociology of medical knowledge. Starting from the premise that all that we know, understand, and believe about the world is related to the social and cultural environments in which we grow up and live, the chapter analyzes how medical knowledge is related to the social backgrounds of physicians and research scientists as well as to the social organizations of which they are a part. This chapter also examines briefly how the social characteristics of patients affect the diagnostic decisions of doctors. Medical treatment, the chapter demonstrates, is not an objective higher-order reality that stands above the real-world machinations of human beings as they go about their everyday lives; rather, it is entirely integrated into that world. Chapter Ten examines the current medical care system and the science upon which it is based through a historical overview of the place of medicine as a world view and practice of relevance to human social behaviour. It also looks at some of the processes through which the medical profession gained the power to define many human behaviours as within its realm of responsibility (medicalization). Here the ways in which the doctor can be seen as a moral entrepreneur are discussed. Chapter Eleven also takes a historical approach. It examines the history, origins, and some of the current issues facing the medical care system. Some of the impacts of the medicare system on the work of the doctor, on the disease profiles of the population, and on the death rates are considered. Chapter Twelve looks at allopathic medical practice as a profession. It discusses medical education in the past and today. Medical mistakes and their handling, along with malpractice, medical markets, and medical subcultures, are also discussed. Chapter Thirteen focuses on two critiques of the contemporary medical care system. The first is the relative dominance of the medical model as compared to other ways of understanding causes and treatments for disease, such as the lifestyle and the environmental/social structural models. The second critique details the extent of sexism and patriarchy in the medical care system. Chapter Fourteen looks at the history and the work of nurses and midwives in social context. It also examines some of the challenges currently facing nurses and midwives in their practice in Canada today. Chapter Fifteen briefly describes the growing importance of various complementary and alternative practices related to health and health care. In addition, it describes in somewhat more detail the philosophies and work practices of chiropractors and naturopathic doctors. Finally, Chapter Sixteen describes and critically analyzes the medical-industrial complex. It pays particular attention to the pharmaceutical industry, the major industry in this complex about which there is significant research.

This third part of the book covers some of what is traditionally covered in a course in the sociology of medicine. It does not, however, discuss hospital structures and functioning or the place of hospitals in society today. Nor does it address in depth issues related to home care. In both cases much more Canadian and other research needs to be undertaken.

Chapter 9

The Social Construction of Scientific and Medical Knowledge and Medical Practice

Learning Objectives

- Both medical practice and scientific knowledge are products of the societies in which they occur. They are also affected by history.
- The modern and Western medical model of disease is only one possible understanding.
- The medical model encompasses a number of value judgements. There is a gap between scientific values and the work of science and that of the doctor.
- Technology seems to have its own imperatives.
- Medical science and practice are infused with cultural understandings such as gender role stereotypes.
- Medical knowledge is both accepted and rejected by different parts of the population at different times.
- Doctor-patient communication reflects broader social structure and cultural issues.

Introduction: The Sociology of Medical Knowledge

Is scientific knowledge universally true? Is scientific knowledge objective? Is medical knowledge based on science? Is medical practice based on science? Given a choice, how can a person decide whether to take chemotherapy and/or radiation or to do visualization, immunotherapy, or something else after a cancer diagnosis? Is chronic fatigue syndrome really just a 'yuppie flu' experienced by spoiled middle-class and upper-middle-class women or is it a 'real' disease? Do allopathic doctors have a 'better' theory of medicine than chiropractic or naturopathic doctors? Does the introduction of a new technology, for example the CAT scanner, occur as the final stage of a process of rational decision-making, including cost-benefit analysis and an evaluation of its efficacy and efficiency? Does medical science reflect cultural attitudes, such as racism, sexism, and homophobia, or is it a neutral and objective endeavour?

This chapter will investigate the sociology of medical science and medical practice. To say that there is a sociology of medical science is to say that it is reasonable to examine how medical and scientific knowledge are determined, created, and constructed by, or at least influenced by, social

Box 9.1   Prozac

One of the most interesting public debates in recent years is the debate over 'personality-changing' drugs such as Prozac (Kramer, 1993). The miraculous nature of this drug's effects on a wide variety of symptoms, coupled with its supposed lack of side effects, has led to disagreement about the ethics of prescribing or refusing to prescribe a drug reputed to make people feel 'better than well'. The availability of Prozac begs the question of whether people ought to take drugs that change their very selves (personalities) to make them 'better than well'. Prozac's existence also raises the question of whether doctors should have the right to prescribe or withhold this powerful 'feel-good' drug. What do you think?

conditions. It is also of value to explore how medical science affects or constructs social conditions. Moreover, in the tradition of conflict theory, it is possible to ask whose interests the present forms of medical knowledge, organization, and practice serve. The meanings and constructions of medical science and practice are also topics for discussion. This approach is consistent with another substantive field within sociology, the sociology of knowledge, described as follows:

> the objectivity of the institutional world, however massive it may appear to the individual, is a humanly produced, constructed objectivity. The process by which the externalized products of human activity attain the character of objectivity is objectification. The institutional world is objectified human activity, and so is every single institution. (Berger and Luckmann, 1966: 60–1)

The argument of this chapter is as follows. Science is humanly produced. It has become embedded in an institutional structure and is maintained through processes of negotiation by some actors who live in a particular time (history) and place (culture, society, strata). Medical practice is based on this socially constructed science and is also influenced by other social forces, such as the particular social characteristics of the medical care labour force and the socio-economic backgrounds from which the members of the labour force have been drawn and within which they continue to live.

Medical and Scientific Knowledge: Historical and Cross-Cultural Context

Positivism, the model of science upon which medicine is based, is described by attributes such as objectivity, precision, certainty (within a specific degree of error), generalizability, quantification, replication, and causality. Its search is ultimately for a series of law-like propositions. These, its formal characteristics, portray science as if it stands over and above the ways of the world. Science, in this view, is outside of culture and social structure. It would follow that the subjects of study, the methods of studying such subjects, the findings and their interpretation, the publication and dissemination of scientific knowledge, would follow the same course everywhere and at every time in history. However, there are many reasons to challenge this assumption.

A number of social theorists and researchers have demonstrated that beliefs regarding scientific objectivity are problematic. Kuhn (1962) has described the historical development of science and how the methods, assumptions, and even the very subject matter of science are infused with cultural categories. Freund and McGuire (1991) have specified the value assumptions of contemporary medicine as: mind-body dualism, physical reductionism, specific etiology, machine metaphor, and regimen and control.

Mind-body dualism is said to have begun with

Descartes, the philosopher who effectively argued the case for the separation of the mind from the body. Descartes's writing and thinking, however, arose out of a context of increasing secularization, which allowed for the separation of the body from the soul/mind. It wasn't until the Christian doctrine determined that the soul could be sent heavenward after death, without the body, that a notion of a secular body, which was accessible to scientific investigation, became possible. Foucault (1975) has described the changes in the eighteenth and nineteenth centuries that allowed the physician to view the patient's body directly through the 'clinical gaze', and not merely indirectly through the patient's verbal descriptions. Specific technical inventions such as the stethoscope gave physicians direct access to bodily functioning. With a stethoscope the doctor could observe, categorize, and explain the patient's body (or a part of the body) without the conscious awareness or involvement of the patient. Dissection of cadavers opened up a new world of patienthood and medicine for description and explanation. Such inventions further entrenched the distinction between the soul/mind and the body as they made the body into a precisely describable and observable empirical entity. .

Physical reductionism emphasizes the physically observable at the expense of other aspects of the individual, such as the mental, sensual, and the emotional. It also leads to a disregard of social, political, and economic causes of ill health.

René Dubos (1959) was the first to write that *the doctrine of specific etiology* is another characteristic of modern medical science. It developed from the discoveries of nineteenth-century researchers such as Pasteur and Koch, who noted the specific effects of particular microorganisms on the body, and it has led to an exaggerated emphasis on the discovery of the 'magic bullet' to cure one specific disease after another. Dubos notes that this emphasis is overly restrictive because it ignores the fact that the very same microorganisms may assault a number of people but only a certain proportion of

these people respond by becoming ill. It is also problematic because it has tended to ignore how a treatment for one disease may lead to side effects that may cause other diseases.

The machine metaphor for the body emphasizes discrete parts, such as individual organs, and their relationship to other discrete parts. Resulting from this are specialization and the removal and replacement of parts of the body, such as heart, kidney, liver, blood, and bone marrow.

Finally, *regimen and control* are an outgrowth of the machine metaphor. They involve the underlying assumption that the body is to be dealt with, fixed, improved. Not only strictly medical procedures but even health promotion policies imply that the body is perfectible and under the control of the individual through such actions as exercise and diet, and by maintaining healthy habits, such as not smoking and consuming alcohol only moderately. An emphasis on the correct number and spacing of checkups reinforces this notion of the perfectible body. Stein has noted how Western, particularly American, medicine has adapted to American cultural values. As he says:

> disease conceptualization and treatment are embedded in the value system of self-reliance, rugged individualism, independence, pragmatism, empiricism, atomism, privatism, emotional minimalism and a mechanistic metaphor of the body. (Stein, 1990: 21)

In an expanded analysis of the foundations of the medical model, Manning and Fabrega (1973) articulate the elements of what they call the *biologistic* view of the body. The biologistic view of the body includes the following tenets: first, organs and organ systems, and their specific functions, are identifiable and observable as discrete entities; second, the normal functioning of the body goes on pretty much the same for everybody unless disturbed by injury or illness; third, people's sensory experiences are universal; fourth, disease and experience of disease do not vary from one culture to another; fifth, bound-

Box 9.2   Do You Know What Causes HIV/AIDS?

What do you think causes HIV/AIDS? What do you do to prevent becoming infected? North American children and adults have been exposed to information about the transmission of HIV in schools and through doctors, public health initiatives, and the mass media. We have been advised to avoid sexual intercourse or needle sharing with an infected person, to use blood that has been screened and determined to be clear of the HIV virus, and to prevent childbirth or pregnancy if infected because the virus is transmitted through bodily fluids. Most of us have heard of the new anti-viral drugs used to maintain life and extend life expectancy in the presence of a diagnosis of HIV/AIDS.

During 2002 in South Africa, 21,000 cases of child rape were reported to the police. In the middle of July a one-week-old baby was raped. Her mother changed her diaper only to find bruising around her genitals and bloodstains on the diaper. This baby was the youngest child in this series of child rapes said to be motivated by the belief said to be prevalent in sub-Saharan Africa that sex with a virgin cures AIDS.

'Week old infant raped in S. Africa', *Toronto Star*, 31 July 2002, A2.

---

aries between self and body and between self and others are obvious and shared; sixth, death is the body's ceasing to function; and seventh, bodies should be seen objectively.

Sociological research allows us to critique all of these assumptions. First, being able to observe organs and organ symptoms depends directly on the tools available for measurement and indirectly on the theories of the body and the level of technology in a given culture. For example, the psychoneuroimmunological system has just been 'discovered' and methods are now being developed to study it as a new system. Awareness of the possibilities of research on the body/mind connection is, in part, the result of the re-establishment of the link between mind and body that has come from the Eastern medical tradition, including meditation in particular. Second, it has become clear that much of the research on the 'normal person' has been on the male person. Thus, less is known about the functioning of the female body (except the reproductive functioning) with respect to a whole range of disease categories such as heart disease. Third, cross-cultural, anthropological, and linguistic studies have shown how people's experiences arise out of their available language. Fourth, cross-cultural research has shown that what is considered disease in one culture may be considered normal in another (e.g., the Japanese have named a new disease category—Karoshi, which is disease and death as a result of overwork). Fifth, contagious diseases such as AIDS raise serious questions about the vulnerable boundaries between people's bodies. Sixth, the definition of death is now very problematic in part because of the possibility that, for instance, 'machines' can keep people alive even when they are 'brain-dead'. Seventh, perhaps bodies should be seen objectively, but that is an impossible value to achieve. The values implicit in the medical model and in the biologistic view of the body reflect particular cultural histories, biases, and predispositions. Medical science and practice are not objective and do not stand above everyday social practices.

Medical Science and Medical Practice: A Gap in Values

There is often a significant gap between published biomedical research and the actual practice of medicine (see Montini and Slobin, 1991). To try to minimize the distance between researcher and practitioner, the National Institutes of Health in the United States, through the Office of Medical Applications of Research, began in 1977 to convene Consensus Development Conferences (CDCs). The Canadian government and medical associations have also initiated this process at times. The goal of these conferences has been to bring together practitioners and researchers, to inform practitioners of the latest scientific findings, to inform scientists of the practical issues facing practitioners, and to work towards the development of timely, national standards of practice.

Unfortunately, the research to date has indicated that the CDCs have little or no effect on physicians' practice. Montini and Slobin show how various differences in the work cultures of clinicians and researchers have served to limit the effectiveness of CDCs for medical practice. These differences relate to distinct *value differences between researchers and practitioners*, including (1) certainty versus uncertainty, (2) evolutionary time versus clinical timeliness, (3) aggregate measures versus individual prescriptions, (4) scientific objectivity versus clinical experience, and (5) constant change versus standards of treatment.

(1) Doctors' work involves patients who want and need an immediate and certain response. Scientific work does not depend on or even expect certainty; rather, probability is the focus. Time-related concerns are considerably different. The practitioner needs at least enough certainty to make decisions about caring for a particular patient at a specific point in time. By contrast, the scientist works within a world of probabilities—thus, uncertainty.

(2) Science does not progress by proof but rather by failing to disprove. There is always caution in drawing conclusions. Scientific truth develops in incremental stages as more and more hypotheses are disconfirmed. However, the clinician must make timely decisions in response to the expressed and observed needs of individual patients.

(3) While the scientist, in working with probabilities, deals in aggregates, the practitioner must deal with the suffering individual. Again, because of the immediacy of the sufferer, clinicians need to rely on what they know from experience to be tried and true. They may at times be uneasy about relegating a given individual to a clinical trial whose outcome is unknown and will likely be unknown for a considerable period of time.

(4) The scientist tries to control all variables in the interest of objective and generalizable findings. The clinician, in contrast, is faced with a unique and changing individual and, usually, subjectively experienced symptoms.

(5) The researcher is aware of continuous change in research findings as new hypotheses are put forward and supported or rejected. The clinician, on the other hand, attempts to practice medicine under the direction and with the support of practice standards that must have a longer life than frequently changing scientific hypotheses.

Medical Technology: The Technological Imperative

New medical technologies continue to be developed, manufactured, distributed, and employed. Among the new technologies are cardiac life support, renal dialysis, nutritional support and hydration, mechanical ventilation, organ transplantation and various other surgical procedures, pacemakers, chemotherapy, and antibiotics. The question that we ask here is: What is the relationship between medical science and this evaluation process that culminates in the use of new technologies? Available evidence suggests that practitioners tend to adopt new technologies before they are evaluated and continue to use them after evaluation indicates they are ineffective or unsafe (Rachlis and Kushner, 1989: 186).

In fact, the introduction of new medical technologies and their use patterns have been shown to be related to four social forces (Butler, 1993). These are: (1) *key societal values*; (2) *feder-*

al government policies (while this study is based in the US, there is no reason to assume that Canadian legislation provides greater safeguards, and, in fact, available evidence indicates that in many ways, e.g., the thalidomide disaster of the fifties and sixties, Canadian regulation may be more lenient); (3) *reimbursement strategies*; and (4) *economic incentives*.

(1) A number of social commentators have described the love affair of North Americans with new technology of all sorts. Enthusiastic optimism rather than realistic caution typifies our attitude to new technology. For example, while we have yet to understand all of the possible constraints to freedom and democracy created by the Internet, plus other threats that may easily result from global electronic communication, it already exists and is in widespread use. Moreover, the development of other new and related technologies continues to precede considerations of and safeguards for social impacts.

(2) In the health area, the federal government, through the Medical Research Council, the Heart and Lung Association, and the National Cancer Institute, quietly funds biomedical research. Taxation policies, free trade agreements, support for education and science, and other federal incentives encourage the discovery of new technologies. Our national medical care system has operated to foster growth and expansion of the use of medical technologies immediately upon their development.

(3 and 4) While there are no definitive studies of the costs of new technology, a variety of studies taken together suggest that 20–50 per cent of the annual increases in health-care costs during the past 20 years or so are the result of progressive innovations in medical technology, including pharmaceuticals. A few new technologies appear to save costs—e.g., cimetidine for peptic ulcers and lithotripsy for the removal of kidney stones. Most new technologies are expensive, however, and add costs to the medical care system. As long as the medical-industrial com-

plex is even partly guided by privatization and the profit motive, the development and dissemination of medical technological innovations will result from market principles rather than planned, rational, and evaluated change strategies. For instance, babies weighing as little as one pound can now be 'saved' at a cost of several hundreds of thousands of dollars per baby through neonatal intensive care for a number of months, and then continuing care for those babies and children with ongoing medical and other needs. By contrast, a low-technology approach to preventing low-birth-weight babies that would include feeding pregnant women nutritious diets and maintaining minimal equitable socio-economic standards (via, for instance, a guaranteed annual wage) for all—a much more effective and efficient strategy for a healthy citizenry—has yet to be implemented.

One of the best examples of the tendency for new technologies to be adopted first and then evaluated later is demonstrated by the case of electronic fetal monitoring. Designed first for use with high-risk births, it was to provide doctors information regarding the health of the fetus during labour. If a fetus showed dangerous vital signs the physician could actively intervene in the labour process by Caesarean section, for example. Electronic fetal monitoring (EFM) was initially made available in the 1960s. By the 1970s EFM and ultrasound were widely available in most hospitals. By the 1980s, 30 per cent of all obstetricians had EFM in their offices to detect prenatal problems. It rapidly became a standard monitoring device, even for low-risk situations. Its widespread use was associated with a growth in the diagnosis of prenatal problems. The Caesarean section rate, at 4.5 per cent of all births in 1965, rose to 16.5 per cent by 1980 and 24.7 per cent by 1988. (C-sections were the most common surgical procedure in US hospitals in 1989.) Studies, moreover, found that the rate varied substantially by region, ethnicity, socio-economic status, and availability of insurance for payment.

Box 9.3   Même Breast Implants: Public Policy, Scientific Knowledge, and Medical Practice

Medical devices range from contact lenses to CAT scanners, MRIs, and hip replacement parts. One of the most controversial of medical devices in recent years is the widely used and accepted silicone breast implant. Information about its side effects and other problems associated with its insertion followed its widespread adoption. Même silicone breast implants are a case in point. Most breast implants have been available on the Canadian market since before 1982 and were thus exempt from federal regulation requiring that manufacturers of new medical devices implanted into the body for 30 days or more submit data on the safety and efficiency of proposed new products.

By 1988 a Public Citizens Health Research Group in Washington released data indicating that 23 per cent of rats injected with silicone developed highly malignant cancers. Questions were then raised in the House of Commons. An article was published in the Canadian scientific journal, *Transplantation/Implantation Today*, presenting the evidence that polyurethanes (of which the Même was constructed) were known to deteriorate in the human body. There was still no direct evidence about the long- or short-term effect of breast implants. A registry of all Canadian women who received breast implants, with a health follow-up, was considered, but it was not implemented. Nicholas Regush, a *Montreal Gazette* investigative health reporter, wrote an article questioning the health effects and legal status of the Même breast implant. Although it had been introduced and used since 1982, not only was there no record of its sale in Canada but there were no safety data on file. A number of women who had received transplants responded quickly to Regush's article, and an organic chemist from the University of Florida called to inform him that he had found 2–4 toluene

diamine, a potential carcinogen, in the Même's polyurethane cover. Research had indicated that 2–4 toluene diamine had caused liver damage, central nervous system problems, blindness, and skin blistering. Despite evidence from several sources that there could be dangers associated with the Même breast implant, active lobbying efforts in both the United States and Canada, and more 'horror' stories from individual women, as well as the active opposition of the (later fired) Health Protection Branch's expert on breast implants, Pierre Blais, the federal government did nothing. In one memo Blais tried to warn his bosses of the hazards of the Même:

In late January 1989, I reported to you that prosthesis coating is made from a common class of commercial polyurethane foam available from various vendors for assorted consumer product applications. Industrial (non-specific) applications of such foams allow broad compositional variations, elevated impurity levels and the incorporation of reactive intermediates of unknown biocompatibility. The safety, efficiency and quality assurance levels of a medical implant based on these foams therefore cannot be demonstrated without testing each implant. (Regush, 1993: 91)

In response to growing concern raised in the House, the Health Minister, Perrin Beatty, appointed a plastic surgeon to conduct an 'independent' review. Her review concluded, on the basis of a number of poorly controlled studies, that the Même could be declared neither safe nor unsafe. It was not until a few years later that the FDA commissioner in the US, on 6 January 1992, declared a moratorium on breast implants. Two days later Benoît Bouchard, at the time Canada's Health Minister, followed suit with a Canadian moratorium. This was almost 12 years after Regush had first raised questions about the safety of breast implants.

The response of the plastic surgeons is instructive. As a group, they retaliated with a $3.88 million campaign lamenting the loss of choice for women. Later, a number of individual and class action suits were filed by women against various manufacturers of breast implants. The women won. More recently, a new story in the long saga with breast implants broke. Dow Corning (US) had filed for bankruptcy, claiming that it couldn't both pay the awards to the women who had sued and remain profitable.

Despite the rapid growth in the use of electronic fetal monitoring, randomized, controlled trials undertaken since 1976 have failed to demonstrate benefits of EFM in comparison with simpler methods of monitoring, such as the stethoscope. Moreover, EFM leads to certain risks for fetus and mother. The safety of ultrasound still remains to be established. In addition, overuse of technology has been estimated at 20 per cent, 17 per cent, and 15 per cent for cardiac pacemakers, gastrointestinal endoscopy, and coronary bypass surgery, respectively (ibid.). McKinlay and McKinlay (1981) provided a model—the seven stages in the career of a medical invention—they argued could be used to explain the dissemination of new medical technologies.

Stage 1: A promising report.
Stage 2: Professional and organizational adoption.
Stage 3: Public acceptance and state (third-party) endorsement.
Stage 4: Standard procedure and observational reports.
Stage 5: Randomized controlled trial.
Stage 6: Professional denunciation.
Stage 7: Erosion and discreditation.

The most important point is that evaluation, which is purported and believed to be the bedrock of scientifically based treatment innovations, occurs at stages 4 and 5, long after the introduction and widespread use of a medical invention.

Medical Science Reinforces Gender Role Stereotypes

Scientific medical knowledge is portrayed as an objective, generalizable, and positive accomplishment. Yet, what is taken to be objective medical science has been shown to reflect fundamental cultural and social-structural beliefs (Clark et al., 1991). Normative categories of social relations, in fact, infuse medical conceptions. Findlay (1993) studied the 10 most highly circulating texts in obstetrics and gynecology in the 1950s in Canada, as well as a representative selection of academic articles from five major obstetrics/gynecology journals and from the *Canadian Medical Association Journal*. Her research showed that physicians' descriptions and understandings of the female body guarded and reflected family values. The publications emphasized the importance of separate spheres for men and women, of stable marriage and family life, and encouraged fertility among women (who were assumed to be white and middle-class). Findlay noted that the essence of the 'normal' woman was to be always potentially fertile. Women's bodies were described largely with respect to fluctuations in their hormones and menstrual cycles. They were described as living to reproduce. As Findlay reports, one influential obstetrician/gynecologist explained: 'The desire for children by the normal woman is stronger than self interest in beauty and figure, stronger than the claims of a career, [while] in the man it is less intense' (Jeffcoate, 1957, in Findlay, 1993). By

Box 9.4   Chronic Fatigue Syndrome: A Diagnostic and Moral Enigma

Perhaps one of the most common complaints that humans suffer is tiredness. Who has not felt tired at one time or another? Most people have suffered a headache at some time. All have experienced vague discomfort or pain periodically. People who visit doctors with symptoms in patterns that include fatigue, vague bodily complaints, and aches and pains have received a variety of diagnoses over the years. They inhabit an area of anomie, of ambiguity. A century ago they might have been diagnosed with neurasthenia or chlorosis; today they may be diagnosed with chronic fatigue syndrome. In the US the oldest epidemic usually included with this realm of symptom patterns is an outbreak of atypical poliomyelitis among hospital workers at Los Angeles County General Hospital in 1934.

Since the early 1980s a series of case studies and epidemiological and psychosocial research have been undertaken on a disease characterized by viral-like symptoms manifest as weakness, exhaustion, and other self-defined symptoms. First officially called Epstein-Barr virus (EBV), it appeared to be associated with serological evidence of recurrent or prolonged infection with this virus. One of the difficulties involved in this diagnosis is that almost everyone has EBV antibodies because they have been exposed to the virus at one time or another. During the same years that the studies were published, the Atlanta Centers for Disease Control investigated an outbreak of a prolonged sickness in over 100 patients near Lake Tahoe, Nevada. EBV antibodies were not particularly associated with this outbreak. A new consensus conference was called and the disease was renamed chronic fatigue syndrome (CFS) and new diagnostic criteria were developed (1988). All diagnostic criteria were patient-defined signs. Later, skepticism resumed in the face of the lack of patho-biological criteria and studies calling CFS a psychiatric disorder emerged. The medical legitimation of CFS is still lacking and people continue both to suffer the symptoms and, at times, to be refused disability insurance.

contrast, the abnormal woman was defined as one who had sexual or reproductive problems.

Emily Martin's *The Woman in the Body* (1987) also instructs us about gender biases in medical conceptions of women's bodies and their functions. She demonstrates how culture shapes what biological scientists see. One interesting illustration of her thesis is how assumptions about gender infuse descriptions of the reproductive cycle and its elements, such as the egg and sperm. For instance, the female menstrual cycle is described in negative terms. Menstruation is said to rid the body of waste, of debris, of dead tissue. It is described as a system gone awry. By contrast, while most sperm are also 'useless' and 'wasted', the life of the sperm is described as a 'feat'. The magnitude of the production of sperm is consid-

ered remarkable and valuable. Whereas female ovulation is described as a process where eggs sit and wait and then get old and useless, male spermatogenesis is described as continuously producing fresh, active, strong, and efficient sperm. While the eggs are swept and drift down the fallopian tubes like flotsam, sperm actively and in a 'manly' and machismo fashion burrow and penetrate.

The Sociology of Medical Practice

Just as medical/scientific knowledge is a social product with social consequences, so, too, is the everyday practice of medicine. Have you ever left your doctor's office only to realize that you had forgotten to tell or ask him/her about something?

Box 9.5   Medicalization and Demedicalization of Homosexuality

In the nineteenth century, homosexuality was defined as a disease. In the past two decades or so it has been demedicalized. The definition of homosexuality as a disease was part of a nineteenth-century trend. As science and medicine were becoming more widely legitimate and as secularization was beginning to occur, behaviours formerly defined as sin became adopted as diseases. The sick were thereby held to be largely blameless. This process was true of drug and alcohol addiction, compulsions, anxiety, and depression, as well as homosexuality.

Besides being a part of the general trend to humanize and secularize behaviour, disease-making in the case of homosexuality had other explanations. Hansen (1988) links the medical 'discovery' of homosexuality to urbanization and the gradual development of self-conscious homosexual communities in large cities whose density of single people enabled single-sex groupings and culture. Parallel to this was the development of a new medical specialty: neurology. Neurologists tended to deal

on an outpatient basis with people with a variety of 'nervous' symptoms. Neurologists were a logical choice for assisting people who were ambivalent about their sexual appetites (ibid., 104–33). It wasn't until 1869 that the first medical case describing same-sex sexual activity was published in Berlin in *Archiv für Psychiatrie und Nervenkrankheiten*. After that, more cases were published in Germany, France, Italy, Britain, and the US. The terms used at this time included 'sexual inversion', 'contrary sexual instinct', and 'sexual perversion'.

Hansen's analysis emphasizes the mutual benefits to doctors and homosexuals involved in the medicalization of homosexuality. The diagnosis provided a name for people and this enabled them to realize that they were not alone. Ironically, then, the labelling facilitated self-conscious acceptance among some, the development and maintenance of alternative homosexual cultures, and, eventually, the modern successful lobbying that led to the demedicalization of homosexuality.

Have you ever left the office unclear about what the doctor has said about your problem/disease, your medication, or something else? Have you ever felt that you 'couldn't get a word in edgewise' in a conversation with your physician? Have you ever asked for a second opinion or been skeptical about a doctor's diagnosis?

Considerable evidence demonstrates that medical knowledge and practice are profoundly affected by social characteristics of both patients and doctors. First, with regard to patients, there is evidence that physicians tend to prefer younger patients and to hold negative images of elderly patients. Elderly patients tend to be seen as both sicker and less amenable to treatment than younger patients. The older patient, 'far in excess of actual numbers, represents the negative idea of

the uncooperative, intractable, and generally troublesome patient' (Clark et al., 1991: 855). Elderly patients are significantly more likely to be treated with digitalis, tranquilizers, and analgesics, regardless of their actual diagnoses. Several studies have looked at the impact of attitudes towards gender on medical diagnosis and treatment. Their findings are contradictory (ibid.; see Chapters Five and Thirteen for more complete discussion of age, gender, and health).

Physicians' attitudes/actions in regard to ethnic characteristics reflect those of the wider sociocultural context of which physicians are a part. For instance, several US-based studies have demonstrated that black patients tend to be referred to specialists less often, are treated more often by doctors-in-training, are more likely to be

Box 9.6   Task Force on Sexual Abuse of Patients

A task force to examine sexual abuse of patients was established by the College of Physicians and Surgeons of Ontario. Its 1991 report documented the significant level of sexual abuse by physicians of patients. In all, the task force documented 303 detailed reports of sexual abuse by physicians and others in a position of trust. Sixteen reports were of the abuse of men; in the remaining 287 cases the victims were women. The actual incidence has been estimated in a few other studies—about 7–13 per cent of physicians have had sexual or erotic contact with patients. A survey of Ontario women found that 8 per cent of Ontario women reported sexual harassment or abuse by doctors.

The consequences of this abuse of power and sexual integrity are known to be far-reaching and include physical symptoms such as abdominal pain, pelvic pain, gastrointestinal tract problems, and headaches, as well as eating disorders and drug and alcohol abuse. The psychological problems include intense anxiety, fear, panic, depression, suicidal feel-ings, loss of trust in the world, difficulty in developing and maintaining intimate and/or sexual relationships, flashbacks, nightmares, and sleep disorders.

In light of these findings, the task force recommended a policy of zero tolerance so that sexual abuse is never acceptable or tolerated. They also recommended education for the public about appropriate physician examinations, awareness of warning signs, education for physicians about how to prevent such behaviour in themselves and how to help patients who have been abused by another physician, and education for the College to encourage it to respond sensitively and effectively to complaints and reports of physician misbehaviour. Various other remedial and monitoring strategies were advocated as well.

The issue of penalties for physicians who have been found guilty of sexual abuse has generated a great deal of controversy, in particular the mandatory revocation of licence for a minimum of five years and a fine of up to $20,000.

Box 9.7   Looking for Health Information on the Internet

Looking for information about health, disease, and treatments on the Internet is one of its most popular reasons for use. There are probably millions of sites dedicated to various health matters, including sites on specific diseases, related goods and services, hospitals and health-care organizations, chat rooms, and on-line support groups. With such a myriad of possibilities, how can one be assured of access to good, valid, and confidential information? What criteria should be used to assess health information? Many librarians, health-care professionals, and interested lay people have developed strategies and checklists to be used in evaluating articles on the Net. The code established by the Health on the Net (HON) Foundation is one indication that a Web site has been evaluated and found trustworthy. The HON code requires that sites that receive this seal of approval include the following: information is to be provided by a trained professional; it is to be confidential; references are to be given where possible; information is clear; contact addresses are available; and the advertising policy is transparent and shown on the site.

How useful do you think these criteria are in the light of medical dominance ? Whose interests might these sites serve? What sorts of knowledge are taken to be valid and reliable?

placed on a ward, and are admitted less frequently to hospital except when they are involuntarily hospitalized for mental health problems. Black patients also tend to receive less aggressive workups and intervention. There are documented differences, too, in the way that physicians treat patients of different class backgrounds. For example, patients with poorer backgrounds are likely given poorer prognosis and less 'state of the art' treatment (see Chapter Six for a more detailed discussion of ethnicity, class, and health). The social characteristics of physicians themselves, including gender, age, professional training, education, and form of practice, have also been shown to influence their work. Some research has shown that female doctors are less likely to dominate in physician-patient discussion and that female physicians tend to spend more time with patients than male physicians (ibid.).

Cultural Variation in Medical Practice

In an intriguing study, Lynn Payer (1988), a journalist, travelled and visited doctors in several countries: the United States, England, West Germany, and France. To each doctor she presented the same symptoms. She also examined morbidity and mortality tables and read medical journals and magazines in each country. Using this casual and commonsensical method, Payer found strong cultural differences in diagnostic trends and patterns that seemed to reflect fundamental differences in history and culture. Both diagnoses and treatments varied from country to country, even under allopathic medical care. 'West Germans, for instance, consume roughly six times as much cardiac glycoside, or heart stimulant, per capita, as do the French and the English, yet only about half as much antibiotic' (Payer, 1988: 38). In general, Payer found that German doctors were far more likely to diagnose heart problems than doctors in other countries. English physicians, by contrast, are characterized as parsimonious. For this reason, Payer describes the British as the accountants of the medical world. They prescribe about half of the drugs that German and French doctors prescribe and perform about half of the surgery of American doctors. 'Overall in England one has to be sicker to be defined ill, let alone receive treatment' (ibid., 41). By contrast, the Americans are spendthrift and aggressive. They have a tendency to take action even in the face of uncertainty. They do not, however, focus on a particular organ. Among the French, most ills are ultimately attributable to the liver.

Payer argued that these patterns reflected the German emphasis on the heart—on romance, in literature and music, for instance; the French focus on the pleasures of eating and drinking; the English preoccupation with rationalizing the national medical care system; and the American emphasis on getting things done and getting on with it. Payer's work suggests, in broad strokes, something of the relationship between culture and medical practice.

Class and Resistance to Medical Knowledge

The way that lay people in the US interpret, accept, or resist 'medical knowledge' is described in relation to a cancer education project developed for a white, working-class, inner-city area that was known as a 'cancer hot spot' because of the relatively high rates of cancer mortality (Balshem, 1991). The problem was believed by the local inhabitants to be largely the consequence of air pollution from nearby chemical plants and occupational exposure of those who worked in the plants. With this belief system in mind, the community rejected 'health education' about cancer. To illustrate the resistance, Balshem, who was working as a health educator at the time, describes the aftermath of her slide show and talk about the cancer prevention possibilities of a diet that is high in fibre and low in fat. Immediately after this talk Balshem asked if there were any questions. She was met with silence. Then she raffled off a hot-air popcorn maker.

People responded warmly, with pleasure. After that, there was silence again. The meeting adjourned and the subtext of the silence emerged. One person talked about her old neighbour (93 years old) who ate whatever she liked and was still alive. Another teased Balshem: 'you mean your husband will eat that stuff; mine sure won't.' Another confessed that the people in the room liked their kielbasa (spicy sausage) too much to eliminate it from their diets. Finally, Balshem was invited to their next church supper for some really good eating. Balshem describes the meeting finale as follows:

> Then, the social climax: I am offered a piece of cake. The offerer, and a goodly number of onlookers, can barely restrain their hilarity. Time stops. Then I accept the cake. There is a burst of teasing and laughter, the conversation becomes easier, the moment passes. We eat, pack our equipment, and leave. (Ibid., 156)

While the general atmosphere of these meetings was amiable, the explicit health messages were ignored or indirectly criticized as impractical and less important than things such as pleasure, family feeling, and 'human' nature in the pursuit of health.

To understand the community and its responses, Balshem engaged in survey research, long open-ended interviews, and focus-group research strategies. One of the findings was that the community members have sharply contrasting attitudes towards heart disease and cancer.

The causes and treatments of heart disease were both fewer and considered more responsive to lifestyle alterations. Cancer was described as the result of a horrible fate. It was seen as caused by almost everything in their environment. Many of the respondents directly denied the scientific views of cancer causation and prevention. In particular, there were 16 direct denials of smoking and 11 direct denials of fat as cancer-causing agents. By contrast, no one questioned the stan-

dard scientific views about the prevention and causation of heart disease. Balshem called this response 'resistance' and explained that:

> maintaining a rebellious consciousness is part of constructing a valued self, valued community, valued life, in a subordinate class environment. Self and community, valuing and supporting each other, process myriad insults, betrayals, and frustrations. Local belief and tradition, it is asserted, are superior, as is local insight into the workings of authority and hegemony. (Ibid., 166)

For an abundance of reasons, class and community solidarity proved to be more important than expert health knowledge, beliefs about disease causation, and prevention strategies.

Despite the power of 'medicalization from above', there is always resistance, or as Cornwell (1984) says, 'medicalization from below'. Calnan and Williams (1992) demonstrate another type of resistance to medical hegemony. They studied lay evaluations of the trustworthiness of doctors with respect to nine specific medical care issues.

In particular they asked whether or not laypersons would unquestioningly accept medical opinion with regard to the following nine interventions: (1) prescription of antibiotics; (2) hernia operation; (3) operation for bowel cancer; (4) prescription for tranquilizers; (5) hip replacement operation; (6) hysterectomy; (7) heart transplant; (8) test-tube babies; and (9) vasectomy. Their findings indicated that in only one case would the majority of respondents accept medical intervention without question: 54 per cent said they would accept antibiotics without question. Yet even here, 41 per cent said they would only accept the doctor's recommendation for antibiotics with an explanation. Moreover, the views of the public regarding all interventions varied according to gender, class, age, and health categories. Table 9.1 shows the survey results for four of the nine medical interventions.

In making their decisions, Calnan and

Table 9.1   Summary of Basic Findings Regarding the Lay Evaluation of Modern Medical
Technology

Doctor's Recommendations	Accept Without Question	Accept With Explanation	Not Readily/ Not At All
Antibiotics			
%	54	41	5
(N)	(239)	(180)	(20)
Bowel cancer operation			
%	29	60	12
(N)	(119)	(249)	(48)
Tranquilizers			
%	8	29	63
(N)	(35)	(120)	(262)
Hysterectomy			
%	20	65	16
(N)	(43)	(138)	(32)

*Numbers may not total 454 for each question due to the exclusion of those who did not answer.

Source: Adapted from Calnan and Williams (1992: 239).

Williams note, respondents were guided by certain fundamental values of their own. A good intervention was characterized in the following ways: as life-saving rather than life-threatening; as enhancing rather than diminishing quality of life; as natural rather than unnatural; as moral rather than immoral; as necessary rather than unnecessary; as restoring independence rather than promoting addiction/dependence; and as giving good value for money rather than being a waste of money.

The lay population knows that medical knowledge does not form a consistent whole. Nor do the different conceptions of medical knowledge necessarily complement one another: 'The medical world is a melting pot of contradictory theories and practices, controversies and inexplicable phenomena about which doctors and lay people are in constant debate' (Bransen, 1992: 99).

Medical Knowledge Becomes Popular Knowledge

Magazines, newspapers, and audiovisual media have long been important as sources of health-related information and attitudes in modern mass societies. These channels are currently being surpassed, however, by information available through the electronic superhighway. Daily updates of scientific/medical news are available through the Internet, where there are probably hundreds of millions of pages of information. Some Web sites are affiliated with major medical institutions or disease-related charities such as the Heart and Stroke Foundation and the Canadian Cancer Society. Many of these are professionally run and present valid, reliable, and current information. Others are unreliable. Privacy and confidentiality are not always protected. Some sites are outdated. Some represent various commercial interests. Some reflect the concerns of special

Box 9.8   Selling Sickness

We have discussed the social construction of illness, disease, and sickness. We have suggested something of the role of capitalism in the unequal patterns of morbidity and mortality and in inequity in the health-care labour market. In a slightly different formulation of medicalization, Moynihan and colleagues (2002) draw our attention to 'disease-mongering' or the corporate construction of disease in the pharmaceutical industry. They point to several examples of disease mongering. Using the case of the discovery of a new drug for baldness, followed by newspaper reports about the growing problem of hair loss and the panic and emotional difficulties said to accompany the problem, as well as the report of the founding of a new International Hair Study Institute as one example, Moynihan and his colleagues make a case for disease-mongering among pharmaceutical companies. The authors describe the ways in which public relations firms, through media reports, created diseases subsequent to the pharmaceutical discovery of drugs for social phobias, irritable bowel syndrome, and osteoporosis.

interest groups. For example, if you investigate any number of disease-specific Web sites for sponsorship you will notice that pharmaceutical companies are often behind-the-scenes financial supporters. The extent to which this 'pharma'-sponsorship colours the information available in favour of one drug or another is as yet unknown but can be hypothesized. The information thus varies in accuracy and accessibility. People interpret information according to their own culture and socio-economic, gender, age, educational, and psychological characteristics.

Recent studies of health information on the Internet paint a fairly pessimistic picture of its validity and reliability. One study set out to find out how people use the Internet by establishing a Web site to provide information regarding cardiology. The researchers found that users were seeking information 'correctly', that is, 95 per cent of those who asked for information asked pertinent questions (Widman and Tong, 1997). Another study evaluated information regarding pharmaceuticals. Here the researchers found that about 50 per cent of the information provided was correct and another 50 per cent was incorrect; 10.4 per cent of the errors were potentially harmful (Desai et al., 1997). In an evaluation of the quality of information regarding how to detect and manage childhood fevers, researchers found that only about 10 per cent of the Web sites providing information on childhood fevers adhered closely to recommendations in peer-reviewed guidelines (Impicciatore et al., 1994). Clearly, these are issues of concern to those who use the Internet for health information. Another recent study of breast cancer sites (Hoffman-Goetz and Clarke, 2000) found inadequacies with respect to validity and reliability of information, presence of references, dated information, dead-end sites, lack of acknowledged ownership, security and privacy protection, widely different reading levels from site to site, and dominance of the English language.

To date the Internet is open, free, and unregulated. There are debates about whether that is the best strategy in the long run. Some researchers and institutions are working to develop indices and software that would provide organization, guidelines, and maps for users. In the meantime, however, technology leads social change and people are running to catch up!

The mass media remain a fundamental source of health information in mass society. Some studies have found that they comprise the most important source of health information for many people. Different people use different types of media, and people use different media for distinct types of information. Wade and Schramm (1969) found that magazines and newspapers were the most important source of health information for those of higher educational background, while the broadcast media were more often used by those with less education.

Moyer and her colleagues (1994) evaluated, over a two-year period, the accuracy of scientific information as it went from original research/medical sources to the various mass media, including newspapers and women's, science, and health magazines. They began with 116 articles in the mass media. Of those, 60 included traceable citations. There were 42 content-based inaccuracies, including misleading titles, shifts in emphasis, treating speculation as fact, erroneous information, omitting other important results, omitting qualifications, overgeneralizing findings, and inaccuracies in personal communications. Women's magazines had the highest percentage of inaccuracies in traceable citations, at 88 per cent. 'Quality' newspapers had the fewest inaccuracies, at 25 per cent.

In addition, readers typically misunderstand at least some of the information they receive through the mass media. Yeaton et al. (1990) surveyed a small sample of college students regarding their understanding of popular press articles on health issues such as surgical alternatives for breast cancer, drug treatment for congestive heart failure, use of starch blockers for weight reduction, dietary cholesterol and heart disease, and skin transplants for burns. The overall rate of misunderstanding was 39 per cent. The fact that this level of misunderstanding exists among college students raises serious questions about the quality of the health information accessible to the average citizen. If information is both inaccurate (to an extent) and misunderstood (to an extent), we have to wonder about the quality of health information that exists among the general population.

Social-psychological and disease status characteristics also influence the use of the media for health information. Kassulke et al. (1993) found that those who use health information tend to be at a low risk for disease and to employ more positive health habits than others. Klein et al. (1993) found that adolescents who were more likely to engage in risky behaviours were more likely to listen to radio and watch music videos. Those who favoured heavy metal bands and who read sports and music magazines were more likely to engage in risky behaviours. In this observational study, risky behaviours included sex, drinking, smoking, cheating, stealing, marijuana smoking, cutting class, and driving illegally.

Evidence also suggests that the journalists who write about science and medicine in the mass media may not fully understand the information they try to convey. They may, for example, misunderstand statistics and sampling issues and relevant scientific issues of research design and measurement, or concepts of validity and reliability. The need to make mass media appealing to the broad public may also inevitably lead to misunderstanding and oversimplification.

Nonetheless, the mass media may have considerable influence on health-related behaviour for the following reasons:

- viewers of mass media campaigns are fairly representative of the general population and include groups that are often difficult to access, such as younger individuals;
- mass media can be relatively inexpensive;
- mass media can have powerful effects, particularly through the use of celebrities;
- mass media have the potential to modify the knowledge of a large proportion of the population at once, and because of the consequent possibilities for social support, in regard to behaviour change, this in itself may increase its effectiveness.

Box 9.9   Mental Illness

There are three major approaches to the sociological study of mental illness. The first is parallel to an *epidemiological approach*. It examines the correlations between various social statuses such as gender, income, education, ethnicity, and religious affiliation and the incidence and prevalence of various diagnoses of mental illness. For example, such studies have found that women are more likely to be diagnosed with depression and men with alcohol and drug dependency. Such research has also found the general population rate of mental illness has been relatively stable over a number of years. Correlational analysis, it must be noted, does not necessarily reflect a causal connection. In fact, consideration of the likely direction of causality from mental illness to income, on the one hand, has given rise to different theoretical perspectives—the *social selection perspective* and the *drift explanation*. The social selection perspective suggests that the presence of mental illness in a person leads that person into downward mobility through such things as the inability to hold a job, finish school, or manage to maintain a successful marriage. Mental illness in a parent tends to lead to a lower socio-economic position for the offspring or a 'drifting' down the social status hierarchy. A social causation explanation examines the ways that aspects of the social structure lead to mental illness. Thus, poorer people not only tend to have more stress in their lives but they also tend to have poorer resources for dealing with stress. The relevance of these theories seems to depend, in part, on the diagnosis. Schizophrenia, for instance, seems to have a significant genetic component.

The second perspective in this field of sociology is that of *labelling theory*. Here the focus is less on predicting and explaining rates of mental illness and more on the meaning and social construction of mental illness, a symbolic interactionist perspective. Mental illness is considered a category or label that has been devised for and attached to people whose behaviour does not conform to everyday norms and yet often is not criminally deviant. The concept 'resid-

ual deviance' captures the meaning of this view of mental illness. All of us at some time or other, this theory would suggest, act in ways that violate norms. It is only when such violation is very noticeable, is repeated, or occurs among less powerful people that it is labelled as a mental illness. The labelling and the treatment themselves, this theory suggests, tend to reinforce the behaviour and the assessment of the individual as mentally ill. Once the label has been applied it is exceptionally difficult for others to separate the individual from it. The third direction of sociological investigation attempts to explain variations in the rates of mental illness by variations in the source, amount, and type of stress. Stress has been associated with a variety of psychosocial manifestations of distress and mental illness such as depression. This perspective also examines how mediating variables, such as self-esteem and social support, along with social structural variables, such as gender, age, education, and income, have been investigated as causes of mental illness.

In Canada, as elsewhere in North America, one of the most significant changes in mental health policy has been the widespread deinstitutionalization of the mentally ill. Institutions specifically for the mentally ill have existed for centuries. By the 1950s institutions in the United States and Canada were housing unprecedented numbers of mentally ill people. Then, both because of the development of pharmaceuticals to control depression and psychosis and to save money, many of these institutions were closed. Along with deinstitutionalization there was a corresponding increase in patients' rights, including the right to refuse treatment. However, deinstitutionalization occurred too rapidly to ensure an adequate level of support in housing, drug-taking, and sociability, among other things. Among the tragic results of the process of deinstitutionalization has been the rapid growth in homelessness, although it must be emphasized that people are homeless for a lot of reasons besides mental illness, such as housing policies (Frankel et al., 1996).

> ### Box 9.10   Non-Disease
>
> The British Medical Journal recently called for an election by readers of the top non-diseases (Smith, 2002). They defined non-disease as a 'human process or problem that some have defined as a medical condition but where people may have better outcomes if the problem or process was not defined that way' (883). The resulting list, in order of non-diseases, follows.
>
> - Aging
> - Work
> - Boredom
> - Bags under the eyes
> - Ignorance
> - Baldness
> - Freckles
> - Big ears
> - Grey or white hair
> - Ugliness
>
> - Childbirth
> - Allergy to the twenty-first century
> - Jetlag
> - Unhappiness
> - Cellulite
> - Hangovers
> - Anxiety about penis size/penis envy
> - Pregnancy
> - Road rage
> - Loneliness

Doctor-Patient Communication

Doctor-patient communication reflects broader social structure and culture. Both physicians and patients embody their own particular spaces as carriers of culture and structure. In a study based on ethnographic fieldwork that involved joining the surgical ward rounds at two general hospitals, Fox (1993) examined the communication strategies used by doctors to maintain authority and power in interaction with surgical patients. When patients tried to ask questions such as why they felt the way they did, how soon they would feel better, and when they could go home, the surgeons tended to ignore them. Instead, the surgeons maintained control by focusing on the success of the surgery with respect to the specific goals of surgery (e.g., absence of infection, minimal scarring) and its specific outcome. Fox demonstrates that ward rounds can be understood as an organizational strategy entered into by surgeons to capture and maintain discursive monopoly. By keeping the discussion focused on surgeon-centred themes, patients have few opportunities to introduce their own views, concerns, or worries.

In another example, a tonsillectomy is a very common surgical procedure, yet there is considerable variation in its use from geographic area to geographic area and from hospital district to hospital district. The proper treatments for tonsillitis are debatable. One of the ways this debate is resolved appears to be along the lines of specialty preferences. For instance, pediatricians tend to favour recurrent use of antibiotics to control flare-ups, whereas otolaryngologists are more likely to prefer the surgical procedure. It appears that the ideology of the specialty is buttressed by scientific research based on clinical trials and published in specialty research journals tending to favour one procedure over another. Although it may appear that economics might drive the preferences for action chosen by each different type of specialist, even in jurisdictions where physicians are on salary these specialty group differences remain. The author of the study suggests that the need to believe in one's own procedure may reflect more than material interests: it may

Table 9.2	Doctors' Strategies for Talking about Sex to Patients

Strategies	Device
DELAYING	• delaying discussion of sex • refraining from answering 'sensitive' questions • acting agitated in the context of delicate terms
AVOIDING	• using vague, indirect, and distant terms • avoiding certain delicate terms • using pronouns
DEPERSONALIZING	• avoiding personal references • using definite articles
TUNING/ADAPTING	• adopting and repeating patients' use of pronouns and their omission of delicate terms

Source: Adapted from Weigts et al. (1993: 4).

reflect the need to protect and promote the hard-earned skills necessary for the long-run success of the specialty (Chow, 1998). One implication of this is that the communication of doctors is limited to their knowledge of their own specialty. A specialist cannot be expected to offer an evaluation of the costs and benefits of different types (based on different specialties) of treatments even though this would likely be in the interest of the health of the patient.

One area of social life around which there is a great deal of ambiguity and ambivalence is sexuality. On the one hand, sex is more openly discussed, portrayed, and symbolized in all of the mass media today than in the past. Acknowledgement of the pervasiveness of sex outside of the strict bounds of monogamous marriage is widespread. Accompanying the 'liberalization' of sexuality, and particularly women's sexuality, is the belief that a satisfactory sex life is an important part of a satisfactory life as a whole. Yet many are still ambivalent about sex and many still believe it to be a shameful duty to be kept secret. Today, people are more likely to consult doctors when dissatisfied with their sexual functioning (Weigts

et al., 1993). Moreover, women's dissatisfaction with their sex life seems to be hidden behind complaints about physical functioning, including such things as vaginal infections and pain during intercourse (Stanley and Ramage, 1984).

It is useful to understand how such ambiguity and ambivalence are manifest in personal relations and in talk between doctors and their female patients. One study of doctors' and patients' talk showed constructions of sexuality were managed in the doctor's office quite 'sensitively' so as to reinforce gender stereotypes about the 'shame' and 'mystery' surrounding female sexuality (see Table 9.2). The strategies used to discuss such 'delicate' matters are best characterized as delay, avoidance, and depersonalization. Reflected in the talk and the silence is the construction of the 'delicate and notorious' character of female sexuality in the context of the possible discourse with an often more powerful and male doctor (Weigts et al., 1993).

Sociological discussion of talk is more than trivial. It is important both theoretically and practically. Delicacy with respect to sexuality, particularly female sexuality, is a major factor in unwanted pregnancies, sexually transmitted diseases, and the transmission of the HIV/AIDS virus in heterosexual populations. To the extent that women remain unable to talk clearly and confidently about their sexuality, about their genital and reproductive health, and about birth control and health and safety devices such as condoms, they may be more likely unable to refuse unwanted and/or unprotected sex.

Summary

(1) Medical knowledge is socially constructed. It reflects cultural values and social-structural locations. It has varied historically and cross-culturally.

(2) Some of the specific values of contemporary medicine include: mind/body dualism, physical reductionism, specific etiology, machine metaphor and regimen, and control. Sociological research provides a critical overview of these medical assumptions.

(3) There is a large and significant gap between the findings of biomedical research and the implementation of the consequences of these findings in medical practice. The values of medical scientists and medical practitioners are, in many ways, at odds with one another.

(4) Available evidence demonstrates that new technologies are usually adopted (even widely) before their safety and effectiveness are established.

(5) One example of the way that medical science is infused with cultural stereotypes is found in the work of Emily Martin, who contrasted the gender stereotypes observed in the descriptions of male and female reproductive systems as described in medical textbooks.

(6) Research shows that medical practice, too, is infused with cultural stereotypes, including those that pertain to age, gender, class, and race.

(7) One cross-cultural study of medical practice by Lynn Payer offers tantalizing evidence as to provocative cultural differences.

(8) There are also significant class differences in the lay understanding and acceptance of medical knowledge.

(9) Lay views of medical practice vary according to gender, class, age, and specific health categories.

(10) Media information about medical knowledge is frequently inadequate or inaccurate.

(11) Medical doctors employ various discursive strategies in an attempt to maintain control over their own definitions of reality in the face of patient questioning.

(12) Medical practice regarding sexuality issues reflects cultural practices and the shame and mystery often associated with human sexuality.

Questions for Study and Discussion

1. Find examples of mind-body dualism, physical reductionism, the doctrine of specific etiology, the machine metaphor, and regimen and control in an on-line medical journal such as the *British Medical Journal* or the *Canadian Medical Association Journal*.
2. Do a search of a major newspaper over a period of at least one year and compare and contrast the understandings put forward of HRT (hormone replacement therapy).
3. What are the advantages and disadvantages of the widespread availability of health-related information on the Internet for the doctor and for the patient?
4. What social, institutional, and organizational forces in the current way that medicine is practised might tend to promote poor communication between patients and doctors?
5. Consider the attitude in your own family to medicine and doctors. What are its characteristics and to what are they related?

Suggested Readings

Berger, Peter L., and Thomas Luckmann. 1966. *The Social Construction of Reality*. Garden City, NY: Doubleday. This is one of the best discussions of social constructionism as a theoretical perspective.

Clark, Jack, Deborah A. Potter, and John B. McKinley. 1991. 'Bringing Social Structure Back into Clinical Decision Making', *Social Science and Medicine* 32, 8: 853–63. A review of literature on the relationships among diagnosis and various socio-demographic characteristics of doctors and patients.

Dubos, Rene. 1959. *The Mirage of Health*. Garden City, NY: Doubleday. A biologist's view of medicine and changes in medicine that is still valuable.

Freund, Peter, and Meredith B. McGuire. 1999. *Health,* *Illness and the Social Body*, 3rd edn. Englewood Cliffs, NJ: Prentice-Hall. An excellent book for describing some of the most important sociological issues regarding health, illness, and medicine.

Martin, Emily. 1987. *The Woman in the Body: A Cultural Analysis of Reproduction*. Boston: Beacon Press. A 'must read' for those with a particular interest in gender, social constructionism, and biology.

Payer, Lynn. 1988. *Medicine and Culture: Varieties of Treatment in the United States, England, West Germany and France*. New York: Holt. A fascinating book written by a journalist about differences in medical culture in different countries.

Chapter 10

Medicalization: The Medical-Moral Mix

Learning Objectives

- Canada has become more medicalized over the last century and a half.
- Medicine, as treatment for illness, has a very long history in the world.
- Hippocrates, a Greek physician from the era before Christ, can be considered one of the founders of what has become the Western view of illness, disease, and related treatment. The Hippocratic Oath of ethical practice is still used today.
- Currently there are debates about whether society is best characterized as increasingly medicalized or demedicalized.
- The process of medicalization has, in many ways, paralleled the process of secularization. Medicine and religiosity or spirituality, over time and across cultures, have often overlapped in that they deal both with matters of life and death.
- There are important critiques of medicalization as a cultural, socio-economic, philosophical, and technological system.
- The contemporary physician can be seen as a moral entrepreneur.
- Medical definitions of reality are powerful.

Introduction

What is the medical response to illness, sickness, disease, and death? We have discussed the processes by which people notice signs and call them illness. What are the processes by which doctors recognize some of these signs, label them symptoms, and provide a diagnosis? How have medical diagnostic categories changed over time? What are the relationships among medicine, law,

and religion? In what sense is medicine an institution of social control? To what extent have medicine's powers of social control been increasing over the past century? What is medicalization? Are women's bodies more medicalized than men's bodies? Do some people resist medicalization? What are the origins of our contemporary medical care system? To what extent is the practice of medicine a science? To what extent is it an art?

Medicine and illness are intertwined; they are

not necessarily co-extensive. Today the definitions and diagnoses of illnesses are made primarily by the medical care system. The signs or symptoms that people pay attention to, and those they ignore, are largely determined by medical definitions of illness. The expectations people have of their bodies, and the way they sometimes communicate by being ill, also depend in part on categories of disease defined by the medical care system.

Some illnesses, however, resist medical definition for a number of reasons. For example, sufferers frequently experience fibromyalgia and chronic fatigue syndrome long before they are able to find a clear diagnosis. Multiple sclerosis is notoriously difficult to diagnose because it lacks clear markers and symptoms, and at times mimics normal though perhaps exaggerated behaviour, such as periodic stumbling, slurring, and tiredness. Alzheimer's cannot be definitely diagnosed until autopsy. At other times, medical diagnosis precedes a person's awareness of a physical problem. High blood pressure, for instance, is often detected only by tests, not by any physical sensations experienced by the person. The point is that sometimes what is defined as a deviant, unusual, or unacceptable feeling, behaviour, or attitude is seen as a medical problem. Sometimes one of these problems may also fall within the realm of religion or law. For instance, AIDS is viewed as a disease by the medical care system. It has also been seen as evidence of sin by some churches in their homophobic focus on 'immoral' sexual behaviour of a person who has been thus diagnosed. Because AIDS can be contagious, AIDS patients may also be subject to legal controls.

A Brief History of Western Medical Practice

At the beginning of written history, medical practitioners and priests in the Tigris-Euphrates and Nile valleys were one. Illness was a spiritual problem. It was regarded as punishment for sins or for violations of the norms of society such as stealing,

blaspheming, or drinking from an impure vessel (Bullough and Bullough, 1972: 86–101). In Egypt under Imhotep, the Egyptian pharaoh who built the stepped pyramid, medicine began to receive some separate recognition. Even here the medical functionaries' roles, by modern Western standards, were strictly curtailed. Medical practitioners could only treat external maladies. Internal illnesses were firmly believed to result from and be treatable through supernatural intervention.

Modern Western medicine appears to have been derived from Greece in the fourth and fifth centuries before Christ and from medieval Europe. In both times, the tie between the body and the spirit, the physician and the cleric, was strong. Early Greeks erected temples in honour of Hygeia, the Greek goddess of healing, and those who were ill sought treatment in these temples. Sometimes they simply slept in them in hope of a cure. Sometimes temple priests acted as physicians and used powers of persuasion and suggestion to heal. Early Greek physicians viewed their calling as holy or sacred.

One of the most important Greek physicians of the time, Hippocrates, perhaps best illustrates this view. He proposed the Hippocratic oath, still subscribed to by physicians today. The first sentence of the oath illustrates both the sense of calling of the physician and the dedication to the gods that medical practice involved:

> I swear by Apollo Physician, by Asclepius, by Health, by Panacea and by all the gods and goddesses, making them my witnesses, that I will carry out, according to my ability and judgement, this oath and this indenture.

The oath further states: 'But I will keep pure and holy both my life and my art' (Clendening, 1960: 1, 5). The Hippocratic oath contains prohibitions against harming the patient, causing an abortion, and becoming sexually involved with a patient. It considers that things said by a patient to a doctor are to be kept confidential and treated as 'holy secrets'. Nevertheless, Hippocrates and the Greek physicians of his time and somewhat later were also distinguished by their efforts to secularize the concept of disease by taking its treatment away from the sole concern of priests and a focus on the supernatural and thereby to make medicine a practice based on repeated, systematic empirical observation. Through this conscientious focus on method, 'Hippocratic medicine achieved a level of excellence never again attained in the subsequent two thousand years, and surpassed only in the twentieth century' (Lewinsohn, 1998: 1262).

Hippocrates is also recognized for the introduction of detailed observational and experimental methodology. The idea of balance that dominated Hippocratic medicine in the fourth and fifth centuries before Christ continues and persists today in a variety of forms. To Hippocrates, health depended on a harmonious blend of humours—blood, phlegm, black bile, and yellow bile—that originated in the heart, brain, liver, and spleen, respectively. Sickness resulted from an imbalance in any of these four humours. Symptoms reflected this lack of balance. Treatment relied largely on the healing power of nature and on the use of certain diets and medicines to return the organism to balance.

There were two types of practitioners, each catering to a different social class. Private physicians cared for the aristocrats. Most large towns, partly for the prestige of having a doctor and partly to serve those who needed medical care, retained public doctors. Both the public and private physicians tended to cater to the wealthier classes. The poor and the slaves usually received an inferior quality of medical care from the physician's assistant (Rosen, 1963).

The Greek period is often thought to have culminated in the work of Galen (AD 130–201). His discoveries were influential for more than a thousand years after his time. Working with the principles of Aristotelian teleology, he thought that every organ had a purpose and served a spe-

cial function. But Galen's greatest contributions were his anatomical and physiological works (his knowledge of anatomy was based on dissections of pigs and apes) and his systematic speculation (Freidson, 1975: 14).

When the Roman Empire collapsed, medicine and other sciences fell into decay and religious scholarship developed greater prominence. There was conflict between two modes of thought: the spiritual and philosophical, in which truth was deduced from accepted religious principles without any reference to the real world, and the empirical, in which truth could only be inferred from evidence based on observation in the real world. Medicine lost much of the scientific analysis and empirical practice developed by the Greeks. Religious dogmatism limited scientific advances by prohibiting dissection and by forbidding independent thought, experimentation, and observation. The only knowledge deemed acceptable was that found in ancient texts and approved by the Church. For medieval Christians, disease was a supernatural as well as a physical experience. Secular medical help and public health measures were criticized as signs of lack of faith. The Church, its liturgies, and its functionaries were believed to be the source of healing; sinning was believed to be the source of illness.

The Church thus influenced the practice of medicine. It also influenced its organization. Medicine was taught in the universities by rote and faith, through the memorization of the canons of Hippocrates, Aristotle, and Galen. The clergy practised medicine, but they were not allowed to engage in surgery or use drugs. These two physical treatments were left to the 'lower' orders. Barber-surgeons treated wounds, did other types of surgery, and cut hair. Even lower than barber-surgeons were the apothecaries, who dispensed medicines. Hospitals, too, were taken over by religious orders, thus coming under the control of the Church.

Medicine itself did not progress much during this medieval period. However, the epidemics of disease and death caused certain new methods of inquiry that were instrumental in the later development of scientific medicine. Faced with a horrendous death rate such as that during the bubonic plague (the Black Death is said to have taken one-third of the population of Europe in the fourteenth century), people began to raise empirical questions about disease. In the first place, it became clear that the plague was contagious from person to person. Second, not all people succumbed to the plague. Questions about the background differences of those who did and who did not fall ill seemed relevant. The bases for quarantine, germ theory, and the case history were laid.

By the eighteenth century scientific medicine was becoming distinguished from religious practice and folk medicine. Available medical knowledge was organized and codified. Many new medical discoveries were made. The universities, particularly in Western Europe and Scotland, became centres of exciting medical advances in both research and treatment. New tools such as forceps and the clinical thermometer were invented. New medicines such as digitalis were made available. Edward Jenner demonstrated the value of the smallpox vaccine. At the same time, the popular climate was confused by the competition among various types of healing. People visited shrines or used the services of a variety of alternative healers. Medical research was inadequately financed, lacked facilities, and had no specialties; the few practising doctors were overworked.

The modern separation of medicine and the Church is the result of a number of social processes. The secularization of the human body as an object of science is a part of this process. This happened in part because of the developing Christian doctrine of the separation of the body and the spirit, a doctrine that paralleled the philosophical discussions of Descartes. One of the results of the separation was that autopsies were allowed. If the body was no longer the house of the soul, then the wholeness of the body

after death was no longer of great importance. Institutional secularization occurred, too, as the Church became separate from the state. Through this process clearer distinctions between disease, deviance, crime, and sin were forged.

The growing belief in the potential power of science and the emphasis on individual rights and freedoms contributed to the development of modern secular medicine, too. In the nineteenth century, particularly the last half, an enormous number of new discoveries occurred. 'The medical literature of those years makes horrifying reading today: paper after learned paper recounts the benefits of bleeding, cupping, violent purging, the raising of blisters by vesicant ointments, the immersion of the body in either ice water or intolerably hot water, endless lists of botanical extracts cooked up and mixed together under the influence of nothing more than pure whim, and all these things were drilled into the heads of medical students—most of whom learned their trade as apprentices in the offices of older, established doctors' (Thomas, 1985: 19). In fact, most of these remedies did more harm than good, with perhaps the exception of morphine and digitalis. Biology moved from the level of the organ to that of the cell, and both physiology and bacteriology were studied at that level. Germ theory emerged. Surgery grew in sophistication along with asepsis and anaesthesia. Figure 10.1 outlines some of the most important discoveries in the history of allopathic medicine.

Medicalization: The Critique of Contemporary Medicine

Medical science became increasingly influential during the period that urbanization, industrialization, bureaucratization, rationalization, and secularization developed. Medical institutions began to increase their powers as agencies of social control. More and more types of human behaviour began to be explained in medical terms. It has been argued that as the medical sys-

Figure 10.1   Making Medical History

−400
- Hippocrates separates medicine from religion and philosophy, treats it as a natural science

−300
- Anatomy and physiology develop in Alexandria

100s
- Asclepiades brings Greek medicine to Rome; bases treatment on diet, exercise, baths, massage

100s
- Ancient medicine culminates with Galen; his influence will last until Renaissance

200s
- Growing Christian religion emphasizes healing by faith

400s
- Fabiola founds first hospital in Western world at Rome

700s
- Arabs develop pharmacology as a science separate from medicine

800s
- Monk-physicians treat the sick in infirmaries attached to monasteries

900s
- Influential medical school founded at Salerno, Italy; students include women

1000s
- Arab physician Avicenna writes the *Canon*, textbook used in medieval Europe

1200s
- Thomas Aquinas describes medicine as an art, a science, and a virtue
- Human dissection practised at Bologna

1300s
- Urine sample first used
- Black Death kills one-third of Europe's population; medicine powerless to stop it

1500s
- First attempts to restrict right to practise to licensed and qualified doctors
- Advances in anatomy and surgery as influence of Galen wanes

1600s
- William Harvey discovers circulation of blood
- Descartes conceives of body as machine and sees medicine as part of developing modern science
- Hôtel-Dieu in Quebec City founded, first hospital in Canada
- Use of microscope leads to new discoveries

1700s
- First successful appendectomy performed
- Guild of surgeons formed in England separate from barbers, with whom they had been joined
- Advances in scientific knowledge begin to be reflected in medical practice
- Edward Jenner proves value of vaccination in preventing smallpox

1800s
- Medical specialties begin to develop

1810s
- René Laënnec invents stethoscope

1830s
- Theodor Schwann shows all living structures made of cells

1840s
- Inhalation anaesthesia discovered
- Edwin Chadwick brings about public health reforms in England

1850s
- Nurses led by Florence Nightingale save thousands in Crimean War
- Dr Elizabeth Blackwell founds New York Infirmary for Women

1860s
- International Red Cross founded
- Joseph Lister introduces antiseptic surgery
- Gregor Mendel develops law of heredity
- Louis Pasteur shows that diseases are caused by micro-organisms

Figure 10.1   (continued)

1870s	1880s	1890s
• Robert Koch discovers tubercle bacillus	• Otto von Bismarck introduces first state health insurance plan in Germany • Sigmund Freud begins to develop psychoanalytic method • Founding of Johns Hopkins medical school introduces systematic medical education in US	• Malaria bacillus isolated • Wilhelm Roentgen discovers X-ray

1900s	1910s	1920s
• The hormone adrenalin is isolated • Flexner Report leads to reform of medical education	• Influenza epidemic kills millions worldwide	• Banting and Best produce insulin for use by diabetics • Iron lung invented • Alexander Fleming discovers penicillin

1930s	1940s	1950s
• Norman Bethune of Canada introduces mobile blood transfusion unit in Spain, continues works in China	• Use of antibiotics becomes widespread • World Health Organization founded	• J. André-Thomas devises heart-lung machine • Discovery that DNA molecule is a double helix provides key to genetic code • Jonas Salk develops polio vaccine • Ultrasound first used in pregnancy

1960s	1970s	1980s
• First state health insurance plan in North America successfully introduced in Saskatchewan despite doctors' strike • Michael DeBakey uses artificial heart to keep patients alive during surgery • Christiaan Barnard performs first heart transplant	• Smallpox eliminated from earth • First baby conceived outside the womb born in England	• Cyclosporin allows full-scale organ transplantation • Nuclear magnetic resonance makes possible more accurate diagnosis • A new disease, AIDS, kills thousands; no cure or vaccine in sight

Source: *Compass* (May 1988): 10

tem's powers of social control increase, so do the religious institutions' powers of social control decrease. Behaviours once viewed as sinful or criminal are now more likely viewed as illnesses.

Alcohol addiction is a case in point. There was a time when drinking too much, too frequently, was seen as a sign of moral weakness, in fact, a sin. Today, however, alcohol addiction is seen as

Box 10.1   Christian Science

Religion and medicine are irrevocably intertwined among several major contemporary religious groups. One such group is Christian Science, founded by Mary Baker Eddy in 1866. Born in New Hampshire in 1821 to a Puritan family, Mary Baker Eddy spent the first 45 years of her life poor and in bad health but committed to the self-study of various medical systems, including allopathy, homeopathy, and hydropathy. She met and was influenced by a hypnotist healer named Phineas P. Quimby.

In 1866 Mary Baker Eddy fell on a patch of ice and was said to have been told by doctors that her life was at an end. Within a week she was well and walking. She claimed that she healed herself with the aid of God and the power of the mind over the body. Overwhelmed by this experience, she told others. She trained students, the first Christian Science practitioners, in a series of 12 lessons for which she charged $100. She wrote *Science and Health with a Key to the Scriptures*, she said, under direct inspiration from God. By 1879 Mary Baker Eddy was able to found a church, the First Church of Christ, Scientist, in Boston. In 1881 she established an educational institution, Mrs Eddy's Massachusetts Metaphysical College. The church grew quickly and by 1902 there were 24,000 church members and 105 new churches. By 1911, the year Mary Baker Eddy died, there were 1,322 churches in Canada, Great Britain, Europe, Australia, Asia, and Africa.

Today the church is worldwide, and each church around the world follows the same lessons and readings at the same time. While there are no ministers, there are practitioners who must graduate with a Christian Science degree. The basis of the philosophy of Christian Science is that sin and sickness are not real but represent the lack of knowledge of God. According to Mary Baker Eddy:

Sickness is part of error which truth casts out. Error will not expel error. Christian Science is the law of truth, which heals the sick on the basis of one mind on God. It can heal in no other way, since the human mortal mind so-called is not a healer, but causes the belief in disease. Then comes the question, how do drugs, hygiene and animal magnetism heal? It may be affirmed that they do not heal but only relieve suffering temporarily, exchanging one disease for another. We classify disease as error, which nothing but truth can heal, and this mind must be divine not human. (Eddy, 1934)

Treatment for sin and sickness involves prayer. Thinking about God and concentrating on God both lead to and constitute healing. Sickness is the result of incorrect, sinful, or ungodly thoughts.

Healing involves changed thought:

To remove those objects of sense called sickness and disease, we must appeal to the mind to improve the subjects and objects of thought and give the body those better delineations. (Ibid.)

Christian Science constitutes an archetypal modern example of the tie between religion and medicine.

a medical problem. Treatment centres for the 'disease' are located in hospital settings, and treatment frequently includes medications and is under the control of the medical profession.

Medical institutions, including hospitals, extended-care establishments, pharmaceutical companies, and manufacturers of medical technology, have grown in importance. A large (and, until recently, increasing) part of the gross national product is spent on health care. Some thinkers call this process 'medicalization'. One definition of medicalization, from the work of Zola (1972), is that it is a process whereby more and more of life comes to be of concern to the medical profession. Zola portrays medicalization as an expanding 'attachment process', with the following four components:

1. the expansion of what in life is deemed relevant to the good practice of medicine;
2. the retention of absolute control by the medical profession over certain technical procedures;
3. the retention of near-absolute access to certain areas by the medical profession;
4. the expansion of what in medicine is deemed relevant to the good practice of life.

In this view, the first area of medicalization is the change from medicine as a narrow, biological model of disease to a broader concern with the social, spiritual, and moral aspects of the patient's life. As well as bodily symptoms, the entire lifestyle of the patient may now be considered of concern to the doctor. For example, some physicians now routinely include in their patients' case histories questions about eating habits, friendships, marital and family relationships, work satisfaction, and the like.

The second component is the retention of absolute control over a variety of technical procedures. A doctor is permitted to do things to the human body that no one else has the right to do. Doctors are responsible for surgery, prescription drugs, hospital admittance, and referral to a specialist or another doctor. Doctors are the gatekeepers to numerous associated services and provisions. The average doctor generates significant health-care costs annually through prescriptions, hospital admittance, treatment costs, and the like.

The maintenance of nearly absolute control over a number of formerly 'normal' bodily processes, and indeed over anything that can be shown to affect the working of the body or the mind, is the third component. Zola argues that the impact of this third feature can be seen by looking at four areas: aging, drug addiction, alcoholism, and pregnancy. At one time, aging and pregnancy were viewed as normal processes, and drug addiction and alcoholism were seen as manifestations of human weakness. Now, however, medical specialties have arisen to deal with each of these. Zola illustrates this point with a discussion of the change in the view and treatment of pregnancy.

> For in the United States it was barely 70 years ago when virtually all births and their concomitants occurred outside the hospital as well as outside medical supervision . . . but with this medical claim solidified [to manage births] so too was medicine's claim to whole hosts of related processes: not only birth but prenatal, postnatal and pediatric care; not only conception but infertility; not only the process of reproduction but the process of sexual activity itself. (Zola, 1972: 77)

The last component is the expansion of what in medicine is seen as relevant to a good life. This aspect of medicalization refers to the consideration of a variety of social problems as medical problems; depression, obesity, criminality, and juvenile delinquency are among those 'problems' that were once moral/religious problems and are increasingly seen as amenable to medical definition and treatment.

The Medicalization of Human Behaviour

Conrad and Schneider (1980) have analyzed the impact of the medicalization process in a number of areas, including mental illness, alcoholism, opiate addiction, delinquency, hyperkinesis, homosexuality, and crime. In all of these they attempt to show how medicine is increasingly an institution of social control. Their research on hyperkinesis (now called ADD or attention deficit disorder and ADHD or attention deficit hyperactivity disorder) provides one specific illustration of the process of medicalization.

Box 10.2   Disease Definition

There are a number of different, competing models of disease. Some classes of disease are virtually assertions about the cause, e.g., cut on finger; others are simply descriptions of visually obvious or verbally presented symptoms, e.g., high blood pressure. Some are classified by site, e.g., diseases of the stomach; some are categories of symptoms, e.g., headache; others are the names of syndromes that include the nature, symptoms, cause, and prognosis, e.g., Tay-Sachs disease. This list of catego-

rizations could be extended. But the point is that disease diagnosis is not a straightforward and unequivocal procedure. Diseases vary fundamentally in their certainty, ranging from the best defined, e.g., major anatomical defects caused by trauma, to those with unknown etiology and variable description, e.g., multiple sclerosis. Given variability in the meaning of disease, it is not surprising that the process of diagnosis is sometimes considered to be an art rather than a science (Blaxter, 1978).

Hyperkinesis is a relatively new 'disease' that has been 'discovered' over the past half-century or so. It is estimated that it affects between 3 and 10 per cent of the population. Although its symptoms vary a great deal from person to person, typical symptom patterns include some of the following: excess motor activity, short attention span, restlessness, mood swings, clumsiness, impulsiveness, inability to sit still or comply with rules, and sleeping problems. Most of these behaviours are typical of all children at least part of the time. In fact, all these behaviours are probably typical of all people at least once in a while. Conrad and Schneider have explained the processes by which these 'normal' behaviours became grouped and categorized as indicators of 'disease'. They argue that hyperkinesis was 'discovered' for a number of sociological reasons.

The first step was the discovery in 1937 by Charles Bradley that amphetamine drugs had a powerful effect on the behaviour of children who had come to him with learning or behaviour disorders. Only later, in 1957, were the 'disorders' to become a specific diagnostic category—hyperkinetic impulse disorder. A national task force in the US, appointed to deal with the ambiguities surrounding the diagnosis of the disorder and its treatment, offered a new name: 'minimal brain dysfunction' (MBD). In 1971 Ritalin, a new drug

with properties similar to those of amphetamines but without the negative side effects, was approved for use with children. Soon afterwards, Ritalin became the drug of choice for children with hyperkinesis or minimal brain dysfunction. MBD became the most commonly diagnosed psychiatric problem of childhood. Special clinics to treat hyperkinetic children were established, and substantial research funding became available for those studying the problem. Articles appeared regularly in mass media periodicals in the 1970s, and many teachers developed a working clinical knowledge of the diagnosis. In short, once the drug to treat the disorder was synthesized, produced, and made available, MBD became a popular disease around which a great deal of lay knowledge and activity was organized.

Three broad social factors aided the discovery of hyperkinesis: (1) the pharmaceutical revolution, (2) trends in medical practice, and (3) government action (Conrad and Schneider, 1980: 157). First, the pharmaceutical revolution led to a great number of drug-related success stories, such as penicillin's success as a widely effective antibiotic and the results of psychoactive drugs in a variety of mental illnesses. Such successes encouraged hope for the potential value of medications in many areas of life. Second, at this time the mortality rate from infectious diseases in children decreased and the possibility of concern with less-threatening disorders emerged. Medical practice consequently began to pay more attention to the mental health of children and to child psychiatry. Third, government publications, task forces, and conferences, along with the activities of the pharmaceutical companies, reinforced the legitimizing of MBD as a new diagnostic category to be managed by the medical profession.

The points made in this analysis are several. First, the behaviour labelled hyperkinetic existed long before the diagnosis. Indeed, such behaviour was, and is, widespread throughout the population. Second, the popularizing of the diagnosis corresponded to its recognition as a 'pharmacologically treatable' disorder. Third, the popularizing process was aided by the entrepreneurial behaviours of government and the drug companies, along with the Association for Children with Learning Disabilities. To conclude, medicalization is seen, in this example, as a process by which a common behaviour becomes codified and defined as entailing certain symptoms that are best managed through medical interventions.

Two other new 'diseases' are PMS (premenstrual syndrome) and menopause. Considerable medical and then critical feminist attention has been paid to these. McCrea (1983) documents the history of the discovery of menopause as a deficiency disease and notes several parallels to Conrad and Schneider's analysis of hyperkinesis. McCrea dates the discovery of the disease to the 1960s when a gynecologist was given more than $1 million in grants by the pharmaceutical industry. Very soon, this gynecologist was writing and speaking about menopause. He described it as a deficiency disease leading to a loss of femininity and 'living decay'. The diagnosis was coupled with a solution—ERT (estrogen replacement therapy). In a recent feminist analysis, Dickson (1990: 18) argued that the 'mounting sales of estrogen are a result of the expanding concept of menopause as pathology.' Still, many argue that menopause is not a 'disease', nor do most women

pass through it with difficulty.

Other recent studies suggest that the lay public, far from being duped by the power and knowledge of medicine, is actually anything but passive or uncritical (Williams and Calnan, 1996). Statistics demonstrate the willingness of the population at large to seek 'medical' help, in the form of complementary and alternative (CAM) care, contrary to that which is suggested by allopathic medicine. Indeed, Eisenberg et al. (1998) found that more than 40 per cent of the US population did so even when well.

The Contemporary Physician as Moral Entrepreneur

During the nineteenth and twentieth centuries the medical model reached its peak. Complete separation of body and the soul/mind, and of Church and state, occurred in these two centuries. In all of its major institutions, society has become more secularized. The modern world has increasingly relied on reason, not faith, as the way to truth. The rationalization of the world is seen in the spread of the money economy, capitalism, the complex division of labour, bureaucratic social organization, technological development, mass production, factory organization, urbanization, and the like. Modern medicine is seen as the practice of a type of science, and the hopes people hold for the benefits of science are unbounded.

Yet, in many ways the physician can be seen partly as a physical scientist and partly as a moral decision-maker. Not only must the doctor work out a diagnosis consistent with his/her understanding of both scientific and medical knowledge as well as the expectations of the patient, but the doctor must also do this within the context of his/her own religious and other values. Diagnosis involves negotiation between the patient, who presents some symptoms and not others, and the doctor, who sees as symptoms things the patient does not notice and disregards

Box 10.3   The Voice of Medicine and the Voice of the Life World

The clinical encounter between doctor and patient has been described as a struggle for the control of discourse between the 'voice of medicine' and the 'voice of the life world' (Mishler, 1984). A number of different studies have shown the voice of medicine tends to dominate in the patient-physician encounter. Physicians ask most questions (ibid.; Waitzkin, 1989). Patients' responses are narrowly circumscribed and when they move off the topic they tend to be interrupted, ignored, or their discussion is redirected to fit the goals of the physician. Nevertheless, patients often persevere in trying to have their stories told (Mishler, 1984). Mishler argues that allowing and even encouraging patients' stories may have two important health benefits—patient satisfaction and physiological control of disease.

some things that the patient sees as symptoms.

A direct link between medical and moral considerations in medical decision-making is described in the work of Talcott Parsons (1951: 428–47; also see Freidson, 1975: 205–77). In his work on the sick role, Parsons argued that medicine legitimates illness through diagnosis, on the condition that the patient plays the prescribed sick role. To be exempted from social responsibilities due to illness and from responsibilities for the condition, the patient is expected (1) to want to get well; (2) to seek technically competent help; and (3) to co-operate with the 'appropriate' helper in getting well. The sick role involves social evaluation and judgement along with physical anomalies.

Freidson's argument elaborates on Parsons's work. Freidson suggests that because medicine is authoritative on what illness is, it creates illness as a social role. And illness, because it is generally assumed to be unwanted and people are expected to want to get well, is a type of deviance from the norms defining 'normal' health. Human, and therefore social, evaluation of what is normal, proper, or desirable is as inherent in the notion of illness as it is in notions of morality. Quite unlike neutral scientific concepts like that of 'virus' or 'molecule', then, the concept of illness is inherently evaluative. Medicine is a moral enterprise like law and religion, seeking to

uncover and control things it considers undesirable (Freidson, 1975: 208).

Illness, in this perspective, is legitimated deviance. The physician, as the labeller of illness, can be thought of as a moral entrepreneur. Calling behaviour illness rather than sin is a moral act. The consequence, for instance, of labelling drug addiction as an illness rather than a moral weakness is that punishment is minimized and moral condemnation is avoided. The addicted person is treated with sympathy rather than with opprobrium. The choice of label is a moral act. It is an instance of what Zola (1972) calls medicalization.

The labelling of an illness is one instance of the moralizing of the physician. Other decisions that must be made by the doctor in the course of his/her work may also be seen as moral decisions. Tuckett (1976) enumerated a number of situations where decisions would have to be made between conflicting demands. Each decision is affected by religious and moral values. The first results from the *conflict between the needs of one patient and the needs of a group of patients*. Sometimes the adequate care of one patient may require the neglect of other patients. The need of an Alzheimer's patient for care 24 hours a day while in a nursing home or hospital may, for instance, have to be balanced against the needs of the ward nurses and other patients for order and their own ongoing care. The administration of experimental chemotherapeutic drugs may lead to suffering or the death of a cancer patient, but can lead to knowledge that will benefit a large number of similar cancer patients at a later date.

A second conflict situation concerns *the allocation of time, resources, and skills among individual patients.* Organ transplantation may be the last resort for many patients who experience organ failure. It is exceedingly costly, however, and there is a limit to the number of transplant surgeons available to carry out the surgery; it also requires intensive, round-the-clock nursing. As well, organs are in limited supply. In this case the doctor may have to choose to allocate resources to one patient rather than another. Some people are likely to die and some to live as a result of the doctor's decision.

A third conflict involves *the choice the doctor must make between the present and the future interests of a patient.* For example, morphine might be the drug of choice for a victim of severe burns because of its pain-killing properties. However, morphine is addictive and in the long run could cause problems for the patient once he or she has recovered from the burns.

A fourth conflict has to do with *meeting the expected needs of the patient versus the needs of the patient's family.* While it may be in the patient's interests to be cared for at home, this may conflict with the interests of the family members. His or her family may see a schizophrenic patient as incapable of self-care. The family may want hospitalization and the patient may reject it. In this situation a diagnosis and treatment plan must consider at least these two sets of interests.

A fifth conflict situation arises *when a physician is unable to help a patient and thus cannot live up to his or her self-perception as a healer.* At times a patient may present a physician with a problem that the physician does not feel is within his or her realm of understanding or expertise, e.g., difficulties with sleep, or alcohol, or with a father, mother, child, or boss. Advice concerning such problems is frequently sought from a general practitioner. Even though the doctor may not see the problem as a medical one or as within his or her official jurisdiction, he or she may, perhaps to satisfy the patient and to reinforce his or her desire to be a healer, look for biological causes and prescribe 'medical' remedies. Oftentimes the remedies for such problems of living are mood-altering drugs.

Sixth, a doctor may experience *conflict between service to the patient and service to the state or some other organization.* Company doctors may be torn between the interests of a patient who wants legitimation for sickness because he or she desires time off work and the interest of the employer. Or the conflict might be between the interests of an insurance company and the interests of an individual. In one of my recent studies of parents whose children have cancer one of the most frequently described frustrations was that parents had to be certified by a psychiatrist before certain insurance companies would give them support for a leave from work.

A seventh conflict results from a *doctor's dilemma in balancing the advancement of his or her career against the interests of patients.* A doctor is unlikely to enhance his status or wealth by serving in a small Inuit village, and yet the members of the village may need the services of the doctor more than do those in urban areas that are often oversupplied with doctors.

An eighth and final conflict is between the *doctor's role as a doctor or his/her role as a church member, a father, a mother, a wife, a husband, a friend, and so on.* For instance, the work of a doctor may frequently involve the provision of birth control to men or women. This may directly oppose the individual religious values of some doctors.

It is important to emphasize that training in ethical decision-making is not a major part of the curriculum in medical schools. By and large, doctors must face difficult moral and ethical decisions on their own. One of the most controversial of such decisions in the late twentieth century and at the beginning of the twenty-first century, following the legalization of abortion, is whether or not to perform abortions. A number of doctors have been killed and wounded in attacks made by opponents to abortion. Doctors may choose to or not to perform abortions, and the availability of abortion varies across North America (Lazarus, 1997). Clearly, this is one serious, even life-threatening, ethical decision that many contemporary doctors have to consider in their medical training and career.

Uncertainty and Medicalization

Uncertainty is a fundamental aspect of diagnosis, prognosis, and treatment. As many have said, medicine is an art as well as a science. While the layperson expects the physician's work to be straightforward, the physician constantly has to make judgements in situations lacking in clarity (Burkett and Knaft, 1974: 82). When faced with an ambiguous situation, or when having to choose to do something rather than nothing, the medical practitioner generally tends towards active intervention (Parsons, 1951: 466–9; Freidson, 1970: 244–77; Scheff, 1963: 97–107). This is another instance of medicalization. Scheff has called this tendency to act in a situation of uncertainty the 'medical decision rule'. Several studies document this rule. Bakwin (1945), for example, reported on physicians who judged the advisability of tonsillectomies for 1,000 school-children. Of these, 611 were judged to need, and subsequently had, their tonsils removed. Another physician examined those remaining, and an additional 174 were selected for tonsillectomies. Finally, 215 children remained. A different physician examined them, and still another 99 were judged to require a tonsillectomy.

In another common treatment, antibacterial drug prescription, a similar tendency towards action in the face of uncertainty is evident. Most sore throats are not sore because of an infection due to strep bacteria (the treatment of which requires antibiotics). Yet the administration of antibiotics, which at times are known to have negative side effects, does not always depend on proof of the existence of strep bacteria.

Clifton Meador (1965) has explored this tendency and has suggested some of the social sources of medical diagnoses. One is that there is no category of illness called non-disease. Because the physician's job is to diagnose illness, not health, all diagnostic categories are for diseases. They omit the very important additional set of categories that would indicate the absence of a suspected disease. Meador suggests that there must be some prevalence of non-tuberculosis, non-brain tumour, non-influenza, and so on.

Sometimes, too, people want diagnosis or medicalization for a condition (Kohler-Reissman, 1989). The problems faced by people with any of the 'new diseases' such as chronic fatigue syndrome, fibromyalgia, tight-building syndrome, and total environmental allergic reactions are not the result of medicalization. Rather, they result from a lack of medical definition, research, and treatment. And so people who suffer from such illnesses are likely to have to search for a physician who will provide them with a medical explanation for their symptoms. Without a diagnosis such sufferers may be without disability pensions, sick-leave provisions, unemployment insurance, and the like. Because allopathic doctors have been given the right by the state to define wellness and illness, people must depend on their signatures for compensation when they feel ill. While a naturopath or an acupuncturist might recognize an illness and even have an explanation for its cause and treatment, because of the 'illegitimacy' of these practitioners (in the policies and procedures of the state and of corporations) their understandings may not be used as the basis for compensation claims.

Several papers on the experience of one of the new diseases of the twentieth century—chronic fatigue syndrome—document how the lack of access to a medical diagnosis can lead to a number of social problems. Chronic fatigue syndrome is a chronic illness with a multitude of changing symptoms and symptoms in changing organs. In the absence of a diagnosis persons suffer from a lack of legitimacy for their suffering. This frequently results in loss of employment, inability to qualify for sick leave or disability benefits, and estrangement from family and friends, among other things. Broom and Woodward (1999) studied people with chronic fatigue syndrome and discovered that there were times when medicalization is particularly beneficial and times when it may not be helpful. The benefit in chronic fatigue is that a diagnosis 'renders meaningful an incoherent and disruptive experience, and opens up possibilities for managing and living with symptoms' (ibid., 376). Yet, interactions with doctors frequently did not help. Situations in which doctors were authoritarian, maintained dominance, and retained control of the information and meanings were found to be 'unhelpful and damaging to health and well being' (ibid., 375).

That diagnostic decision-making is not always in the direction of active intervention has been discussed by Szasz (1974) and Daniels (1975). Szasz examines the concept of malingering, cases in which a person's claim to be ill is not accepted by the medical diagnostician. Daniels suggests that in some settings, such as the military, a person's claim to be ill is more likely to be rejected than in others. There is, however, an ironic possibility that a person who claims to be ill and who absents her or himself from military service, for example, may be seen as having another special kind of particularly stigmatizing illness—a psychosomatic illness. This general tendency towards medicalization or active intervention depends on the labels and categories of illness available, the social characteristics of physicians, the social and economic situation in which the diagnosis occurs, and the demographic characteristics of the patient. Sudnow (1967), in a study of hospital emergency rooms, has

shown that the age, social background, and perceived moral character of patients affect the amount of effort made to attempt revival of the patient when signs of 'clinical' death are detected.

In *The Sanctity of Social Life* (1974), Crane provides additional evidence that physicians respond to social variables in treating the chronically and terminally ill. In making a prognosis, they consider the extent to which patients are able to relate to others. The 'treatable' patient is one who is most capable of interacting with others. The social status of the patient, while not as important as the ability to interact, is nevertheless an important consideration. Crane notes considerable differences among physicians of varying specialties in terms of the types of decisions made with regard to treatability. The social status of the affiliated hospital in which the medical practitioner works apparently affects his or her judgement in predictable ways. For instance, physicians in more prestigious institutions tend towards active intervention when compared with those in less prestigious ones.

Medicalization has been described as a unilateral and non-problematic process generated by the powerful medical establishment. Lay people, however, may also either resist or encourage medicalization. A growing field of study is lay epidemiology, which is beginning to demonstrate the pervasiveness of lay beliefs about symptoms, their causes, and treatments (Gabe and Calnan, 1989; Hunt et al., 1989; Kaufert, 1988; Walters, 1991, 1992, 1994).

The critique of medical practice is not only at the macro level of systems. A number of sociologists have investigated the patient-doctor relationship by means of observation, recording, transcription, and analysis of the verbal interaction between doctors or between doctor and patient. Waitzkin's (1989) work is one example of this type of study, which tries to link the relationship between personal troubles and social issues (Mills, 1959). Observations showed how doctors interrupt, question, and in a variety of ways direct

Box 10.4   Causes of the Decline of Medical Dominance

Extrinsic

(beyond the direct control of the medical profession)

1. Changing nature of the federal-provincial funding and accountability relationships
2. Changing legislative climate re the practice of the profession
3. Changing status/legitimacy of other providers of health-care services
4. Changing nature of doctor-patient relationship due to education of citizens, influence of mass media, etc.
5. Growth of risk society and with it critical uncertainty about truth claims of science, technology, and medicine
6. Changes in cultural conceptions of the body and responsibility for the body
7. Shifts to chronic disease
8. Shift of ethic from cure to care
9. Growth in focus on spirituality and wholism

Intrinsic

(amenable to change by the profession)

1. Patient/physician ratio leading to oversupply in some places and undersupply in others
2. Fragmentation within medicine along with growth in medical elites (e.g., university-based physicians/scientists)
3. Increasing specialization
4. Wide variations in standards of care

the conversation as they desire it to go. Their greater power in the interaction, as the providers of the definition of the problem (diagnosis) and treatment, allowed doctors to direct the verbal interaction into technical areas and away from social issues. When patients raise issues about their lives, doctors, Waitzkin found, tended to question and interrupt so as to redirect the attention to technical/medical solutions. Thus, what might otherwise be seen and responded to as social issues deserving and requiring social, political, and economic response became smaller matters amenable to medical intervention. In this way, the doctor forestalls political/economic analysis and critique and operates as an instrument of social control in support of prevailing social practices. Waitzkin's observations supported the following three propositions: '(i) that medical encounters tend to convey ideologic messages supportive of the current social order; (ii) that these encounters have repercussions for social control; and (iii) that medical language generally excludes a critical appraisal of the social context' (Waitzkin, 1989: 220).

Mishler's (1984) work reinforces the observations and interpretations offered by Waitzkin. Again, through the analysis of detailed transcriptions of doctor-patient interaction, Mishler documents attempts by patients to raise 'voice of the life world' (the everyday, largely non-technical problems that patients carry with them into the medical encounter with doctors) and doctors' tendency to respond through the 'voice of medicine' (the technical topics of physiology, pathology, pharmacology, and so on). Mishler, too, noted that doctors use conversational strategies such as interruption, questioning, and topic-changing to maintain control of the doctor-patient interviews.

Box 10.5   Neonatal Resources and Outcomes

New and high levels of technology do not necessarily result in better health or lower rates of mortality. The United States has more neonatologists and neonatal intensive-care beds per person than Canada, Australia, and the United Kingdom. However, the US continues to have higher rates of low-birth-weight babies as well as deaths among newborns. The US has 6.1 neonatologists for every 10,000 live births as compared to Canada and Australia with 2.6 and the UK with 0.67. Yet 1.45 per cent of newborns in the US as compared to 1 per cent in other countries had a very low birth weight (less than 1,500 grams). The US also had a higher rate of babies born at less than 2,500 grams. The high rate of teenage pregnancy in the US plays a part in the excess in low-birth-weight babies. Aside from death and disease, low weight at birth is implicated in a number of cognitive, behavioural, and mobility disabilities. In addition, the crude death rates were higher in the US. Such differences may be related to the fact that, unlike other countries studied, the US does not have universal health insurance (only 78 per cent of women have health insurance), nor does it offer free advice regarding family planning, birth control, or prenatal and perinatal care.

Source: Janne Janice Hopkins, 'High level of resources for neonatal intensive care does not give better outcome', *British Medical Journal* 324 (2002): 1353. Available at: <www.bmj.uk>.

Medicalization and Demedicalization

The link between health and illness and morality is a universal phenomenon (Freidson, 1970, 1975). Religion, medicine, and morality are frequently connected. This integration may become a problem, however, in a complex industrialized society such as ours, in which the medical and the religious institutions are separate. The official perspective is that doctors deal with physiologically evident illnesses, while the clergy and the courts deal with moral concerns. The jurisdictions are believed to be distinct. Yet, the doctor is accorded a good deal more power, prestige, and influence in our society than the clergyman or average lawyer. This power is granted in part because the doctor's work is seen as altruistic, related to the service of others, and impartial (see Parsons, 1951, and Chapter Nine for further discussion). In fact, however, as we have demonstrated, the doctor makes moral judgements in ever-widening spheres of life (Illich, 1976; Zola, 1972; Conrad, 1975).

Physicians tend to act in the face of uncertainty, to diagnose disease and not non-disease, to consider social characteristics of patients in their diagnoses and treatments. In a variety of ways the job of the doctor is to label or 'create' a definition of illness for the person who consults the doctor.

A central aspect of the work of a physician is the diagnosis of illness. Illness is not an objectively defined physiological occurrence independent of cultural meanings, but involves social, moral, and physical considerations. Various physical states do exist. Whether they are called health or illness does not depend directly on the physical states, but rather on the evaluation of the states by those who label them.

A number of people would argue that demedicalization is more characteristic of the contemporary society than medicalization (Fox, 1977). There is evidence that the power of the medical model to determine how we think about health and illness has recently declined. Other types of health-care providers are challenging the dominance of the physician in the medical labour force. The prevalence of the medical model's way of thinking about health, illness, and treatment has been criticized frequently (Carlson, 1975; Foucault, 1973; Illich, 1976; Freidson, 1975). Increasing expenditures on the provision of medical care have not meant an increase in the level of good health in the population. The new disease profile, which demonstrates the prevalence of chronic illness, mitigates the pervasive power of the medical model.

Implicit in Freidson's argument about the dominance of the medical profession is the notion that it has control over (1) the content of care, (2) clients, (3) other health occupations, and (4) policy (Coburn et al., 1997). Many have argued that allopathic medicine is declining in power due to the proletarianization of the profession and the decreasing gap in education between physicians and patients (ibid., 2). Others disagree. Coburn and his colleagues have recently examined this question and concluded that 'the state in Ontario is increasingly controlling both the context, and, more indirectly, the content of medical care. Physicians' fees, incomes, numbers,

and modes of representation have all been affected' (ibid., 18). This has occurred largely through resource allocation. The boundaries of medical practice are increasingly critically examined and constrained by the state through (1) an increased reliance on health planners, health economists, evidence-based medical practice, and epidemiologists in the conceptualization of appropriate and inappropriate medical treatments via such things as cost/benefit and health outcome measures; and (2) an increasingly legitimated critique of the scientific basis of much of allopathic medical practice. The state has been able to 'cut through' dealing with an increasingly hierarchical medical profession, i.e., a profession controlled via its colleges, professional associations, and other medical elites (such as specialists, and physicians at university hospitals). While medical professionals still comprise the most powerful occupational group in the overall medical system, as compared to their own previous position they have decreased in dominance.

Williams and Calnan point to larger cultural changes that are implicated in threats to medical

---

Box 10.6   Fundamental Contradictions in the Canadian Health-Care System

There are several contradictions inherent in the Canadian health or medical care system (Williams et al., 2001). The first is that it does little to produce health. Instead, it provides treatment for illnesses on the basis of one person at a time. Inequity, poverty, poor or no housing, poor sanitation, inadequate education, unemployment, hazardous work, gender inequality, and other social factors are important causes of disease. They are best addressed by social and health policies involving investment in housing, guaranteed annual incomes, full employment, and the like. Investing in the medical system, in some senses, perpetuates these social problems to the extent that money is spent on the medical

cure of the individual and not on the recovery of social justice. Moreover, the dominance of the medical model of defining and solving problems individualizes social issues that might better be understood as community or government responsibilities.

The second contradiction is that medicare reinforces the historically organized dominant political interests and relationships (ibid.). It supports allopathic medicine, hospitals, and the pharmaceutical industry. It also supports the relations of power and inequity in the medical system, in the medical division of labour, and in the hospital and pharmaceutical industries. In ways, it serves to protect doctors and the prevailing ideologies of allopathic medicine.

dominance. In particular, they are persuaded that 'the lay public are not simply passive and dependent upon modern medicine, nor are they necessarily duped by medical ideology and technology. Rather, in late modernity, a far more critical distance is beginning to open up between modern medicine and the lay populace' (Williams and Calnan, 1996: 1617). Contributing to this view that, in today's postmodern society, the medicalization thesis is overstated is the growth of social reflexivity—a process through which people now think about truth(s) as relative: 'a chronic feature of late modernity' is 'a never ending cycle of reappraisals and revisions in the light of new information and knowledge' (ibid.). As more and more people pay attention to various mass media and as these media reflect constantly critical and changing views of various aspects of social and cultural life, such as science, technology, and medicine, they tend to become more knowledgeable about issues that relate to health, illness, and medical care. The experience that everything constitutes a risk for some disease or misfortune—even the sunshine now causes skin cancer—leads the populace to be cynical, uncertain, and skeptical of esoteric knowledge, science, allopathic medicine, and claims to objectivity and truth. Thus, culture may be becoming demedicalized.

Summary

(1) The definition and diagnosis of illness today are largely the result of the labelling activities of the medical profession. The medical profession labels 'deviant' and 'normal' feelings and bodily signs and symptoms, and these definitions become reality for social actors.

(2) The chapter gives a brief overview of the relationship between medicine and religion through history.

(3) Over the past two centuries, medicine has become a distinct discipline. Definitions of sin, crime, and illness have changed. Some criminal or sinful behaviours are now viewed as illnesses, e.g., drug and alcohol addiction.

(4) Through medicalization, medicine has increasingly become an institution of social control. Medicalization is characterized by four components: movement from a narrow view of disease to a broader one; control by the medical profession over a variety of procedures; the almost exclusive access of doctors to do things to the human body; and the ability of the medical profession to identify certain social problems as medical problems.

(5) The physician is not only a scientist but also a moral decision-maker. Medicine can legitimate the illness it diagnoses on the condition that the patient adopts the 'sick role' prescribed by the doctor. Medicine defines what is deviant from health and also how the patient is to react to that definition. Illness is legitimated deviance insofar as it has been identified by the physician and the appropriate steps are taken by the patient to get well.

(6) Doctors also make other moral decisions such as: the allocation of resources, choosing between the present and future interests of the patient, and balancing the needs of the patient versus those of his family.

(7) Medicalization has also caused doctors to take medical action in situations of uncertainty.

(8) Medicalization can be observed in the microsituation of verbal interaction between the patient and the physician.

(9) More recently, there is evidence of a decrease in medicalization.

Questions for Study and Discussion

1. Take one behaviour that has been seen both as moral/immoral and as wellness/disease and elaborate on the consequences of each diagnosis or definition of reality.

2. Have you any experience of the integration of religion into medicine or medical practice or of medical issues into the practice of religion? For example, does your place of worship (if this is a relevant concept to you) have services related to prayer for healing? Discuss.

3. Examine a search engine for Web sites on a controversial 'disease' mentioned in the text (e.g., ADHD). Critique the information available from the conflict or feminist theoretical perspective.

4. After examining a major national newspaper for medical stories over the past year or so, what do you think are the major challenges to medical dominance today? Don't forget that you should be able to trace this on-line fairly easily.

5. Evaluate the notion that doctors tend to act in the face of uncertainty.

Suggested Readings

Conrad, Peter, and Joseph W. Schneider. 1980. *Deviance and Medicalization: From Badness to Sickness*. St Louis: Mosby. A classic text on the problem of medicalization of health and social problems.

Freidson, Eliot. 1975. *The Profession of Medicine: Study in the Sociology of Applied Knowledge*. New York: Dodd Mead. A primary text for those interested in medical power.

Mishler, Elliot. 1984. *The Discourse of Medicine: Dialectics of Medical Interviews*. Norwood, NJ: Ablex. This work provides insight into interviews between doctors and patients.

Scheff, Thomas J. 1963. 'The Role of the Mentally Ill and the Dynamics of Mental Disorder', *Sociometry* 26 (June): 463–83. An explanation of the 'medical decision rule', which advocates action in the face of uncertainty.

Waitzkin, Howard. 1989. 'A Critical Theory on Medical Discourse: Ideology, Social Control, and the Processing of Social Context in Medical Encounters', *Journal of Health and Social Behavior* 30 (June): 220–39. An exposition of the 'politics' of the doctor-patient encounter.

Zola, Irving. 1972. 'Medicine as an Institution of Social Control', *Sociological Review* 20: 487–504. One of the most important explications of medicalization.

Chapter 11 *Medical Practitioners, Medicare, and the State*

Learning Objectives

- The first Canadian 'medical' system was composed of the various medical and religious institutions of the many Aboriginal peoples.
- The health of early settlers to Canada was severely threatened in a number of ways.
- Some of the first public health measures adopted in Canada resulted from the cholera epidemic brought to Canada first in 1832.
- Initially, medical practitioners from widely different backgrounds competed with one another for patients.
- Homeopathy was the first profession to be legalized and to establish its own licensing board. Soon after other groups did the same
- The development of medicare had both supporters and detractors.
- Tommy Douglas played an important role in the development of medicare in Canada.
- Medicare has had an impact on the class-based utilization rates of medical service.
- Medicare has had mixed consequences for medical practice and for doctor morale.
- Medicare is currently, and has been in the past decade or so, experiencing significant threats to public financing.

Introduction

What is the history of the medical profession in Canada? Have allopathic doctors always been dominant in the provision of medical care? What is the relationship between the state and physicians and how does it affect the practice of medicine in Canada? How did medicare develop? How successful has medicare been in broadening and equalizing access to the medical care system for all Canadians? Has the change in accessibility led to changes in the overall health of the population or in the distribution of health in the population? What is privatization and is it relevant to a thorough understanding of our health-care system today? What are the implications of trends towards restructuring and downsizing the health-care system? These are among the questions that will be addressed in this chapter.

Box 11.1   Medicine Among the Aboriginal Peoples of Ontario

In the seventeenth century, at the time of the arrival of the Europeans, the Native peoples of Ontario were divided into two linguistic groups: the Algonquian and the Iroquoian. A study of Iroquoian bones dug from a burial mound near Kleinburg, Ontario, revealed that the Native peoples (around the year 1600) suffered from such well-known diseases as arthritis, osteomyelitis, and tumours. Evidence of a hole in a skull revealed the skill of a local surgeon. Some treatments devised by the Aboriginals, when the cause was obvious, were empirical and rational. Internal conditions of unknown cause were often attributed to supernatural origins such as (1) the breaking of a taboo, e.g., mistreating an animal or showing disrespect to a river, (2) ghosts of humans, which craved company, (3) the evil ministrations of a menstruating woman, or (4) unfulfilled dreams or desires.

The Native peoples believed that everything in the world had a spirit or a soul, including animals, trees, rocks, the sky, lakes, and rivers. Thus, every-thing in the world was to be respected. In some Aboriginal cultures all young people, especially males, were expected to search for a vision or a dream as a guide through life. To achieve this goal it was customary to spend at least a week alone without food. Hungry, lonely, and full of transient concerns, the young person would generally have a vision, which was then interpreted by the medicine man or father. Medicine men were both the spiritual leaders and healers. They were able to cast out spells, predict the future, recover lost objects, diagnose and treat disease, and bring rain. Some were also magicians and jugglers.

A practical armamentarium of medicines evolved, which included treatments for widely different medical problems, from fractures and wounds to freezing and frostbite, burns and scalding, rheumatism, arthritis, urinary problems, fevers, intestinal disorders, cancer, blood poisoning, and toothaches. Some of the herbs and plants used by the Native peoples continue to be used today.

Source: Holling (1981).

Early Canadian Medical Organizations

The first Canadian medical 'system' was composed of the various medical/religious institutions of the many groups of Aboriginal peoples. Each of these groups had its own culturally unique definitions of what constituted health and what constituted illness, its own pharmacopoeia, and its own preferred types of natural and supernatural interventions. Since these peoples handed down their traditions orally, the only written accounts are from white settlers, priests, explorers, and traders. These writers tell us that medicine men or shamans were frequently called upon to diagnose and treat various types of injuries and disease.

Shamans, and other Aboriginal peoples, too, developed a number of very effective botanical remedies, such as oil of wintergreen, and physical remedies, such as sweat lodges and massages.

Canada's Aboriginal peoples are known to have used over 500 different plants as medicines. Some were chewed and swallowed, some drunk in herbal teas, some boiled and the vapours inhaled, some infused and even poured as medicine into the patient's ear. At times plants were used for ritual purposes only. For example, thorny or spiny plants were sometimes used to ward off evil spirits or spirits of disease and death. At other times the value resided in the pharmacological effectiveness of a particular plant for a particular symptom or disease. A

Box 11.2   Canada's Cholera Epidemic

The worldwide epidemic of cholera reached Canada for the first time in 1832. Apparently Irish immigrants, who were escaping the potato famine and the beginnings of cholera in Ireland, were already affected when they set forth for Quebec City and Montreal. The boats they travelled on were built for 150 but carried as many as 500 passengers. Such unsanitary circumstances invited the spread of the virulent and contagious disease. It attacked apparently healthy people, who could die within a matter of hours or days. It erupted in a number of symptoms, including severe spasms and cramps, a husky voice, sunken face, a blue colour, and finally kidney failure as various bodily processes collapsed. Doctors could do virtually nothing to help their patients. Although there were various theories associating the disease with dirt and filth, its cause was not understood.

When it realized the nature of the calamity before it, the Canadian government established a Board of Health with a mandate to inspect and detain ships arriving in Canada from infected ports. A Quarantine Act was passed in February 1832 and remained effective until February 1833. Another Act provided a fund for medical assistance to the sick immigrants and to help them to travel to their destinations when they had sufficiently recovered.

In the spring of 1832 Grosse Isle in the St Lawrence, which was directly in the path of ships arriving from Europe, was established as a place of quarantine. All ships were stopped for inspection. Distinctions were made between ships arriving from infected and non-infected ports. Those from infected ports were required to serve a quarantine period, while the ships with ill passengers were thoroughly cleaned and those who were diseased were disembarked and treated; those who died were buried there. Some of the government actions were very unpopular because they restricted individuals' freedoms, which resulted in riots in various locations throughout the country. Crowds burned down some cholera hospitals.

Cholera invaded Canada at three other times—in 1834, 1852, and 1854. While statistics are not entirely reliable, it is estimated that as many as 20,000 people died in all the epidemics.

Sources: Bilson (1980); Heagerty (1928: vol. 1); Marks and Beatty (1976).

famous example of a plant with specific and now scientifically substantiated medicinal benefit was the scrapings of white bark of cedar, which is rich in vitamin C, for the treatment of scurvy. This was taught to Jacques Cartier by Aboriginal peoples. By today's medical standards, there seem to have been pharmacologically useful treatments for a wide variety of symptoms such as wounds, skin eruptions, gastrointestinal disorders, coughs, colds, fevers, and rheumatism.

The health of the early settlers in Canada was continually assaulted. Even before they arrived, immigrants faced grave dangers from the over-crowded conditions on the boats in which they came to Canada. These densely packed quarters greatly increased susceptibility to the spread of contagious diseases. Pioneer life, too, was fraught with hazards. The winters were often extremely cold. The growing season was short and difficult. Accidents occurred frequently as people cleared the bush for timber and for farmland, roads, and buildings. Accidents also occurred on the rapidly flowing waterways. The building of roads, canals, and railways was extremely dangerous. Epidemics of smallpox, influenza, measles, scarlet fever, and cholera decimated the population from time to time. Childbirth in pioneer conditions was often dangerous for both mother and child (Heagerty, 1928). Local midwives, a few doctors trained in Britain and the United States, and travelling medical salespeople performed most medical treatment. Other treatments were based on folk remedies or on mail-order medicines.

The Origins of the Contemporary Medical Care System

The origins of the type of medical practice dominant today can be traced back to nineteenth-century Canada. At that time a wide variety of practitioners were offering their services and selling their wares in an open market. Lay healers, home remedies, folk cures, and other kinds of medicines were all medical options available to the population. Whisky, brandy, and opium were used widely as medicines, as were various types of patent concoctions. Medicine shows were common from the 1830s and 1840s.

Most of the first allopathic medical practitioners in New France were either barber-surgeons from France, who had received primitive training as apprentices, or apothecaries who acted as general practitioners dispensing available medicines. Barbering and surgery both required dexterity with a knife: they were handled by the same person because of the ubiquitous practice of bleeding as a treatment for a wide variety of ailments. Surgery was only practised on the limbs and the surface of the body. Internal surgery almost always resulted in death because bleeding and sepsis were not yet either successfully treatable or preventable. Two other common treatments were purging and inducing vomiting. Among the first doctors in Upper Canada were army surgeons; there were also some civilian physicians. Homeopathic doctors and eclectics (practitioners who used a variety of treatments) worked alongside allopathic practitioners. Lay-trained midwives delivered babies in the home, and other lay-trained persons performed surgery and set bones. No one type of healer was predominant.

Although the first medical school was established in Canada in 1824, theories about disease were still varied and not scientifically based. The first involvement of the state in this hodgepodge of medical practices was in 1832; it occurred because advance warning had been received of the possible arrival in Canada of immigrants with cholera. The government immediately appointed a Sanitary Commission and a Board of Health, which issued directives for the protection of the people. Infected people were quarantined. Contaminated clothing was burned, boiled, or baked. Private burials were ordered. Massive outbreaks of cholera in 1832 and 1854 necessitated the establishment of a quarantine station at Grosse Isle on the St Lawrence for ship passengers who were infected and thus not allowed to enter Canada. Both Montreal and Quebec adapted buildings to isolate disembarking passengers who had cholera. Public ordinances, which received the force of law in 1831, prevented the sale of meats from diseased animals and appointed civil authorities to inspect dwellings for their state of cleanliness. Early public health measures primarily emphasized quarantine and sanitation. Later the government became involved in other types of public health efforts. These included the Public Health Act of 1882 of Ontario, which was soon adopted in the rest of the country, the Food and Drug Act, the Narcotics Control Act, the Proprietary and Patent Measures Act, and the establishment of hospitals and asylums.

The Efforts of Early Allopathic Physicians to Organize

In spite of the primitive state of their medical knowledge, numerous attempts were made by allopathic doctors, dating from 1795, to have legislation passed that would: (1) prohibit any but allopathic practitioners from practising; (2) provide the allopaths with licences under which they

Box 11.3   The Flu Epidemic of 1918

In the fall of 1918 Canada's population was about 8 million. About 60,000 people had died in World War I. Between 30,000 and 50,000 died during the fall, as a result of the dreaded flu epidemic sweeping much of the world. Apparently the flu came to Canada on a troopship, the *Anaguayan*. One hundred seventy-five of the 763 soldiers on board took ill. The ship was quarantined at Grosse Isle. Yet the disease was passed on to Canadians. By the end of September it was clear that Canada had a serious problem. The epidemic spread quickly. New York and Massachusetts were hit. It spread up and down from the US into Canada and vice versa. It also spread westward along the railways and highways. It was attributed to Spain and called the Spanish flu, not because it started there but because, as Spain was neutral in the war, it was easy to attribute it to the Spanish.

It was unique because it tended to hit young adults and often kill them. Previously, the flu had tended to affect both the very old and the very young. The flu epidemic attacked one in six Canadians. Schools, auditoriums, and various halls were opened as temporary hospitals. Children were left without parents. Quarantines were imposed. Public meetings were forbidden. Partly because of the impact of the flu, the need to establish a federal health authority was acknowledged. The bill to institute such a department received first reading in March 1919, and the new department became operational that fall. But quarantines did not seem to work. Many people thought that quarantine was unjust. Others just did not believe that it worked because they saw people succumbing who had been very careful, while others, less careful, remained disease-free.

Because quarantine did not seem to work, other measures were introduced. Laws were passed to ensure that people wore masks. But the laws differed. In some municipalities those who were caring for the ill were required to wear masks. In others, anyone who was in contact with the public was expected to wear a mask. Alberta required that anyone outside the home had to use a mask. Yet masks proved as ineffective as quarantine. Rather than boiling and sterilizing them frequently, and certainly between wearings, people allowed the trapped germs to spread and multiply in the moist, warm environment inside the mask.

Most homes had their own trusted preventive measures and treatment. Mothballs and camphor in cotton bags worn about the neck were common. Travelling medical salespersons reaped profits from the salves and remedies they sold. Alcohol and narcotics were prescribed.

Losses to business were enormous. People were too sick to shop or were afraid to venture into the stores for fear of catching the disease. Many staff, too, were off sick. Theatres and pool and dance halls suffered heavy losses. Some 10,000 railway workers were off at one time. Ice storms, blizzards, and below-zero weather had never exacted so heavy a toll as this epidemic. Telephone companies were heavily over-extended, both because people were relying on the phone rather than leaving the house and because so many employees were away sick. The insurance industry was one of those most heavily hit. Apparently some companies dealt with more flu claims than war claims. All in all, Spanish flu had an enormous effect on Canadian society.

Sources: Dickin McGinnis (1977); Heagerty (1928: vol. 1); Pettigrew (1983).

could practise; and (3) control admittance to allopathic practice. The allopathic practitioners often had high social standing in the new colony. In the English-speaking areas, they were usually British immigrants and often ex-military officers (Torrance, 1987). Generally, they moved in the highest social circles, married into important families, stood for Parliament, edited influential newspapers, and provided care for the wealthier classes (Gidney and Millar, 1984). In small towns outside Toronto, allopathic practitioners were often among the most important businessmen, church leaders, and town politicians. In 1852 an informal group of these men established the *Upper Canada Journal of Medical, Surgical and Physical Science*.

The allopathic doctors expressed frustration with their working conditions. They claimed they were under-rewarded and under-esteemed because of the competition from 'irregulars' and because of 'quackery' and the disorganized state of the medical schools. Many of the 'irregulars' were also educated, and because they did not engage in the heroic measures of the allopaths, such as the application of leeches, bloodletting, and applying purgatives, they were less likely to cause harm. But the allopathic doctors thought of them as uneducated, ignorant imposters who ruthlessly and recklessly administered untried, untested methods with dangerous results.

In fact, even at this time, the 'irregular' doctors exhibited considerable strength and organizational skills. In 1859 homeopathy was the first profession to be legalized and to establish a board to examine and license practitioners. The eclectics were successful in consolidating their own board in 1861 (ibid.). Perhaps because of their relative success in organizing themselves, the homeopaths and eclectics and other heterodox practitioners were 'contemptuously lumped together by the established profession as "empirics"' (Hamowy, 1984: 63). *The Upper Canada Journal* denounced homeopathy as 'so utterly opposed to science and common sense, as well as so completely at variance with the experience of the medical profession, that it ought to be in no way practiced or countenanced by any regularly educated practitioner' (quoted ibid.). Opposition to the eclectics was equally passionate. They were called 'spurious pretenders' and seen as embodying a contin-

uous and strong threat to 'true science'.

Competition within the ranks of the allopaths, largely between 'school men' (the university-trained and affiliated practitioners) and the Upper Canada practitioners (Gidney and Millar, 1984), prevented the unified stance necessary for the establishment of standards of education, practice, and licensing. In 1850 the 'school men' held more power. By 1865 they had conceded some of their authority to the elected representatives of the ordinary practitioners. In the same year (1865) these ordinary practitioners succeeded in passing self-regulatory licensing legislation. This was revised in 1869 under the Ontario Medical Act to create the College of Physicians and Surgeons of Ontario. Much to the surprise of the 'regular' or allopathic physicians, both homeopaths and eclectics were included under the same legislation. Homeopaths continued to be represented by the College until 1960. Eclectics were excluded in 1874.

This 1869 legislation gave the practitioners, via their representatives on the College, control over the education of medical doctors. Proprietary (privately owned) medical schools were founded, but they were rapidly affiliated with universities in order to grant degrees. The power struggles between the university-based doctors and the practitioners continued.

In Lower Canada the attempts to define and limit the work of physicians were complicated by the tensions between French and English doctors. The College of Physicians and Surgeons of Lower Canada, formed to regulate practitioners, was created in 1847. In 1849 legislation was passed to allow automatic incorporation of anyone who had been engaged in practice in 1847.

The competition and infighting that characterized much of the medical care system in the nineteenth century had receded by the beginning of World War I (Coburn et al., 1983). The year 1912 marked a turning point in the position of allopathic practitioners. The Canada Medical Act, which standardized licensing procedures across

Canada, was passed. Finally, by this time a patient who sought the services of an allopathic practitioner had more than a 50 per cent chance of being helped by the encounter. The passage of the Canada Medical Act coincided with another important event. The momentous Flexner Report, *Medical Education in the United States and Canada*, sponsored by the Carnegie Foundation and the American Medical Association and financed by the Rockefeller philanthropies, was published in 1910. The Flexner Report severely criticized the medical systems of Canada and the United States. It advised the elimination of the apprenticeship system, the standardization of entrance requirements to medical schools, and the establishment of a more rigorous scientific program of study. It recommended the closing of many medical schools, particularly the proprietary ones, because they did not meet the criteria of scientific medicine.

Flexner's report radically changed medical education in the US and Canada. McGill University and the University of Toronto were the only schools in Canada given very high ratings. The medical schools in Halifax and London moved rapidly to become affiliated with Dalhousie University and the University of Western Ontario, respectively. Medical education began to be taught as a scientifically based, scholarly field under the aegis of universities.

The Flexner Report had a significant impact on the organization of Canadian medical education and the practice of medicine for the next half-century. The report enhanced the legitimacy of science as the basis of clinical practice. It reinforced the importance of empirical science with its emphasis on observation, experimentation, quantification, publication, replication, and revision as essential to medical-scientific research. It emphasized the importance of the hospital for the centralized instruction of doctors-to-be and the use of medical technology for standardization in diagnosis and treatment. By the 1920s the hospital-based, curatively oriented, technologically

sophisticated medical care system that Canadians know today was firmly established.

One important side effect of the report was that the schools that were closed were primarily those that educated women and blacks. Thus the closing of the proprietary schools further entrenched the position of white, middle- and upper-class males in medicine.

A Brief History of Universal Medical Insurance in Canada

Mackenzie King first suggested a system of universal medical insurance in 1919 as part of the Liberal Party platform; it was recommended regularly by organized labour after the end of World War I (Walters, 1982). Later, universal medical insurance was proposed at the Dominion-Provincial Conference on Reconstruction in 1945. At this time, the provinces opposed the federal initiative, favouring free-market health insurance. In 1957 the federal government introduced the Hospital Insurance and Diagnostic Services Act, which provided for a number of medical services associated with hospitalization and medical testing. The federal government was to pay 50 per cent of the average provincial costs.

In 1961, the federal government appointed a Royal Commission on Health Services. The Commission, under Supreme Court Justice Emmett Hall, recommended that the government, in co-operation with the provinces, introduce a program of universal health care. The result was the Medical Care Act of 1968. Finally implemented in 1972, the new universal medical insurance scheme was to cover medical services, such as physicians' fees, not covered under the previous Hospital Insurance and Diagnostic Services Act. The scheme had four basic objectives. (1) *Universality*. The plan was to be available to all residents of Canada on equal terms regardless of such differences as previous health records, age, lack of income, non-membership in a group, or other considerations. The federal gov-

Box 11.4   Time Line: The Development of State Medical Insurance

Germany and Western Europe introduced social welfare insurance, including health insurance, in the 1880s.

New Zealand introduced social welfare insurance, including health insurance, in the early part of the twentieth century.

Great Britain introduced national health insurance in 1948.

Canada

1919 Platform of the Liberal Party under Mackenzie King includes medicare.

1919 End of World War I: organized labour began what was to become an annual statement by the Canadian Congress of Labour concerning the importance of national health insurance.

1919–20 Talk of medicare in the US: several states passed medicare legislation that was later withdrawn.

1934 Canadian Medical Association appointed a Committee on Medical Economics, which produced a report outlining the CMA position in support of national health insurance, with several provisos.

1934 Legislation passed for provincial medical insurance in Alberta. Government lost power before it could be implemented.

1935 British Columbia introduced provincial medical insurance legislation. Despite public support via a referendum, this legislation was never implemented because of a change in government.

1935 Employment and Social Insurance Act, including a proposal for research into the viability of a national medical insurance scheme, was introduced.

1942 Beveridge Report on Britain's need for a National Health Service published in Great Britain—the subject of much discussion in Canada.

1945 Dominion-Provincial Conference on Reconstruction included proposals for federally supported medical insurance. Conference broke down in the wake of federal-provincial dispute.

1947 Saskatchewan implemented hospital insurance.

1951 A Canadian Sickness Survey completed. It demonstrated income differences in illness.

1958 Hospital Insurance and Diagnostic Services Act passed.

1962 Saskatchewan CCF/NDP government introduced provincial medical insurance; Saskatchewan doctors' strike.

1962 Royal Commission, headed by Justice Emmett Hall, appointed to investigate medical services.

1966 Federal legislation for state medical insurance passed.

1968 Federal legislation implemented.

1971 All provinces fully participated in medicare.

1972 Yukon and Northwest Territories included in federal legislation.

1977 Federal government changed the funding formula with the provinces—Established Programs Financing Act (EPF).

1984 Canada Health Act reinforced the policy that medical care to be financed out of the public purse (penalties for hospital user fees and physician extra-billing).

1987 Ontario doctors' strike.

1990 Bill C–69 freezing EPF for three years, after which future EPF growth was to be based on GNP minus 3 per cent.

1991 Bill C–70 passed to freeze EPF for two additional years before new formula (–3 per cent) came into effect. Made it possible for federal government to withhold transfer payments from provinces contravening the Canada Health Act.

1999 Throughout the nineties, medical care deteriorates across the country. Hospitals close; patients at times are turned away from emergency; emergency-room waiting increases dramatically. Nurses, doctors, and other health-care workers strike in various actions. Increased evidence of a two-tiered medical system appears.

2000–3 There were increasing debates between the federal government and the provinces on health-care funding. The provinces blamed 'the crisis in medicare' on the lack of sufficient federal funding and the federal government, in turn, chastised the provinces for misspending. A number of investigations and reports were solicited, including the Alberta-sponsored report by former federal cabinet minister Don Mazankowski and the federal reports by Senator Michael Kirby and former Saskatchewan Premier Roy Romanow. Each report was received in a flurry of contradictory political discourse.

ernment stipulated that at least 95 per cent of the population was to be covered within two years of the provincial adoption of the plan. (2) *Portability*. The benefits were to be portable from province to province. (3) *Comprehensive coverage*. The benefits were to include all necessary medical services, as well as certain surgical services performed by a dental surgeon in hospital. (4) *Administration*. The plan was to be run on a non-profit basis.

The Canada Health Act of 1984 added *accessibility* to make five principles. The costs for the new plan were to be shared 50/50 by the federal and provincial governments. They were also to be shared in a way that would serve to redistribute income between the poorer and the richer provinces.

Government soon faced increasing financial pressure as health-care costs grew. Physicians who felt they were not paid enough 'extra-billed' their patients. When a critical level of frustration and complaint was reached, the government appointed Emmett Hall again to chair a committee to re-evaluate medicare. In 1980, Hall reported to the federal government that unless extra-billing was banned, Canada's universal health-care system was doomed. In response, but amid much controversy, the Canada Health Act, which limited the provinces' right to permit extra-billing, was passed.

The Canadian Medical Association filed a lawsuit against the federal government, claiming: (1) that the Canada Health Act went beyond the constitutional authority of the federal government; and (2) that it contravened the Charter of Rights and Freedoms by prohibiting doctors from establishing private contracts with their patients. The Ontario Medical Association, the largest and most vocal provincial group, representing about 17,000 physicians, challenged the Act in court. The Ontario government passed the Health Care Accessibility Act (Bill 94) in June 1986 in response to the federal legislation, thus making extra-billing illegal. Members of the Ontario Medical Association staged a 25-day strike in protest, but eventually had to back down when the government refused to capitulate. Public opinion was decidedly against the strike action, and many doctors went back to work even before it was officially over. There have been many other doctors' strikes across the country from British Columbia to Labrador and Newfoundland. Doctors have continued to protest their incomes, working conditions, and the state of medical care for Canadians, among other things. There is widespread evidence of the dissatisfaction of doctors with the medical conditions across the country.

Factors in the Development of Medicare in Canada

Today, Canada's health-care system, usually called medicare, is predominantly publicly financed and privately delivered by a combination of funds and policies established at the federal level and operational decisions executed at the level of the provinces and territories. It is considered a national system because its fundamental principles are federally based and federal funding reflects, in part, adherence to these principles. The federal government is also responsible for direct health service delivery to specific groups, including veterans, Aboriginal Canadians on reserves, military personnel, inmates of federal penitentiaries, and the RCMP. In addition, the federal government's health-related responsibilities involve health protection, promotion, and disease prevention. It is important to note that the system relies primarily on the services of family and general practitioners, who comprise 60 per cent of physicians practising in Canada and are essentially the gatekeepers to the rest of the system, including specialty care, hospital admission, diagnostic testing, and prescription drugs. Doctors are generally paid on the basis of fee-for-service. Most work in solo or group practice and share on-call work responsibilities. Some physicians work for community health centres, in group practices, or for corporations, and some of these are paid by salary or some alternative mode of payment. The situation in Quebec is an exception to this. Quebec established its own study of health care, the Castonguay-Nepveau Commission in 1965. This Commission established prevention as a priority area and decided that health-care services would be offered under one roof in CLSCs—local community service centres. Doctors were to work together with other health-care providers in this type of group and community setting. Many physicians and others rejected this model. Some CLSCs were founded but health care continues to be offered in a patchwork of organizational forms similar to the rest of Canada (Armstrong and Armstrong, 2003).

Most hospitals are run as private non-profit corporations overseen by a community board, voluntary organization, or municipality. Although funded in large part by government, hospitals operate independently so long as they stay within budget. Besides hospital and physician services, the provinces also pay for some or all of such goods and services as prescription drugs, dental and vision care, and assistive devices for the elderly and welfare recipients. Complementary and alternative care is largely financed out-of-pocket or by medical insurance for those who have such coverage.

The development of medicare over the last half-century in Canada was influenced positively or negatively by a number of significant social forces. The most important of these are: (1) the widespread movement in Western industrialized societies towards rationalized bureaucratic social organization and monopoly capitalism; (2) the spread in Western Europe and beyond of social welfare legislation in public education, old age pensions, family allowances, unemployment benefits, and medical care insurance; (3) the benefits to the medical profession in maintaining fee-for-service, cure-oriented, hospital and technologically based medical practice; (4) the interests of the life and health insurance companies in perpetuating their share of a profitable market; (5) the interests of the drug, medical, and hospital supply companies in continuing to develop their increasingly profitable markets; (6) the interests of the urban labour unions and farm co-operatives in social welfare benefits for their members; and (7) the charismatic qualities and dedication of individuals such as Tommy Douglas, who had both a position of power at the 'right' time in Saskatchewan and a commitment to universal medical care. Each of these will be discussed in turn.

First, the movement towards state medical insurance in Canada must be seen as part of a widespread trend in Western industrialized nations towards rationalization and bureaucratization in the context of monopoly capitalism. It

Box 11.5   Tommy Douglas

Tommy Douglas is one of the most important figures in the development of a universal state-supported medical care system. He was born in Scotland in 1904 and immigrated with his family to Winnipeg when he was just a boy. An incident in his own life stands out because it was often said to have provided the motivation for his determined fight for medicare. Before coming to Canada, Douglas injured his knee in a fall. As a result of the injury he developed osteomyelitis and was forced to undergo a series of painful operations. Despite these operations, osteomyelitis recurred while he was living in Winnipeg. The doctors in Canada felt that amputation was necessary. However, while Douglas was at the Children's Hospital in Winnipeg in 1913, a famous orthopedic surgeon, Dr R.J. Smith, became interested in his condition. Dr Smith took over the case and saved his leg. He did not charge the far-from-wealthy Douglas family. As Douglas says of this experience, 'I always felt a great debt of gratitude to him, but it left me with this feeling that if I hadn't been so fortunate as to have this doctor offer his services gratis, I would probably have lost my leg.'

In addition to this personal experience, Douglas was moved by the social conditions in Winnipeg in the early twentieth century. Unemployment was high. People lived with a great deal of uncertainty and were able to afford only the barest of necessities. These conditions made a lasting impact on Douglas. He was also sensitive to and strongly opposed to the discrimination and prejudice based on ethnic and racial differences that he saw around him in Winnipeg.

He acted out his commitment by first becoming a Baptist minister in 1930 and then by becoming a parliamentarian. In 1932 he joined the Labour Party. In 1935 he was nominated as the Co-operative Commonwealth Federation (CCF) candidate for the Weyburn federal riding in Saskatchewan and was elected to the House of Commons. He was re-elected in 1940. From 1944 until 1961, Tommy Douglas was Premier of Saskatchewan, the leader of the first Socialist government in Canada. He worked towards economic security for the farmer, full employment for the urban worker, and the development of natural resources. Tommy Douglas promised that socialism would provide health and social services and lift taxation from the shoulders of the people and place it upon the 'fleshy backs of the rich corporations'.

By January 1945, free medical, hospital, and dental care was provided in Saskatchewan for 'blue card' pensioners and indigent people. Treatment for mental disorders and polio was made free to all. A school of medicine was opened at the University of Saskatchewan to increase the supply of doctors. Geriatric centres were built to provide care for the chronically ill elderly. Canada's first district-wide medical insurance program was established at Swift Current, where 40 doctors served a population of 50,000 people. This was financed by a family payment of $48 per year and a land tax. Thus Swift Current became a testing ground for a provincial program.

By 1 January 1947, Douglas introduced the Hospital Insurance Plan. The premium at the time was $5 per person and $10 per family. At the end of 1947, the *American Journal of Public Health* stated that 93 per cent of the population of Saskatchewan was covered by the new scheme. The only exceptions were some remote northern communities.

In 1959 Douglas announced the introduction of medicare, which was to be based on five basic principles.

1. Medical bills would be prepaid and patients would never see a doctor's bill.
2. The plan would be available to everyone regardless of age or physical disability.

3. The plan would accompany improvements in all areas of health service.
4. The plan was to operate under public control.
5. The legislation was to satisfy both patients and physicians before it went into effect.

A few days after Douglas stepped down in 1961 as Premier of Saskatchewan, the medical bill passed. In 1962 the Saskatchewan doctors' opposition to the government medical scheme intensified. A strike followed the announcement that the Act was in force. The strike lasted 23 days, during which time the government kept medical services in operation by flying doctors over from Britain.

The Saskatchewan plan soon became the basis for a Canada-wide plan. In 1964 Prime Minister Lester Pearson announced that the federal government would give financial aid to any province that had a satisfactory medicare system. By 1969 most of the provinces were participating in the plan, with 50 per cent of the costs covered by the federal government.

Tommy Douglas re-entered federal politics and remained a member of the House of Commons from 1961 to 1979, first as the leader of the New Democratic Party, which had been formed in 1961 by a coalition between labour and the CCF.

Sources: McLeod and McLeod (1987); Shackleton (1975); Thomas (1982); Tyre (1962).

was not until the twentieth century that the work of the physician came to be highly regarded as the most effective form of medical care. With the development of antibiotics to treat bacterial infections and neuroleptic drugs to treat the psychosis associated with various forms of emotional despair and mental illness, the efficacy of the doctor became firmly established in the public mind. Along with the increase in legitimacy of allopathic medicine, medical practice itself began to alter as hospitals changed from being institutions for the dying and the indigent into being the doctor's place of work. Medical specialization increased and medical and paramedical occupations grew in number. All of this growth and development served to enmesh the physician within enormous bureaucratic structures.

The once-familiar physician with his little black bag is being replaced by a complex 'health-delivery system' centered in a proliferating number of large, urban-based bureaucratic settings, such as university medical centers, hospitals, community health centers and health maintenance organizations. (McKinley, 1980)

Bureaucratic organization is technically efficient. It is also suited to capitalist development because it assists in organizing the expansion and maintenance of control over profit necessary for capitalist accumulation.

Second, the introduction of medicare in Canada must be seen in the context of the spread of similar policies in the Western industrialized world. The first legislation was passed in Germany in the 1880s. By the time Britain first introduced universal medical insurance in 1912 (to be formally established as the universal National Health Service in 1948), much of Western Europe, as well as New Zealand, had already pursued this course. Talk of medicare and the passage of legislation in support of medicare (which was later withdrawn) occurred in the United States by 1919–20. From 1919 until the introduction of comprehensive state-sponsored medical care in Canada a half-century later, both federal and provincial governments made various attempts to draft legislation to implement medicare.

Third, the medical profession has had an impact on the timing and the nature of medicare. In 1934, the Committee on Medical Economics

Box 11.6   Impediments to the Development of State-Sponsored Medical Care in Canada

1. The traditional division, early in the century, between the urban industrial labour force and the farmers, and the consequent inability of these two working-class groups to form a unified labour lobby in favour of medicare.

2. The strengthening and unification of the Canadian Medical Association in 1920 with the appointment of Dr T.C. Routley as leader, which gave the CMA a unified voice with respect to the conditions under which medicare might be acceptable.

3. The extensive representation of medical doctors in local, provincial, and federal politics and departments of health gave physicians the power to voice their individual views regarding medicare.

4. Through the British North America Act, 1867, the responsibility for health rested with the provinces.

5. Opposition of Canadian Roman Catholics to state medical insurance.

6. Regional, ethnic, occupational (labour/farmer) heterogeneity of Canadian society retarded the development of social democratic policies.

7. Steady growth of private insurance companies, especially during the fifties and sixties. Medical insurance became an increasingly common fringe benefit in collective bargaining agreements.

8. Repeated opposition of the Canadian Life Insurance Officers Association, the Canadian Chamber of Commerce, and the Canadian Manufacturers' Association to state medical insurance. (Walters, 1982)

of the Canadian Medical Association completed a report that described the characteristics of the ideal medical insurance scheme. At this time the CMA expressed support for state medical insurance provided that: (1) it was administered by a non-political body of whom the majority would be medical practitioners; (2) it guaranteed free choice by physicians of their method of payment; (3) it provided for medical control over fee scheduling; and (4) it allowed for compulsory coverage up to certain levels of income (Torrance, 1987). Following World War II, after the return of economic growth when most patients were able to pay their bills either independently or through private medical insurance, the majority of the profession opposed medicare. The strongest statement of the opposition of the doctors to state medical insurance was the 23-day strike in 1962 by about 800 of Saskatchewan's 900 physicians.

Fourth, the life and health insurance companies, through the Life Insurance Officers Association, opposed medicare. They argued that the role of the state was to provide the infrastructure for the development of such things as transportation and communication. State-sponsored medical insurance was to be limited to those who could not pay for their own policies and to assist in payment for catastrophic illnesses. The insurance companies were already making a profit and wanted to continue to do so.

Fifth, the drug, medical, and hospital supply companies and their representative body, the Canadian Manufacturers' Association, opposed government intervention in medical financing.

Sixth, the labour unions and farm co-operatives advocated national medical insurance. Except in the case of Saskatchewan, however, they did little actively to bring about state medicare.

Seventh, the importance of individuals such as Tommy Douglas cannot be overlooked. He was

Table 11.1   The Use of Medical Care Services before Medicare (1950–1), by Income Level

Rate per 1,000 Population	Adults	Children	All Persons
Low income	508	368	474
Medium income	524	536	540
High income	528	581	544
Higher income	571	663	588

Source: *Medicare: The Public Good and Private Practice. A Report by the National Council of Welfare on Canada's Health Insurance System*, 1982: 10, Table 1, Catalogue no. 82–3267. Reproduced with permission of Minister of Supply and Services, Canada, 1989.

especially dedicated to the principle that medical care be accessible and available on a universal basis. He owed his well-being and perhaps his life to the fact that a physician operated on him without fee and saved his leg from amputation when he was a boy. Partly as a result of this personal experience, and also, of course, because of his socialist beliefs, Douglas made medicare a fundamental plank in his CCF platform (see Box 11.5).

The Impact of Medicare on the Health of Canadians

The most important goal of medicare was the provision of universally accessible medical care to all Canadians regardless of class, region, educational level, religious background, or gender. To what extent has this goal been reached? Before the introduction of medicare there was a positive and clear relationship between income level and use of medical services. Low-income groups visited the doctor over 10 per cent less often than did high-income groups (see Tables 11.1 and 11.2). After medicare this pattern was reversed: lower-income groups are now more likely to visit the doctor (28.8 per cent versus 14.8 per cent).

In spite of the equal availability of health care to people of all classes and the disproportionately greater use of medical care facilities by the poorer classes, health continues to vary by class.

People of the lower classes still live shorter lives and have more days of disability during these shorter lives. The health of those of lower income and education in Canadian society continues to be poorer than that of those of higher socioeconomic status (see Chapter Six for a detailed examination). Obviously, health results from more than accessibility to medical services. Moreover, some medical services require out-of-pocket expenditures that are not always affordable to every Canadian. In a system that relies so heavily on drugs and yet does not insure the out-of-hospital cost of drugs, it is impossible to claim universality.

In a sense, much of Canada's health-care system is already private. 'Most hospitals and other institutions are owned by a wide variety of organizations, not by the state. Most doctors are in private practice and most services such as home-care are purchased by the government from other organizations. However, although some of the government money currently goes to for-profit institutions, most tax dollars go to nonprofit providers' (Armstrong and Armstrong, 1996: 187). Approximately 70 per cent of health-care funds come from the public sector; 30 per cent are from the private sector. There are many new incentives across the country for the developing private health-care sector. For instance, 'Canada's capital city, where public health care

Table 11.2   Distribution of Insured Health Services among Canadians in Different Income Groups after Medicare (1974)

Income Quintile	Medical Care Program	Hospital Insurance Program	Both Programs
	%	%	%
Lowest	28.8	33.1	31.7
Second	22.0	23.9	23.3
Middle	18.0	17.2	17.4
Fourth	16.4	13.4	14.4
Highest	14.8	12.4	13.2

Source: *Medicare: The Public Good and Private Practice. A Report by the National Council of Welfare on Canada's Health Insurance System*, 1982: 23, Table 4, Catalogue no. 82–3267. Reproduced with permission of Minister of Supply and Services, Canada, 1989.

and sacred trust are the two terms federal politicians most dearly love to combine, has two provocative new "health" enterprises' (Gray, 1998: 165). In Ottawa there are 13 walk-in family medical clinics that offer service 12 hours every day. A medical services company, Your Family Medical Centres (YFMC), which has recently been added to the Alberta Stock Exchange, runs all of these. In return for 32 per cent to 34 per cent of their gross earnings, physicians are provided with examination and treatment facilities, equipment, nurses, receptionists, and a billing service. The other new private service is a lab that does urine testing at between $50 and $950, depending on the number of tests desired. This urinalysis is supposed to indicate a person's vulnerability to genetic disorders such as Alzheimer's disease and the ongoing effectiveness of cancer treatment during treatment. Many of these tests are not covered by medicare. There are similar stories of privatization across the country, such as the growth in laser surgery to correct vision, cosmetic surgery, and the like.

In addition, a survey by the Institute of Clinical Evaluative Services in Ontario of some 1,150 health-care providers, including cardiologists, cardiac surgeons, internists, family physicians, and hospital managers, indicated that 53 per cent of the hospital executives and 80 per cent of the physicians had been involved in the care of a patient who received preferential access to treatment. Those most likely to have been favoured in these ways included relatives and friends, high-profile public figures, and patients and families who were well informed, aggressive, or likely to sue. It is important to note that most of this preferential treatment was given for elective rather than necessary care (www.ices.on.ca).

As well, many costs associated with the use of the allopathic medical care system are not covered. To visit a doctor, one must often be able to afford transportation, take time off work, understand how to make an appointment, and speak the language necessary for making an appointment. Following the doctor's orders also frequently involves costs that may not be manageable to the non-working or working poor or those receiving unemployment or social security benefits. One study of access to medical treatment services among the working poor (Williamson and Fast, 1998) found that a significant minority of people failed to have a pre-

---

Box 11.7   The Canadian Medical Care System: A Qualified Success

Mhatra and Deber (1992) state that 'the Canadian health care system can be considered a qualified success.' Canadians are, by and large, satisfied with and even proud of their system; it provides universal and comprehensive coverage to good effect and at a cost comparable to that of other advanced industrial nations. Among the qualifications to success, Mhatra and Deber point to a growth in physician supply in excess of population growth; limited innovation in the hospital sector; possible overuse of certain drugs (especially for the elderly); some types of tests and some surgical procedures; inadequate provision for quality control of drugs and of independent physician practice.

Today, claim Mhatra and Deber, there are two major challenges to Canada's health-care system: access to technology and broadening understandings of health predictors. First, with respect to tech-

nology there is evidence that certain high-technology procedures (e.g., magnetic resonance imaging) are more easily available elsewhere, particularly in the US, than in Canada. This claim is debatable, however, because some evidence suggests both overuse in the US and an appropriate level of use in Canada. Second, health today is seen in broader terms than equitable access to medical care. Many health determinants are outside the broad areas of the provision of medical care and include such important issues as education, housing, racial and gender equity, environmental protection, and traffic safety. Canada's ability to address these challenges to health equity depends on the Canadian economic trend, demographic predictions, federal-provincial disputes, and ideological disputes about medical services. Until and unless these concerns are dealt with, equitable access to health in Canada will continue to be elusive.

---

scription filled in the previous year (40.0 per cent) or failed to obtain physician services (37.7 per cent). Most of those who did not fill a prescription (74.8 per cent) reported that this was because they were unable to afford it. The reasons for not going to a physician when sick included thinking that one would get better without a doctor; that the doctor would prescribe unaffordable medication; that transportation was impossible or too difficult; that doctors had not been helpful in the past; that they did not have time; that they did not like going to the doctor; that they were too emotionally drained; that they could not get an appointment; that they could not afford child care. This study did not include homeless persons or those who do not speak the language of the majority in their community. The rates of non-utilization of medical services are likely to be even higher among these groups.

The Impact of Medicare on Medical Practice

According to Naylor (1982), before the Great Depression, from approximately 1918 to 1929, doctors made more than four times the average Canadian salary. The Depression had a devastating effect on all incomes. In the period of recovery in the 1940s, doctors' salaries averaged about three times the national average. By 1989, with various private insurance schemes in place, doctors made about 3.7 times the average Canadian salary. Initially, medicare gave a dramatic boost to doctors' salaries. In the early 1970s doctors' salaries were approximately 5.2 to 5.5 times the national averages. Wage and price controls, which were introduced in the mid-1970s, retarded the expansion of physicians' salaries during that period.

The number of doctors in Canada grew

Box 11.8   Forces That Favour and Oppose the Continuation of Medicare as a Publicly Funded System

Those that favour public funding	Those that oppose public funding
Many in the medical profession	Political parties on the right wing of the
Pharmaceutical industry	spectrum, e.g., Canadian Alliance
Hospitals	Pro-business groups such as the C.D. Howe
Employers in unionized sectors	and the Fraser Institutes
	Some members of the medical profession

Source: From A. Paul Williams, Raisa Deber, Pat Baranek, and Alina Gildiner, 'From Medicare to Home Care: Globalization, State Retrenchment, and the Profitization of Canada's Health-Care System', in Pat Armstrong, Hugh Armstrong, and David Coburn, eds, *Unhealthy Times: Political Economy Perspectives on Health and Care in Canada* (Toronto: Oxford University Press, 2001), 7–30.

much more quickly than the population and continues to do so. Between 1968 and 1978 the number of doctors grew by 50 per cent, the population by 13 per cent. The physician-to-population ratio has been narrowing for more than a century. In 1871, there were 1,248 citizens to every physician; by 1951 the ratio was 1:976; and by 1981 the ratio was 1:652. This trend continues, as does the increasing number of specialists. Table 11.3 shows that the growth rate in the number of doctors over the 1986–92 period varied substantially from province to province. Saskatchewan and Newfoundland, for example, had growth rates of less than 1 per cent, while the Northwest Territories and Yukon saw an almost 5 per cent increase. Table 11.4 indicates that from 1980 to 1992 the country's population as a whole was growing approximately 1 per cent per year whereas the number of doctors was growing by 3 per cent per year.

As the physician-to-population ratio changes, some areas and regions may experience an excess of doctors and others an insufficient number. An oversupply of doctors could be a factor in the hypothesized decline in doctors' salaries and in a decrease in power and prestige. It could also lead to excess rates of surgery, pre-

scriptions, or other unnecessary medical interventions. Even successful treatments may be accompanied by harmful side effects. An under-supply of physicians, by contrast, can lead to unnecessary suffering and lengthy travel or waits to see a physician.

The involvement of the state in the practice of medicine has resulted in a number of changes in the actual work of the doctor. These include changes in (1) working conditions, (2) the degree of control over patients and over other occupations in the medical field, (3) self-regulation in education, licensing, and discipline, and (4) the actual content of the work (Coburn et al., 1987). Charles (1976) has documented the ways that universal medical care insurance has altered the medical profession through increased administrative, economic, political, and social constraints. The controls of which Charles writes have increased since her publication.

With respect to administrative constraints, Charles was chiefly referring to the increased bureaucratic surveillance of the actual practice of individual physicians through the computerized account systems detailing the number of patients seen and the medical problems diagnosed in a given period of time. The government, through this

TABLE 11.3   Average Annual Growth Rate of Active Civilian Physicians for Canada and the Provinces, 1986–1992

	Number of Physicians 1986	1992	Average Annual Growth 1986–1992 (%)
Newfoundland	847	892	0.87
Prince Edward Island	174	173	–
Nova Scotia	1,536	1,759	2.29
New Brunswick	853	1,024	3.09
Quebec	12,564	14,534	2.46
Ontario	16,881	20,473	3.27
Manitoba	1,856	1,995	1.21
Saskatchewan	1,423	1,493	0.80
Alberta	3,650	4,441	3.32
British Columbia	5,736	6,953	3.26
Yukon	29	38	4.61
Northwest Territories	46	61	4.82
Canada	45,595	53,836	2.81

Source: Statistics Canada, *Health Reports* 4, 2 (1992).

Table 11.4   Growth Rate of Population and Physicians

	Population	Physicians
Growth Rate 1980–6	0.9%	3.4%
Growth Rate 1986–92	1.4%	2.8%
Growth Rate 1980–92	1.1%	3.1%

Source: Statistics Canada, *Health Reports* 4, 2 (1992).

bureaucratic control, became able to investigate individual doctors whose practices varied substantially from the norms. The privacy of the independent entrepreneur was effectively eliminated through the powers of this bureaucratic surveillance.

Certain financial constraints resulted. While the salaries of physicians continued to increase under universal medical care, it was no longer possible for all individual doctors to reach the salary levels they might desire. The Quality Service Payment Formula dictated the maximum number of weekly 'units' of service that could be provided by an individual physician without jeopardizing the quality of patient care. Doctors whose weekly incomes were regularly higher than the designated quota were then subject to closer examination by a Medical Review Committee.

The question of what proportion of the resources of a society should be dedicated to medical care, essentially a political concern, is the third area of constraint noted by Charles. One effect of universal medical care insurance is that physicians' fees are now negotiated between the provincial government and the provincial medical association. The government needs to keep down medical care costs and to ensure universal availability of service. It must also seek to minimize inequity among different medical care personnel within a global budget that includes hospitals and extended-care facilities, drugs, and expensive new technology. All of this is then bal-anced against the need or desire of physicians for a certain standard of living.

The final constraint noted by Charles is social. One such example is that in order to pro-vide equitable medical care to people all across Canada, even in remote and isolated areas, gov-ernments may implement quota systems that would allow doctors to practise in a given area only if their services were needed as determined by a standardized physician-to-population ratio.

Nor are doctors immune from stress. A recent study of doctors, based on a national rep-resentative sample of 2,584 Canadian physicians, indicates a significant amount of stress associated with the profession (Richardson and Burke, 1991). Some two decades or so after the intro-duction of medicare, doctors felt stressed by the number of hours they worked and by the addi-tional hours spent 'on call'. Third in importance for male doctors was the stress that resulted from trying to maintain a decent income. While most physicians surveyed said they were quite satisfied with medical practice, they also tended to find it somewhat or very stressful. They responded that they tended to be satisfied with treating and help-ing patients, feeling needed, and successfully meeting the challenges of medicine (Table 11.5).

Medical practice is a source of stress for med-ical students, interns, and residents as well. The University of Calgary's Department of Surgery studied stress among residents in surgery in 1992, 1994, and 1996 and found that most of the residents felt that their stress level was moderate to substantial. The most important causes of stress among these doctors were consistent pres-sure, overload, working conditions, and an ill-defined work role (Buckley and Harasym, 1999). In the 1996 cohort, for example, the following is the rank order of the stresses:

1. lack of time for personal life
2. oral and written examinations
3. information overload

Table 11.5   Stress and Satisfaction among Physicians

Sources of Stress	Females Rank	Males Rank
Time 'on call'	2	2
Total hours worked	1	1
Medicare paperwork	7	7
Office management problems	10	11
Need to maintain own knowledge	3	5
Life and death situations	4	6
Counselling non-medical problems	12	13
Profession-government relations	5	4
Need to maintain an adequate income	6	3
Uncertainty about diagnosis or treatment	8	8
Delays for patients admitted to hospital	13	12
Co-ordinating services	9	10
Threat of malpractice litigation	11	9

Source: Adapted from Richardson and Burke (1991: 1181).

4. time demands of research
5. sleep deprivation
6. financial hardship
7. fear of being incompetent
8. time demands of being on night call
9. OSCAR (the hospital computing system)
10. unco-operative hospital staff
11. insecurity over future career opportunities
12. resident and staff conflicts. (Ibid., 220)

The Impact of Medicare on Health-Care Costs

Clearly, health-care costs as a portion of GNP have increased during the period from about 1960 to the present (see Table 11.6). In 1991 Canadians spent about $67 billion on private and public health care, an average expenditure of $2,474 for every citizen (*Canada Year Book*, 1994: 128). Health-care expenditures passed $100 billion in 2001 and the forecast for 2002 was $102.5 billion (*Health Care in Canada 2002*, at: www. cihi.ca). This averages out to about $3,300 per person. It does not include private expenditures such as extended health-care insurance, prescribed or over-the-counter drugs, and dentistry. Private expenditures per household were $1,357 in 2000 (ibid.). Moreover, those in the highest income groups spent more than three times as much on health care as those in the lowest (taking family size into consideration). Figure 11.1 shows total health expenditures in Canada for 1999 by the sources of funding, while Figure 11.2 indicates where the billions of dollars were spent.

The federal government has been withdrawing from the health-care field amid great debates with the provinces. This is despite the fact that the federally sponsored National Forum on Health recommended both national home care and pharmacare programs in addition to the present medicare system. In the meantime the federal government, a number of provincial governments, and other organizations are studying the 'crisis' in medicare and making various proposals. Recent examinations of this crisis include the Romanow Report and the report by Senator Michael Kirby, among others. Some of the proposals favour an expansion of services offered universally and others favour a retrenchment of service offerings. As long as medicare is subject to the fortunes of changing political parties and their accompanying ideologies it will be vulnerable. The provinces and territories manage their own health-care systems, educational programs, and health personnel and certification. Provinces vary in respect to the numbers of programs in addition to the basic medicare services offered. Some, for instance, provide additional benefits, including psychologists, dentists, optometrists,

Table 11.6   Total Health-Care Costs, as a Percentage of Gross National Product (GNP), Canada, 1960–1994, and Selected US Figures

Year	Health-Care Costs as % of GNP US	Health-Care Costs as % of GNP Canada
1960		5.6
1961		6.0
1962		6.0
1963		6.1
1964		6.1
1965		6.2
1966		6.2
1967		6.5
1968		6.8
1969		6.9
1970	7.5	7.3
1971	7.7	7.5
1972	7.9	7.4
1973	7.8	7.1
1974	8.1	7.0
1975	8.6	7.5
1976	8.7	7.4
1977	8.8	7.4
1978	8.8	7.4
1979	8.9	7.2
1980	9.5	7.5
1981	9.7	7.6*
1982	10.5	8.4*
1985	10.5	8.5
1987	10.9	8.8
1988	11.1	8.7
1989	11.9	8.9
1990	12.2	9.4
1991	13.2	9.9
1992	–	10.2
1993	–	10.1
1994	–	9.8

*Provisional.

Sources: Health and Welfare Canada, *National Health Expenditures in Canada 1970–1982* (Ottawa, 1982); ibid. (Ottawa, 1984), 9, figure 3 (Cat. no. 84–2094); Statistics Canada, Cat. no. 82–221–XDE.

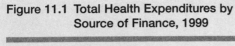

Figure 11.1 Total Health Expenditures by Source of Finance, 1999

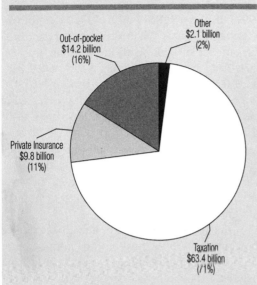

Note: 1999 is used here rather than forecasted data for 2000 or 2001. The 'other' component of private-sector financing included such items as non-patient revenue including ancillary operations, donations, and investment income.

Source: Commission on the Future of Health Care (2002: 24).

Figure 11.2   Total Health Expenditures by Use of Funds, 1999

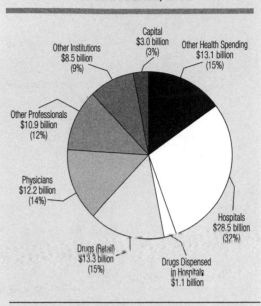

Source: Canadian Institute for Health Information, Statistics Canada.

chiropractors, and podiatrists, as well as home care, drugs, and general preventive services. Many Canadians pay for private insurance plans for additional services.

What, then, is the impact of universal insurance on physician use in Canada as compared with the US? Overall, Canadians of all classes are more likely to visit a physician than Americans are. This difference is minimized but not eliminated among the elderly, who in the US have medicare available to them. However, there are no significant differences between Canada and the US with respect to hospital admission rates or length of stay. In addition, there are greater class disparities in the US than in Canada—the poor in

the US visit the doctor less often, yet once they have made an initial visit they tend to have a higher number of visits and to stay in the hospital, once admitted, longer than those of the higher class levels (Hamilton and Hamilton, 1993). Still, medical care on average is more expensive in both Canada and the United States as compared to other OECD countries (Figure 11.3).

The portions of the medical care dollar in the years between 1960 and 1994 devoted to expenditures on medical institutions, physician services, other professional services, drugs and appliances, and all other health-care costs have varied, but the highest level of expenditure was in the hospital sector, followed by physicians and then drugs (Table 11.7). The rest of the health-care dollar went to other professional services and costs. Now, despite significant numbers of hospital closures, hospitals continue to account for the

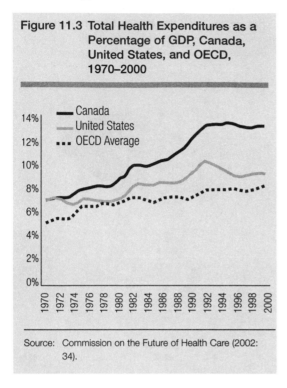

Figure 11.3 Total Health Expenditures as a Percentage of GDP, Canada, United States, and OECD, 1970–2000

Source: Commission on the Future of Health Care (2002: 34).

highest component of the spending. This was 32 per cent in 2001. However, spending on pharmaceuticals (15 per cent) has displaced spending on doctors (14 per cent) as the second highest expenditure (Figure 11.2). In 1960 doctors received 16.6 per cent of total health-care expenditures while 14.2 per cent of total expenditures were on drugs. In 1994 doctors accounted for 14.2 per cent and pharmaceuticals for 12.6 per cent. Clearly, the impact of pharmaceutical use, along with the costs of drugs, is an important cost factor in the health-care system (CIHI, 2002).

The 1990s saw dramatic changes in the medical care system across the country. Elected on a platform that involved eliminating the deficit, the federal Liberal government withdrew specifically earmarked funding to the provinces for medicare with the introduction in 1996 of the Canada Health and Social Transfer (CHST), which over the next several years meant less money to the

provinces but with fewer strings attached. There have been dramatic decreases in the numbers of hospitals across the country (Tully and Etienne, 1997). Between 1986–7 and 1994–5 the number of public hospitals declined by 15 per cent, and the number of beds in these hospitals was cut back by 11 per cent. The number of staffed beds per 1,000 people has declined from 6.6 to 4.1. The number of outpatient visits has increased at the same time as the number of in-patient visits has decreased. In the context of the control of hospital costs, necessary because of federal transfer cutbacks along with provincial decisions, many hospitals across Canada posted negative annual growth in expenditures despite population growth.

Cuts in the hospital sector already seem to be showing effects in the health of the population. A retrospective before/after cohort study that included 7,009 infants born by uncomplicated vaginal delivery between 31 December 1993 and 29 September 1997 in a Toronto hospital compared the rate of hospital readmission among newborns born before and after the implementation of a supposedly cost-saving early-discharge policy. Before the early-discharge policy was implemented the mean length of stay was 2.25 days. Following the initiation of the policy the mean stay decreased to 1.62 days. Deleterious effects of the new policy were observed in the higher rate of readmissions—11.7 per cent as compared to 6.7 per cent. The most frequent cause of readmission was jaundice (Locke and Ray, 1999). In that healthy infants are one of the best predictions of a healthy population, this finding warrants serious attention.

The cost of medical care, along with the provision of other social services, has been front and centre in political debates during the years since the implementation of medicare. It is fair to say that the issue is now critical—and has been dramatized by physician and nurse strikes, the closing of numerous hospitals through regionalization and debt, government caps on funding,

Table 11.7   Percentage Distribution of Health Expenditures, Public and Private

	Hospitals	Other institutions	Physicians	Other professional services	Drugs and appliances	All other health costs
1960	37.9	5.7	16.6	7.4	14.2	18.2
1965	42.7	6.1	16.0	6.6	13.3	15.3
1970	45.0	7.2	16.6	5.7	12.5	13.0
1975	44.4	9.7	15.7	6.0	10.7	13.5
1980	40.9	11.6	15.2	6.9	10.8	14.6
1981	41.2	11.4	15.0	6.8	11.0	14.6
1986	39.6	10.3	15.8	6.7	13.4	14.2
1987	39.2	10.3	16.0	6.8	13.9	13.8
1988	38.9	10.5	15.7	6.9		
1989	38.6	10.6	15.5	6.9		
1990	38.2	10.7	15.2	7.0		
1991	38.8	9.5	15.4	8.5	11.6	16.1
1992	38.2	9.7	14.9	8.4	12.0	16.5
1993	37.8	9.7	14.4	8.4	12.3	17.2
1994	37.2	9.7	14.2	8.5	12.6	17.4

Sources: *Canada Year Book*, 1994; Statistics Canada, Catalogue no. 82–221–XDE.

globalization accompanied by the political focus on the level of deficit in the government financing, the expanded free trade agreements, and a variety of other initiatives designed to restructure the provision of medical care.

Using a model of analysis focusing on the inherent contradictions in a capitalist welfare state, Burke and Stevenson (1993) provide a critique of contemporary Canadian strategies for controlling costs and redesigning health services. They argue that the political economy of health care must be studied in relation to the wider national political economy. Furthermore, they suggest, current policies suffer from several biases, including (1) *therapeutic nihilism* (a critique of the medical model used to cut back on the various essential medical services without provision for an alternative); (2) *healthism* (a model that attaches

health not only to medical services but also to various other issues, such as lifestyle), which can be used by the state to provide it the discursive space to claim that almost every expenditure has a health-enhancing effect and thus specific 'medical' care is less important; and (3) *the discourse of health promotion*, which can easily be 'captured by neoconservative forces to further an ideology favouring decentralization, flexibility, the intrusive state, individual responsibility, and the sanctity of the family' (ibid., 70). All of these forces are in fact evident in the federal government's health emphases over the past two and a half decades, beginning with Marc Lalonde's 1974 report, *A New Perspective on the Health of Canadians*.

There are various proposals for cutting costs. A first set of proposals includes user fees, extra-billing, co-insurance, and deductibles (suggested usually by the medical profession, often with state support). However, a number of researchers have found that such strategies do not work to control costs but rather serve to decrease equali-

Table 11.8   Incentives of Various Funding Systems

Funding System	Incentive
Fee-for-service	• Provide more service
Global funding	• Keep within the budget • Provide less service
Fee-for-service with hard cap, Equity funding, Reallocation	• Provide more service • Reduce cost per service
Capitation	• Keep people healthy • Avoid expensive service • Provide less service

Source: Closson and Catt (1996: 87).

ty of access to care, deter use by the poor, and redistribute the burden of paying for health care from taxpayers to sick people (Barer, Evans, and Stoddart, 1979; Stoddart and Labelle, 1985).

A second set of proposals concerns controls over the supply of physicians and hospitals through limits on immigration of foreign physicians, on enrolments in medical schools, and on residency positions, monitoring of physician billing, hospital and bed rationalization and closings, decreasing budgets, and contracting out of services to the private sector. The problems associated with such provisions are that they are largely ad hoc and will, without explicit planning, inadvertently result in the dismantling of universal medical care. Table 11.8 shows the relationship between the type of funding system and service incentives. Table 11.9 shows the growth in health expenditures in various categories from 1996 to 1999. Despite the widely cited weakening of the public medicare system across the country, expenditures as a proportion of the gross domestic product increased slightly in 1998–9.

Table 11.9   Health Expenditures, by Type

	1996	1997	1998	1999*
	$ Millions			
Health expenditures**	75,274.3	78,909.5	83,955.0	89,017.0
Hospitals	25,496.5	26,024.7	27,638.4	28,631.1
Other institutions	7,495.7	7,714.3	8,045.1	8,492.4
Physicians	10,705.6	11,132.3	11,686.9	12,198.6
Other professionals	8,977.3	9,724.0	10,239.6	10,733.9
Drugs: prescribed and non-prescribed	10,252.2	11,306.0	12,385.2	13,490.9
Other expenditures	12,347.0	13,008.3	13,959.7	15,470.0
	% of gross domestic product			
Health expenditures**	9.0	9.0	9.3	9.3

*Preliminary data.
**Health expenditures include spending by federal, provincial, and local governments, workers' compensation board.

Source: Canadian Institute for Health Information, National Health Expenditure Trends, 1975–2000.

Table 11.10   Private-Sector Health Expenditures, by Source of Finance and Use of Funds, Canada, 1999

	Private Sector				Private Sector as Percentage of Total Goods and Services
	Households (Out-of-pocket)	Private Insurance	Total	Public Sector	
	($000,000)			($000,000)	
Professional Services:					
Dental care	2,870	3,508	6,378	397	94
Vision care	1,701	428	2,129	218	91
Other services	717	482	1,199	546	69
Health-Care Goods:					
Prescribed drugs	2,302	3,387	5,680	4,418	56
Over-the-counter drugs	1,641	—	1,641	—	100
Personal health supplies	1,575	—	1,575	—	100
Other health care goods	178	$50	228	435	34
Total	10,984	7,855	18,839	6,014	76

Note: 'Other services' include expenditures for chiropractors, massage therapists, orthoptists, osteopaths, physiotherapists, podiatrists, psychologists, private-duty nurses, and naturopaths. 'Personal health supplies' include items used primarily to promote or maintain health (e.g., oral hygiene products, diagnostic items such as diabetic test strips, and medical items such as incontinence products). 'Other health care goods' include hearing aids and other medical appliances.

Source: Commission on the Future of Health Care (2002: 25).

A third set of proposals involves recognition of the increase in alternative models of health care (homeopathy, nurse practitioners, chiropractic), the introduction of alternate physician payment schemes such as MSAs (medical savings accounts), capitation, and salary, health promotion education, and publicly financed competition between types of health-care practitioners. Capitation is a system in which funding is given to service providers to take responsibility for the health of a specific number of people in a population, i.e., per patient annual payment to a physician. 'The goal in a capitated system is to keep the population healthy so that they will not require expensive services' (Closson and Catt, 1996). There is a relationship between the type of funding system and service incentives as proposed by Closson and Catt. Even in the midst of a universal medical care system, dental and vision care and prescription drugs are private expenditures. Table 11.10 portrays the breakdown in the source of expenditures for health-care services that fall outside of the universal medicare system for many.

Summary

(1) The chapter provides an overview of the history of medicine in Canada. Aboriginal peo-

ples had medicine men and shamans who used a wide variety of effective herbal remedies. Early Canadian settlers relied on a variety of treatments provided by midwives, local doctors, travelling salesmen, and mail-order dispensers of remedies. During the nineteenth century the government started to institute public health measures to deal with cholera and to license allopaths, homeopaths, and others.

(2) The implementation of universal medical insurance in Canada, which was completed in 1972, was the conclusion of a long, uphill battle, yet that battle has continued to the present day.

(3) There are several explanations for the development of medicare in Canada. Two of the most important are: movement in Western industrialized societies towards rationalized bureaucratic social organization and monopoly capitalism and the spread in Western Europe and beyond of social welfare legislation.

(4) The main goal of medicare in Canada was to provide equal health care to all Canadians, thus enhancing the general health of the population. To some extent, this goal has been reached; people in low-income groups visit physicians more often. Health, however, continues to vary by class.

(5) Medicare has also had an impact on medical practice: doctors' salaries increased dramatically, but have since levelled off. The ratio of doctors to population in Canada continues to decrease. Working conditions, control over other occupations in the medical field and over clients, self-regulation in education, licensing, and discipline, and the actual content of the work have all undergone significant alterations. As well, the medical profession is now under increased administrative, economic, political, and social constraints.

(6) Health-care costs as a portion of Canada's GNP have, since the introduction of medicare, increased. However, medicare seems to have controlled potentially spiralling costs of medical care. The greatest growth in medical expenditures until 1982 was in institutions; from 1982 to the present, the cost of drugs has represented the greatest growth in the health sector. In spite of some deinstitutionalization policies, the growth in the pharmaceutical sector is likely to continue as the population ages. Moreover, the elderly disproportionately consume pharmaceuticals. Again, as this population expands, drug costs can be expected to continue to grow. The cost of medical care is currently at the centre of a number of political debates regarding the provision of a universal social safety net.

(7) There are continuing debates about the successes and failures of medicare.

Questions for Study and Discussion

1. Compare the cholera and flu epidemics in early Canada.

2. Describe and critically analyze the organizing efforts made by the early allopathic doctors.

3. Explain in detail why some forces supported the development of a nationally funded medical care scheme and others rejected it.

4. How has medicare altered the health of Canadians?

5. How has medicare altered the work of doctors?

6. Evaluate the medicalization/demedicalization debate.

7. Debate the public/private issue with respect to medical care in Canada today.

Suggested Readings

Armstrong, Pat, and Hugh Armstrong. 2003. *Wasting Away: The Undermining of Canadian Health Care*, 2nd edn. Toronto. Oxford University Press. Together and separately, the Armstrongs have contributed immensely to our understanding of medical care from a critical and social scientific perspective.

Charles, Catherine A. 1976. 'The Medical Profession and Health Insurance: An Ottawa Case Study', *Social Science and Medicine* 10: 33–8. A useful critique of the impact of government financing on health-care work.

Dicken McGinnis, Janice P. 1977. 'The Influence of Epidemic Influenza: Canada', Canadian Historical Association, *Historical Papers*. One of several useful accounts of the flu epidemic of 1918.

McLeod, Thomas H., and Ina McLeod. 1987. *Tommy Douglas: The Road to Jerusalem*. Edmonton: Hurtig. This book (and the other sources mentioned in Box 11.5) gives the reader an understanding of the contribution Tommy Douglas made to Canadian health care.

Mhatra, Sharmila, and Raise B. Deber. 1992. 'From Equal Access to Health Care to Equitable Access to Health: A Review of Canadian Provincial Health Commissions and Reports', *International Journal of Health Services* 22, 4: 645–68. Explains in some detail why Canada's medicare system is a qualified success.

Chapter 12 | *The Medical Profession*

Learning Objectives

- Medical practice is considered to be a profession.
- There are three somewhat different theories of professionalization (occupation, process, ideology).
- The medical profession has consolidated its position through the subordination, limitation, and exclusion of other types of health-care providers.
- Norman Bethune and Banting and Best are important Canadians in the history of medicine in this country.
- Medical education has changed substantially over the past few centuries.
- Medical students tend to be from relatively high socio-economic backgrounds.
- The proportion of female and visible minority medical students is increasing.
- Medical responsibility and clinical experience are among the values that doctors learn during their education.
- There are several useful critiques of contemporary medical education.
- Some of the critical issues in medical organization and practice today are autonomy, control, authority, technical and moral mistakes, and practice norms and variations.

Introduction

'Society expects a formidable array of virtues and abilities in its doctors: technical competence, mastery of medical knowledge, sensitivity to the "whole patient", communicative ease and skill, wise judgement, compassion and professional integrity' (Gallagher and Searle, 1989).

Why is the occupation of the physician thought to be a profession? What is a profession? How do physicians fit into the whole medical care system? Are doctors losing or gaining power, prestige, and income? Does membership in a professional occupation guarantee a high moral calling and a dedication to service? Do all doctors learn all that must be learned in medical school? How do doctors handle mistakes or conflicts? To whom are doctors accountable? These are among the questions that interest medical sociologists. The purpose of this chapter is to analyze the work of the physician as a profession and to describe the process of medical education in the context of Canadian society, both today and in the past. The chapter will examine the division of labour and medical practice, the issues of social control and autonomy within the profession, ideas about physicians' networks and their cultural environment, their handling of mistakes, and medical education.

The 'Profession' of Medicine

The idea that medicine is a profession is relatively new. Yet in the last half-century or so, the medical doctor has become the archetypal professional. Medicine is generally thought to be the model profession, not only by theorists of occupations and professions, but by the lay public and by those other occupational groups aspiring to reach the 'heights' of professional status.

There are three distinctly different ways to think about professions and professionalization. First, professions can be considered occupations that have certain specific characteristics or traits. Second, professions can be viewed as the result of processes of occupational change over time. Third, it is possible to consider the notion of the profession as ideology.

Profession as Occupation: The Trait Approach

The view of the profession as a particular type of occupation is called the *trait approach*. William Goode (1956, 1960) thought that professions were special occupations that embodied two basic characteristics: (1) prolonged training in a body of specialized, abstract knowledge; and (2) a service orientation. Goode broke these two characteristics down further and described the traits of a profession as follows (1960).

1. It determines its own standards for education and training.

2. There are stringent educational requirements.
3. Practice often involves legal recognition through some form of licence.
4. Licensing and admission standards are determined and managed by members of the profession.
5. Most legislation with respect to the practice of the profession in question is shaped by the profession.
6. The profession is characterized by relatively high power, prestige, and income.
7. The professional practitioner is relatively free of lay control and evaluation.
8. The norms of practice enforced by the profession are more stringent than legal controls.
9. Members are more strongly identified and affiliated with their profession than members of other occupational groups.
10. Members usually stay in the profession for life.

The characteristics of the medical profession in Canada today are somewhat similar to those suggested by Goode. Physicians themselves largely determine what constitutes appropriate subject matter for the study and practical experience of physicians-in-training. Medical schools have some of the most stringent admittance criteria of any educational programs. In addition to grades, many medical schools consider the personal qualities of the applicants, such as their ethical views, behaviour, self-presentation in an interview, ability to work with others as a 'team' player, their leadership abilities, and, increasingly, whole-person communication skills (Kendall and Reader, 1988). The profession, too, determines licensing and admittance standards. Medicine is characterized by the relatively high power, prestige, and income of its professional practitioners. Physicians are largely controlled via various committees and organizations, such as the College of Physicians and Surgeons, which are composed

Box 12.1   Canadian Medical Association Code of Ethics

The Code of Ethics of the CMA includes 43 statements of principle under eight different headings. The following are the 'General Responsibilities' and 'Responsibilities to Society'.

General Responsibilities

1. Consider first the well-being of the patient.
2, Treat all patients with respect; do not exploit them for personal advantage.
3. Provide for appropriate care for your patient, including physical comfort and spiritual and psychosocial support, even when cure is no longer possible.
4. Practise the art and science of medicine competently and without impairment.
5. Engage in lifelong learning to maintain and improve your professional knowledge, skills and attitudes.
6. Recognize your limitations and the competence of others, and, when indicated, recommend that additional opinions and services be sought.

Responsibilities to Society

29. Recognize that community, society and the environment are important factors in the health of individual patients.
30. Accept a share of the profession's responsibility to society in matters relating to public health, health education, environmental protection, legislation affecting the health or well-being of the community and the need for testimony at judicial proceedings.
31. Recognize the responsibility of physicians to promote fair access to health care resources.
32. Use health care resources prudently.
33. Refuse to participate in or support practices that violate basic human rights.
34. Recognize a responsibility to give the generally held opinions of the profession when interpreting scientific knowledge to the public; when presenting an opinion that is contrary to the generally held opinion of the profession, so indicate.

Source: Canadian Medical Association (1999).

primarily of practising doctors. Their own norms, incorporated in the Code of Ethics (Box 12.1), are more exacting than the law although they are not necessarily strictly enforced. A doctor's identity as a person is tied to his or her occupation. This affects all other aspects of his/her life, including family life. Generally, a career in medicine is a lifetime career.

Goode's view of professions has a number of limitations. First, it is based on an acceptance of the viewpoint or ideology put forward by the professional group itself. The ideology of a particular occupation cannot help but be self-serving. Second, it ignores the fundamental importance of the power of the professional group. It is this power that enables it to maintain the prevailing ideology both internally and in society at large. Third, this analysis does not take into account the changes in the profession over time; it assumes that the peak of professionalism is portrayed by the traits of the profession as they are described by its members. Fourth, it ignores the relationship between the profession and the rest of society—the state, the economic and political structure, and the social organization of society. In brief, the trait approach ignores the historical development of the profession and its place in society.

Table 12.1   Profession as Process

Non-Profession		Profession
Very little, very simple concrete education or training not associated with a university.	EDUCATION	Complex, abstract, esoteric, lengthy education associated with university.
Anyone can call themselves a	LICENSING	Profession itself determines eligibility and continuously evaluates ongoing suitability to maintain professional status.
Each person for himself or herself and to his or her own benefit.	CODE OF ETHICS	Altruism, higher calling, collectivity orientation and identity.
Each person for himself or herself and to his or her own benefit.	ASSOCIATION	Organized group encompassing most people actively pursuing the profession.
State-based laws to control individual behaviour and discipline.	PEER CONTROL	Professional association determines standards of education, professional activity, and disciplines members in violation.

Profession as Process

The second view of professions is as a *process* through which various occupational groups may progress or hope and aspire to progress over time under various conditions (see Table 12.1). Within this perspective there are those who accept the ideological view put forward by the profession; but they see the traits such as those described by Goode (1960) as the end points of a pattern of forward growth. Wilensky's (1964) work is representative of such an approach.

The steps to becoming a professional in this perspective are as follows: first, the members of the occupation engage in full-time work; second, they establish a relationship with a training/education program; third, they establish an association; fourth, they gain legal status; and fifth, they construct a code of ethics. This approach brings a historical perspective to the concept of the profession. It also has the advantage of showing that occupations can be seen as falling along continua with respect to the degree of professionalism they incorporate. Underlying this model, as well as the trait approach, is an acceptance of the view that the profession is a more desirable and higher calling than other occupations.

Johnson's (1972, 1977, 1982) model of the professions bridges the process and the ideology approaches in what we can call *the power analysis approach*. Johnson describes professions with respect to process, too, but he focuses on how occupational groups become professions as they increase in power. He discusses the theoretical explanations for the power of professions and sees power as the ability of the professional practitioners to define 'reality' in an increasingly broad way, and even to define the 'good life' for their clients.

From this viewpoint the fundamental characteristic of a profession is the ability of the group to impose its perspective and the necessity of its services upon its clients. Professional power arises out of the uncertainty in the relationship between the client and the professional; this uncertainty stems from the social distance between the two parties. Three crucial variables determine the degree of power held by a profes-

Box 12.2   Specialization

Another characteristic of the contemporary medical care system is extensive specialization. Recently, the *Globe and Mail* advertised vacancies in all the following positions, many of which did not exist only a few decades ago. These were all advertised under the heading **Hospital, Medical and Social Services**.

Psychologist
Ultrasound Technologist
Pharmacist
Staff Occupational Therapist
Cardio-Pulmonary Perfusionist
Speech Pathologist
Manager of Nursing Practice
Executive Assistant (to the President)
Independent Community Living Worker
Administrative Coordinator, Regional Geriatric Program
Histology Manager

Clinical Nurse Specialist
Information Systems Coordinator
Research Assistant
Registered Technologist
Health Science Librarian
Physiotherapist
Director of Plant and Engineering Maintenance
Nurse Manager
Supervisor, Accounts Payable
Psychiatrist
Executive Assistant
Medical Officer

Coordinator, Community Mental Health Program
Director of Pediatrics and Obstetric Nursing
Kinesiologist
Nuclear Medicine Technician
Social Worker
Manager, Nursing Practice
Chaplain
Ultrasonographer
Director, Sexual Assault Care Centre
Audiologist

sional group: (1) the more esoteric the knowledge base of professional practice and the less accessible this knowledge is to the lay public, the greater the power of the profession; (2) the greater the social distance between the client and the professional when the professional is, for instance, of a higher income level and social class than the client, the greater the power of the profession; and (3) the greater the homogeneity of the professional group in contrast with the heterogeneity of the client group, the greater the power of the profession.

Esoteric knowledge is important because the less accessible the knowledge is to a wide spectrum of the population, the greater the power of the professional group compared to the potential client group. Social distance refers to the relative prestige of the occupation within the labour force, the income of the practitioners, and even the relative class background from which the practitioners are typically drawn as compared to

average societal members. The more heterogeneous the consumer group, the more likely they are to be disorganized and unable to work together to protect their interests. On the other hand, the more homogeneous the professional group, the more they are able to organize to attain their ends. The power differential is greatest when a heterogeneous client group must deal with a relatively homogeneous professional group.

Johnson's model overlaps part of the process model in that he articulates some of the bases upon which professional power varies. His work is also related to the trait approach to professions in that the power of the profession is in its ability to persuade others of its 'higher traits' (or ideology).

Subordination, Limitation, and Exclusion in the Medical Labour Force

The medical profession successfully consolidated its position as the provider of medical care by restricting the scope of the work of other types of practitioners. According to Willis (1983), whose research was carried out in Australia, the allopathic medical profession achieved the level of dominance it has come to enjoy by three distinct processes. The first is *subordination*. This refers to the process whereby potentially or actually competing professions come to work under the direct control of the doctors. Nursing is as an example of this process, because the practice of nursing has been severely restricted and constrained so that the primary legal position of nurses today is subordinate to the medical profession (see Chapter Fourteen).

The second process is called *limitation*, and is illustrated by such occupations as dentistry, optometry, and pharmacy. Such occupations are not directly under the control of the allopathic practitioners, but they are indirectly controlled through legal restrictions. The process by which pharmacy came to be subordinate to medicine is a case in point. In the nineteenth century, pharmacists operated as primary caregivers. They prescribed medicines to patients who came to them for help, particularly to the poor and doctorless. In many ways the roles of the pharmacists and the doctors overlapped at this time because most doctors made and dispensed their own drugs. When the pharmacists became self-regulating in 1870–1, they agreed on an informal compromise with the doctors. Pharmacists gave up prescribing, and doctors gave up dispensing drugs. Today the profession of pharmacy is attempting to expand pharmacy's care into the community, especially through educating and communicating with the public. One of its particular mandates is the reduction in drug-related problems (over-medication, drug overdose, drug interactions, and side effects) among the elderly (Battershell, 1994; Muzzin et al., 1993; Muzzin, 2001).

The third process, *exclusion*, is the process whereby certain occupations that are not licensed and therefore are denied official legitimacy come to be considered 'alternative' practices. The

Australian example given by Willis (1983) is that of the chiropractors. However, chiropractors in Canada have an ambiguous position today. (See Chapter Fifteen for a thorough discussion of this issue.) Perhaps a better Canadian example would be naturopaths. Because naturopathic medicine is based on a different model of science than allopathic medicine and is not yet the subject of sufficient (traditional scientific) research confirming its effectiveness, it is not considered a mainstream medical practice and its practitioners are not funded under medicare.

There have been significant changes in the legal status of complementary and alternative health-care practice across the country in the last decade or so. In Ontario, for example, the Regulated Health Practitioners Act came into effect. This landmark legislation restricts allopathic monopoly by delicensing all health-care professions. Consumers can now choose the form of health care they desire although they may have to pay privately for such alternative services. Alternative practitioners are allowed to advertise. By this Act medicine is limited to 13 clearly defined or 'controlled' acts (such as surgery or prescribing drugs). These controlled acts are 'activities which might harm patients, leaving all other health care activities (those presumably which would not cause harm) free to be carried out by any health practitioner' (Coburn et al., 1997: 12). Twenty-four health professions are regulated under the Act, including speech pathology, chiropractic, dental hygiene, dentistry, massage therapy, medical laboratory technology, medical radiation technology, medicine, midwifery, nursing, occupational therapy, optometry, pharmacy, physiotherapy, psychology, and respiratory technology. Others, such as homeopaths, acupuncturists, herbalists, and reflexologists, are unregulated. Both regulated and unregulated professions have the right to practice. Regulated professions have their own administrative colleges with independent self-governing powers and are responsible to the Ministry of Health.

Regulated practitioners may do only what their colleges permit. Unregulated practitioners can do anything, as long as it is legal.

Profession as Ideology

An *ideology* is a group of descriptive and prescriptive beliefs used to explain and legitimize certain practices and viewpoints. The notion that professionalism is an ideological concept was raised first in the writings of Everett C. Hughes (1971). He criticized the trait approach, which was the standard of the time, because it was based on the assumption that what the medical profession said about itself—its ideal image—was an accurate representation of the profession. Hughes noted that this was a biased representation because physicians, as well as offering a valuable service to others, were rewarded generously both by their status and by their income.

Parsons (1951) adopted the prevailing ideology of professionals when he argued that a profession has the following characteristics: (1) *universalism*, (2) *functional specificity*, (3) *affective neutrality*, and (4) a *collectivity orientation*. In this view a physician is expected to apply universalistic, scientifically based standards to all patients. Physicians are not to differentiate between patients or their treatments on the basis of social differences such as gender, education, income level, or race, for instance. All patients are to be provided with the same level of care, for the same level of disease, according to universally applied standards. The work of the physician is also functionally specific to the malfunctioning of the human body and mind. Functional specificity requires that the physician not offer advice to a patient on non-medical matters such as real estate or choice of a career, but restrict advice to the precise area of health and disease. The doctor is expected to refrain from emotional involvement, in other words, to be affectively neutral. When medical issues are involved (or are believed to be involved), the physician has extraordinary access to intimate knowledge of the social and emotional life as well as the body of the patient. The physician is permitted special access to the private sphere of the patient's life on the assumption that his or her duties will be performed in an objective and emotionally detached manner. The doctor is expected to express concern and exhibit a 'good bedside manner', while, because of his or her special knowledge of the body and life of the patient, he or she is also expected to be impartial and unemotional in judgement and treatment. Finally, the physician is expected to exhibit a collectivity orientation, that is, to provide service to others out of a sense of calling to the profession and an altruistic desire to serve others. Self-interest, whether expressed in terms of financial rewards or other aspects of working conditions, is not appropriate within the ideology of medical practice.

Freidson views professionalism as ideology, as is suggested by the title of his book, *The Profession of Medicine* (1975). The profession of medicine refers both to the occupational group, which is composed of medical practitioners, and to the statements made by doctors as they 'profess' their work. In Freidson's model, medicine's claim to professional status rests on three assertions made by physicians: first, medical knowledge is complex, detailed, and difficult; second, medical work is based on the findings of objective science; and third, as professionals, doctors can be trusted to put the welfare of the public ahead of their own welfare.

This view is ideological—and it has served the medical profession well. Through the perpetuation of such a view the public has come to believe that doctors are 'morally superior' individuals who deserve to be trusted, to dominate the practice of medicine, to hold a monopoly in the construction, maintenance, and spread of what is taken to be official 'medical knowledge', to control standards for their training, and to discipline their errant members themselves.

This ideological position is widely challenged today in the wake of increasing costs

Box 12.3   Norman Bethune

Norman Bethune, born in 1890 in Gravenhurst, Ontario, became a prominent Canadian thoracic surgeon who served in three wars and distinguished himself as a surgeon on three continents.

Bethune came from a family with high standards and widely recognized achievement. His great-great-grandfather, Reverend John Bethune (1751–1815), built Canada's first Presbyterian church in Montreal. One of his sons, John Bethune (1791–1872), became Rector of Montreal and Principal of McGill University. Two other sons, Alexander and Angus, also achieved prominence in their chosen professions: Alexander became the second Anglican Bishop of Toronto; Angus became a successful businessman, helping head the two great Canadian fur-trading companies in Canada, the North West Company and the Hudson's Bay Company. Angus's son, Norman (Bethune's grandfather), was educated in Toronto and learned surgery in Edinburgh before returning to Toronto to become one of the co-founders of Trinity Medical School in 1850. Norman himself was one of three children of Elizabeth Ann Goodwin and Malcolm Bethune.

Bethune worked in a number of jobs, as a lumberjack and as a teacher, teaching immigrants how to read. From 1909 to 1911 he was registered in pre-medical studies at the University of Toronto. Just before his third year of medicine, Bethune joined the Royal Canadian Army Medical Corps. After he was wounded at Ypres he returned to Canada to complete his medical degree by 1916. In 1923 he married Francis Penney Campbell, with whom he had a stormy and ambivalent relationship. They were divorced and later married again. In 1927–8 Bethune succumbed to tuberculosis and was treated at Trudeau Sanatorium in New York. As a result of his experience of illness, Bethune developed an interest in thoracic surgery and went into practice with Dr Edward Archibald, a renowned thoracic surgeon at the Royal Victoria Hospital in Montreal. Here Bethune engaged in research on tuberculosis. During this time he invented a variety of surgical instruments that were widely used in North America.

Bethune is, however, best known for his political activities. Nearly 70 years ago, in 1936, Bethune tried to establish a state-supported medicare system for Canadians. He organized a group of doctors, nurses, and social workers, called the Montreal Group for the Security of People's Health. Outraged at the refusal of the Canadian Medical Association to support plans for socialized medicine, he sailed for Spain at the outbreak of civil war in October 1936 to aid in the struggle against the Nationalist forces of General Franco. In Spain he devised a method to transport blood to the wounded on the battlefields.

As a professed Communist, it was almost impossible for Bethune to remain in Canada. When war broke out in China, Bethune decided to help in the fight for communism. Medical treatment was needed. With funds donated by the China Aid Council and also from the League for Peace and Democracy, Bethune purchased much-needed medical supplies. He arrived in Yannarv in 1938 and quickly moved to the front lines in the mountains of East Shanxi. Travelling with the Eighth Route Army, he devoted his remaining years to fighting fascism and saving the lives of the soldiers who stood for the cause he, too, believed in. His fame reached China's political leaders. Summoned to meet Chairman Mao Tse-Tung, Bethune convinced the leader of the need for surgical knowledge in the front lines of the Chin-Cha'a-Border Region.

Bethune founded a medical school and model hospital that would later be renamed the Norman Bethune International Peace Hospital. He had placed his mark in history's pages as a great surgeon and humanitarian.

Bethune died in China of septicemia on 12 November 1939.

Sources: Gordon and Allan (1952); Shephard (1982); Stewart (1977).

Box 12.4   Asymmetry in the Medical Encounter

The idea that the clinical relationship between the doctor and the patient is asymmetrical has been assumed and investigated since Parsons's early work on the sick role. This situation is inherently paradoxical. Patients, on the one hand, are expected to use their own common sense to decide whether or not to seek medical help. On the other hand, once they have decided there is something wrong that needs to be diagnosed they are expected to give their own judgement away. Any response from the patient, such as doubt or questioning of the diagnosis, 'undermines the patient's grounds for seeking professional medical help in the first place' (Pilnick, 1998: 30).

In the case of chronic illnesses, however, patients frequently come to know more than their own doctors about how their bodies respond to various medications or other life changes (such as nutrition) made in the interest of managing the illness. Increasingly, patients with chronic diseases join self-help groups, read newsletters, visit Web sites, and monitor, often with those close to them, their varying levels of symptoms. Pilnick describes how, in a situation in which parents and children regularly visit a clinic for chemotherapy and other treatments associated with childhood leukemia, the parents become experts, in their relationship to the pharmacists, as they are highly involved in the determination of dosage (which varies according to body weight and blood levels, among other things). Even though the parents are often in a position to know more than the pharmacists about their particular child's responses to medication protocols, the pharmacists still tend to have interactional dominance. As Pilnick says, 'since the pharmacist has a particular task to accomplish (handing over the medications) and the patient or carer has visited the pharmacist primarily to receive this medication, for the pharmacists to direct or "dominate" the encounter is perhaps the easiest method to ensure that this is brought about swiftly and successfully by both parties' (ibid., 49).

without parallel improvements in life expectancy or health quality, mounting evidence of doctors' mistakes, and rising rates of malpractice suits. Moreover, in the wake of the 'debt crisis' the future growth of the increasingly specialized occupation of medicine is likely to be curtailed. During the late eighties and well into the nineties hospitals were closed across the country and home health care was to be expanded. The federal government appears to be increasingly supportive of what has come to be called health promotion and disease prevention. Alternative health-care providers such as midwives have become legitimized, with their own colleges, in various parts of the country. Moreover, midwives have recently been granted a degree of professional autonomy. Challenges to the exclusive rights of allopathic doctors to dispense medical care are evident in a variety of ways.

The first blow to the Canadian popular belief in the altruism of the medical profession arose at the time of the 1962 doctors' strike in Saskatchewan. A more recent and equally dramatic demonstration was the strike over extra-billing by many Ontario doctors in 1986. Still, it needs to be emphasized that in a recent Gallup poll (1999) doctors were ranked as ethical and honest by 62 per cent of the respondents. This percentage was higher than that for police officers, engineers, university professors, and even clergy (Buske, 1999c).

Doctors appear to be becoming increasingly militant in their fight for what they consider to be improved health care and health-care funding.

Strikes, lawsuits against the government, and limitations in access to service were among the job actions taken by doctors in British Columbia, Quebec, Alberta, and Manitoba in the latter part of the twentieth century and into the twenty-first century (Sibbald, 1998).

A Brief History of Medical Education in North America

After 1800 a growing number of proprietary medical schools (profit-making institutions that were generally owned by doctors who also served as teachers) began to open in North America. The quality of the education they offered was poor. They were usually ill equipped for teaching, but then medical theory was still very simple (Wertz and Wertz, 1986: 137). Bleeding, the application of leeches, and the ingestion of purgatives to cause vomiting were still the treatments of choice. At this time people were as likely to be harmed as helped by the prevalent and accepted methods of cure.

The most advanced medical training of the time was in Europe, especially France and Germany, where medical research was well supported. Louis Pasteur's germ theory, proposed in the mid-nineteenth century, had a remarkable effect on medicine and provided the basis for the discovery, classification, and treatment of numerous diseases. By the end of the century German physicians had made significant discoveries in the world of medical science, too. Rudolf Virchow described a general model of disease development based on cellular pathology (1858), and Robert Koch discovered the bacillus for anthrax (1876), tuberculosis (1882), and cholera (1883). Because of these exciting developments in European medical science, American doctors began to cross the ocean for their education and training. Approximately 15,000 American doctors studied in German-speaking universities from approximately 1870 to 1914.

European training soon became a symbol of status among Americans. Those with such training were able to establish more prestigious and specialized practices than American-trained doctors. By the beginning of the twentieth century, medical research was well funded by the Carnegie and Rockefeller families. The United States began to move ahead as a leader in the development of scientific and medical resources.

Medical education, too, was radically revised and upgraded at the beginning of the twentieth century. The Flexner Report, published in 1910, reviewed medical education in the US and Canada. Sponsored by the Carnegie Foundation, Abraham Flexner visited every medical school in the two countries. Only three American medical schools, Harvard, Johns Hopkins, and Western Reserve, were given approval. The others were severely criticized and were characterized as 'plague spots, utterly wretched'. Flexner's observations about Canadian medical schools were very similar to those regarding the American schools. As he said:

> In the matter of medical schools, Canada reproduces the United States on a greatly reduced scale. Western University (London) is as bad as anything to be found on this side of the line; Laval and Halifax Medical Colleges are feeble; Winnipeg and Kingston represent a distinct effort toward higher ideals; McGill and Toronto are excellent. (Flexner, 1910: 325)

According to the report, 90 per cent of practising doctors lacked a college education, and the vast majority had attended inadequate medical schools (Wertz and Wertz, 1986: 138). Flexner recommended that medical schools consist of full-time, highly educated faculty and be affiliated with a university. He suggested that laboratory and hospital facilities be associated with universities. He recommended the establishment of admission standards. Medical education, he argued, should be at the graduate school level. However, the effects of the Flexner Report were not as devastating to Canadian schools as to the American schools because Canadian medical schools had already been limited and controlled in their growth. In addition, there were far fewer proprietary schools in Canada. Proprietary schools were gradually closed, and medical education was slowly upgraded. The large American foundations donated monies to Canadian medicine and a scientifically based practice became well established.

By the mid-1920s the medical profession in America had clearly established itself as a leading profession. Its standards for training had been improved and were considered excellent. Medical research had reached great heights. The power of the doctor as a healer and as a scientist was widely assumed.

Medical Education in Canada Today

The first Canadian medical school, established in 1824 with 25 students, was at the Montreal Medical Institution, which became the faculty of medicine of McGill University in 1829 (Hamowy, 1984). By the turn of the century six other university medical schools had opened their doors—Toronto, Laval (Montreal and Quebec City campuses), Queen's, Dalhousie, Western, and Manitoba. There has been a decline since 1983 in the number of students admitted to the first year of medical school. In 1983, the peak year, 1,887 students were admitted. By 1997 only 1,577 students were admitted to medical schools in Canada, in spite of population growth and aging. This represents a 30 per cent decline in the number of first-year positions per 100,000 Canadians (Buske, 1999a: 772). Still, the number of physicians per population has continued to grow as a result of the high rates of immigration of physicians.

The process of becoming a doctor requires three different steps: an undergraduate education in science and/or arts, graduate study leading to the MD, and a minimum one-year internship in which the graduate MD works in a hospital or clinic under the supervision of practising doctors. During the internship year students write qualifying exams through the Medical Council of Canada, after which a licence to practice medicine is issued by any one of the provincial medical licensing bodies. Many doctors continue after the internship to specialize in family practice or any of a number of different specialties recognized by the Royal College of Physicians and Surgeons of Canada. Today 17 Canadian universities grant an MD degree and there are new programs opening in northern Ontario and in northern British Columbia.

Box 12.5   Sir Frederick G. Banting and Charles H. Best

Banting and Best are known for their discovery of how to extract the hormone insulin from the pancreas. This made possible the treatment of diabetes milletus, a disease in which an abnormal buildup of glucose occurs in the body. In 1923 Banting was a co-recipient of the Nobel Prize for physiology and medicine for his research and the development of insulin.

Banting's interest in medicine was aroused as the result of a childhood incident. One day, while on his way home from school, he stopped to look at two men who had just begun the first row of shingles on the roof of a new house. As he watched, the scaffolding on which they stood suddenly broke. The two men fell to the ground and were badly injured. Banting ran for the doctor, who arrived in a matter of minutes. 'I watched every movement of those skilful hands as he examined the injured men and tended to cuts, bruises, and broken bones. In those tense minutes I thought that the greatest service in life is that of the medical profession. From that day it was my greatest ambition to become a doctor.'

He studied at the University of Toronto and became committed to his idea that insulin, a hormone secreted by certain cells within the pancreas, would cure diabetes. However, Banting's qualifications as an investigator of carbohydrate metabolism were limited. He needed an assistant.

Realizing Banting's dilemma, Professor J.J. Macleod at the University of Toronto mentioned to his senior class in physiology that a young surgeon was carrying out research on the pancreatic islets and the isolation of the antidiabetic hormone. Two students, C.H. Best and E.C. Noble, had previously been engaged in experimental studies of diabetes and had an understanding of carbohydrate metabolism as well as the specific skills required to perform the necessary tests. Both were chosen assistants for a period of four weeks each. They tossed a coin to decide who would work the first four weeks and Best won. Mr Noble never did return to assist Banting. Best became his permanent assistant. Banting and Best made a good team. Their skills complemented each other. The younger man's knowledge of the latest biochemical procedures complemented the surgical skills of the older man.

On 16 May 1921 Banting and Best were given 10 dogs and the use of a laboratory for eight weeks. Their first task was to ligate the pancreatic ducts of a number of dogs. The next step involved trying to produce experimental diabetes. Many animal rights' activists argued against the use of dogs in Banting and Best's experiments. However, Banting adopted a very caring attitude towards these 'assistants'. He made sure the dogs were always spared unnecessary pain.

By 21 July 1921 a depancreatized dog and duct-tied dog with a pancreas were available.

Banting opened the abdominal cavity of the latter dog, removed the shrivelled pancreas, and chopped it into small pieces. This mass was ground up and saline was added. Banting and Best administered 5cc intravenously to the depancreatized dog. Samples of blood were taken at half-hour intervals and analyzed for sugar content. The blood sugar fell and the clinical condition of the dog improved.

On 11 January 1922, after months of research to perfect the extract, Banting and Best were ready to experiment with a patient. The first patient was a 14-year-old boy suffering from juvenile diabetes. When he was admitted to the Toronto General Hospital he was poorly nourished, pale, weighed a meagre 65 pounds, and his hair was falling out. A test for sugar was strongly positive. He received daily injections of the extract. An immediate improvement occurred. The boy excreted less sugar, and he became brighter, more active, and felt stronger. This 14-year-old boy was the first of many children who were helped by the discoveries of Banting and Best.

In 1923, Banting and Professor Macleod jointly received the Nobel Prize in physiology and medicine for their investigations into and research on insulin, the active principle of the Islands of Langerhans of the pancreas and regulator of the sugar level in the blood. Macleod received this joint recognition for sharing his laboratory facilities and for finding Best as a collaborator for Banting. Macleod insisted on the verification of the initial work and the repetition of certain controlled experiments. However, Macleod did not create the serum. Banting was somewhat annoyed that Best did not receive any recognition or award for his work, so he divided equally his share of the award money ($40,000) with Best. Furthermore, Banting always assigned 'equal credit' for the discovery of insulin to his friend and assistant, Best.

Sources: Bliss (1982, 1984); Castiglioni (1941); Stevenson (1946); *Academic American Encyclopedia*, vol. 3 (1980: 71); *Colliers Encyclopedia*, vol. 3 (1973: 602); *Encyclopedia Britannica,* vol. 3 (1976: 134).

Table 12.2   First-Year Enrolment in Canadian Faculties of Medicine by Sex, 1957–8 to 2000–1

Year	Men	Women	Total	% Women
1957–8	925	86	1,011	8.5
1961–2	890	116	1,006	11.5
1966–7	1,040	152	1,192	12.8
1971–2	1,242	359	1,601	22.4
1977–8	1,224	602	1,826	33.0
1981–2	1,144	737	1,881	39.2
1987–8	929	815	1,744	46.7
1991–2	969	806	1,775	45.4
1996–7	791	807	1,598	50.5
2000–1	809	954	1,763	54.1

Source: Adapted from *Canadian Medical Education Statistics, 2001*, Association of Canadian Medical Colleges, at: <www.acmc.ca>.

Medical students have been and continue to be drawn from middle- and upper-middle-class family backgrounds (Kirk, 1994). There has been a significant change in the proportion of women graduating from medical school: 6 per cent of all graduates in 1959 and 44 per cent in 1989 were women (Williams et al., 1993). By 1990, women comprised almost 50 per cent of all medical students. Since 1996, as shown in Table 12.2, women students have outnumbered males (CIHI, 2002: ix). Also, as Figure 12.1 indicates, first-year enrolment declined somewhat over the 1980s and 1990s. Financial concerns are still among the top three reasons mentioned by students who considered and then rejected medical school education (Colquitt and Killian, 1991). Tuition increased from 1998–9 to 2001–2 by 39 per cent to an average of $6,554 per year (ibid.). Nevertheless, applicants to medical school today exceed the available spaces by a 13:1 ratio (ibid., 19).

Although more women are entering medical school, their incomes are still, on average, considerably smaller than those of male doctors.

Nevertheless, they are significantly greater than those of either male or female nurses. The incomes of both male and female doctors are still relatively high.

The Process of Becoming a Doctor

The most influential and complete sociological studies of medical education were done in the 1950s and 1960s. The two most notable were the studies done at the University of Chicago by Howard S. Becker and others: *Boys in White: Student Culture in Medical School* (1961), and at Columbia University by Robert K. Merton and his colleagues, *The Student Physician: Introductory Studies in the Sociology of Medical Education* (1957). Each in its own way contributed to our knowledge of the socialization of the physician. Each explained some of the processes whereby young men (and some young women) pass through one of the most rigorous, busy, lengthy, and pressured educational programs and come to

Figure 12.1   First-Year Enrolment in Canadian Medical Schools

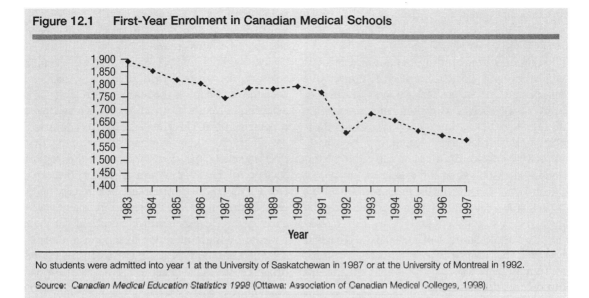

No students were admitted into year 1 at the University of Saskatchewan in 1987 or at the University of Montreal in 1992.

Source: *Canadian Medical Education Statistics 1998* (Ottawa: Association of Canadian Medical Colleges, 1998).

adopt the values, norms, skills, and knowledge expected of a medical doctor.

Becker and his colleagues observed and spent time doing participant observation with medical students during their years of medical education at the University of Kansas Medical School. These researchers noted that the major consequences of medical school were that physicians-in-training became aware of the importance of two dominant values: *clinical experience* and *medical responsibility*. These two dominant values then guided and directed the strategies used by the medical students to manage the potentially infinite workload involved in learning all that had to be known before graduation. Clinical experience essentially refers to the belief that much of medical practice is actually based on the 'art' of determining, from complex and subtle interpersonal cues and in interaction with the patient, the nature of the disease and the appropriate treatment. More important than either abstract knowledge based on medical school lectures or book or general scientific knowledge, clinical experience was considered a fundamental aspect of good doctoring.

Along with clinical experience, doctors-in-training were impressed by the notion of medical responsibility. By this Becker and his colleagues stressed the 'enormous' moral responsibility of the life-and-death decisions that frequently confronted doctors in practice.

These two values were the most important aspects of learning. They served to enable the medical students to choose, from the masses of detail presented in books and in lectures, what actually had to be learned. The notion of clinical experience guided the selection of facts that had to be memorized to pass the examination. It tended to lead the students to disregard basic science and focus on classes where they were provided with practical information of the sort that was not typically found in medical textbooks. Furthermore, the focus on medical responsibility tended to result in an emphasis by the student on interesting cases that involved life-and-death medical judgements rather than on the more common and mundane diseases. It also tended to guide the choice of specialties. The most desired specialties frequently were those with the potential of saving patients (or killing them), such as surgery and internal medicine.

Merton and his colleagues described medical education and socialization as a continuous process by which medical students learned to think of themselves as doctors and in so doing absorbed sufficient knowledge to feel comfortable in their new role. Accordingly, two basic traits were developed: the ability to remain emotionally detached from the patient in the face of life-and-death emergencies, great sorrow or joy, or sexuality; and the ability to deal with the inevitable and constant uncertainty. Fox (1957) observed three sources of uncertainty. The first occurred because it was impossible to learn everything there was to learn about medicine and its practice. The second stemmed from the awareness that, even if the student was able to learn all the available medical knowledge, there would still be gaps because medical knowledge was itself incomplete. The third and final source of uncertainty arose from the first two: the uncertainty resulting from distinguishing between lack of knowledge on the part of the student and inadequacy in the store of medical knowledge.

Over time, disease and death ceased to be frightening, and emotional issues came to be seen as medical problems. The researcher elucidated the processes by which the students learned, in the face of enormous amounts of information, what they would be quizzed about and thus what they had to know to pass their courses and to graduate. *Boys in White* also described the conversion of the early idealism of the new student to the cynical stance held by students in later years. When graduation approached, the original commitment to helping patients and practising good medicine tended to return.

Medical education has been shown to be sexist both in textbooks and in clinical examples used in classroom lectures (Giacomini et al., 1986; Zelek et al., 1997). In the past an unwritten quota system governed the admittance of women into medical school (Woodward, 1999). In fact, the practice of medicine has in many ways been shown to be built around a masculine prototype (Zelek et al., 1997). A great deal of scientific research, the basis of medical practice, has also used the male body as the norm (McKinlay, 1996). Sexism is currently being addressed in a variety of programs in medical schools across the country.

There is a new awareness developing that doctors reflect the heterosexism of the rest of society and that lesbians and gays may not always receive the most appropriate health care as a result (Simkin, 1998). Doctors, too, may experience the heterosexism and homophobia of their patients. A study done via telephone interviews with 500 randomly selected Canadians in a large urban centre asked whether or not the respondents would be willing to consult gay, lesbian, or bisexual (GLB) physicians (Druzin et al., 1998); 11.8 per cent said they would refuse to see a GLB family physician. The two most common reasons were the belief that such doctors would be incompetent and that the respondent would feel uncomfortable. Men and older people were more likely to express discriminatory opinions. Attention to teaching students about larger and broader diversity issues than gender and sexual orientation is one of the contemporary challenges in health care and in medical education.

Getting Doctored

Shapiro (1978), in one of a number of autobiographical accounts of medical school, has critically evaluated his own experiences of becoming a physician in a book entitled *Getting Doctored*. In this analysis the two most important features of medical education are the concepts of *alienation* and the *authoritarian personality*. Alienation is evident in the relationships of medical students to one another, in the relationships of doctors, interns, and residents towards one another, and in the approach of the medical student to studies, medical school, and pharmaceutical companies

---

Box 12.6 Success in Medical School

What are the characteristics of individuals that lead to success in medical school? According to a meta-analysis of articles located through Medline, OVID, Web of Science, and Psychlit, among other sources, these are the highlights (Ferguson, 2002). Previous academic performance accounts for 23 per cent of the variance in competence in medical practice. General cognitive ability is a moderate predictor of success. There is little research on the value of learning styles, personal statements, or references in predicting success in medical school.

Source: Eamonn Ferguson, David James, and Laura Madely, 'Factors associated with success in medical school: systematic review of the literature', *British Medical Journal* 324 (2002): 952–7.

---

and other related institutions. The authoritarian personality, which breeds alienation, is experienced at most stages of medical education, and later in medical practice. Karl Marx described four types of alienation—the alienation of labour or productive activity, alienation from the product of labour, alienation of people's relationships with others around them, and alienation from life.

Alienation of labour is seen throughout the medical care system, from the workers at the top down to those at the bottom. Shapiro provides numerous examples of alienated labour in medical school. These include: fierce competition between medical students, an enormous workload, and little direction regarding what out of the mountains of information is most relevant. 'Students, especially in the early stages, spend extraordinarily long hours at study without any assurance that they have mastered what is necessary' (Shapiro, 1978: 29). Shapiro uses the phrase 'doc around the clock' to encapsulate the doctor's experience of being tied to medical work.

Alienation from the product of labour exists when the worker does not feel that the product of his or her labour is a true reflection of his or her self and values. The way that doctors learn to talk about patients and their illnesses provides some illustrations of their lack of identification with patients. Patients were called 'crocks' when their complaints were believed to be psychsomatic.

They were described as having 'two neurons' when they were believed to be lacking in intellectual functioning or were unco-operative (ibid., 168)

Alienation of relationships, too, is repeatedly evident in Shapiro's description of medical school. One set of interpersonal strategies will be used to illustrate this. Competition is a central feature of the interpersonal interaction of physicians-in-training. There is widespread fear of failure. Students compete for rank in class. Students vie for the best internships and for the position of chief resident. Shapiro's personal critique of medicine may be idiosyncratic but it is not unique to him.

Conrad (1998) analyzed four autobiographical studies of medical school and practice. His findings parallel those discussed previously.

- 'Medical training was set up in a way that discouraged and often prevented such caring.' (340)
- Doctors' clinical perspective focused almost entirely on the disease rather than the illness.
- Doctors are not taught how to talk to patients.
- 'Medical school does an excellent job at imparting medical knowledge and technique, but it is inadequate in conveying humane and caring values.' (343)
- 'Technological medicine, with its disease orien-

tation, myriad lab tests, complex interventions, and "fix-it" mentality, pays scant attention to teaching about doctor-patient relations.' (343)

- Medical students' life of long hours, sleep deprivation, excessive responsibility, and (arrogant) superiors inhibits the growth of compassion and empathy.

Despite the constraints on doctors, many, both individually and together, work on social justice issues. One example of a group of doctors who are organized to aid global social justice is Doctors without Borders. There are also doctors who are trying to further social justice causes within Canada. The Coalition of Physicians for Social Justice is one such group. Formed five years ago to protest the inequities in the newly proposed universal drug plan in Quebec, they have protested poverty as a cause of ill health as well as the limitation in access to medication among vulnerable groups in Quebec, including seniors, single parents, and welfare recipients (Gagnon, 2002; www:cmaj.ca).

Organization of the Medical Profession: Autonomy and Social Control

Physicians are self-regulating. This means that through their organizations they decide what constitutes good medical practice, determine the requirements for training a physician, set standards of practice, and discipline colleagues who depart from these standards. The way that practice is organized, its locus of activity, and the payment modality all affect the regulatory power.

The profession has established two major control bodies, the College of Physicians and Surgeons and the Canadian Medical Association. The federal and provincial governments recognize both of these organizations. Both attempt to define expectations of medical behaviour, to improve standards of performance, and to protect the status and economic security of their members.

The Canadian Medical Association is an amalgamation of the provincial medical associations. Physicians with membership at the provincial level also have membership at the national level. The CMA represents physicians as a national lobby group. The provincial bodies negotiate with the respective medical care plans for fee scales and other matters of relevance to the practice of medicine. The situation is somewhat different in Quebec. Here two organizations—the Federation of General Practitioners and the Federation of Medical Specialists of Quebec—created to defend the 'social, moral, and financial' interests of their members, negotiate collective agreements with the provincial government (Collège de Médecins du Québec, 1999, personal communication). The College of Physicians and Surgeons has bodies in each province whose responsibility it is to oversee the practice of medicine in the province in the interests of protecting the public. The Medical Act describes the powers and responsibilities of the College. These include such things as the designation of the qualifications required for medical practice, the certification of specialists, and the investigation of professional incompetence or misconduct.

The Medical Act requires that the Medical Council of Canada be responsible for the licensing of qualified medical practitioners, for supervising what these practitioners do, and for preventing unqualified practitioners from practising. Thus, the provincial colleges have the power to eliminate from the register all those who are convicted of certain offences. And while practitioners may appeal the judgements of the Medical Council in court, the view of the Council is almost invariably upheld. The courts thereby have in fact declared that the profession is the proper judge of the actions of its colleagues (Blishen, 1969: 81).

Autonomy and power are crucial characteristics of an occupational group that claims to be a profession. As Freidson (1975: 71) says, 'The most strategic distinction [between a profession and any other occupation] lies in legitimate organized autonomy—that a profession is distinct from other occupations in that it has been given the right to control its own work.' Doctors themselves determine the terms (1) of admittance to medical school, and (2) of licensing to practice once medical school, internship, and residency are completed. As professionals they hold 'sacred' their right to control their own work without outside interference.

Freidson (1975) described the way in which the self-regulating doctors' institutions depend on the type of practice in which the doctors are engaged. Freidson distinguished among doctors practising alone, colleague networks, large group practices, and university clinics. Those who practise alone enjoy the greatest freedom from outside control. Pure forms of solo practice are generally quite rare. Solo practice, however, is still lauded as the ideal model of the entrepreneurial professional who is free from control: the doctor treats the patient privately and confidentially, without the interference of colleagues, insurance companies, governments, or any other outsiders. This patient-doctor relationship is described as a 'sacred trust'. Assurance of competence by the physician in private practice is based primarily on the assumption of adequate recruitment policies, educational programs, and licensing procedures. The ongoing day-to-day control of practice ultimately rests with the individual practitioner.

Various kinds of colleague networks, including the very common network of independent practitioners who share on-call times, are more tightly controlled and are potentially more vulnerable to continual scrutiny of colleagues. Those who work in group practices and clinics are probably most subject to collegial surveillance, as well as observation by administrators and paramedical practitioners. But even in this situation, most of the day-to-day practice of medicine in the office is primarily under the control of the practitioner and his or her colleagues.

One of the primary sanctions used against behaviour deemed inappropriate by professional colleagues is ostracism by not referring patients or by denying certain privileges, such as hospital privileges. This is only useful to the extent that the particular medical practitioner is dependent on colleagues and hospitals for practice. Specialists are usually colleague-dependent to a greater extent than are general practitioners, because access to these specialists by patients can only occur through the medical referral system. Ostracism is only of limited effectiveness in actually changing the inappropriate behaviour because the more the practitioner is isolated, the less is his/her behaviour under surveillance (Blishen, 1969); as Freidson argues, 'observability of performance is a structural prerequisite for regulation' (Freidson, 1975: 157). The number of doctors in solo practice is decreasing. A 2001 survey by the College of Family Physicians found that 25 per cent of family doctors were in solo practice as compared to 31 per cent in 1997. Solo practitioners tend to be more common in the inner cities than in rural areas. Seventy-four per cent of family doctors work in group practices that include sharing office space (92 per cent), staff (91 per cent), expenses (85 per cent), patient records (82 per cent), and on-call duties (75 per cent). Some group practice also involves different specialties working together, including complementary and alternative medicine (CAM) practitioners and other types of health-care providers, such as nurse practitioners and audiologists working within the allopathic model (CIHI, 2002: 61).

The mode of practice also relates to how doctors in Canada today are paid. About $13 billion is spent on the services of doctors. Most receive at least some of their income from fee-for-service payments. Ninety per cent of those surveyed recently by the Canadian College of Family Physicians were paid by fee-for-service, 14.9 per cent were paid by salary, and 1.9 per cent were paid by capitation or the number of patients in the practice (ibid.). Some doctors are paid by more than one method.

Box 12.7   The Robert Latimer Case

On 24 October 1993 a 12-year-old girl was killed by her father. He had put her in his truck and piped carbon monoxide into it. She fell asleep and died. Tracy weighed 40 pounds or so and functioned at approximately the level of a three-month-old. She could not walk, talk, or feed herself. She was apparently in almost constant pain, had undergone numerous major surgeries, and was scheduled for more. Still, according to the brief presented by the Crown at her father's second trial, 'Tracy enjoyed outings, one of which was to the circus, where she smiled when the horses went by. She also responded to visits by her family, smiling and looking happy to see them.'

Robert Latimer was charged and convicted of second-degree murder in 1994. In 1995 he lost an appeal to the Saskatchewan Court of Appeal. In 1996 the case went to the Supreme Court. A new trial was recommended because of jury interference. He was, however, found guilty of second-degree murder again in 1997. This time the judge made 'a constitutional exemption' in that he rejected the mandatory 10-year imprisonment in favour of two years' imprisonment, one of which was to be spent in the community. In 1998 the Saskatchewan Court of Appeal rejected the judges' recommendation and upheld the mandatory life sentence with no parole for 10 years. In 1999 Robert Latimer went again to the Supreme Court of Canada. The Court heard the appeal in 2001 but upheld the 10-year mandatory life sentence with no parole for 10 years.

The various decisions reflect the widespread division in the Canadian population about whether or not Robert Latimer's deed should be considered murder and punished in a traditional sense or whether, because it was motivated by compassion, it should be forgiven. Disability rights activists were particularly involved in arguing that the act should be considered a murder. Numerous important civil and parental rights issues are raised by this case. Should the courts abide by the spirit or the letter of the law? Would a decision supportive to Robert Latimer legitimate other 'mercy killings' of disabled children? Would it endanger the sanctity of life of disabled people or other people who cannot speak for themselves? Would it eliminate mandatory sentences in more general terms? What do you think the arguments, on both sides, are?

Source: <http:www.cbc.ca/news/indepth/background/latimer_robert.html>.

Oswald Hall's early studies of the medical profession showed how important the network of personal contacts was to professional control. For instance, the prestige of the hospital at which the internship is carried out significantly affects the future practice and subsequent level of income and prestige of the physician. The first appointment was particularly symbolic because it was 'a distinctive badge' and 'one of the most enduring criteria in the evaluation of his status' (Hall, 1948: 330). Hall noted also how the major hospitals were organized in a hierarchy of status: intern, resident, and other staff members of varying ranks. Each is a step up in prestige and power. There were also differences in status between hospitals due to such social considerations as the class and ethnicity of the patients who populate the hospitals.

Many of the clinical decisions made by doctors are explainable in the context of the network of medical contacts. Class, ethnicity, and educational background of the doctor affected the type of colleague networks and hospitals of which he/she was part, and these in turn affected the type of practice taken up (Hall, 1946). Practice is also known to be affected by a number of physician characteristics, including gender, age, area of specialization, quality and time of training, ongoing involvement in the professional community, and practice setting (see Clark et al., 1991, for a review of various studies describing the effects of these issues on variations in physician practice). Coleman et al. (1957) noticed how the adoption of new drugs depended on the position of the doctor within a network of colleagues: the most closely integrated physicians were most likely to prescribe the new drugs first.

The practice of medicine is observed and regulated within the setting of the hospital. But access to the hospital is not equally available to all medical practitioners. Considerations other than medical expertise are known to affect doctors' hospital privileges. Oswald Hall has shown how networks based on friendship, ethnicity, religion, and social class influence which students enter certain hospitals as interns and residents, and who obtains hospital privileges. Appointments are not made on the basis of technical superiority. Those appointed must be technically proficient, but after that level of competence is reached, other factors take precedence over sheer proficiency. At this level personal factors play a part in determining who will be accepted (Hall, 1948: 332).

Most hospitals have several committees that guard standards of medical practice. The 'credentials' committee scrutinizes the qualifications and experience of the physicians who want to practise in the hospital and specifies the kinds of professional activities they are allowed to undertake. The 'tissue' committee studies the tissues removed by surgeons and evaluates whether or not particular operations were warranted. The 'medical audit' committee reviews medical records and pre- and post-operative diagnoses. And the 'medical records' committee evaluates the records kept by physicians (Blishen, 1969: 78). Roman Catholic hospitals also have 'medico-moral' committees to ensure that Catholic morality prevails, particularly with respect to matters concerning the 'sanctity of life'.

Recent analyses suggest that today the power and autonomy of the physician within the hospital are severely restricted. Doctors used to be the only gatekeepers to the hospital system: they determined which patients, medical colleagues, and various paraprofessionals would be admitted. Now hospital administrators, many of whom are graduates of university-based hospital administration programs, are the pivotal figures in organizing the hospitals (Wahn, 1987). Today doctors function as the middle managers whose work is likely to be constrained, organized, and directed by the hospital administrators (Coburn et al., 1997).

This new occupational group of hospital administrators is generally responsible to the government for containing costs, as well as to the board of directors of the hospital. The board of directors is composed of representatives of the doctors, nurses, and others who work primarily in the hospital, along with members of the community. Provincial hospital commissions, employing large numbers of financial experts and hospital administration specialists, including a few physicians, evaluate the budgets and monitor the performances of every hospital. At times hospitals have adopted measures recommended by the commission that have been contrary to the interests of the medical personnel (Wahn, 1987: 427).

Hospital administrators are guided by different primary goals than doctors are. They are chiefly concerned about managing the organization in a rational and efficient manner and eliminating 'unnecessary' services and costs so as to balance the hospital budget. This, of course, does involve satisfying the goals of promoting and maintaining good, safe, and efficient medical care. But these medical goals must be met in the context of rationalizing services and balancing the interests of many specialty groups who work within the hospital.

Wahn explains some of the specific processes that affect the work of the doctors in the hospital. He mentions one hospital in which the demands for financial cutbacks were used to force doctors in the emergency ward, despite their opposition, to accept salaries because the fee-for-service expenses were too high. He discusses another situation in which the neurosurgeons at a particular hospital were ordered to schedule surgery every day rather than simply on one day of the week (which had been the norm) in order to maintain the department's services (nursing and so on) at a consistent level. The doctors opposed this because it meant, among other things, that they had to make hospital calls on the weekends. The doctors' wishes were ignored for the 'greater good'—the efficient running of the hospital.

Despite the potential importance of hospital committees for the maintenance of health-care standards, they do not always do their job as well as might be expected. There is some evidence from an American study that smaller hospitals are not as likely to control standards as effectively as large hospitals (Blishen, 1969: 77). Informal controls actually operate in all hospitals, so that doctors' reputations may be spread by word of mouth by any member of the medical, paramedical, or administrative staff. The effectiveness of gossip as social control is probably greater in a small hospital in a small community than in a large hospital in a large community, and yet the effectiveness of this control has not been widely documented.

Coburn et al. (1997) have argued that the medical profession has, in part, declined in power via the imposition of state control through restratification. In particular, 'in recent years, the state has introduced changes in the structure and functions of the self-regulatory college, has intervened with a number of cost controlling mechanisms—denying funding for new technologies, tightening controls on insured service, and promoting explicit guidelines for medical decision-making' (ibid., 17). The autonomy of the medical profession is a fragile and complex matter and the threats to that autonomy are very real.

The Management of Mistakes

Mistakes happen to all of us. They happen both on and off the job. They are an inevitable part of life. Which student has ever received 100 per cent on all tests, essays, and exams? Which teacher has never made an error in adding or recording marks? Doctors are no exception: they also make mistakes. But when doctors make mistakes the results can be devastating—they can result in death or serious disability for the patient. One question Marcia Millman asks in her book, *The Unkindest Cut* (1977), is how do doctors handle their mistakes? Millman carried out her research for two years at three university-affiliated hospitals. She was a participant observer working with doctors at all status levels. Because these hospitals were teaching hospitals attached to universities, their standards can probably be considered above average.

Millman's work highlights three basic points. First, *the definition of what constitutes a mistake is variable*. In fact, the old joke that the operation was a success but the patient died has a basis in fact. Results that patients interpret as mistakes are not necessarily considered mistakes by doctors. And doctors in different specialties may have different understandings of what constitutes a mistake. Actions that would be considered reprehensible in an attending physician are considered permissible in an intern who is, after all, 'just learning'. The point here is that there is no universal standard of perfect or imperfect medical practice. Norms are worked out in practice.

Second, while the designation among doctors of what constitutes a mistake is problematic, *some results of medical practice are considered undesirable enough to warrant investigation*. One example would be an unexpected death during surgery. When such an outcome occurs, Millman notes, doctors tend to use two mechanisms for

Box 12.8   Medical Practice Is Inevitably Error-Ridden

An interview study of 40 doctors' interpretations of what constitute mistakes in their work demonstrated the 'anguish of clinical action and the moral ambiguity of being a clinician' (Paget, 1988). Mistakes, the interviewed doctors noted, are absolutely inevitable in the work of the doctor. Mistakes are intrinsic to medical decision-making: they are essential to the experience of doctoring. Clinical practice involves risks because it requires the application of finite knowledge to specific situations with their own limitations of responses, settings, and patient-doctor communication. Doctors are often not 'to blame' or incompetent. Medicine by its very nature is an essentially 'error-ridden activity'. Because of the method of interpretive understanding based on interview data, Paget was able to describe medical practice with an empathy for doctors. As she says, 'mistakes are complex sorrows of action gone wrong' (ibid., 131).

The doctor knows that she/he is making decisions based on some but not all of the information available. Moreover, even if the doctor has all the available information, it may not be enough to diagnose or treat a disease. Medical practice inherently encapsulates a degree of uncertainty. Yet it usually results in, even requires, action. Paget's work enables us to see the definition of mistakes from the perspective of the practising clinician. Based on open-ended interviews and using a phenomenological approach, she shows the everyday struggles of doctors who make decisions in an error-ridden climate. The following quotations illustrate how doctors talk about mistakes.

Well, all mistakes are relative. They're relative to the setting in which they are made, and they're relative to the intent of the physician.

I think, dealing with mistakes . . . I think, we see mistakes all the time. But the errors are errors now, but weren't errors then.

This characteristic of medical work was less problematic a half-century ago. Today, however, when treatments can be dangerous, the potential for deleterious results from mistakes has grown enormously. Irreparable mistakes are inevitable: they occur, in spite of good intentions, good education, and care.

---

dealing with it: (1) neutralization, and (2) collective rationalization. As Millman says:

By neutralization of medical mistakes I mean the various processes by which medical mistakes are systematically ignored, justified or made to appear unimportant or inconsequential by the doctors who have made them or those who have noticed that they have been made. (Millman, 1977: 91)

Thus, an action that results in harm to a patient can be ignored, or it can be justified because of the intricate nature of the surgery involved or because it was the patient's fault for not informing the physician of a drug reaction. In justifying themselves, doctors may emphasize unusual or misleading clues; or they may focus on the patient's unco-operative attitude or neurotic behaviour. Even though 'doctors may have differences and rivalries among themselves with regard to defining, blaming, and acting on mistakes, all doctors will join hands and close ranks against patients and the public.' The assumption made is, 'there but for the grace of God go I' (ibid., 93). In the face of mistakes, doctors will tend to band together to support one another and to explain the behaviour leading up to the 'mis-

Box 12.9   Accountability of the Medical System

Lisa Priest, a reporter for the *Toronto Star*, with support from the Atkinson Foundation, wrote an important series of articles in the fall of 1997. In the articles she documented medical mistakes in hospitals and in practices across the country. She also explained how difficult, indeed, often impossible, it was to get information about individual hospitals and doctors and about rates of side effects from prescribed drugs and mortality from specific surgeries per hospital or per physician. In a variety of ways Priest documented the lack of control over or knowledge about their medical system that Canadian patients have, in short, the lack of accountability of the system to those who pay for and depend on it. She contrasted this to the hospital and doctor report cards regularly published for citizens of some jurisdictions. She revealed the presence and the work of Britain's Audit Commission, a sort of health-care police that traces and publishes mistakes. This commission is legislated to review the 'economy, efficiency, and effectiveness of Britain's National Health Service' (Priest, 1997b: A26). It is independent of the government or any other special interest group and has thus been successful both in making people aware of some of the inadequacies of the system and in effecting some changes. For example, there is now a published Patient's Charter in which hospitals are rated on a 0–5 star rating system with respect to 59 indicators. In addition, a patients' association, partly subsidized by the government, has published a book entitled *Best Doctors of Britain*. In Scotland, already, 'patients are finding out exactly which hospitals by name have the best five-year survival rates for patients with cancer of the ovaries, breast, lung, and large bowel courtesy of Britain's National Health Service' (Priest, 1997c: A33).

Lisa Priest asked a number of questions in her series of articles on quality control and accountability in health care.

1. Should hospitals be rated? Other countries are doing it, so why shouldn't Canada?
2. What is more important, doctors' rights to privacy or patient safety?
3. Should patients know the complication rates, death rates, and readmission rates for procedures and operations by surgeons in the hospitals where they are performed?
4. Would 'scorecard medicine' help ensure that doctors whose skills are slipping would be tossed out or forced to shape up?
5. Are hospitals too soft on surgeons?
6. What should happen when dramatically different rates for particular surgeries or drugs appear in this country's hospitals?
7. Should we set 'volume' standards for doctors performing surgeries?
8. Should the sickest patients have priority for treatment?
9. Should it be easier for hospitals to fire doctors whose skills are inadequate? Should there be a mandatory monitoring process for such doctors performed by an outside body? Are doctors' reputations being protected at the expense of the public?

take' as blameless or at least as being as logical as possible given the circumstances.

The third point of Millman's work is that *hospitals have instituted formal mechanisms for dealing with mistakes, for using errors as a source of education, and for investigating culpability.* The Medical Mortality Review Committee, one such mechanism, met monthly to discuss deaths within the hospital and to review each death in which there may have been some possibility of error or gener-

Box 12.10   Errors in Infertility Treatments

There have been a number of obvious errors made in fertility clinics. Three of the most obvious cases involve a situation in which black twins were born to a white couple and two cases of twins in which one was black and the other one white.

Mistakes such as these raise many ethical and legal issues. To whom should the children belong? Is maternity more important than paternity in these cases? Is maternity more important than ethnicity? Should a black couple undergoing fertility treatment at the same time as any of the above cases and having identifiable genetic links be given the babies? Or should the woman who carries and bears the baby 'own' the baby?

Source: Owen Dyer, 'Black twins are born to white parents after infertility treatment', *British Medical Journal* 325 (6 July 2002): 64.

al mismanagement. The fundamental yet unspoken rule governing such a review was that it was to be 'a cordial affair'. Even though the atmosphere may sometimes be slightly strained, and the individual physician whose decisions are being reviewed may be embarrassed, rules of etiquette and sociability were stringently enforced. All members of staff who had a part in the mistake used the committee meeting as an opportunity to explain to the others how each was individually led to the same conclusion. Emphasizing the educational aspect of the event rather than its legitimate investigatory nature also minimized the discomfort level.

Technical and Moral Mistakes

Bosk's (1979) work on mistakes among doctors adds another dimension to the analysis already discussed. Bosk studied the ways surgeons and surgeons-in-training at a major university medical centre regulated themselves. He noted that the medical centre's hierarchy is structured and managed so that those at the bottom levels are more likely to have to bear the responsibility for mistakes than those at the top.

There were, he noted, *two different kinds of mistakes—technical* and *moral*. Technical mistakes are to be expected in the practice of medicine, and colleagues are normally forgiven them. They are viewed as an inevitable part of medical work and are seen as having definite value in that they often motivate improvements in practice. People are expected to learn from their technical mistakes. Moral mistakes, however, are severely reprehensible. They constitute evidence that the physician or physician-to-be does not belong as a medical colleague (as a member of the team, or a team player). Moral errors that demonstrate an unco-operative attitude, unreliability, or a lack of responsibility to patients are more serious. Moral errors are not as easily forgotten or forgiven because the person who made them is believed to be unsuitable as a doctor.

Practice Norms and Variations

A study by Wennberg (1984) showed that different colleague networks develop different sets of beliefs, norms, and practices regarding specific diseases and the appropriate treatment for them. Wennberg compared rates of hospitalization and surgery in the states of Iowa, Vermont, and Massachusetts and found tremendous variations from state to state and within states. He then divided the different areas into what he called 'hospital markets' or hospital service areas (populations using one hospital or a group of hospitals). He found that different hospital service areas had highly variable rates of all measures of hospital and

Box 12.11   Medical Error

The medical system, as all systems, is mistake-ridden. However, under-reporting of mistakes is common. In the US the under-reporting is said to be 50 to 96 per cent per year (Lawton and Parker, 2002). This is partly because of the culture of medicine that in many ways reflects the capitalist economies of the West. It is a culture that emphasizes professional autonomy, collegiality, and self-regulation. Such an individualized system does not easily foster shared responsibility and the opportunity of learning from mistakes. Rather, it encourages denial, fear, and blame. In addition, there is an increasingly litigious population and numerous lawyers ready to take medical error cases.

Estimates are that 80 per cent of the accidents with hazardous technologies are the result of human error (ibid.). This may reflect the biases of reporting. Although doctors and other health-care personnel are clearly often at 'the sharp end' of the system (ibid., 16) the failure may actually often be attributable to action or inaction further down the line. It may, for instance, be due to faulty machinery. In the absence of systematic reporting of errors, improving the quality of health care is hampered.

Many patients feel unsafe. A recent poll in the US found that 42 per cent of the respondents disagreed with the proposition that the current health-care system had made adequate provisions to prevent medical mistakes. A further 42 per cent said that either they had personally experienced a mistake or a close friend had (Vincent and Coulter, 2002). The majority of complaints stem from problems in communication. Miscommunication can lead to misdiagnosis and mistreatment. It may even lead to death. Yet consultations with doctors average less than 10 minutes. This is insufficient for many patients to feel they have an opportunity to get their point across.

The medical profession has traditionally relied on the method found most unhelpful in reducing errors—'shame and blame of individuals with accusations of incompetence, unprofessionalism, and unworthiness to treat patients' (Liang, 2002: 64). The first step in changing this is to educate physicians regarding the appropriate focus of quality improvement systems. 'Physicians cannot claim full credit for a positive patient outcome; rather, it is a team effort involving a minimum of physician, nurses, administrators, and the patient' (ibid.).

Nor should doctors take all of the blame. In the airline industry, for example, it is not only the pilot who is held responsible for the safe outcome of a flight but also the air traffic controllers, the maintenance people, the stewards, and the ground staff. It is the system that is held accountable.

The most extreme case of medical 'error' to come to light in the recent past is that of a British doctor, Harold Shipman, who has been found to have murdered at least 215 of his patients and to have done so without any suspicion being directed towards him for a very long time. He was caught only when he crudely altered the will of his last victim in a way that apparently made detection inevitable. It has been suggested that the doctor was addicted to pethidine. He may have also been addicted to murder.

But how did these murders go undetected for so long? How did he manage to get corroborating signatures from other doctors on certificates of cremation? Donna Cohen has suggested that he was able to avoid detection, in part, because of prevalent ageism. She argues that because the elderly are more likely to die of all sorts of conditions, people tend to ask fewer questions when a death is unexpected or unexplained. All of the people killed by Shipman were at least middle-aged, 82 per cent were women, and many had been healthy.

Sources: Lawton and Parker (2002); Vincent and Coulter (2002); Liang, (2002); Cohen, (2002).

surgery utilization. For instance, he noted that the rate of hysterectomy (among all women under 70) varied from 20 per cent in one market to 70 per cent in another. The rate of prostatectomy varied from 15 per cent in one market to 60 per cent in another. Tonsillectomy rates varied from 8 per cent to 70 per cent in two different markets. In trying to explain these wide differences, he examined the roles played by (1) illness rates, (2) insurance coverage, (3) access to medical services, (4) age distribution, (5) per capita hospital bed ratios, and (6) physician-population ratios. None of these factors made a significant impact on the utilization of hospitals or surgery. Wennberg concluded that the differences must be due to subjective variations in the practice styles of physicians in each area.

Rachlis and Kushner (1994: 5) have illustrated how the productivity of doctors varies substantially from area to area. For example, they note that radiation oncologists in Toronto have 50 per cent fewer patients than those in Hamilton and that those in Hamilton see 50 per cent fewer patients than those in Halifax. Part of the difference is due to research responsibilities and part to the expansionist role of radiation oncologists— from the technical (as is common in Britain) to whole-patient management (as is common in the US). Within the Canadian medical care system there is considerable treatment variation from place to place. Rachlis and Kushner note the following findings: (1) a person is three times as likely to receive a tonsillectomy in Saskatchewan as in Quebec; (2) county-by-county rates for coronary bypass surgery vary 2.5 times throughout Ontario; (3) the length of stay for hospitalized heart attack patients ranges from 6.6 to 12.9 days (within just one province).

According to John P. Bunker (1985), such variation occurs because medicine is an art and not a science, and therefore a great deal of uncertainty is involved in the practice of medicine. Most surgery, possibly 85 to 90 per cent, is not for life-threatening problems but for conditions of discomfort, disability, or disfigurement. Moreover, in most cases the benefits just about equal the risks. Surgery is equally likely to improve the health, comfort, and lifespan of the patient as it is to cause an increase in morbidity. There are no clear differences in mortality rates in different hospital markets. Hospitalization or surgery rates are not correlated with declines in either the mortality or morbidity rates.

Wennberg, Bunker, and Barnes (1980) studied seven different types of surgery, including hysterectomy, tonsillectomy, gall bladder surgery, prostatectomy, hemorrhoidectomy, but in this case they compared Canada, the United Kingdom, and different locations in the United States. Generally, the rates were highest in Canada and lowest in the United Kingdom. The authors suggest that while such differences have enormous implications for costs, and for morbidity and mortality rates, they are not the result of malpractice but occur because diagnostic and treatment procedures are not perfect. Norms of practice develop out of colleague and network interaction. Comparative studies of medical care in Canada and the US demonstrate how economic and socio-cultural phenomena influence practice. For example, US physicians generally use more invasive procedures and fewer evaluative and management techniques (Welch et al., 1996). There are lower levels of cardiovascular service for the elderly in Canada than in the US and these differences increase as people age (Verrilli et al., 1998). Canadian physicians are more likely to take age into account when suggesting invasive cardiovascular procedures or dialysis. There are also large differences in the availability of certain technologies. In 1992, Canada had 1.3 open-heart surgery units per million whereas the US had 3.7 units per million (ibid.). Whether these differences result in improved health, quality of life, or longevity is not clear, however. Hospital and clinic routines play a part in determining styles of practice. As Horowitz (1988: 29) states:

In medicine there are few certainties. There are more questions than answers. There are few truths. And everything is changing. Most of the

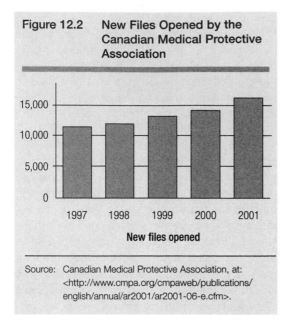

Figure 12.2   New Files Opened by the Canadian Medical Protective Association

New files opened

Source: Canadian Medical Protective Association, at: <http://www.cmpa.org/cmpaweb/publications/english/annual/ar2001/ar2001-06-e.cfm>.

time, the best we can hope for is the best judgement based on the best available facts and the particular circumstances.

Malpractice

One of the fastest growing types of social control of medical practice is the malpractice suit (Table 12.3). Malpractice insurance policies are now taken for granted as a necessity, and fees for malpractice insurance are growing substantially. One Canadian estimate is that the rates of malpractice suits have tripled over the past 15 years and that the amount of the awards has quadrupled (Figure 12.2). Twice as many lawsuits against doctors today are successful than was the case 15 years ago. Most complaints originate in hospitals or other health-care institutions. The provincial/territorial licensing bodies are required by law to examine all complaints against their members that are brought to them. The Canadian Medical Protective Association (CPMA) investigated 2,495 such cases in 2001 (http://www.cmpa.org/cmpaweb/publications/english/annual/ar2001/ar2001-06-e.cfm). Figure

12.2 and Table 12.3 indicate the extent and kinds of activity that the CPMA is involved with on behalf of medical practitioners.

As a consequence of these trends, doctors are now spending at least $200 million annually on insurance for claims of injury alone. In 1994 family doctors paid an average of $1,500, while those in the high-risk specialties of anaesthetics and obstetrics paid $17,000. This rate is still, however, not close to the insurance malpractice rate in the US. The Canadian doctors' 'insurance company', the Canadian Medical Protective Association, which was established in 1913 by an Act of Parliament (www.cmpa.org/english/whatis-e.cfm), grew financially from a base of $24.5 million in assets in 1983 to $614 million at the end of 1992. The growth in the numbers of complaints in the later 1990s suggests that this figure is likely considerably higher today. Growing at about $100 million a year, membership fees are running at about 30 per cent above total expenses (Rachlis and Kushner, 1994: 305). The membership of over 50,000 doctors represents the vast majority of the medical profession in Canada.

Canadians reported just under 15,000 new medico-legal concerns in 2001 to the Canadian Medical Protective Association. This is an increase of 5 per cent over 2001. There were 1,308 new legal actions initiated against CMPA members in 2001, approximately equivalent to a risk of one new legal action for every 27 members. Legal cases usually average three to four years before they are settled. In 2001, 6 per cent of the judgements were in favour of the doctors, 2 per cent in favour of patients, 32 per cent led to settlements before trial, and 60 per cent involved a withdrawal by the plaintiff before trial (http:www.cmpa.org/cmpaweb/publicatons/english/annual/ar2001/ar2001-06-e.cfm).

Summary

(1) The medical profession can be thought of as an occupation, a process, a power group, or

Table 12.3   Canadian Medical Protective Association, Canada, 1997–2000

	2000	1999	1998	1997
New files opened	14,168	13,531	11,738	11,462
Files closed	13,386	11,874	10,194	13,970
Miscellaneous inquiries	3,636	3,473	2,971	2,748
Patient-related inquiries	7,304	7,044	6,034	6,015
Threats (of medico-legal difficulty)*	882	940	842	588
Legal actions commenced	1,337	1,354	1,339	1,399
Legal actions proceeding to trial				
— judgement for plaintiff	37	31	21	22
— judgement for defendant physician	97	103	86	86
Legal action settled	408	396	332	374
Threats settled	32	49	50	43
Legal action dismissed/discontinued/abandoned	827	902	824	770
Inquests	88	93	66	67
College (licensing body) matters	2,279	2,067	2,116	2,078
Hospital matters	234	233	211	207
Billing matters	275	229	221	135
Criminal matters arising from medical care	12	20	17	15
Human rights matters arising from medical care	15	20	8	13
Membership	60,099	58,722	57,948	56,899
Educational sessions	305	205	240	220

*Beginning in 1998 this figure includes members named but not in contact with the CMPA by 31 Dec.

Source: Canadian Medical Protective Association, at: http://www.cmpa.org/cmpaweb/publications/english/annual/ar2001/arpics/p06_thenumbers>.

an ideology. There are certain strengths and limitations to each of these descriptions and it is possible for them to overlap.

(2) As an occupation, medicine has two basic characteristics: prolonged training in a body of specialized, abstract knowledge and a service orientation. However, the view of profession as occupation accepts the profession at its own valuation and ignores the power of the group, changes over time, and the relationship between the occupation and the rest of society.

(3) As a process, the medical profession can be seen as developing over time. Members engage in full-time work, establish a training/education program, belong to an association, gain legal status, and construct a code of ethics. The members of the occupational group must have esoteric knowledge and social distance from the rest of the population and must be more or less homogeneous.

(4) As an ideology, the medical profession holds descriptive and prescriptive beliefs that explain and legitimate certain practices and

viewpoints. The ideology includes: universalism, functional specificity, affective neutrality, and a collectivity orientation. An effective ideology allows physicians to dominate and monopolize the field.

(5) Today, there are three steps to becoming a doctor: an undergraduate education, graduate study leading to the designation MD, and a minimal one-year internship. Medical students generally come from middle- and upper-middle-class family backgrounds. Physicians-in-training become aware of two dominant values: 'clinical experience' and 'medical responsibility'. Medical students learn emotional detachment and the ability to deal with inevitable and constant uncertainty; they also encounter alienation and may develop authoritarian personalities.

(6) Power and autonomy of the medical profession have been somewhat curtailed by the emergence of hospital administrators who direct and organize doctors' activities. Physicians are also governed by provincial Colleges of Physicians and Surgeons and the Canadian Medical Association.

(7) Doctors make mistakes. The definition of what constitutes a mistake is variable; doctors use two mechanisms for dealing with undesirable mistakes: neutralization and collective rationalization. The formal mechanism hospitals have instituted to deal with mistakes is the Medical Mortality Review Committee. There are two kinds of mistakes: technical, which are to be expected and are normally forgiven, and moral mistakes, which may indicate that the person who made them is somehow unsuitable to be a doctor.

(8) Different colleague networks within the medical field develop different sets of beliefs, norms, and practices regarding specific diseases and their appropriate treatment. Variations in medical practices indicate that medicine's diagnostic and treatment procedures are not perfect.

(9) Medical malpractice and complaints against doctors appear to be growing.

Questions for Study and Discussion

1. Assess the different views of the meaning of profession and the processes of professionalization with respect to allopathic doctors.

2. What are the characteristics of a good doctor? Critically examine the list of responsibilities mentioned in the Canadian Medical Association Code of Ethics. Use your own experience to do so.

3. Explain the reasons for the socio-demographic backgrounds of medical students today. Do you expect that this will change? Why or why not?

4. Compare the alienation of labour described by Shapiro with that of some work in which you have been employed.

5. Explain the distinction between technical and moral mistakes. Is this difference relevant for any other occupation? Discuss.

Suggested Readings

Becker, Gary, et al. 1961. *Boys in White: Student Culture in Medical School*. Chicago: University of Chicago Press. A classic example of participant observation research, with a focus on observing students becoming doctors.

Goode, William J. 1956. 'Community within a Community: The Professions', *American Sociological Review* 22 (Apr.): 194–200. Goode's statement provides the starting point for the sociological study of the medical profession.

Gordon, Sidney, and Ted Allan. 1952. *The Scalpel, The Sword*. Toronto: McClelland & Stewart. A fascinating introduction to Norman Bethune's life and contribution.

Johnson, Terence. 1972. *The Professions and Power*. London: Macmillan.

_____. 1977. 'Industrial Society: Class, Change and Control', in R. Scase, ed., *The Professions in the Class Structure*. London: Allen and Unwin, 93–110.

_____. 1982. 'Social Class and the Division of Labour', in A. Giddens and G. Mackenzie, eds, *The State and the Professions: Peculiarities of the British*. Cambridge: Cambridge University Press, 182–208. Johnson offers a dynamic assessment of the profession of medicine.

Merton, Robert K., George Reader, and Patricia Kendall, eds. 1957. *The Student Physician: Introductory Studies in the Sociology of Medical Education*. Cambridge, Mass.: Harvard University Press. Provides insight into professional training for doctors.

Willis, Evan. 1983. *Medical Dominance: The Division of Labour in Australian Health Care*. Sydney: George Allen and Unwin. Compare Willis's findings with your estimate of the dominance of allopathic medicine vis-à-vis other types of health-care providers.

| *The Medical Care System: Critical Issues*

Learning Objectives

- The medical model is based on different assumptions from those of the lifestyle or environmental/social-structural models.
- The medical model is dominant in contemporary society.
- There is evidence of the decline of medical dominance.
- Health promotion and prevention provide alternative visions of the best way to invest in health.
- Modern societies have been called 'risk' societies.
- There is evidence that medical practice has been and continues to be sexist.
- There are important debates with respect to the trends towards privatization in the medical care system.
- Women's health has recently become a specific focus for medical research.
- The unequal distribution of doctors across the country is a significant concern today.
- Models of care are changing and the use of home care is growing.

Introduction

What is wrong with the medical care system today? Is it underfunded? Is it too expensive? Would it be better if it were privatized? Is it poorly organized? Is it too 'high-tech'? Will there be enough money for medicare to support the aging Canadian population? Do we overemphasize treatment and neglect prevention? Should home care be supported under the Canada Health Act? Is there any justification to the charge that medicine is a sexist institution? These are the sorts of questions that will be addressed in this chapter.

This chapter will focus on three main critiques of the medical care system. The first centres on the notion that the contemporary medical care system is dominated by the 'medical' model of health and illness (see Table 13.1). We will discuss the various characteristics of this model, the value of alternatives to the medical model, such as environmental and lifestyle models, and

Table 13.1 Models of Disease Causation

Medical Model	Environmental/ Social-Structural Model	Lifestyle Model
Disease is an objectively measurable pathology of the physical body, which is the result of the malfunctioning of parts of the body. Cure is through chemo-therapeutic, surgical, or other 'heroic' means. Hospitals, as places for the practice of high-tech medicine, are of primary importance.	Disease is best understood as the result of social-structural inequalities in class, gender, race, ethnicity, and environmental conditions such as air and water pollution, dangerous and stressful work, harmful organization of major societal institutions such as the family and education.	Disease is best understood as the result of individual behaviours based on decisions about such things as 1. exercise 2. stress management 3. diet 4. smoking 5. substance use and abuse 6. sexual habits 7. seat belt use, speed limit observance, and the like

Typical 'Health' Problems in Each Model

Coronary heart disease	Poverty	Smoking
Respiratory disorders	Unemployment	Alcohol addiction and abuse
Cancer	Pollution	Drug addiction and abuse
Sexually transmitted diseases	Family violence	Unsafe sex
AIDS	Sexual abuse	Poor dietary habits
Arthritis	Unsafe and unhealthy working conditions	Lack of exercise
Mental illness	Homelessness	Poor stress management
Hypertension	Poor wages	Unsafe driving habits
Multiple sclerosis	Racism, sexism	Equipment or appliances that are unsafe
Diabetes	Underemployment	
Colitis	Lack of adequate child care	
Alzheimer's disease	Lack of readily available and safe birth control	
Burns		
Influenza		
Pneumonia		
Broken limbs		

the adequacy of the medical model with respect to the changing demographic profile of Canadian society and the epidemiological data on the causes of diseases. The second critique concerns sexism in medicine and in the experiences of health and illness. The third major issue is the changing balance between public and private funding in health care. A fourth critical issue is the distribution of physicians across the country. This is discussed briefly at the end of the chapter.

The Medical Model

The medical model is based on the assumption that disease is an objectively measurable pathology of the physical body that results from the malfunctioning of parts of the body. All diseases are eventually explainable through a close analysis of the biological components of specific individual human beings. The first implication of this model is that the most significant advances against disease are through scientific investigations, in the laboratory and the clinic, of the individual human body. The second is that the search for causal mechanisms should focus primarily on the pathological alterations within the cells of the body. The third is that disease is considered undesirable and abnormal. The fourth is that disease, being undesirable, is to be eliminated as quickly and completely as possible with as powerful means as necessary.

The limitations of the medical model are best clarified through comparison with competing models—the environmental/social-structural model and the lifestyle model. The environmental/social-structural model focuses on causes of disease that lie outside the individual organism. In this model, disease is best understood as the result of a complex of social-structural inequalities revealed by such relationships as those between disease and class, gender, ethnicity, environmental pollutants and contaminants, dangers in the workplace, and stress. These inequalities are also evident in the personal difficulties resulting from how, in certain circumstances, the family, sexuality, and education engender human suffering leading to illness. Whereas this model is not able to cure disease in the individual, at least not as quickly or heroically as allopathic medicine, and certainly not with the 'magic bullet' of a pill or surgery, it can be used as a basis for planning programs of disease prevention or health promotion, programs that in the long run should decrease the burden of disease on the population.

The third model is the lifestyle model. In this model the individual is not just a body, but must be considered in the context of his/her whole life. Here disease is understood as the result of individual actions based on personal decisions regarding such things as (1) exercise, (2) stress management, (3) diet, (4) smoking, (5) substance use and abuse, (6) sexual behaviour, and (7) other behaviours such as using a seat belt or observing the speed limit. As in the medical model, the individual is the source of both the problem and the cure. Unlike the medical model, however, individual choice and free will, rather than biological malfunctioning, are viewed as the immediate causes of illness. Both treatment and prevention require a change in lifestyle.

No one of the three competing models is in itself sufficient to explain, prevent, or cure all disease. All three models are useful and valuable. Each addresses a particular problem. A complete medical care system would include some aspects of all three models. A basic problem with the contemporary Canadian medical care system has been the over-reliance on the medical model at the expense of the other two. Disease prevention, in spite of increasing formal recognition, has received relatively little financial support. The largest expenditure of the medical care system is and has been on hospitals—60 per cent of the whole budget, when all institutions, including homes for special care and others, are included (see Chapter Eleven for a detailed discussion of this issue). Acute-care hospitals alone use $25.7 billion annually, about one-third of the total health-care budget (*Canada Year Book*, 1999: 118). Chapter Eleven has described the expenditures on various medical professionals. Clearly, the greatest proportion is spent on allopathic physicians. All these expenditures are for services provided primarily within the medical model. Only a very small percentage of the total health expenditure is used for disease prevention and health promotion or for interventions that would fit within the environmental and lifestyle models. Financially, then, the medical model currently dominates the system.

This reliance on the medical model is particularly problematic because of the limited relevance of the notion of cure to the most significant diseases in modern society, namely the degenerative, chronic diseases. As discussed, the chief causes of death today are heart disease, strokes, and cancer. These tend to be diseases of middle and old age and are usually chronic rather than acute. As the Canadian population ages, these and other chronic conditions will become more prevalent and the relevance of the medical model, and the cure that it seeks, will decrease. On the other hand, the importance of long-term care and patient education increases and the crucial role of socio-economic inequities in the causes of and treatment for disease continues.

In addition, medical intervention has enabled many people to live who would previously have died. Some are able to live fully independent lives. Others, such as premature and underweight babies, are kept alive for many months in hospital by surgery, drugs, complex technology, constant care, and intravenous feeding only to die. Some advances in medical care have meant longer life for many other severely disabled people who can only be kept alive with intensive nursing care but cannot be cured by medicine. Such medical interventions may lead to a controversial issue—decrease in actual quality of life.

The Decline of the Medical Model: Demedicalization

In spite of the many successes of modern medical practice in individual cases, involving such miracles as heart transplants, heart-lung transplants, artificial heart transplants, in vitro fertilization, and the like, there is widespread evidence that the biomedical model of illness is rapidly losing support. In *A New Perspective on the Health of Canadians* (1974), then Health Minister Marc Lalonde considered the ways morbidity and mortality are the result of a complex of factors, including biological host factors such as genetic

heritage; environmental conditions, including both physical and social-economic environments; and 'self-imposed' factors such as cigarette smoking and excessive alcohol and drug consumption. Lalonde's work has made an important impact on Canadian government policy and has influenced the World Health Organization and numerous nation-states as well.

This approach is called 'health promotion' and is defined as the process whereby people can increase control over and improve their health (see Table 13.1). According to Health Minister Jake Epp's 1986 report, *Achieving Health for All: A Framework for Health Promotion*, the mechanisms for addressing health problems are (1) self-care, or the decisions individuals take in the interests of their own health; (2) mutual aid, or the actions people take to help one another; and (3) the development of healthy environments. The report suggests three ways to implement this approach: by fostering public participation, by strengthening community health services, and by co-ordinating public health policy (see Figure 13.1). Health promotion and disease prevention continue to be a part of the official federal government health strategy. The provinces, however, have jurisdiction over the health-care system and expenditures within it. Given fiscal restraints and sizable populations of already sick people in need of the use of the system's hospitals and doctors, the actual investment in health promotion is limited.

Strategies for implementing this approach are diverse: they include media promotion, health education, health advocacy, community development, and community economic development (*Health Promotion*, 1987: 7–10). Media promotion includes the production and distribution of all sorts of materials such as videos, slide shows, pamphlets, posters, and the like; these are designed to be used in community centres, schools, libraries, hospitals, and at health fairs to improve the public's general awareness. For instance, if a community identifies unemployment as a significant cause of health problems,

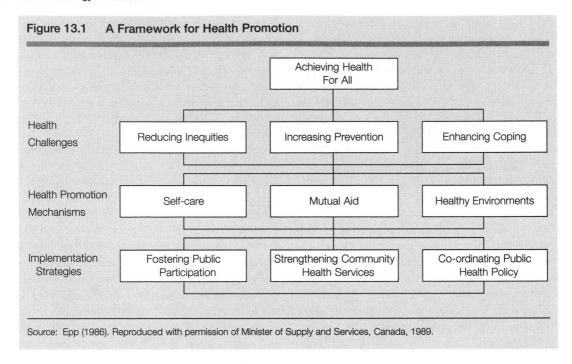

Figure 13.1   A Framework for Health Promotion

Source: Epp (1986). Reproduced with permission of Minister of Supply and Services, Canada, 1989.

they might undertake the publication of a brochure to be sent around to local doctors suggesting that the doctors refer unemployed patients to self-help political action groups and employment counselling agencies.

Among its targets, health education includes schools, communities, and health professionals, and involves many different types of popular education techniques, partly modelled on the work of Paulo Freire. Freire and his colleagues approached Brazilian peasants wherever they gathered—on the streets, at market, in their homes. Freire taught the people empowerment through literacy. So, too, the goal of health education is empowerment through knowledge.

Health advocacy involves lobbying for social policies and laws that promote health. Legislation, for example, covers smoking and non-smoking policies, lead-emission controls in automobiles, and workers' right to know the names and effects of potentially hazardous products with which they work. Health advocacy

means taking a stand on health issues: seeking controls on pollutants that cause acid rain would be a case in point.

Community development and community economic development work to mobilize a community around an issue so that the members of the community work together to reach the goals they have defined for themselves. Credit unions, community banking schemes, and co-operatives are examples of community economic development.

Canadian society has changed a great deal over the past century, as has the rest of the Western industrialized world. Most Canadians now live in cities: in fact, 30 per cent live in the three largest Canadian cities. Over 90 per cent of all Canadians in the labour force work for others, the majority in service, trade, and financial institutions. The medical care system has become a medical-industrial complex and includes the pharmaceutical industry, hospitals and long-term care institutions, and the medical supplies (e.g., from bandages to CAT scanners) and affiliated food and laundry industries. Large bureaucracies administer different parts of the system. They include, among others, medical and hospital administrators, managers and planners, government health ministries, and local health units with jurisdiction regarding reportable and communicable diseases. In addition, there are diverse medical care workers, including nurses, pharmacists, dentists, chiropractors, allopathic doctors, and others. In the midst of such complexity, the role of the medical practitioner as the guardian and definer of health and illness has diminished (Coburn et al., 1997). Fiscal restraint, competition from alternate and lay healers, and unionization among nurses and other medical care practitioners have also served to diminish the dominance of the doctor in the medical system and in so doing have diluted the force of allopathic medicine as an ubiquitous and pervasive institution of social control.

Changes in government policy reflect wider trends in Canadian society. One important trend is the *women's movement*, which has led to the radical alteration of many aspects of contemporary life—increased numbers of women in the labour force, legislation for equal pay for equal work and equal pay for work of equal value, increased divorce rates, decreased fertility rates, and so on. Of particular relevance to demedicalization are issues in women's health.

Among the earliest thrusts of the movement was the demand for knowledge and information about women's bodies. And among the most important publications in the area of women's health was the contribution of the Boston Women's Health Collective, *Our Bodies, Our Selves* (1971, 1996). With the women's health movement, women were primed to ask questions and demand second opinions. They became aware of the deleterious effects that medicine had had on both the mental and physical health of women. They documented the prevalence of extensive and unnecessary hysterectomies and excessive and sometimes debilitating prescriptions of mood-altering drugs and tranquilizers. They became aware of the devastating, long-term side effects of using drugs that had been inadequately tested, such as thalidomide and DES (diethylstilbesterol), and the defects of various birth control devices. Some women sued major manufacturing and pharmaceutical companies as well as their doctors. Millions of women called for natural childbirth, for the Leboyer method of immersing the baby in warm water immediately after birth, for home births, for various types of non-medicated, non-interventionist birth procedures. They taught one another how to do internal exams. They formed self-help and consciousness-raising groups to enable them to be more powerful and to have more autonomy in their individual dealings with doctors. In many ways the women's movement challenged the power of medicine to speak with authority about most aspects of women's lives. The recent legalization of midwifery in many provinces is just one of the successes of the several-decades-old women's movement.

A second important trend is the *changing disease profile*. In the past most illnesses were either minor and self-limiting or acute and fatal. Much illness today is chronic. Chronic illness is expected to last a long time, even over a lifetime, with intermittent remissions and exacerbations of symptoms. One consequence of the changing disease profile is the high rate of long-term institutional care and increasingly long-term home care accompanied by reliance on pharmaceuticals and other medical devices. Chronic illnesses require management by the patient as well as care, at times, by others, including family members, friends, and medical professionals. While medical research continues to play an important role in chronic illness, actual medical practice often plays only a minor role. Figure 13.2 shows the changing patterns of disease prevalence among adult Canadians of some of the more common chronic health problems and disabilities. Table 13.2 illustrates the lack of correspon-

Table 13.2		Comparison of Federal Funding for Disease-Specific National Strategies				
Disease	Actual Deaths (1997)	Number of Canadians Living With	Potential Years Life Lost	New Cases Per Year	National Strategy	Health Canada Funding
Cancer	58,703	1,100,000	924,000	137,000	National strategy began in 1998, no dedicated funding	$600,000–700,000/year through cancer secretariat
HIV Infection	626	50,000 (HIV + AIDS)	Estimated 25,000 to 40,000	2,119 (HIV)	Dedicated funding since 1998	$42.2 million/year
Diabetes	5,699 direct 25,000 through complications	1,200,000 to 1,400,000 (estimated)	25,000	60,000	Dedicated funding beginning in 1999	$115 million over 5 years
Breast Cancer	5,500	100,000 (estimated)	94,000	19,500	Dedicated funding since 1992, renewed 1998 to 2003	Canadian Breast Cancer initiative, $7 million/year

Source: *Cancer Care in Canada* no. 3 (Summer 2002): 1.

dence between the financial investments made by the federal government and the health burdens of three diseases with significant morbidity—cancer, HIV, and diabetes. This table raises the important question of whether or not disease-based research investments should be commensurate with the numbers of people who suffer the particular disease.

About four million Canadians of all ages are currently living with a disability expected to be of over six months' duration and causing restriction or lack of ability to perform normal activity (*Canada Year Book*, 1997: 113). These include disabilities affecting mobility, agility, vision, hearing, and speaking. In addition, as the population continues to age, so, too, the proportion of people with physically disabling chronic illnesses increases (Tables 13.3 and 13.4). Unreported in Tables 13.3 and 13.4 is the prevalence of those who suffer from emotional problems. The National Population Health Survey of 1994–5

estimated that about 5.6 per cent of Canadians over 18 (7.3 per cent female and 3.7 per cent male) recently suffered a major depressive disorder. In numbers, this constitutes some 1.1 million Canadians. Anxiety and phobic disorders are generally found to be even more frequent in community surveys (Bland et al., 1988). These data suggest that chronic mental suffering and disorder also make a significant contribution to the suffering of the Canadian population.

Chronic illness is predicted to be an increasingly significant component of the overall disease profile (Angus, 1984). According to Fries (1980), who has studied the changing disease patterns since 1900, by the year 2050, if present trends continue, the average life expectancy will be 85 plus or minus 12 years. Fries calls this maximum life expectancy the biological wall. By the year 2021 those over 65 are expected to comprise 17 per cent of the population, and by 2031, 20 per cent of the population. The most elderly (over

Figure 13.2   Changing Patterns of Disease

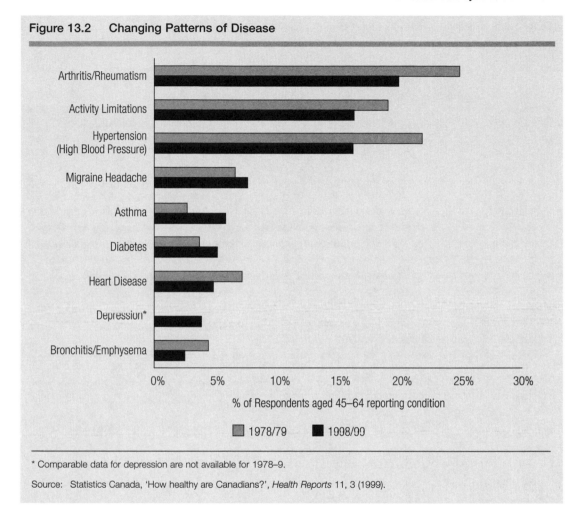

% of Respondents aged 45–64 reporting condition

■ 1978/79   ■ 1998/99

* Comparable data for depression are not available for 1978–9.

Source: Statistics Canada, 'How healthy are Canadians?', *Health Reports* 11, 3 (1999).

85) population is projected to grow even more rapidly than the total over-65 age group. This is particularly significant because the older the age group, the greater the incidence of chronic illness and associated frailty.

According to Mustard (1987: 26), 'the main concerns of health care services will be caring for an older population that is losing, at a varying rate, the vitality of its organ systems, and caring for individuals with the mental health problems that affect all age groups.' In this situation the most important role for the medical system 'will

be to provide efficient, effective and supportive care to an aging population' (ibid., 27). Canada does not appear to be making progress in a shift away from hospital-based services and curative medicine to community-based primary care and health promotion.

A third important trend is the *growing awareness of the importance of prevention* in minimizing and/or eliminating the major 'killers' in Canada today. A review of mortality trends in various age groups in Canada documents that the most frequent causes of mortality—heart disease, cancer,

Table 13.3   Persons with At Least One Disability, 1991

	All ages	15–24 years	25–44 years	45–65 years	65 years and over
Persons with at least one disability	3,795,330	266,135	917,172	1,163,149	1,448,874
Household	3,533,089	263,601	895,345	1,138,187	1,235,955
Institution	262,241	2,533	21,827	24,962	212,919
Men	1,734,051	133,034	449,054	582,221	569,742
Household	1,644,955	131,168	436,155	569,001	508,631
Institution	89,097	1,866	12,899	13,221	61,111
Women	2,061,279	133,101	468,118	580,928	879,132
Household	1,888,135	132,433	459,191	569,187	727,324
Institution	173,145	668	8,928	11,741	151,808

Note: 'Disability' is defined as any restriction or lack of ability to perform an activity in the manner or within the range considered normal for a human being not fully corrected by a technical aid and lasting or expected to last six months.

Source: *Canada Year Book*, 1997, 113, from Statistics Canada, *Health and Activity Limitation Survey, 1991*, Catalogue no. 82–602.

Table 13.4   Nature of Disability, 1991

	Any disability	Mobility	Agility	Seeing	Hearing	Speaking	Other	Unknown
	% of population							
Canada	17.0	10.4	9.6	2.7	5.3	1.5	5.6	1.0
Newfoundland	10.9	7.4	6.4	1.9	3.4	1.1	3.2	0.3
Prince Edward Island	19.3	12.1	11.1	3.0	6.3	1.7	6.4	0.7
Nova Scotia	23.8	14.9	14.3	3.2	7.3	1.7	6.7	1.2
New Brunswick	19.6	11.8	10.4	3.2	7.1	2.1	7.2	0.5
Quebec	13.7	8.4	7.8	2.4	3.4	1.4	4.7	0.8
Ontario	17.6	11.2	10.1	2.9	5.4	1.5	5.9	1.0
Manitoba	19.4	11.7	11.2	3.5	7.2	1.5	5.3	0.7
Saskatchewan	20.0	11.4	10.7	3.6	7.0	1.9	6.7	1.4
Alberta	18.7	10.6	9.3	2.6	6.2	1.3	6.0	1.5
British Columbia	18.0	9.8	9.9	2.5	6.7	1.6	5.6	1.5
Yukon	12.1	5.3	5.4	0.9	4.4	0.8	3.8	1.2
Northwest Territories	14.0	6.2	5.5	1.6	5.3	0.9	4.5	0.9

Note: See Table 13.3.

Source: *Canada Year Book*, 1997, 114, from Statistics Canada, *Health and Activity Limitation Survey, 1991*, Catalogue no. 82–602.

respiratory disease, accidents, suicide, and violence—are amenable to reduction through social, structural, environmental, and lifestyle changes (Trovato and Grindstaff, 1994).

A fourth significant component is the *focus on cost-containment*. Health-care costs have grown. Aside from the US, which spends 12 per cent of its GNP on health care, Canadian expenditures, at just under 10 per cent, are the highest in the world. Yet, several countries have better health records in spite of less expenditure and older populations (Manga, 1993). The infant mortality, life expectancy, and mortality rates from chronic conditions are clearly poorer in the US, which is characterized by greater proportional medical expenses per capita than Canada. Canada continues, however, to spend more of its GNP on medical care than most. Only three OECD countries spent more in 1998—the United States (12.9 per cent, Switzerland, 10.4 per cent, and Germany 10.3 per cent (CIHI, 2002: 29). The demand for health care, in fact, can grow expansively and almost endlessly because the 'theoretical' end product of medical care—good health—is always elusive.

There is debate about whether or not the changing demographic profile will significantly increase the financial costs of medical care. In this context future predictions are that there will be an increasingly significant decline in the transfer of federal funds for health to the provinces. Thus the monies available for this aging population are already decreasing. On the other hand, the benefits of medicine are not seen as increasing as rapidly as the costs. Social policy researchers have made us aware that the great benefits to health that occurred at the end of the nineteenth century and at the beginning of the twentieth century were largely the result of public health measures, not medical measures. The present government emphasis on lifestyle changes, health promotion, and disease prevention hearkens back to the success of the early public health movement.

The new focus on health promotion and the social and environmental causes of illness is not without negative implications. The very articulation and mobilization of support for a model of illness that would be broader than the medical model could ultimately be used to delegitimize the differences between health and sickness and even to normalize sickness and consequent suffering. If the notion of 'health' becomes too broad it can no longer be addressed in health-related public policy. Moreover, the themes elaborated as aspects of the newer health promotion trends such as 'disease prevention, health promotion, iatrogenesis, individual and community empowerment, social networks, and family and home care can as easily become ideological justifications for the privatization, deregulation and constriction of health services, with all that implies for the quality and equality of care' (Burke and Stevenson, 1993: 54).

Risk Society

Some would argue that the contemporary shift to health promotion adds a number of new problems that challenge a healthy society. The notion that everything causes cancer is now a truism. Many have commented on the fact that we are confronted with new risks every day. Water, air, and land are polluted with carcinogens whose effects are still hotly debated (Epstein, 1998). The underside of health promotion and disease prevention—a positive goal in its own right—is the resultant anxiety about myriad life choices, from the first meal of the morning (shall I have strawberry jam with red dye, toast made of wheat heavily sprayed with pesticides and grown in soil treated with fertilizers, and butter from cows who accumulate toxins in the food chain?) to the last decision before bed (should I leave my window open to allow the fresh air in, or is the air too polluted?). Eating, sleeping, breathing, exercising, and loving (and hating) have become decisions made by many in the context of health benefits and health costs.

Sexism and Patriarchy in Medicine

Both sexism and patriarchy are prevalent in the medical care system. Sexism is the tendency to construct and act on stereotypes based on gender. Thus, for example, women who suffer from migraine headaches are likely to be seen by the medical profession as neurotic, whereas men with the same set of symptoms are likely to be seen as victims of severe occupational demands (MacIntyre and Oldman, 1984). Recent research has shown that doctors may be even more 'blinded' by the sex of men than of women and that they are now six times as likely to make stereotypical assumptions about men as about women as patients (Groce, 1991). Such different views are partly the result of sexist attitudes held by doctors (Fisher, 1986), which are reinforced by medical texts (Martin, 1993; Findlay, 1993), pharmaceutical advertisements, and the portrayal of disease in the mass media (Rochon-Ford, 1986; Clarke, 1992a, 1992b). Patriarchy is male dominance over women. Examples can be seen throughout society, in the positions held by men in the family, in the schools, in sexual relations, in work, and elsewhere. Patriarchy is also evident in the generally superior position held by men in the medical labour force and in the power of male health providers over female patients.

Sex and the Medical Hierarchy: A Brief History

That there have always been women healers in society is documented on stone tablets, carved in relief on ancient walls, and told in legends of ancient Egypt, Sumeria, Greece, and Rome. The notion that only men can be doctors and that women healers must be different and subservient is relatively recent. The drive to exclude women from positions of rank in the medical labour force is coincidental with the drive towards professionalization.

At first women and men were both involved in the practice of medicine. In a number of European countries women from powerful families often ran convents (Mumford, 1983). In most large religious institutions the infirmarian offered her services as physician, pharmacist, and health teacher. Herbs for medicinal purposes were grown and cared for in the gardens of the religious. Often, particularly in large convents and abbeys, nuns provided nursing services.

The famous medieval medical school in Salerno in the eleventh century accepted both men and women as medical students and as teachers. In fact, one of the best-known medical school teachers in the eleventh century was a female, Trotula. She taught medicine and wrote an important gynecological-obstetrical treatise that became a major reference work for centuries. In addition, she co-authored medical books with her husband and son. In the fourteenth century, Roman women from important families could remain single and work as doctors or professors. This was true also in the other major schools in Italy and in the Muslim world—Cairo, Baghdad, Cordova, Toledo, and Constantinople (ibid., 27). Jewish women physicians were widely accepted in Italy and France, and one woman ran a large medical school in Montpellier in the 1320s. Women doctors were even more common, yet no less important, in Germany. There is evidence, too, that women were practising in the Netherlands.

Attempts to exclude women from practising medicine apparently began in earnest in Britain in 1412, when Cambridge and Oxford universities sent a petition to Parliament outlining the dangers of allowing 'ignorant and unskilled persons' to practise medicine and surgery. The result was the near-exclusion of women from the practice of medicine. At that time there were very few educated male physicians either. In 1512 Henry VIII set out to centralize state power. One strategy was the passage of the Medical Act of 1512, which prohibited undesirable and uneducated persons from doing medical work. Women comprised one of the categories of undesirables—

they were believed to be causing grievous harm in the name of healing. Medical practice was restricted to those who were licensed by bishops. This effectively excluded women from practising medicine, though they could be midwives under a great deal of control from local churches. However, Henry VIII's dictum and the influence of the bishops were limited to London. In the countryside men and women continued to work side by side in the medical field.

The Roman Catholic Church was particularly alarmed at the declining birth rate and the 'breakdown' of the family. Seeking to bring these trends under control, the Church fathers began to write about witchcraft (which was, at that time, associated with healing) and its potential for spreading sin and evil. The most important work on witchcraft was the official Catholic text written by two German monks, Kramer and Sprenger—*Malleus Maleficarum* or *The Hammer of Witches* (Ehrenreich and English, 1973, 1978). Many of the people who were named witches, persecuted, and put to death were female healers and midwives, especially those of the peasant population. The *Malleus Maleficarum* declared that women were particularly likely to be witches because they were especially vulnerable to consorting with the devil in a sexual way. Lust was believed to be insatiable in women. Entry into a coven was said to involve sexual intercourse with the devil. In addition, helping and healing were in themselves evidence of witchcraft because they demonstrated a lack of faith. The Christian was supposed to accept sorrow and pain as a visitation from God, not seek to be healed.

Witch-hunting in Europe spanned approximately four centuries; between 1479 and 1735, about 300,000 people were put to death as witches. Most of these were women. Some have argued that the campaign against witches was primarily a campaign against women (Ehrenreich and English, 1973). Most of their crimes were related to their roles as healers and midwives.

Midwives were particularly vulnerable to

attack as witches because they had access to what were considered to be prized witchcraft materials—newborn babies, placentas, and umbilical cords. In addition, it was thought particularly important to prohibit women from attending childbirth: no baby should be allowed to die unchristened, but midwives could not conduct a christening. For a time, women healers either 'went underground' or left the field entirely. Later they resurfaced quietly, primarily as nurses attached to monasteries and hospitals.

Then in the middle of the nineteenth century in the United States, one woman, after numerous unsuccessful attempts, was granted admittance, after the support of a student referendum, to the medical school at Geneva, New York. Elizabeth Blackwell graduated as a medical doctor in 1849 with honours in all courses, except, ironically, in the one course in which she was forbidden to enroll: 'Women's Diseases'. Later she established the New York Infirmary for women and children.

By the 1850s Canadian women, too, began to ask for admittance to medical schools. As late as the 1880s, the few women practising medicine in Canada had received their training outside Canada. In 1883 women's medical colleges affiliated with Queen's University and the University of Toronto were established to provide medical instruction to women. By 1895 women could take examinations at medical schools of their choice (Roland, 1988).

The Medical Labour Force in Canada Today

Both sexism and patriarchy prevail in the Canadian medical labour force at all levels of care: administrators, physicians, nurses, nurses' assistants, clerical workers, and housekeeping staff. The higher the prestige, income, and power of the occupation, the smaller the percentage of females working in it. The medical profession is largely male. The nursing profession is largely female. Below these two levels is the service sector, made up of various technicians, orderlies, nurses' aides, nurses' assistants, and domestics. This sector is also largely female and poorly paid. Put in simplest terms, males predominate in the most prestigious, powerful, and highest-paying professions and have relegated females to the less prestigious, less powerful, and less remunerative semi-professions. This situation is illustrative of patriarchy. It is worth adding that the proportion of visible minorities is also likely to be highest in the lowest ranks of the health-care system.

The Medical Profession

In the 20 years in Canada from 1969–70 to 1989–90, the proportion of female medical students grew from 12 per cent to 44.4 per cent and later to 50 per cent and more, as was discussed in Chapter Eleven. It may be argued, however, that during this same period the prestige and power of Canadian doctors compared to other workers in the health-care field had declined. The growing proportion of women in the medical schools and in subsequent medical practice cannot, therefore, necessarily be taken as indication of a decline in sexism.

Within the medical profession women continue to be concentrated in certain 'female' specialty areas (Lorber, 1984) such as pediatrics, family medicine, and gynecology (Kirk, 1994). In general, these offer the lowest levels of financial reward and the least prestige. Women are also underrepresented in the upper echelons of medicine, in medical school faculties, and within the hierarchies of medical schools (Ackerman-Ross and Sochat, 1980). The average salary of all doctors in Canada in 1990 (full-time) was $102,370, while the average salary of male doctors was $111,261. Comparatively, lawyers made $76,966, chemical engineers $56,073, and professors $62,064 on average (Armstrong and Armstrong, 1996: 164). By contrast, the average salary in 1990 for (mostly female) graduate nurses was $33,510 and, for nursing assistants, $25,000 (ibid., 175). Similar differences by sex

are evident among other health-care providers, such as osteopaths and chiropractors (men made $58,645 and women made $35,680), and in optometry (men made $61,625 and women $33,600) (Statistics Canada, 1985).

Moreover, women physicians, as other women workers, are vulnerable to sexual harassment in medical school, in practice with patients, and with colleagues. In fact, a study published in the *New England Journal of Medicine* and co-authored by Dr Susan Phillips of Queen's University found that 40 per cent (422 of 1,064) of Ontario female family physicians had experienced sexual harassment, primarily from male patients (Graham, 1994: 14). Women physicians, the study states, are particularly vulnerable in private practice because they often must examine patients alone in their offices.

Nursing

The professional status of doctors has been achieved and is continued through the dominance of male physicians. Medicalization is a process that has been largely invented and perpetuated by male thinkers, scientists, and practitioners. The dominance of males in the medical care system has been maintained through the relegation of female medical care workers, such as nurses and nurses' assistants, to relatively powerless and poorly remunerated positions.

Nursing was and is a female job ghetto. Moreover, within nursing, males are more likely to become administrators and to hold positions of power. The percentage of male nurses with a higher education than the basic diploma is only very slightly larger than the percentage of female nurses with higher education. Yet, although men only have a slight edge in educational background, they have a higher percentage in the upper echelons of nursing than women do. (These figures give a conservative estimate of male power and potential power in nursing because the entry of males into nursing in any numbers is fairly recent; thus, male nurses will likely tend to be younger and to have had less time in which to be promoted on average than female nurses.)

In 1996 there were about 55,000 physicians and 264,305 professional nurses practising in Canada (*Canada Year Book*, 1999: 118–20). Yet expenditures for physicians comprised 14.7 per cent of the medical care budget, while 7.1 per cent was spent on all other workers. Thus, although there are more than 4.5 times as many nurses as physicians, nurses and their colleagues received only one-half of the total expenditures of physicians.

Two explanations are given for the division of labour by sex in health care (Navarro, 1975). The first is the socio-economic roles of the family in society, and of men and women within the family. The main function of the male in the family is to be the breadwinner, and therefore he is an active member of the labour force. The female's function is largely the maintenance of the labour force through her husband and the reproduction of the labour force through her children. Because of this division of labour within the family, the employer pays for the work of one and often receives the benefits of the work of two. The male worker receives financial remuneration, which he can then share as he sees fit. The reward for the female is considered to be the 'emotional satisfaction' she derives from caring for her family, as well as the financial support provided by her husband.

The second reason for the division of labour by sex is the economic utility for capital owners of having a 'reserve army', a temporary and readily available cadre, of workers. In periods of high employment and production, or during war or other periods when the labour force requires additional workers temporarily and at short notice, women can be brought out of their homes and given additional work in the paid labour force. However, because women are still seen as primarily responsible for and rewarded by the family and domestic sphere, their jobs tend to be marginal to the paid labour force and poorly

rewarded in terms of income, status, and working conditions.

Women's Health: A New Focus

There is, however, a new focus on women's health and on research into women's health under the aegis of the United States and Canadian governments. According to the *Women's Health Office Newsletter*, men's bodies have been considered normative for major research trials such as myocardial infarction. Drug use and reactions have been tested on the bodies of young men. Women's bodies have seldom been studied in major investigations of significant causes of morbidity and mortality because women's bodies are known to function, in part, cyclically due to reproduction-related processes. This has been believed to complicate testing and analysis. Nevertheless, the under-representation of women in these studies has resulted in significant gaps in knowledge. To redress this lack, new research efforts are being addressed to women's health issues and women's bodies are being studied along with those of men.

The following are some of the most important reasons cited for the new focus on women's health: women comprise 52 per cent of the population; women use disproportionately more medical care services than men; women have ongoing health problems associated with their reproductive systems; some diseases affect women and men differently and at different rates. Men and women have different risk factors and require different interventions. Women's multiple roles may affect their health. Women are usually gatekeepers and custodians of health care for the entire family; a woman's health affects the health of her family. Women live longer than men and have more chronic illnesses than men, and thus it is hoped that addressing women's health needs alongside those of men may contribute to new paradigms of understanding (*Women's Health Office Newsletter*, 1994: 17).

Box 13.1   The Registered Nurses Association of Ontario Responds to the Events at the Hospital for Sick Children and the Grange Inquiry

'The Grange Inquiry was the highest-priced, tax-supported, sexual harassment exercise I've ever encountered', said Alice Baumgart, the Dean of Nursing at Queen's University. The Registered Nurses Association of Ontario agreed, and in a little booklet called *The RNAO Responds* they explain why. This next section will summarize its arguments.

The arrest of Susan Nelles exemplified sexist bias for a number of reasons.

(1) The police and others jumped to the conclusion that the unprecedented number of deaths, 36 between 1 July 1980 and 25 March 1981 on wards 4A and 4B at Toronto's Hospital for Sick Children, were the result of murder. They neglected to investigate the possibility that the theory of digoxin overdose was questionable because digoxin is notoriously difficult to measure. It is normal to find some digoxin after death, and there is some evidence that digoxin levels may increase after death. No control groups were used for the baseline data.

(2) Once the police and hospital officials decided that the deaths were due to murder, they neglected to examine systematically all the possible sources of digoxin 'overdoses'. They failed to consider that the drugs might have been tampered with in the hospital pharmacy; or in the manufacturing or distributing branches of the pharmaceutical companies; or administered secretly by any of a number of other hospital personnel who had regular access to wards such as physicians, residents, interns, dieticians, lab technologists, or even a member of the general public who might unobtrusively have entered the hospital on a regular basis. Instead, the focus of suspicion was immediately placed on the most powerless people in the system—the nurses. Because, according to the first analysis, Susan Nelles appeared to have been the only nurse on duty for a

number of suspicious deaths, she was questioned. When she asked to see a lawyer before answering questions, the police assumed that she was guilty and arrested her. The case against her was strengthened because she apparently had not cried when the babies died. Both aspects of her behaviour—asking to see a lawyer, which was, of course, responsible adult behaviour, and her failure to cry—violated sex stereotypes; thus her behaviour was taken as evidence that Nelles must be guilty.

Other sources of bias in the investigation were evident.

(3) The focus was on individuals within the bureaucratic system (the hospital) rather than on the malfunctioning of the system itself.

(4) The media were accused of biased and sensationalized reporting of unfounded allegations and suspicions. As criminal lawyer Clayton Ruby stated, the media, when reporting on the inquiry, ignored their usual rules of fairness and thus held some responsibility for the damage done to reputations.

(5) Justice Grange tended to assume that a nurse was responsible for the murders and to disregard other evidence. He also disregarded the evidence that tended to raise questions about whether or not the 'excess' digoxin could have resulted from measurement error or some alternative explanation.

(6) The television coverage overemphasized the putative guilt of the nurses. The cameras tended to zoom in on the nurses' faces or hands as they were giving evidence, but rarely seemed to focus on those of the police or the lawyers. Such camera work emphasized discomfort of the nurses and encouraged a picture of them as probably guilty.

Among the issues that were raised for nurses by the events at Sick Children's and the Grange Inquiry are the following.

(1) Nurses have little status or authority within the hospital. Yet they are held responsible or accountable for their work.

(2) In contrast to the continuing low status of nurses, their clinical roles have grown for three reasons: (a) the increased number of critical-care patients in hospitals; (b) the increased number of specialists involved with each individual patient; and (c) the increased use of technology, all of which the nurse must co-ordinate.

(3) The Associate Administrator: Nursing—the highest level in the nursing echelon—was three administrative levels below that of the senior management of the hospital. Nurses thus had no access to the most senior levels of hospital management.

(4) Nurses are expected to be generalists and to move easily from one part of the hospital to another and from one type of care to another. They are expected to perform duties at night that they are not permitted to perform in the day, because during the day only the doctor is thought to have the ability to perform them.

(5) The bureaucratic structure, the assumption that nurses are generalists, and the low level in the hierarchy held by top nursing administrators limit the opportunities for nurses' advancement. In addition, nurses suffer from burnout, job stress, low job satisfaction, and the like.

(6) The events surrounding the inquiry also reinforced the notion that the 'feminine' skills of nurturing and caring are much less important than the 'masculine' skills of curing and analysis.

(7) It became clear that the image of nursing was infused with negative stereotypes and myths, similar to the negative stereotypes of women in society.

By articulating the issues, publishing the book, lobbying various levels of government, and dealing with the hospital bureaucracy, nurses are beginning to make some changes. Destructive as the events at Sick Children's were, the outcome for the nursing profession in the long run may be hopeful.

Source: Registered Nurses Association of Ontario (1987).

This new focus on women's health has the potential of contributing to either an increased or a decreased medicalization of women's bodies. As the number of women scientists and medical practitioners increases, and as long as women become more vocal and more powerful—as they have with respect to two major women's health issues, breast cancer and midwifery—women's health issues and female-defined medical concerns may be increasingly addressed without medicalization.

Women as Hidden Healers

Recently the analysis of the division by sex of the medical labour force has been expanded from the formal medical care system to the informal, from the discussion of health care in the paid labour force to health care in the unpaid labour force (see, e.g., Graham, 1984). Just as earlier feminists focused attention on the essential place of domestic labour in the economy, feminist scholars have re-examined the contribution made in the home to the health field. They are finding that women have always been carers and healers: they have cared for their children and other family members during times of sickness; they have provided information about health and healing remedies. Regardless of how pivotal this caring work is, the role of women as invisible healers, negotiators, and mediators has long been overlooked.

Women's health work in the home involves most of domestic life. It includes cooking, cleaning, and providing a secure, warm, and stable

Figure 13.3   Provincial-Territorial Hospital and Home-Care Expenditures ($ millions), 1980–1 to 2000–1

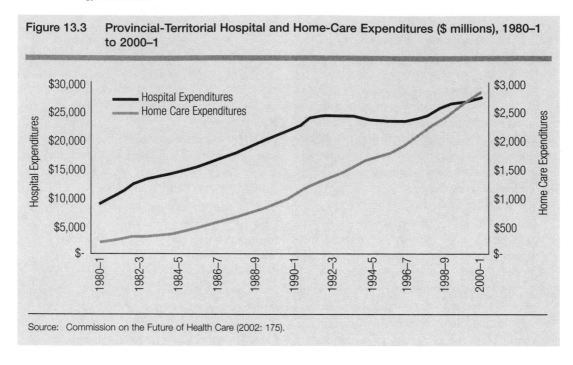

Source: Commission on the Future of Health Care (2002: 175).

home environment. It involves feeding others with adequate nutrients, clothing the family in seasonally appropriate garments, and providing soap and water and the other necessary accoutrements to good hygiene. Women also provide a social/emotional environment conducive to good mental health. Women are usually responsible for teaching other family members about the ways and means of maintaining and promoting health and preventing illness, both by example and by giving information. They also usually decide when medical intervention is required, make relevant appointments, and see that family members are able to keep the appointments.

Women's health work takes place when all family members are healthy and also when they are not. Because fewer people are kept in institutions and because an increasing number of diseases are chronic rather than acute, health care in the home is becoming more demanding. It may prevent women from maintaining or seeking outside employment. It may be a serious threat to

the woman's own mental or physical health. As with other domestic work, women's health-care work in the home has been overlooked and underestimated. Studies are only now being published documenting the nature, experience, and extensiveness of domestic health labour. It is important to note that women and men who provide home health care often speak about its benefits to their lives along with the costs. It is also noteworthy that home health-care costs have increased dramatically over the past two decades, as Figure 13.3 indicates.

The impacts of some of the decreases in hospital beds and nursing have been taken up by the private sector and in particular by women's health-care work. Canada's Health Monitor 1998 survey found that 20 per cent of Canadians care for family members at home or elsewhere. Almost two-thirds of the informal caregivers (63 per cent) care for one person, 22 per cent care for two, and 9 per cent care for three or more. Seven per cent of these caregivers said they themselves needed care (Buske, 1999b: 1427). The vast majority are women.

The increase in public home-care expenditures over the years from 1975–6 to 1997–8 is substantial. However, this is still a small proportion of total health-care expenditures. In 1975–6 home-care expenditures were 0.65 per cent of the total public health expenditure; in 1997–8 they were 3.98 per cent of the total expenditure (www.hc-sc).

The Medicalization of Women's Lives

Every stage of a woman's life has been subject to medical scrutiny. Pregnancy and childbirth, which many would argue are natural events, are seen as occasions for medical intervention. From the 'diagnosis' of pregnancy to the delivery itself, medical care dominates women's experience of childbirth. Births take place (usually) in hospitals, in high-tech delivery rooms, amid glaring lights in sterile conditions, and in an equally sterile emotional atmosphere, with anaesthetics to dull pain, surgery to speed delivery (whether Caesarean section or merely episiotomy), forceps to change the position of the baby, and fetal monitoring to check on the progress of the baby. Women at puberty may experience menstrual cramps or irregularity; doctors give them pills to help. Some women have noticed that they feel differently at different times during their monthly cycles. Mood and physiological changes such as depression and breast swelling have been diagnosed as PMS or premenstrual syndrome. Hormones are used to smooth out the emotional ups and downs and the physical discomforts. Menopause has been defined as a deficiency disease. Again hormones are prescribed. Many types of contraception are available only from physicians—the 'pill', the IUD, the cervical cap, and the diaphragm. Indeed, most types of contraception are for women. It is women, usually, who are to take responsibility, with the help of their doctors,

for preventing pregnancy. Wherever abortions are legal, doctors perform them. Even old age, a condition experienced by women more than men, is generating new medical specialties—geriatrics and geriatric psychiatry.

Deborah Findlay's (1993) work demonstrates that it is impossible to separate socio-cultural norms regarding the good and bad woman from the conceptualizations made by obstetricians and gynecologists regarding female physiology, pregnancy, and labour. Rather than being characterized by objectivity, as medical science claims to be, Findlay demonstrates how 'objectivity' in medical science is better characterized as a resource that has enabled physicians to define and regulate the social world of women by surveillance and labelling of some body behaviours as normal and others as pathological (Findlay, 1993). It is not that medical science sometimes errs and bias creeps in. On the contrary, Findlay argues that medical science is integrally rooted and bound up in socio-cultural categories of gendered normality and deviance.

Women's emotions, too, are frequently medicalized. The oppressive experience of living in a sexist society characterized by unequal access to opportunities and rewards in the family, the society, the economy, and the political sphere is bound to result in some costs, emotional and otherwise, to women. Yet they are likely told that 'it is all in your head', and are prescribed counselling, psychiatric treatment, and mood-altering psychotropic drugs. As well, there are numerous historical examples of sexism in the social construction of medical diagnoses and treatment. In the nineteenth century, middle- and upper-middle-class women were described as weak and as vulnerable to their reproductive systems. The belief was that each individual human organism had only a fixed and limited amount of energy. Because the provision of an heir for her husband was thought to be a middle-class or upper-class woman's most important role in life, women were admonished not to seek education or to work, either inside or outside the home. Sickly, weak, and hysterical, they were expected to rest—to lead a life of invalidism.

Ill health became a virtue, a sign of the refinement of middle-class women. Good health, by contrast, came to indicate a coarser makeup. Art and popular literature presented the female heroine as frail and pale, and thus beautiful. To achieve this desired look, women drank vinegar and took arsenic (*Ideas*, 1983). Not only were doctors telling women that they were basically sick, but a whole patent medicine industry developed to deal with the problem. The following advertisement illustrates how women's lives were defined as inherently diseased.

> Lydia E. Pinkham's vegetable compound—the only positive cure and legitimate remedy for the peculiar weaknesses and ailments of women. It cures the worst forms of female complaints—that bearing down feeling, weak back, falling and displacement of the womb—inflammation, ovarian troubles. And it is invaluable to the change of life. Dissolves and expels tumours from the uterus at an early stage and checks any tendency to cancerous tumour. Subdues faintness, excitability, nervous prostration, exhaustion—and envigorates [sic] the whole system! (Ibid., 4)

Women were taught that they were controlled by their reproductive systems. A gynecology textbook used by Canadian doctors in 1890 states, 'Women exist for the sake of their wombs' (Mitchinson, 1987). Women's natural physical processes were seen as potential diseases. Menstruation required rest. Pregnancy and childbirth required medical treatment. Menopause, as the symbolic end to the meaningful life of women, was expected to leave women depressed. Masturbation was evil, so heinous that the only appropriate cure was a clitorectomy. In fact, this was a very popular medical procedure and was used to treat almost anything considered 'unfeminine' (Barker-Benfield, 1976). Because of the

central role of women's reproductive systems, women were advised to forgo education. It was thought that it would deplete the body of the vital energy required for pregnancy, childbearing, and lactation, which were, after all, the most important functions of women. The medical indications for 'ovariotomies' (the removal of the ovaries) included a wide variety of behaviours and attitudes, including:

> troublesomeness, eating like a ploughman, masturbation, attempted suicide, erotic tendencies, persecution mania, simple cussedness, and anything untoward in female behaviour. (*Ideas*, 1983: 6)

If they were not subjected to gynecological surgery, women who were suffering were sometimes prescribed the 'rest cure'. This involved isolation in a dark room, eating a bland, boring diet of soft foods, and receiving no company except the nurse and doctor. This sensory deprivation was for the purpose of resting the brain or inducing the cessation of thought—thinking, after all, was the cause of the problems in the first place.

In the nineteenth century Charlotte Perkins Gilman was prescribed this rest cure and became famous when she published a description of the misery of her domestic life with its myriad restrictions. In *The Yellow Wallpaper* (1899), Gilman described how she just about 'went crazy' under the prescribed regime, until she realized that to heal herself she had to leave her husband and her upper-class domestic life and pursue a career in writing and feminist leadership.

In contrast, working-class women were expected to work constantly and hard even while bearing many children. Employers did not give them time off for pregnancy and childbirth or for any illness, 'feminine or not'. A day's absence, in fact, could cost a woman her job. The lives of working-class women were exceedingly hard. They commonly worked every day of the week, and even until midnight. Industrial accidents and occupational hazards were ubiquitous. Contagious diseases always attacked the crowded tenement flats of the poor first. There was no cult of invalidism here.

A number of feminist social commentators have noted that the social/sexual control effected through gynecological surgery and the rest cures prescribed by male medical doctors in the nineteenth century have been extended today by other means: women today receive psychotherapy, tranquilizers, and anti-depressants to keep them in their places and to help them cope with the tribulations of life in a sexist and patriarchal society.

Cooperstock and Lennard (1987) have documented the ways in which tranquilizers, one tool used by psychiatrists and general practitioners, are often used by women as aids in helping them cope with their 'assigned' and 'expected' social roles. In this study, women themselves talked of taking tranquilizers: (1) to help manage their feelings of exhaustion, busyness, and stress resulting from child-bearing and child-rearing responsibilities; (2) as an aid in minimizing their feelings of anxiety and upset because they lacked time to be themselves and to do what they wanted as independent human beings (e.g., write); and (3) to enable them to continue to live with their husbands and families under situations of grave unhappiness, but without options. Two illustrations follow:

> I take it to protect the family from my irritability because the kids are kids . . . I'm biding my time. One of these days I'm going to leave kit and kaboodle and walk out on him. Then maybe I won't need any more Valium.

> I would like to be off in Australia somewhere, writing. You know, do my own work. But having to stop the writing to get the supper on, it irritates me. And there are so many irritations during the day. But I cannot change the situation because of my family. (Ibid., 319)

A number of types of gynecological surgery are still used today. In fact, obstetricians and gynecologists claim to be 'the spokesmen for women's health care' (Scully, 1980: 15). Many women consult obstetricians or gynecologists for any woman's 'problem' and for routine prenatal and postnatal care, childbirth, abortions, birth control prescriptions, insertions, and fittings, and care during menopause.

Diana Scully (1980) examined, through a participant-observation study, the work of these specialists, and published the results in *Men Who Control Women's Health: The Miseducation of Obstetrician-Gynecologists.* She showed how the male-dominated profession is infused with sexist ideas, dating back to the struggle engaged in by obstetrics and gynecology to legitimate its place in the world of medicine in the nineteenth century. Among residents and interns women are seen as objects whose fundamental purpose is to provide teaching and learning material for future obstetricians and gynecologists. Female medical students are underrepresented in the specialty as compared with other medical specialties.

Michelle Harrison, in her autobiography, *A Woman in Residence* (1982), documented this through her personal experience as a resident in obstetrics and gynecology. Harrison described case after case of the prevalence of sexism; of the desire to get things done quickly, according to medically defined bureaucratic protocol; of the too frequent use of surgery; and of the preference for working with unusual cases. All this frequently takes place while the experiences of the individual woman—her questions, her desires, and her particular situation—are ignored. No matter whether the issue was birth control, childbirth, a D&C (dilation of the cervix and curettage of the uterus), a hysterectomy, or some other medical procedure, Harrison was able to document from personal experience the aggressive practices of the obstetricians/gynecologists.

A number of researchers have shown that rates of hysterectomies are excessive (see Fisher, 1986, for a review of the literature). The American Medical Association, through research it sponsored, has placed the hysterectomy and the D&C as coming second—after surgery on the knee—in unnecessary surgical procedures (Scully, 1980: 17). Some have noted that this increase in women's surgery follows a decline in birth rates; consequently, physicians need to find new work opportunities. One of the best predictors of the rate of hysterectomies in a population is the number of ob/gyn surgeons who are paid on a fee-for-service basis.

The definition of a diseased womb is indeed a very broad one. What is an acceptable level of symptomatology (irregular bleeding, fibroid tumours, menopausal flush or flash) in one area is unacceptable to some doctors and thus to their patients in another area. As John Bunker (1970, 1976) has noted, there are twice as many surgeons in the US in proportion to the population as there are in England and Wales. There are also more than twice as many hysterectomies relative to the female population.

A hysterectomy terminates the production of some necessary hormones. Pharmaceutical companies have busily synthesized artificial hormones that can be administered to women after they have had the uterus removed. This raises another possible explanation for the increased rates of hysterectomy—the pharmaceutical industry's need for profit. Through drug salesmen and expensive advertising, doctors and medical students are led to believe that a cure for the 'side effects' of the hysterectomy caused by lack of hormone production can be remedied simply through the prescription of a synthetic product.

Explaining the Medicalization of Women's Lives

Scholars have described the many ways that the contemporary medical system tends to medicalize women's lives and experiences. Women are a population at particular risk from medicalization for birth control, pregnancy, childbirth, the new reproductive technologies, menstruation, premenstruation, menopause, their physical appear-ance, and the whole realm of women's emotional well-being and stability. There is no medical specialty of doctors trained to work on men as there is for women—obstetricians and gynecologists. Men's life stages and life cycles, relatively speaking, have hardly been noticed or studied, yet men have been the chief subjects in medical research and the establishment of medical norms.

Doctors and women patients of certain classes have together 'generated' and 'marketed' certain types of diseases associated with the very facts of women's lives, such as pregnancy and childbirth, contraception, menstrual cycles, menopause, weight, and various types of unhappiness (Reissman, 1987). In so doing, they have served the short-term needs of one another. Physicians have been able to grow in power and authority, and their incomes have risen. In return, women have been provided with relief from pain and acknowledgement of their special needs for rest, mood-altering chemicals, freedom from unwanted burdens, and the like. The cost to women has been their lack of knowledge about their own bodies and lack of power to determine what actions they should take. The solution is not to repudiate medicine entirely. Rather, claims Reissman, the solution is to change the proprietorship, production, and utilization of scientific knowledge.

For certain problems in our lives, real demedicalization is necessary; experiences such as routine childbirth, menopause, and weight in excess of cultural norms should not necessarily be defined in medical terms, and medical-technical treatments should not always be seen as appropriate solutions to these 'problems'. For other conditions where medicine may be of assistance, the challenge will be to differentiate the beneficial treatments from those that are harmful and useless (ibid., 118).

Sexism Today

Doctors in Canada and the US are responding to charges of sexism by a commitment to address the concerns that women, both inside and outside of the profession, have expressed. For example, in 1987 the Ad Hoc Committee on Women's Health Issues of the Ontario Medical Association (OMA) reported to the OMA that women's health issues are unique to women and require special care and thought. The report made a number of recommendations that would require the OMA to take an active stance in defining women's health issues and in changing medical practice, medical education, and research investment so as to better address the concerns of women physicians as well as women patients (*Report to the OMA Board of Directors*, 1987).

The Private/Public Debate

Canadians cherish medicare as a social benefit in society that is an important part of their identity. In an era of free trade and a general move to the right in the politics of the Western developed world, all sorts of features of the 'social safety net' are threatened. Despite medicare's place in the hearts of Canadians it is in the process of being undermined—while public expenditures for health care are rapidly declining, private expenditures are up. Most Canadians think of our health-care system as a public system. In fact, it is a publicly funded private system—95 per cent of Canadian hospitals, for example, are private, non-profit entities (Cloutier-Fisher, 2000). Family physicians, the main gatekeepers to the system, are private entrepreneurs. These facts minimize public control and maximize the control of the professionals and doctors in the system. A partly privatized two-tiered system is a reality. Private per capita health-care expenditures averaged $482 in 1991, $491 in 1992, and $502 in 1993. There has been a dramatic change in the split between private and public financing of health care. Canadians spent an average of $606 on private health care and $1,761 in taxes used for health care in 1991. By 1997, the average Canadian spent $790 privately and $1,737 in taxes for health care. Thus, between 1991 and 1997 private expenditures grew by 30 per cent,

while the tax expenditure decreased by 1.6 per cent (Fuller, 1998: 6).

A significant component of the cuts to health care associated with the increase in private expenditures is the result of shorter hospital stays. This not only means fewer beds but fewer nurses, nurses' aides, orderlies, cleaners, launderers, chefs, kitchen help, and so on. It also means that a family member frequently has to stay home from work to care for a sick relative who is released from hospital sooner. Thus, too, a whole variety of expenditures, such as for dressings, drugs, and numerous pieces of medical furniture (such as a cane or wheelchair), have to be incurred privately. Nevertheless, because of (or in spite of) their advocacy of downsizing social and health services, many governments are being elected and re-elected. The Ontario Ministry of Health Annual Report (1992–3), in breathtakingly positive prose:

> celebrated the fact that hospitals in the province have been able to control costs at the same time as the number of patients treated actually increased—thanks to shorter stays and more day surgery and other out-patient services. (Armstrong and Armstrong, 1996: 66)

One of the most recent possible consequences of downsizing in the health-care system is the case of SARS in Ontario. The Ontario Conservatives fired five senior health scientists in the months before the outbreak. Then, when the syndrome was noted in Toronto, the provincial government had to scramble to find the necessary assistance ('Ill-planned cuts hurt SARS fight', 2003).

When medicare was introduced doctors were already in private practice. With medicare they began to receive public funding for their privately organized work. They began, under medicare, to be paid for each service they performed. They were not amenable to capitation or salaries.

The fact that physicians are essentially private practitioners who are financially supported by tax dollars has led to some difficulties and

Figure 13.4   Acute-Care Facilities in Canada, 1999–2000

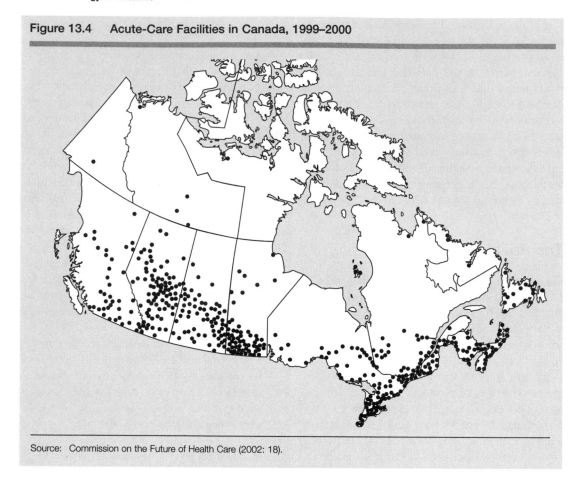

Source: Commission on the Future of Health Care (2002: 18).

inadequacies in the Canadian system. For instance, attracting and retaining doctors in rural settings has been a long-standing problem in Canada (Barer and Stoddart, 1999; Crichton et al., 1997; Kasperski 2001). For example, consider the locations of acute-care facilities across the country shown in Figure 13.4 and the variation in reported unmet health-care needs across the provinces and territories in Figure 13.5. In 2000, towns under 10,000 in population accounted for 22.2 per cent of the population, yet they were served by only 10.15 per cent of the doctors (Hutton-Czapski, 2001). A Decima poll recently found that 26 per cent of Canadians living out-side of major urban centres reported difficulty in finding a family doctor (Kasperski, 2001). It may be argued that there is a fundamental mismatch between those who become doctors and the needs of remote and rural communities. Most of those who are accepted into medical school have grown up in urban areas and are trained in urban medicine (Barer and Stoddart, 1999). They are not prepared for the heavy workloads, isolation, or the minimal access to clinical and educational supports that they experience in small towns and in the country (Kasperski, 2001). Currently many rural doctors cannot find replacements. There is a predicted shortage of family doctors and doctors willing to work in rural areas (Rachlis et al., 2001). Today in most provinces any doctor can set up a practice anywhere. The chronic and geographically specific shortage of doctors threatens to worsen. The fee-for-service remuneration system is favoured by doctors because of their desire for independence and autonomy (Angus and Manga, 1990; Wanke et al., 1996). However, it is incompatible with a process that would ensure an even distribution of doctors across the country.

There is evidence of inequity in services across provincial boundaries as the provinces try to manage medicare. For instance, women in British Columbia have a significantly higher five-year survival rate from breast cancer, as shown in Figure 13.6. Large variations in both public and private expenditures for health care are also evident, as shown in Figure 13.7. The increase in public home-care expenditures over the years from 1975–6 to 1997–8 is substantial (Figure 13.8). However, this is still a very small proportion of the total spent on health care even though most health-care work takes place in the home. Figure 13.9 shows the decline in hospital admissions in the latter part of the nineties. Figure 13.10 indicates the parallel decline until 1999 in the average length of hospital stay for Canadians over 65. Figure 13.11 shows the number of general practitioners or family physicians and specialists per population from 1980 to 2001.

Home Health Care

All medical care used to take place in the home. In the past century, however, hospitals, doctor's offices, and clinics became the favoured places for medical care. These locations and health-care providers working within the medical model were supported financially and in numerous policy and legal initiatives under the Canada Health Act. Some dramatic changes in the last few decades have moved substantial amounts of care back out of the hospitals, clinics, and doctors'

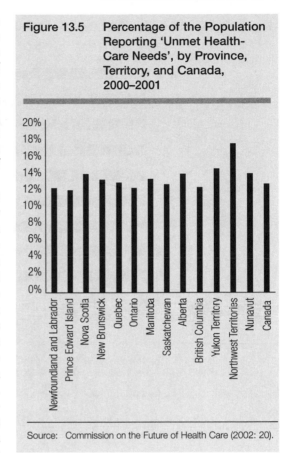

Figure 13.5   Percentage of the Population Reporting 'Unmet Health-Care Needs', by Province, Territory, and Canada, 2000–2001

Source: Commission on the Future of Health Care (2002: 20).

offices. Now home medical care may involve complex tasks such as that provided when a person is recovering from surgery, dialysis, and intravenous therapies, as well as routine monitoring of frail elderly people living on their own, those with mental illnesses whose medications need monitoring and who themselves need support, and even palliative care for people dying at home. Among the reasons for the rapid growth in the services offered at home are the deinstitutionalization of the mentally ill, the closing of hospitals, the disproportions of both specialists and general practitioners across the country, the availability of many new drugs to treat diseases that formerly required surgical or other hospital-

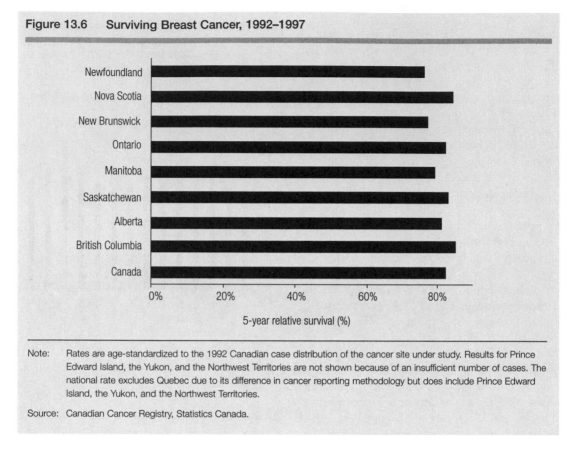

Figure 13.6   Surviving Breast Cancer, 1992–1997

Note: Rates are age-standardized to the 1992 Canadian case distribution of the cancer site under study. Results for Prince Edward Island, the Yukon, and the Northwest Territories are not shown because of an insufficient number of cases. The national rate excludes Quebec due to its difference in cancer reporting methodology but does include Prince Edward Island, the Yukon, and the Northwest Territories.

Source: Canadian Cancer Registry, Statistics Canada.

based treatments, and the growth in the proportion of elderly people, including the frail elderly, living alone.

The types of care provided in the home can be classified into three different categories (Romanow Report, 2002: 173). The first is the provision of professional services such as nursing, occupational and physical therapy, and speech therapy. The second is the provision of personal care such as bathing, toileting, feeding, and the like. The third is homemaking services, including housecleaning, laundry, and meal preparation.

According to the Romanow Report the future of health care is likely to include increases in the care provided at home. Among the pro-

jections from this report are the following:

1. new developments in medications, technology, and various treatments that make home care feasible and preferable to hospital care;
2. new models of primary health care that include teams of different types of care providers to work in concert and thus offer support to those in their own homes;
3. increasing numbers of elderly people who prefer care in their own homes and communities;
4. the stresses and strains experienced by those who presently must provide care for family members, neighbours, and friends even in the face of costs to their own health, employment, and nuclear families;

Figure 13.7 How Much We Spend Per Capita

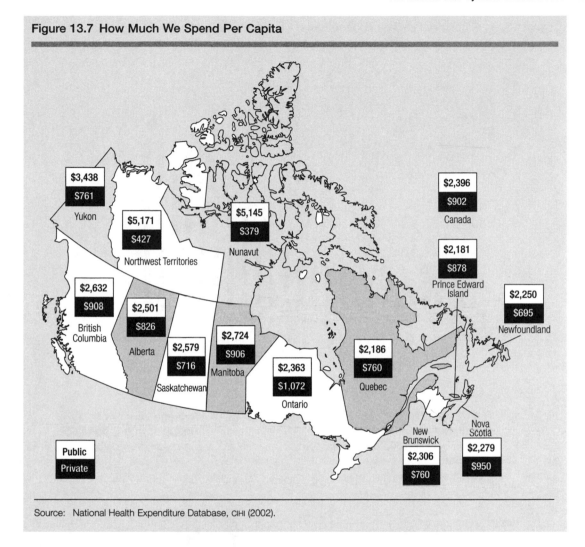

Source: National Health Expenditure Database, CIHI (2002).

5. the projected continuing trend towards early discharge from hospital;
6. the fact that home care saves dollars even while it may provide a more satisfactory milieu for care. (Ibid., 176)

Unfortunately, home care is presently financed differently across the country—some provinces include some services; other provinces include others.

Summary

(1) Two main critiques of the contemporary medical care system are that it is dominated by the medical model of health and illness and that there is a great deal of sexism in medicine and in the experiences of health and illness. Implications of the medical model are: advances against disease only happen through scientific investigation, the

Figure 13.8   Public Home-Care Expenditures, Canada, 1975–6 to 1997–8

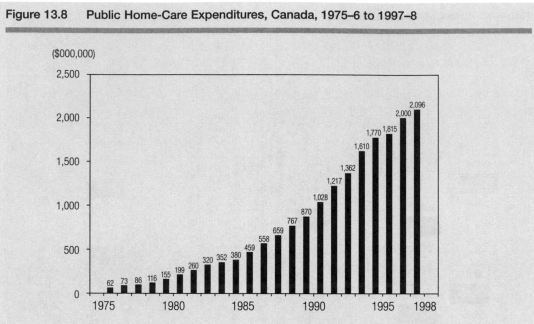

Source: Health Canada, at: <www.hc-sc.gc.ca/datapcb/datahesa/E_home.htm>.

Figure 13.9   In-patient/Acute-Care Admissions, Age Standardized (number per 100,000 people), Canada, 1994–1999

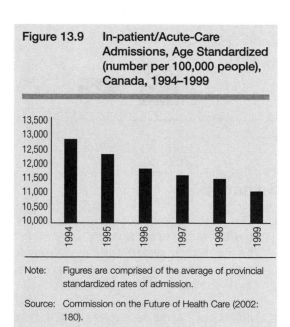

Note: Figures are comprised of the average of provincial standardized rates of admission.

Source: Commission on the Future of Health Care (2002: 180).

Figure 13.10   Average Length of Hospitalization, Ages 65+, Canada, 1994–1999

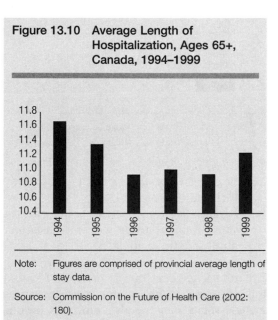

Note: Figures are comprised of provincial average length of stay data.

Source: Commission on the Future of Health Care (2002: 180).

Figure 13.11   Total Number of General Practitioners/Family Physicians and Specialists per 100,000 Population, 1980–2001

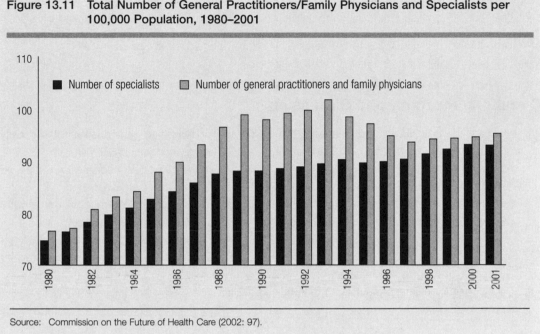

■ Number of specialists   ☐ Number of general practitioners and family physicians

Source: Commission on the Future of Health Care (2002: 97).

focus being on the pathological alterations within of the body. Disease is considered an undesirable and abnormal functioning within the individual.

(2) Two models that compete with the medical model are the environmental/social-structural model, which focuses on the causes of disease that lie outside the individual organism, and the lifestyle model, which focuses on understanding disease as the result of actions based on personal decisions regarding lifestyle.

(3) A complete medical care system would include something of all three models. The Canadian medical system almost exclusively relies on the medical model, which has limited relevance to cures for the most significant modern diseases: those that are chronic. Medical intervention has enabled many people to live who would previously have died, thus increasing the burdens of chronic illness and chronic disability.

(4) The Canadian government has moved to a broader vision of disease causation and treatment. Federal and provincial health ministries currently emphasize disease prevention and health promotion strategies through media advertising, health education, and community development.

(5) There are large differences between males and females in income and power in the medical labour force today. Women can be seen as hidden healers through their role in the family. Deinstitutionalization and the increasingly chronic nature of many diseases will intensify the burden of home-based caregivers.

(6) New trends in Canadian society include the women's movement, which has demanded knowledge and information about women's bodies and has discovered the negative effects that medicine has had on women's physical and mental health. Another trend is

the changing disease profile. The main concerns of health-care services in the future will be caring for an older population and for individuals with mental health problems

(7) The balance between public and private in the medicare system is increasingly in favour of the private.

(8) Significant inequities exist in the distribution of physicians in Canada today.

Questions for Study and Discussion

1. What are the advantages and disadvantages of each of the three models of disease enumerated in this chapter?

2. Take the *Framework for Health Promotion* offered by Epp and explain how it might work with respect to a particular disease or condition.

3. Assess McKnight's study, as reported by Rachlis and Kushner, in light of a parallel or similar situation in your experience at university.

4. Which is safer: cigarette smoking or contraceptive use? Explain.

5. What evidence do you observe of a society increasingly concerned with risk?

6. Assess the claim that medical practice is sexist in light of your own experience.

7. Assess newspaper coverage of the private/public investment in health care.

8. What is your opinion about the role of profit-making in the provision of health for Canadians?

Suggested Readings

Boston Women's Health Collective. 1996. *Our Bodies, Our Selves*, 25th Anniversary Edition. New York: Simon & Schuster. An important document for women's health movements around the world.

Culane, Dara Speck. 1987. *An Error in Judgement: The Politics of Medical Care in an Indian/White Community*. Vancouver: Talon Books. An older book but still a classic illustration of research regarding critical issues in Aboriginal health issues.

Ehrenreich, Barbara, and Deirdre English. 1973. *Witches, Midwives and Nurses: A History of Women Healers*. Old Westbury, NY: Feminist Press. A work of great value in understanding women's health issues from a feminist perspective and over time.

Findlay, Deborah. 1993. 'The Good, the Normal and the Healthy: The Social Construction of Medical Knowledge about Women', *Canadian Journal of Sociology* 18, 2: 115–33. Canadian research deftly examining the social construction of gendered medical thinking and practice.

Lorber, J. 1984. *Women Physicians, Careers, Statuses and Power*. New York: Tavistock. A description of women doctors and their work from a sociological perspective.

Chapter 14 | *Nurses and Midwives in the Changing Health-Care System*

Learning Objectives

- Some sort of nursing has always existed.
- The history of nursing is associated with the history of religion in Canada.
- Some of the issues facing nurses today include sexism, managerial ideology, hospital organization, and financial cutbacks.
- Florence Nightingale is important in the history and present practice of nursing.
- Nursing is facing challenges in its attempt to become autonomous.
- Midwifery has very recently become regulated in a number of provinces in Canada.
- There are, however, still major impediments to the widespread acceptance of midwifery for birthing women and their families.
- There is good evidence as to the safety and effectiveness of midwifery.

Introduction

Nurses are a fundamental part of the modern medical care system. Hospitals, long-term care institutions, and many doctors' offices could not function without the essential work of nurses. Nurses and nurse practitioners are often responsible for the health of remote communities on a day-to-day basis. Midwives, who have long helped women give birth and continue to do so in about 80 per cent of the world, have been given legal status in some Canadian provinces for maternity care and birth. What are the sociological forces that continue to affect the recruitment, retention, employment venues, and quality of working life of nurses? Who are the nurses and midwives—in Canada today and historically? What is the relationship of the work of the allopathic doctor to these other health-care providers? Do doctors compete with nurses or do they work in different spheres? Can the work of the nurse be seen as 'separate but equal' to the work of the doctor? Are midwives' rates of mother and infant mortality higher than those of obstetricians and gynecologists? These are among the questions addressed in this chapter.

Nursing: The Historical Context

Some form of nursing has always been available for sick people, even if it was only unskilled assistance such as help with feeding and being made comfortable. Usually nursing was women's work, an extension of domestic responsibilities (O'Brien, 1989). Today, nursing is a complex paraprofessional occupation mostly taking place in hospitals run by rigidly hierarchical bureaucracies segregated 'according to sex and race, power and pay, specialty and education' (Armstrong et al., 1993: 11), and equipped with complex technology (about 80 per cent of all Canadian nurses work in hospitals). The duties of the hospital nurse are extremely varied and specialized, and clearly are limited within a complex division of labour. Some nursing roles, such as those in the coronary care unit (CCU) or the intensive care unit (ICU), involve highly skilled medical management and quick decision-making in operating sophisticated machinery. Thus, one nurse in an ICU or CCU may spend her/his working hours monitoring and recording the readouts on a series of machines that are keeping a patient alive. Another, working in a psychiatric clinic, may spend her/his days in group and individual therapy, where the tasks involve listening and communicating on an emotional level with patients. But wherever nursing is taking place, it is usually under the jurisdiction of a physician. There are interesting exceptions, however, such as occupational nursing in which nurses work in industry as on-site caretakers for minor injuries and sickness, including emotional stress caused by such things as work burnout, and also develop and administer workplace wellness programs.

The rise of Christianity led to distinctive roles for nurses. Healing and caring for the sick came to be thought of as acts of Christian charity, and nursing became a full-time occupation for the sisters of the Church: they worked with the sick, founded hospitals, and provided bedside care. Commitment to the sick was an acceptable role for devout Christian women because it was an occupation controlled by the Church. Nursing sisters were known to refuse the orders of doctors, and even to refuse to work for certain types of patients when such work violated their Christian convictions.

Military nursing, too, has a long history. Evidence suggests that as early as the thirteenth century the Knights of St John of Jerusalem admitted women into their order so that they could nurse the wounded. In the seventeenth century the Knights of Malta maintained a type of nursing service in their hospital at Valetta. Two knights were assigned to each of the towns surrounding the harbour. Each pair of knights had four nurses 'to assist them in their rounds', their duties being to carry supplies to the sick and the poor, to see that the physicians appointed to visit them attended to their duties, and to ensure that patients received the proper care and medicine (Nicholson, 1967: 16).

After the Protestant Reformation of the sixteenth century, nursing disappeared as a respectable service for devout Christian women in countries where the Catholic Church and its organizations were destroyed. Those who could afford it were doctored and nursed at home. Hospitals were built, but they were primarily for the poor and indigent, and were filthy, malodorous, and overcrowded. They usually lacked clean water and adequate drainage. The beds were seldom changed. Patients shared the same dirty sheets. It was not realized that fresh air was healthy and so windows were frequently boarded up. Germs spread and multiplied in such a filthy and airless atmosphere.

Women working in these hospitals were those who had no choice—the poor, infirm, and old, sometimes patients who had recovered. At this time a stereotype emerged of the nurse as a drunken, poverty-stricken old woman who lived and ate with the sick. Hospitals were considered places to go to die, or to go to when there was no other choice. Frequently they were infested with rats, had contaminated water supplies, and were inhabited by patients with contagious diseases such as cholera, typhoid, and smallpox: it is no wonder that the mortality rate, even among the nurses, was often very high (frequently as high as 20 or 30 per cent).

Marie Rollet Hébert is thought to have been the first person to provide nursing care in what is now Canada. She and her husband, a surgeon-apothecary, worked together to help the sick from the time of their arrival in Quebec in 1617. Later, nursing sisters, members of various religious orders, emigrated to what are now Quebec City and Montreal, established hospitals, and treated those wounded in the wars. These nurses were more like doctors than modern nurses; they made and administered medicines and performed surgery. They administered the hospitals and the missions they founded.

By the eighteenth and nineteenth centuries, epidemics of smallpox, influenza, measles, scarlet fever, typhoid, typhus, and tuberculosis threatened the health of the people. In response, nursing sisters from various orders established hospitals as places where the sick could be segregated and cared for. Still, the hospitals were used especially by the homeless and poor. Over time the hospital system expanded. Today, it has become a place for all classes of people when they are acutely ill and need the specialized, and often high-technology, services offered by doctors, nurses, and others.

Nursing Today: Issues of Sexism, Managerial Ideology, Hospital Organization, and Cutbacks

Nurses comprise about two-thirds of all medical care providers. Altogether there were 232,000 RNs working in Canada in 2000, or 754 per 100,000 citizens. As Table 14.1 shows, the proportion of nurses in the population increased substantially from 1965 to 1989 but then began to decrease. This decline in the ratio of nurses to population has been noticeable in Ontario in recent years, as Figure 14.1 illustrates. In Ontario, the population increased by 25 per cent from 1981 to 1997 while the number of registered nurses increased by 12 per cent and the number of registered practical nurses increased by only 2.6 per cent. According to an independent study commissioned by the Canadian Nurses' Association, a severe shortage of nurses is predicted in the next decade. The combined effect of an aging nurse workforce, a decline in young people entering the field, and an aging population is an estimated shortage of between 59,000 and 113,000 nurses by 2011 (*The Canadian Nurse*, 1998: 15).

More than 80 per cent of nurses work in health-care institutions—hospitals and long-term care institutions (Abelson and Strohmenger, 1983: 13). Table 14.2 indicates where nurses in recent years have been employed. Nursing was the fourth largest category in the female workforce in 1996 (*Women in Canada*, 1995: 76). A minority of registered nurses in Canada are male, but their numbers are growing (Trudeau, 1996). In 1985 about 2 per cent of RNs were male; by 1995 about 4 per cent were male. Males tend to be overrepresented in psychiatry, critical care, emergency care, and administration. There tend to be few in such specialties as maternal/newborn care, pediatrics, and community care. Male nurses, on average, are older than female nurses. This may reflect the fact that nursing tends to be a second career for male nurses.

Critical analysis of the work of the contemporary nurse tends to follow one of four lines: (1) the patriarchal/sexist nature of the content of the work and of the position of the nurse in the medical labour force; (2) the managerial revolution in nursing practice today, (3) the impact of the bureaucracy of the hospital on the working life of the nurse; and (4) the impact of cutbacks on the numbers of nurses and the quality and safety of nursing work.

Table 14.1   Population per Active Civilian Physician and Registered Nurse Employed in Nursing, Canada, 1901–1998

Year	Population per physician*	Population per nurse**	Year	Population per physician*	Population per nurse**
1901	978	19,014	1989	535	115
1911	970	1,284	1992	530	122
1921	1,008	410	1993	523	123
1931	1,034	506	1994	530	125
1941	968	441	1995	536	127
1951	976	325	1996	543	130
1961	988	258	1997	546	131
1971	805	146	1998	541	134
1981	652	119			

*Based on census data.

**Registered nurses for 1941 to 1975; census figures for 1931 (graduate nurses) and earlier years (nurses). Excludes Newfoundland prior to 1961; excludes Yukon and Northwest Territories prior to 1941. The 1921 figure includes nurses-in-training. Figures for 1981 and 1989 include only nurses registered during the first four months (three in Quebec) of the registration period and registered in the same province in which they work or reside.

Sources: Statistics Canada, *Historical Statistics of Canada*, 2nd edn (Ottawa: Minister of Supply and Services, Series B82–92, 1983); Health and Welfare Canada, *Health Personnel in Canada* (Ottawa, 1991); Statistics Canada, *Registered Nurses Management Data*; Canadian Institute for Health Information.

Sexism

Sexism is ubiquitous in the medical labour force. Doctors have usually been men and nurses have usually been women. The role of the nurse, in fact, the origin of the word, refers to female functions. Nursing comes from the Latin *nutrire*, and means to nourish and suckle. Both historically and today, nursing refers both to a mother's action in suckling or breast-feeding her baby and to the act of caring for the sick. Because the earliest nurses were nuns working for the glory of God, nurses have long been called sisters. The very concepts of caring, nurturing, feeding, and tending to the sick are inextricably tied up with ideas about women (Reverby, 1987; Growe, 1991). The few men who train or are educated to be nurses usually end up moving up the administrative ladder.

Florence Nightingale's views of nurses and their training reinforced a subservient, feminine image of the nurse. It was her view that while nurses could be trained in some of the detailed duties of bedside care, the most fundamental aspects of the nursing occupation could not be learned. Just as it was impossible to train a person to be a mother, it was impossible to train a woman to nurse. The components of a woman's character, her selfless devotion to others, and her obedience to those in authority could not be learned or taught. Entrance requirements to nursing schools thus traditionally included an interview in which these nebulous characteristics were evaluated.

Fine-tuning was still necessary, but it could only be managed if the woman was first of all 'successful as a woman'. One of the first hospitals to train nurses according to the Nightingale model, the New England Hospital for Women and Children in Boston, included among the requirements for admission 'that an applicant be between 21 and 31 years old, be well and strong, and have a good reputation as to character and disposition, with a good knowledge of general housework desirable' (Punnett, 1976: 5).

This sexism in ideology is reflected in differences in pay, authority, responsibility, prestige, and working conditions between men and women. Physicians have the advantage over nurses in all of these respects. The nurse has responsibility for carrying out the doctor's orders, but no authority to change them when they are incorrect.

Most nurses in a hospital work shifts. Their working conditions are problematic in a number of ways: (1) their working hours are rigid; (2) night and evening shift work is regularly required; (3) they are often restricted in their work to a hospital; (4) they are at risk because of the occupational health and safety conditions in hospitals (Walters, 1994; Walters and Haines, 1989); (5) their workloads are excessive (Walters and Haines, 1989); (6) they are, because of underfunding, often forced to do housekeeping and other non-nursing work (Stelling, 1994). Thus, sexism restricts women to an occupational ghetto, and that ghetto provides them with few rewards and little or no authority (Warburton and Carroll, 1988).

Managerial Ideology in Hospitals

The second critical issue today is the managerial ideology in hospital management systems. This ideology is the outcome of a historical trend that reflects the development of the money economy, bureaucracy, capitalism, and rationalization. Managerial ideology assumes that it is the job of managers to run organizations as efficiently as possible so as to provide adequate service at minimal cost. In Canada hospitals are still funded chiefly through the public sector; federal and provincial funding provides operating grants; local municipalities also provide funds as do local

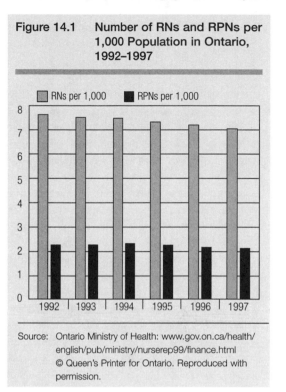

Figure 14.1   Number of RNs and RPNs per 1,000 Population in Ontario, 1992–1997

Source: Ontario Ministry of Health: www.gov.on.ca/health/ english/pub/ministry/nurserep99/finance.html © Queen's Printer for Ontario. Reproduced with permission.

fundraising initiatives. They are run under the jurisdiction of provincial government authorities. Hospital managers are accountable to boards and the boards to the provinces. They are faced with limited financial resources and the necessity of setting priorities within the context of extensive cost-cutting by governments. Payments for nursing services must compete with needs for cleaning, equipment upkeep, purchase of new and increasingly expensive technology and pharmaceuticals, as well as payments to the many other hospital personnel, including occupational and physical therapists, social workers, staff physicians, and others.

Several rationalized management systems have been developed for use in hospitals. One is case mix groupings (CMGs)—a technique for detailing the specific tasks and the time each task takes with reference to the average patient with a

Box 14.1   The Story of Florence Nightingale

The story of the transition of hospital nursing from a duty performed out of charity and for the love of God, or by poor women who had no option, to an occupation requiring training must begin with the story of Florence Nightingale. She revolutionalized nursing work and laid the foundations for the modern, full-time occupation of nursing. 'On February the 7th, 1837, God spoke to me and called me to his service.' Another time she wrote, 'I craved for some regular occupation, for something worth doing instead of frittering away my time with useless trifles' (Bull, 1985: 15). This statement has been taken to be a reflection of her motivation to serve the sick despite years of opposition by her wealthy mother and sister and the pleas of several ardent suitors.

Nightingale was born into a wealthy English family in 1820. The upper-class Victorian woman was expected to marry, and to provide heirs for her husband, to run his household, and to be a decorative companion at social events. Ideally, her days would have been taken up with organizing the servants and governesses in the household, perhaps engaging in some fancywork, and meeting with other women concerning some charitable cause. As has been said, nursing at that time was for the most part done by the indigent. It most certainly was not a 'suitable' occupation for someone of Nightingale's social standing.

Nevertheless, she was committed to making something special of her life in the service of God. Her first experience of the kind of service God might be calling her to occurred one summer when the family was holidaying at their summer place, LeaHurst, in Derbyshire. Nightingale met and helped a number of poor cottagers, taking them food, medicine, and clothing. Later she nursed her sick grandmother and an orphaned baby. When she learned of a school for the training of nurses located in Germany, the Kaiserwerth Hospital, she visited it.

Her father, having seen Nightingale refuse suitors, read and study mathematics late into the night, and maintain her fervent commitment to God's call, finally weakened. Two rich, aristocratic friends, Sidney and Elizabeth Herbert, supported Nightingale and spread the word that she was England's leading expert in matters of health. When a director was required for a nursing home, the Institution for the Care of Sick Gentlewomen in Distressed Circumstances, the Herberts recommended Nightingale. She accepted the position and turned the nursing home into a very good and well-run hospital.

Slightly more than one year later, after she had gained invaluable experience in running the hospital, Sidney Herbert, who was then Secretary of War, asked Nightingale to go to Turkey to nurse British soldiers injured in the Crimean War. The war, to that point, had been disastrous for the British. They had been unprepared. There were widespread shortages of equipment, food, bedding, and medical supplies. The soldiers were expected to live on mouldy biscuits and salt pork. They slept in the mud in clothes and blankets that were stiff with blood and crawling with lice. There was no water for washing, and all the drains were blocked. Almost every man had diarrhea, but there were neither diets nor special medicines to relieve it (ibid., 35). There were no hot drinks, because the necessities for lighting a fire were not available.

Nightingale was asked to recruit, organize, and take a group of 40 nurses into this chaotic and squalid situation. She advertised in London and beyond, but was only able to find 38 women, some of whom were religious sisters, with the qualities she required. Nightingale and her staff set out for the Crimea. She laid down strict orders to be followed: all were to be considered equal; all were to obey her. They were to share food and accommodation. All wore uniforms comprised of grey dresses and white caps.

Nightingale and her nurses arrived at the Barroch Hospital in Scutari ready to work and armed with financial resources. They were met with hostility by the doctors, who refused to let them see patients and offered all 38 women only six dirty, small rooms (one of which had a corpse in it). They were given no furniture, lighting, or food. Nightingale had experienced much opposition in her life; she was prepared to wait. She told her nurses to make bandages, and offered the doctors milk puddings for the patients. These tasks seemed 'suitable' for women, and so the doctors accepted the milk puddings. Less than one week later there was another battle and a huge number of casualties. The doctors, overwhelmed by the enormity of the disaster and the tasks that lay ahead of them, and reassured that the nurses were willing to obey (they had waited) and that they could provide 'feminine services' (make milk puddings), asked the nurses to help out.

Nightingale ordered food, cutlery, china, soap, bedpans, and operating tables. Her nurses sewed clean cotton bags for straw mattresses. Men were hired to clean the lavatories and basins. The floors were scrubbed for the first time in anyone's memory. Soldiers' wives were recruited to wash clothes and bedding. Still the mortality rate did not decline significantly. Nightingale, who knew far more than the doctors about the importance of fresh air, cleanliness, and clean water, had the plumbing inspected. The pipes were blocked and the water supply contaminated. Once this was cleaned out the mortality rate dropped dramatically.

Nightingale was viewed as a heroine both within the hospital and without. Within the hospital she was known as 'the lady with the lamp'. She offered all kinds of services, even banking and letterwriting, to her patients. At the end of the war the grateful soldiers dedicated one day's pay to her for the establishment of the Nightingale School of Nursing and the Nightingale Fund. Outside the hospital, at home in Britain, she was heralded as the most important woman of her time. There were at this time no female judges, MPs, or civil servants. No woman had ever taken charge of an institution. Florence Nightingale was a heroine to Britain and to the Western world.

Her greatest achievements were in public health reform. Her writing and lobbying in this area continued long after she returned from the Crimea even though she spent the rest of her life, essentially, bedridden. It has been suggested, in fact, that Nightingale's work was the beginning of modern epidemiology. Her work is also thought to have provided the model for the early training of nurses. Eventually, after several unsuccessful attempts, the first nursing school, on the Nightingale model, was established at the General and Marine Hospital in St Catharines, Ontario, in 1874. A few years later the Toronto General (1881) and Montreal General (1880) hospitals were established. Nursing students often comprised almost the whole staff of these hospitals (Jensen, 1988).

The long-term effects of Nightingale's work on the practice of nursing are often considered to have been equivocal, however (Reverby, 1987). On the one hand, she herself exhibited enormous strength and commitment, and was able to garner extensive personal power as a leader in epidemiological research models, in health-care policy, in the management of hospitals, in military nursing, and as the most important role model for the secular occupation of nursing in her society. On the other hand, she ensured that the women who worked as nurses for her were taught to be handmaidens to doctors and to be 'mother-surrogates' to patients. Even though Nightingale studied hard to become educated and rejected her own assigned gender role, she expected her nurses to be subservient, obedient, and docile in their relationships with medical doctors.

Nursing, under Nightingale, was to be a woman's job. Only women had the necessary character and qualities. While carving out a respectable occupation for women, she also reinforced a ghettoized and subordinated female labour force that is still in place today. This model of nursing supported the traditional stereotype of the physician as father figure and the nurse as mother.

Table 14.2   Number of RNs by Place of Work, Canada, 1997–2000

	1997	1998	1999	2000
Hospital	**145,467**	**142,043**	**142,752**	**148,366**
Hospital (general, maternal, pediatric, psychiatric)	137,933	134,927	135,691	141,332
Mental Health Centre	3,912	3,586	3,606	3,636
Nursing Stations (outpost or clinic)	956	938	863	805
Rehabilitation/Convalescent Centre	2,666	2,592	2,592	2,593
Nursing Home/Long-Term Care	**27,828**	**26,987**	**26,685**	**26,094**
Community Health	**25,561**	**26,194**	**27,610**	**28,830**
Home Care Agency	9,818	9,992	9,055	8,644
Community Health/Health Agency	15,743	16,202	18,555	20,186
Other Place of Work	**28,312**	**29,380**	**29,140**	**28,655**
Business/Industry/Occupational Health Office	3,298	3,407	3,549	3,621
Private Nursing Agency/Private Duty	2,096	2,084	1,991	1,739
Self-employed	1,641	1,793	1,893	1,858
Physician's Office/Family Practice Unit	5,865	5,881	5,729	5,622
Educational Institution	5,329	5,007	4,926	5,023
Association/Government	3,484	3,581	3,755	3,889
Other	6,599	7,627	7,297	6,903
Not Stated	**2,645**	**3,047**	**2,263**	**467**
Canada	**229,813**	**227,651**	**228,450**	**232,412**

Source: Canadian Institute for Health Information (CIHI), *Canada's Health Care Providers*, 2002.

particular diagnosis. Productivity and cost-effectiveness are the goals. Nurses must try to work within the specified time limits and still provide adequate nursing care to the patients. Case mix groupings are a set of mutually exclusive categories that can be used for describing patients' clinical attributes. Patients within a particular CMG are believed to require roughly equivalent regimens of care and hence are believed to consume similar amounts of hospital resources (May and Wasserman, 1984: 548).

Case mix grouping assumes that all patients with a particular medical condition will require similar medical treatment (e.g., childbirth by Caesarean section, or chemotherapy with stage-one lung cancer). A cost is then assigned to the nursing care required by the typical patient with that specific diagnosis. Each of the patients in the hospital is accorded a particular time/cost value. Nurses, nursing assistants, orderlies, and other medical care personnel can then be assigned to various wards for specific lengths of time to provide predefined services.

According to Campbell (1988), such rationalization has numerous deleterious effects on the working lives of nurses. In many ways such a system demeans the authority of the nurse and diminishes her powers of decision-making. Individual patient needs are not assessed in a holistic way, as a result of experience gained during the practice of the art and science of nursing, but by a predetermined, quantified, and remote system. Nurses know that individual patients always vary from the norm in some way or anoth-

Box 14.2   The Doctor-Nurse Game

Leonard I. Stein's paper 'The Doctor-Nurse Game' (1987) describes one strategy used by doctors and nurses to manage the contradictory position of the doctor who may have more power and authority and the nurse who frequently has more information and knowledge, both about particular patients and their health and well-being on a day-to-day basis while in the hospital, and about hospital routines and common medical practices. This contradiction is especially acute when the doctor in question is a resident, intern, or new graduate. Stein's point is that nurses frequently make suggestions to doctors about how to treat certain situations and cases but that such suggestions must be handled with great subtlety and caution and even disguised. The object of the game is for the nurse to make recommendations to the doctor, all the while pretending to be passive. On the other hand, the doctor must ask for advice without appearing to do so. A typical scene would proceed as follows:

Nurse A: Mr Brown has been complaining of pains in his legs for more than six hours today. He appears to be quite uncomfortable.

Doctor G: Is this a new symptom for Mr Brown or is it recurring?

Nurse A: Mr Brown complained of a similar pain last week when he was admitted. He was given xxxx and it seemed to diminish.

Doctor B: OK. Let's try xxxx. What dosage did he require to get relief?

Nurse A: 3 m/hour.

Doctor G: OK. xxxx, 3 m/hour, nurse, please.

Nurse A: Thank you, doctor.

As Stein indicates, the game plan is taught to the nursing students at the same time as they learn the other aspects of nursing care. Doctors usually start to learn once they actually begin to practise in a system with nurses.

---

er. Yet time for each patient has been allocated by the classification system. The nurse, then, is constrained, by virtue of the time available to her, to behave to all patients, regardless of their individual differences, within certain predefined strictures. Not only is such a requirement destructive to the morale of the nurse, but also it may be dangerous or harmful to the patient.

Staffing assignments based on the information provided by the CMGs do not allow for the fact that, just as patients differ from the norm, so, too, do nurses. For instance, a small nurse may need help in turning a large patient. Turning may be required hourly. Yet, if the assignment has not considered such characteristics of staff/patient interaction as relative size, it cannot predict costs accurately. In this case the smaller nurse will have to get the assistance of a larger nurse, a nursing assistant, or an orderly. Finding the person to provide such assistance will take additional time; the person who provided the assistance will have to deduct the time taken from his/her total time available for care. A generous allotment of flexible time could enable the nursing staff to manage such situations. However, such flexibility does not exist in the climate of cost-containment that typifies the contemporary hospital system. For nurses, the outcomes of such management systems include decreased job satisfaction, burnout, and stress (Conley and Maukasch, 1988). For patients, the outcomes can include poor quality of care, slower recuperation, and, ultimately, greater long-term susceptibility to ill health.

Beardwood and Walters (1999) argue that these new managerial techniques, combined with restructuring and downsizing in hospitals and in the medical care system more generally, are reducing the autonomy of nurses and making it increasingly difficult to meet the standards of their profession. At the same time, government policies are making it easier for patients to complain about the services they are receiving. Complaints, when made, are made by individuals or family members usually against individual nurses. This model of 'accountability' obfuscates the conditions and systems within which the nurse works and highlights her individual responsibility as opposed to the inadequacies of the health-care system. The new managerialism has also exacerbated differences and polarized groups such as RNs and RPNs, degree against diploma nurses, management against staff nurses.

Bureaucratic Hospital Organization

The third area for the critical analysis of the nursing profession today is related to the effect of the hospital's bureaucratic structure on nursing. Opportunity consists of the available career expectations, ambitions and goals, and the probability of reaching these (Kanter, 1977). The structure of opportunity within the organization is determined by rates of promotion, locations for promotion, jobs that lead to promotion, and the like. People who have little opportunity tend to: (1) have lower self-esteem and sense of self-determination, or lack confidence in their ability to change the system; (2) seek satisfaction outside of work; (3) compare themselves with others on the same organizational level rather than with people on a higher level; (4) limit their aspirations; (5) be critical of managers and those in powerful positions; (6) be less likely to expect change; and (7) be more likely to complain (ibid.).

Opportunities for nurses are severely lacking in modern hospital organizations. The structure of promotion in the hospital limits vertical mobility for nurses. The major option open to a nurse with aspirations is to leave nursing and become an administrator. The first step would be to become a head nurse on a ward, with day-to-day responsibility for the running of the ward and for managing a team of nurses, nurses' aides, and

orderlies. Further movement up the system takes the nurse further and further from the actual practice of nursing.

Power is the capacity to mobilize resources (ibid.). Power includes the discretionary ability to make decisions that affect the organization, the visibility of the job, the relevance of the job to current organizational problems, and opportunities for promotion. Nurses, by these criteria, have very little organizational power.

The arrest of Susan Nelles on 25 March 1981 for the murder of four infants at the Hospital for Sick Children in Toronto exemplifies powerlessness as responsibility without authority. Even though physicians and others were routinely on the ward and were also frequently involved with patients, it was a nurse who was first suspected and charged. Furthermore, many nurses (and others) were incensed by the fact that the televised hearing showed that the Grange Inquiry treated doctors differently from nurses—dramatically so. Doctors, on the assumption that they were innocent, were questioned with deference and respect. Nurses were questioned under the assumption of guilt and suspicion. 'It was as if the police assumed, if it wasn't this nurse who committed the crime, which nurse was it?' (Wilson, 1987: 27). Through this and other incidents, nurses discovered that they were the first to be blamed but had little respect or authority within the hospital system.

Cutbacks

Today, cutbacks represent a grave threat to the public nature of the health-care sector and have had significant effects on hospitals. The overall number of beds in hospitals has already declined but hospitals are actually treating more patients (Rachlis and Kushner, 1994), hospital patients are sicker (Stelling, 1994), and medications and treatments are more frequent and more complex. Thus, nurses report that they are increasingly overworked, and frequently they have to work overtime, without pay, just to get their work done and the patients and charts ready for the next shift. Jobs are being eliminated or made insecure; nurses are being laid off and those who remain must work harder, under worsening conditions, with decreasing opportunity to provide the care they are trained to provide (Armstrong et al., 1993). More than half of the nurses working in Canada in 1999 worked part-time and many of those who are considered full-time workers only work on an irregular basis. Moreover, a growing number of registered nurses work for more than one employer (Armstrong and Armstrong, 2003).

Major changes in health-care services, such as financial withdrawal, aging populations, increasingly advanced technology, and restructuring, have all changed the world of nurses in recent years. The nursing profession is extremely vulnerable to such changes in the socio-economic and political environment because nurses are usually paid via the government or government-financed institutions. The federal government has withdrawn billions of dollars in transfer payments to the provinces. This has caused 'the Quiet Crisis in Health Care', according to the nursing profession, which has recommended that the federal government devote $40 million annually to recruitment, retention, and research regarding nursing in Canada for the next five years. At the same time, the number of days spent in hospital and the number of beds available declined over the 1990s. The length of hospital stay decreased from 8.2 to 6.4 days. These cuts have been accompanied by an increase in the proportion of the population over 65, a group almost twice as likely to be hospitalized as those under 65.

Nursing shortages may be associated with an increased rate of infections contracted in hospital (Taunton et al., 1994). Both patients and physicians in Ontario feel the staffing is inadequate and adversely affects the health of patients. Several coroners' juries, as a result of unnecessary deaths, have recommended 'safe' ratios of trained nurses at various places in the hospital. Still the Canadian Nurses' Association (CNA) has pub-

lished a report on the supply and demand for nurses in Canada to 2011 indicating a shortage of from 59,000 to 113,000 registered nurses by 2011. This projection took into account (a) the age distribution of registered nurses, (b) the current number of nurses, (c) ages of students in nursing schools, and (d) population growth predictions. With respect to the age distribution the research found that the average age of nurses and of students in training is increasing. There has been a large decline in the number of nursing graduates, from almost 9,000 in 1991 to 4,599 in 2000. The population predictions would suggest there will not be a sufficient number of nurses in 2011, even given the slight increase in recruitment to schools of nursing since this report was made public (Planning for the Future: Nursing Home Resource Projections, June 2002, at: www.can-nurses.ca).

According to a 1998 Task Force on Nursing, nurses in Ontario face a number of barriers to providing quality patient care, including:

- heavy workloads because of more seriously ill patients in hospital coupled with decline in staff-patient ratios and diminution of front-line supervision;
- focus on task-specific versus holistic care for patients, leading to poorer patient care and increased stress for nurses;
- lack of a 'nursing voice' on boards and senior management teams;
- elimination of full-time jobs (about 50 per cent of RNs and RPNs now have full-time work and the remaining 50 per cent are casual and part-time workers, which has resulted in some nurses working two or more jobs to make ends meet for their families).

In addition, a recent study has documented that nurses are currently experiencing a great deal of job strain as a result of many factors, especially overwork, understaffing, and excessive overtime (http://www.chmonline/story2.asp?ArticleID=50

6). Figure 14.2 indicates the change in the number of registered nurses per population in Canada from1980 to 2001, while Figure 14.3 shows the variation in nurses per capita by province for 2001. Both across time and from one location to another, fairly wide variations have occurred in the proportion of nurses to population.

Nursing as a Profession

Nurses have been striving in many ways to reach professional status. They have done this through: (1) increasing educational requirements; (2) forming their own 'college' to handle questions of practice and the discipline of members; (3) carving out a body of knowledge that would be separate from that used by other medical care workers; and (4) emphasizing the special qualities and skills that nurses have and that physicians do not have.

Over 30 years ago, Freidson (1970: 49) argued that nursing was a paramedical occupation, as were the occupations of laboratory technicians and physical therapists, because of four characteristics they all shared: (1) the technical knowledge used by the paramedical occupations is usually developed and legitimated by physicians; (2) the tasks of paramedics are usually designed to help physicians fulfill their more 'important' duties; (3) paramedics usually work at the request of the physician; and (4) they are accorded less prestige than the medical profession. Despite the efforts of nursing organizations to gain greater autonomy and full professional status for their members, these characteristics have not changed over the past three plus decades. The medical profession is unique in the sense that no other profession has such a bevy of supportive occupational groups enabling it to do its work. While lawyers use members of other occupational groups regularly, these groups (e.g., accountants, real estate agents, court clerks, bailiffs, and so on) are not considered paralegals.

The modern occupation of nursing has developed out of the context of a historical subservience to the medical profession. Nursing tasks, roles, rights, and duties have arisen to serve the needs of physicians in patient cure and care. From the day that Florence Nightingale and her nurses in the Crimea first waited to nurse until the doctors gave the orders, nurses have waited on doctors. Contemporary nurses, in an effort to enhance their position in the medical labour force and/or to achieve the status of a profession, have taken a number of job-related actions. Krause (1978: 52) lists these:

1   the shift to university training;
2.   the takeover of physicians' dirty work;
3.   the use of managerial ideology;
4.   taking control of technology;
5.   unionizing.

The Shift to University Training
Nurses used to be 'trained' while they worked in hospitals for a period of several years and took classes outside of their work as well. For several decades the most popular program for training registered nurses has been the community college. There is no question that the Canadian Nurses' Association wants all nurses to have a baccalaureate in nursing. The Bachelor of Science in Nursing degree program is designed to increase the credibility of the nurse by providing a theoretical background and greater training in critical thinking as it applies to nursing practice.

The Canadian Association of University Schools of Nursing and the Registered Nurses Association of Ontario are attempting to put a unique focus on nursing education and training. Indeed, there are also 11 different possible specialty certificates for graduate nurses. Nurses with particular types of advanced training can be licensed as nurse practitioners now in Alberta, Newfoundland, and Ontario. The nurse practitioner role has been expanded and includes many responsibilities that were once the sole

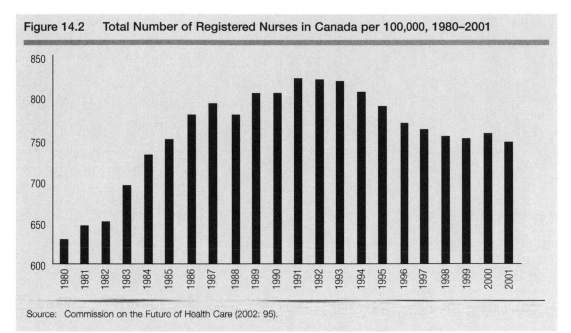

Figure 14.2   Total Number of Registered Nurses in Canada per 100,000, 1980–2001

Source: Commission on the Future of Health Care (2002: 95).

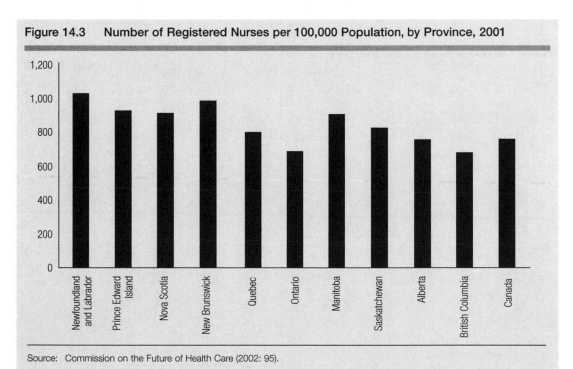

Figure 14.3   Number of Registered Nurses per 100,000 Population, by Province, 2001

Source: Commission on the Future of Health Care (2002: 95).

purview of doctors as Box 14.2 describes (CIHI, 2002). Nurses are being encouraged through education to engage in critical thinking, independent decision-making, research, and leadership. However, the structures in which they work usually limit their ability to do so. Thus, while there is a definite move towards requiring a university degree in order to practise, there is still no significant change in the hospital authority structure (Armstrong et al., 1993). Even nurses with PhD degrees are not able to claim professional autonomy vis-à-vis the physician. Nevertheless, twice as many people are applying to nursing programs than there are available places (CIHI, 2002).

Several creative initiatives have been designed to address other critical health shortages. For instance, the Saskatchewan Indian Federation College recently started a one-year program to assist Aboriginal students to prepare for nursing. The next step will be to prepare a full nursing degree program (ibid.).

Taking Over the Work of the Physician

Nurses have taken over some of the 'dirty work' of physicians, including such routine tasks as monitoring blood pressure, setting up intravenous infusions, and giving medications. At the same time, they have passed some of their own 'dirty work' down the line to registered nursing assistants, e.g., making beds, bathing, feeding, and other actions for the personal care of patients. Both of these shifts have been attempts to shore up the relative importance of nurses in the medical labour force: they have accepted some of the higher-status tasks of physicians and rejected some of their own less desirable tasks. Still, the presence of nurses on the ward makes important differences in the health of patients even after they leave the hospital. One study found a positive relationship between the number of nurses on a ward and a higher level of independence, less pain, better social functioning, and greater satisfaction with care for discharged patients.

Managerial Ideology and Nursing

Managerial ideology applied to nursing has led to a multitude of divisions within the occupational group. These include divisions among nurses by specialty (e.g., intensive-care nurses, pediatric nurses), divisions by type of training (hospital- or university-based training), and divisions by level of responsibility (head nurse, staff nurse). Furthermore, registered nurses have divided the occupations below them in the medical labour force into various classes of subordinates; even while trying to maintain control as the governing body over various types of registered nursing assistants. Below these groups are nursing aides or assistants. The impact of managerial ideology is noticeable both in the increase in the introduction of such efficiency measures as CMGs and other means of speeding up the delivery of nursing care and in the 'ideological subordination' of nurses to the interests of the organization or hospital rather than to the patient or the nursing community (Warburton and Carroll, 1988).

Rejecting High-Tech Medicine

Nurses in Canada are seeking advancement for their occupation in part through an anti-technology ideology. Rather than emphasizing their skill and expertise in handling new technologies, nurses are rejecting the value of the medical model and arguing that medical care should be based much more broadly on holistic care, health promotion, and disease prevention. They emphasize the importance of their caring approach versus a curing approach. This argument is particularly persuasive given the current demography of illness, i.e., the increasing rates of chronic illness and the aging population. 'Expanded rehabilitation-nursing services will be required, due to an increase in chronic illness and stress-related health problems, and will necessitate expanded community health teaching and counselling services' (Kirkby, 1986: 14). The following statement of nursing ideology illustrates some-

Box 14.3   Mistakes and Complaints

'Vocabulary of complaint' is a term used by Turner (1987) in his analysis of the ways that nurses express the stress and frustration they experience in their working lives because of rigid bureaucratic organization, the prevalent managerial ideology, sexism, and relative powerlessness in the medical labour force. According to several pieces of research, such resistance to working conditions tends to be expressed indirectly through addiction to drugs and alcohol (it is estimated that approximately 10 per cent of all nurses are affected), burnout (which is evidenced in the high rate of turnover among nurses and the high rate leaving nursing altogether), and over-compliance (Milgram, 1974). There is some evidence that nurses have been willing to follow doctors' orders even when they could be detrimental to the health and well-being of the patient.

Turner coined the term 'vocabulary of complaint' because he noted a split in nursing discourse between complaint and compliance. As nurses learn the formal public vocabulary of nursing and its ideology, they also learn a less public and defensive discourse of complaint whereby they are able to manage some of their frustrations.

While the official occupational ideology specifies how in principle tasks are to be accomplished, the vocabulary of complaint outlines methods of survival on the job which have the consequences of delegitimizing the authority of the formal structure of operations within the bureaucracy. (Ibid.)

The vocabulary of complaint serves to provide nurses with some sense of shared culture and solidarity to set against their lack of autonomy and authority, coupled with excessive responsibility. Such vocabulary includes the notion that not only do nurses have a unique and special knowledge base and skill with respect to health care, but also that doctors and their medicines can be downright destructive to patients. The second theme of the vocabulary is one that delegitimizes the hierarchy and authority system in the hospital. The third serves to diminish the idealism of the new nurse through the description of nursing as poorly rewarded, emotionally and physically burdensome drudgery. Unfortunately, from the perspective of change, such a vocabulary serves as a safety valve for the frustrations, and this wards off any attempts at real institutional or collective change.

thing of this trend. 'Nurses need to function in the roles of caregiver, teacher, counsellor and patient advocate. Nurses also coordinate the health care provided by many health care professionals' (ibid.).

Unionization

Unionization has had a positive effect on at least one particular aspect of the status of nursing—income. Paradoxically, however, unionization has also served to proletarianize nurses and to establish their position as members of the skilled working class who work for wages. More research

needs to be undertaken on the short- and long-term consequences of the unionization process.

In 1939 a group of Quebec City nurses negotiated the first employment contract. By 1945, the British Columbia nurses' professional association assisted in unionizing the nurses of the province. Almost 20 years later nurses in the rest of the country took the course of unionization. By 1980 nurses in each province were represented by two provincial organizations—a professional body and a nurses' union. In 1981 both of these—the union and professional association—became national organizations (Jensen, 1988).

Table 14.3   A Comparison of the Responsibilities of a Nurse Practitioner and Family Practitioner

	Family Practitioner	Nurse Practitioner
Health assessments	yes	yes
Illness prevention	yes	yes
Health promotion	yes	yes
Education and support for self-care	yes	yes
Diagnosis and treatment	yes	only acute and minor injury
Primary reproductive care	yes	a few exclusions in the case of surgery
Palliative care	yes	all but initial treatment
Supportive mental health care	yes	all but acute/chronic
Co-ordination and provision of rehabilitation services	yes	all but referrals
Co-ordination and referral to other health-care services	yes	all but hospital admission
Supportive care	yes	yes

Source: Adapted from Way et al. (2000).

Nurse Practitioners

Nurses with a bachelor's degree in nursing and additional training to a level at least parallel with a master's degree have been working as independent practitioners in many Western countries for many decades. For a period of time nurse practitioners were being trained in Canada as 'physician extenders'. These courses were terminated for a period in the last part of the last century but are now being redeveloped. Originally, nurse practitioners were to work especially in primary care with children. Today NPs focus more on holistic and preventive care with individuals, although in the United States they can order and interpret diagnostic and laboratory tests and prescribe medications (http://www.allnursingschools.com/faqs/np.php). In the United States, NPs also work independently in a number of areas of specialization, including acute care, community health, family gerontology, home health care, infectious disease, neonatal health, occupational health, oncology, pediatrics, primary care, psychiatric/mental health, and rural, school, and women's health. The numbers of NPs are increasing in Canada along with the diversity of their placements, but NPs are more thoroughly integrated into the health system in the US at this point in time. Generally, nurse practitioners fulfill many of the same roles as family physicians, as is indicated in Table 14.3.

Currently, other nursing specialties are being developed, including parish nursing, school nursing, nursing informatics, forensic nursing, and legal nurse consultants (http://www.allnursingschools.com/faqs/np.php).

Midwifery

Have you thought about your own experience of birth? Have your parents told you about it? Was your father in the delivery room with your mother? Did your mother have any surgical intervention when she gave birth to you? Do you know anyone who has given birth at home or in an institution other than a hospital? Are you aware of the sorts of services that midwives offer to the mother and father before, during, and after the birth? What is the legal status of the midwife in Canada?

The final section of this chapter describes the history of midwives, their work, and their contemporary situation. The term 'midwife' comes from Old English and means 'with the women'. The French translation is *sage-femme*, or 'wise-woman'. Essentially, the work of the midwife is to assist women as they prepare for and give birth and as they learn to care for their new offspring. Midwives have usually practised their work in the home, where the woman is surrounded by her friends and family. Birth in this environment is seen as a natural event, much like sleeping, eating, and relating sexually.

Thus, midwives tended not to use artificial or mechanical means to assist with birth because of their assumption that birth was fundamentally a natural event. For instance, a midwife would predict a breech birth (upside down, feet or buttocks first presentation) through a manual examination. Massage of the fetus in the uterus would be used to turn the baby for a normal delivery. Manual manipulation rather than forceps would be used to move the baby down the birth canal. Pain would be handled by rubbing the back, shoulders, and neck of the woman in labour, and with encouraging words. The woman in labour would be relaxed and comforted by the familiar atmosphere and the presence of a person or persons with experience.

A brief overview of the history of midwifery is necessary for understanding its position in Canadian society today. Birthing assistance has almost always and everywhere been the responsibility of women. The practice of midwifery can be traced to ancient history. The Bible includes a number of references. Exodus 1:15–22 is one example: two midwives, Shiprah and Puah, refused to obey the orders of the King of Egypt that all male infants be put to death. The written work of classical Greek and Roman physicians such as Hippocrates and Galen documents the prevalence of midwives. Male physicians were summoned only when special difficulties developed (Litoff, 1978). Until the Middle Ages, women who had themselves given birth were acceptable attendants at other births.

Up to the fourteenth century, midwifery flourished in Europe. Then came the witch hunts in which women healers of all sorts, and particularly midwives, were put to death. Midwives were especially vulnerable because of their close association with the placenta, which was believed to be an essential ingredient in witchcraft. By the end of the fifteenth century, witch-hunting had declined. In Britain, and soon elsewhere in Europe, midwives gained formal legitimacy under the Medical Act of 1512. This Act was to be administered and enforced by local churches. Licensing depended on the good character of the aspiring midwife and required that she be hardworking, faithful, and prepared to provide service to both rich and poor whenever it was needed. She was also forbidden to use witchcraft, charms, or prayers that were not dictated by the Church. Men were not allowed to be present at birth (ibid.). Then in 1642, the College of Physicians gained authority to license midwives. For the next 300 years the legitimacy, recognition, and power of the male midwives, now obstetricians, grew in England and Europe while those of female midwives declined.

In the last quarter of the nineteenth century, British midwives made numerous attempts to gain legitimacy and recognition as an autonomous professional group. In 1893, a committee of the British House of Commons reported on the significant rate of maternal and infant mortality. They attributed these deaths to poorly trained, unregulated midwives and recommended that midwives be registered (Eberts, 1987).

Most doctors rejected this suggestion because they argued that midwives did not have the necessary training. The Royal British Nursing Association supported the proposal to create a new occupational category: obstetric midwives or nurses.

Public opinion in favour of midwifery seemed to be growing. By the early part of the twentieth century, midwives in Britain were legitimized through regulation. With the establishment of the National Health Service in 1948, midwives were employed as a form of public health nurse. In 1968, legislation in Britain expanded the role of the midwife.

The earliest mention of midwifery among Euro-Canadian women appears in a deed in the Montreal archives, which reveals that the women of Ville-Marie, in a meeting held on 12 February 1713, elected a community midwife named Catherine Guertin. Also, in the English settlement of Lunenburg, Nova Scotia, Colonel Sutherland, the Commander, wrote to the British government in 1755 asking that two pounds per year be paid to the two practising midwives. There are apparently no other regions in Canada where midwives were on government salary (Abbott, 1931).

Until the mid-nineteenth century, most births in Canada took place at home in the presence of midwives (Oppenheimer, 1983), although from this time on home births were frequently attended by physicians. From 1809 until 1895 the legal position of midwives was uncertain and changeable. Whenever midwives did not pose a threat to the work of allopaths they were allowed to practise; but where they did compete with allopaths, primarily in the cities and among the middle and upper classes, there were attempts to restrict them (Wertz and Wertz, 1977; Barrington, 1985; Ehrenreich and English, 1979; Biggs, 1983).

Statistics indicate that in 1899 midwives attended about 3 per cent of all Ontario births and doctors attended 16 per cent (Biggs, 1983).

However, as the legal status of the midwife was questionable, the number given for midwife-attended births is probably an underestimate. Over the duration of most of the nineteenth century, apparently, midwives garnered a significant amount of community and media support. The *Globe* newspaper opposed a medical monopoly of childbirth until 1895, when a bill to reinstate licensing of midwives was vehemently defeated in the legislature. At this juncture the *Globe* reversed its position (ibid).

In the last part of the nineteenth century and on into the twentieth century, the importance of the doctor's exclusive right to attend births grew. In Canada, presently, legislation ensures that midwives are qualified to practise in some provinces but not in others. Once legislation comes into effect the term 'midwife' is protected and the practice of midwifery by those who are unlicensed is illegal, just as it is illegal for someone who is unlicensed to practice medicine. Most provinces have consumer advocacy groups working for midwifery legislation. To date, midwives are licensed in a number of provinces, including Ontario (1994), Alberta (1998), British Columbia (1998), Manitoba (1994), and Saskatchewan (1999). Nova Scotia is currently studying midwifery legislation. Quebec has now established a College of Midwives. The government of the Northwest Territories has agreed that certain policies should govern midwifery practice. It is estimated that about 400 midwives are practising across the country (www.ucs.mun.ca/~pherbert/number8.html;www.cmbc.bc.ca/docs/what_is.html).

Midwives in jurisdictions without enabling legislation risk prosecution if anything goes wrong. Just as social conditions contributed to medicalization in general (see Chapter Ten), they also affected the changing status of midwives; but elements of sexism and patriarchy were additional factors in the conflict between the male-dominated and the female-dominated occupations.

Issues in the Practice of Midwifery

In addition to sexism and patriarchy, other social forces responsible for the contemporary pattern of high-tech, hospital-based, interventionist-oriented, physician-attended births include: (1) bureaucratization and hospitalization, (2) the profit motive, (3) the public health movement, (4) the emphasis on safety and pain relief in childbirth, (5) the campaign for ascendancy waged by physicians.

Bureaucratization and Hospitalization

Before 1880 hospital care was almost entirely for the poor and those suffering the wounds of war. The York Hospital, later to become Toronto General Hospital, opened in 1829 as the first real hospital in Ontario. It was established to treat the veterans of the War of 1812 and destitute immigrants. The first institution for women who needed care during childbirth, the Society for the Relief of Women During Their Confinement, was established as a charity in 1820. It provided the services of midwife-nurses and doctors, and also clothing and food for the mother and child. In 1848 the first hospital, the Toronto General Dispensary and Lying-In Hospital, was established to provide care for destitute women and a place for training medical midwives. Around the beginning of the twentieth century a concerted effort was made to centralize medical care in the hospital. With this move came the further consolidation of hospital births by male midwives or obstetricians. By 1950, Canadian midwifery had all but disappeared.

Concern with modesty spread the belief that decent people did not have their babies at home. Childbirth literature of the time emphasized the complicated, scientifically managed birth event. The new techniques, including the induction of labour, anaesthesia, and the use of mechanical and surgical tools, further entrenched the notions that (1) the hospital was the only place for this potentially complex and dangerous birth procedure, and (2) the skilled hands of the equipped and trained obstetrician were the only ones appropriate for

delivery. This belief was supported further by the fact that the majority of new immigrants who began to populate the cities used midwives. Middle- and upper-class women tried to distance themselves from the poor and immigrant women and from their typical childbirth practices. This, too, reinforced the growing belief in the appropriateness of the hospital as the place of choice for childbirth.

World War I had an impact on the growth of scientifically managed hospital births. Childbirth came to be described as a dangerous process, and women, with war casualties fresh in their minds, were increasingly concerned to deliver their babies in a safe environment. Many were impressed with the physicians' argument that infant and maternal mortality rates could only be substantially decreased when childbirth was recognized as a complicated medical condition (Litoff, 1978). The growth of hospitals provided additional beds. Automobiles and roads cut down the time it took to get to the hospital after labour contractions had started.

Profits for Doctors

Physicians themselves had a lot to lose if midwives were given free rein to practise. According to Biggs (1983), midwives (in about 1873) charged approximately two dollars per birth, whereas male doctors charged five dollars. Biggs quotes from a Canadian letter in the *Lancet* in which the writer expresses the view that the doctors should have a monopoly over birth, at least in part because they have to invest so many years and so much money in their education. As she states, physicians felt that they should be 'protected most stringently against the meddlesome interference on the part of old women', and that the amount of money lost through the competition with midwives would constitute a 'decent living for [his] small family' (ibid., 28).

The Public Health Movement

During the last half of the nineteenth century and into the twentieth century, Canada, along with the rest of the Western industrialized world, witnessed a dramatic decrease in mortality rates. Research has emphasized the important roles played by improvements in nutrition, birth control, and sanitation in this decrease. The decline in maternal mortality rates corresponded to the general decrease in mortality and coincided with the increasing prestige of the physician and the growing belief that medicine could cure all ills. All these developments furthered the move to obstetrician-centred, hospital-based births.

The Emphasis on Safety and Pain Relief in Childbirth

Another element in the move to birth taking place in hospitals was women's search for relief from the pains of childbirth. The desire to alleviate these pains can best be seen against the backdrop of the gender roles and fashions of the nineteenth century. Among the causes of such pain were the cultural constraints on middle-class women, which demanded a certain delicate beauty. This could best be achieved by wearing boned corsets that constricted their waists, rib cages, and pelvises. Sensitivity to pain was considered feminine, and thus women's pain threshold tended to be low. Women were encouraged to see themselves as fragile, sickly, and weak. For middle-class women at the turn of the century, comfort during birth came to mean the obliteration of consciousness through 'twilight sleep'. Since twilight sleep (a combination of morphine and scopolamine) could be monitored more effectively in the hospital, women sought to give birth in hospital.

Precautionary measures, including the enema and shave, were developed to preserve hygienic conditions and prevent puerperal fever. Forceps were developed in the nineteenth century; their use became standard because they could speed the birth process if it were slow. A Caesarean section, a potentially life-saving procedure to be used when labour was ineffective or the pelvis too small, became a frequent and even dangerously overused procedure. By the 1930s there were real safety advantages, including blood transfusions and antibiotics, in treating problematic births at the hospital. Yet as Barrington (1985) ruefully points out, much of the necessity for blood transfusions and antibiotics resulted from hospital-caused infections and doctor-caused hemorrhages.

The Campaign for Ascendancy Waged by the Physician

Doctors described midwives as 'dirty, ignorant and dangerous' (Biggs, 1983: 31). Devitt (1977) quotes a midwife's statement, from 1906, that the obstetricians thought of her as the 'typical old, gin-fingering, guzzling midwife with her pockets full of forcing drops, her mouth full of snuff, her fingers full of dirt, and her brains full of arrogance and superstition'. Biggs (1983) quotes a doctor's view of midwives from the *British American Journal of Medical and Physical Science*:

> And when we consider the enormous error which they [midwives] are continually perpetuating and the valuable lives which are frequently sacrificed to their ignorance, the more speedily some legislative interference is taken with respect to them, the better the community at large.

Physicians gained ideological superiority over midwives by portraying their own work as scientific, and buttressed by safe and efficient tools such as forceps, all of which would improve the likelihood of safe birth for mother and infant. Given that physicians were educated men from good families and were coming to have high status, social power, and also often much political influence, it is no wonder that they were successful in promulgating the view that their births were the best births.

The Present Status of Midwives

Worldwide, midwives deliver approximately 80 per cent of babies today. The North American situation is different, largely because of the presence and historical success of allopathic doctors, including obstetricians. In the past quarter-century or so the women's movement has been powerfully critical of the medical profession for denying the autonomy of women. It has also spearheaded a movement for women's rights over childbirth. Romelis (1985) discussed five specific components of this movement, including groups advocating (1) natural childbirth, (2) the Leboyer method, involving gentle birthing and immersion in water, (3) alternative in-hospital births, (4) home births, and (5) non-hospital birth centres. The role of midwifery fits within this movement, and is also part of a movement that abhors an unthinking reliance on modern hospital practices, such as 'invasive diagnostic procedures, induction and acceleration of labour, reliance on drugs for pain, routine electronic fetal monitoring, dramatically increasing Caesarean-section rates, and separation of mother and baby after the birth' (ibid., 185).

The increasing legitimacy of midwifery reflects both the strategies taken by the state to control health-care costs (e.g., in Ontario midwives are now on salary through the provincial government) and the increasing political influence of women's groups on state policy (Bourgeault et al., 1998). The shift in attitude also reflects the type of service offered by the midwife, who provides a minimum of 44 hours of care, education, and support both prenatally and postnatally. 'Appointments last 45 minutes and conversations are encouraged. In the obstetrician's office, sometimes you would wait 45 minutes to be seen for five minutes, and they're talking to you as they're backing out the door to see the next patient. . . . At the midwife's it was the reverse. You wait five minutes for a 45-minute appointment' (Sarick, 1994: A6). Although a few midwives have always practised in Canada, recently there have been moves to require legislation to ensure that midwives are qualified to practise.

A 1996 study of 3,470 women attended by midwives noted the following: (1) fewer episiotomies (8 per cent as compared to 50 per cent with physician-attended births); (2) less frequent anaesthesia (5 per cent as compared to 30 per cent with physician-attended births); (3) lower cost (primarily because 40 per cent of midwife-attended births occurred at home); and (4) more frequent breast-feeding (95 per cent of those women who had the assistance of midwives were successfully breast-feeding at six weeks) (www.ucs.mun.ca/pherbert/number8.html). The impact of this shift to midwifery on the medical specialty of obstetrics is yet to be determined, but a number of controversial issues remain to be sorted out, including payment inequity between midwives and obstetricians, home birth safety, and malpractice responsibility.

Summary

(1) Some sort of nursing function has always been associated with illness and treatment. Florence Nightingale was the founder of the contemporary system of nursing care. She led a handpicked team of 38 nurses to serve in the Crimean War. Nightingale pioneered sanitary practices and caused the mortality rate to drop. She also provided many other services for the patients.

(2) Although Nightingale established nursing as an important profession in society, she did so by reinforcing a ghettoized and subordinated female labour force. The view of nursing as a woman's job is still in place today.

(3) Critical analysis of the work of the contemporary nurse tends to follow one of three lines: the patriarchal/sexist nature of the content of the work and the low position of nursing in the hierarchy of the medical labour force, the managerial revolution in nursing practice, and the impact of the hospital bureaucracy on the working life of the nurse.

(4) Nursing associations have been striving to reach the status of a profession by increasing

educational requirements, forming licensing bodies, attempting to carve a body of knowledge separate from that of physicians, and emphasizing nurses' special qualities and skills. However, some argue that nursing is a paramedical occupation, not a profession, because the technical knowledge that nurses use is created, developed, and legitimated by physicians, the tasks nurses perform are less 'important' than those of doctors, and nursing has less prestige than the medical profession.

(5) Midwifery is based on the belief that birth is a natural process, and therefore the use of artificial or mechanical means to interfere with birth is avoided. Midwives have almost always been women. Attempts by midwives to gain legitimacy have been met by rejection because doctors argue they do not have the necessary training, and because their presence threatens the work of allopaths.

(6) The social conditions that allowed allopathic practitioners to achieve a monopoly of the childbirth process also contributed to the contemporary pattern of high-tech, hospital-based, interventionist-oriented, physician-attended births. These social conditions include patriarchy and sexism, bureaucratization and hospitalization, the profit motive, the association of the medical model with the success of the public health movement, the growth in measures for safety and pain relief, and the campaign for ascendancy waged by the physician.

(7) While the legal status of midwives is still ambiguous in some provinces, it is changing. With legal recognition of midwifery in some provinces, salary and workload levels have been established and institutionalized as part of the health-care delivery system.

Questions for Study and Discussion

1. What social forces affect the work of nurses today?
2. What organizational challenges do nurses face today?
3. How do you evaluate the move to increase the status of nursing? In other words, are nurses 'professionals' or 'paraprofessionals'?
4. In what ways can nursing be seen to suffer from sexism today?
5. Critically evaluate case mix grouping.
6. What is the position of midwifery in your province?
7. Do you favour the use of a midwife for yourself or your partner in pregnancy and childbirth? Explain your decision.

Suggested Readings

Armstrong, Pat, Jacqueline Choinière, and Elaine Day. 1993. *Vital Signs: Nursing in Transition*. Toronto: Garamond Press. The working situation of Canadian nurses from a critical perspective.

Beardwood, Barbara, and Vivienne Walters. 1999. 'Complaints against Nurses: A Reflection of the New Managerialism and Consumerism in Health Care?', *Social Science and Medicine* 48, 3: 363–74. A useful analysis of relationships among work structures, working conditions, and work satisfaction.

Biggs, C. Lesley. 1983. 'The Case of the Missing Midwives: A History of Midwifery in Ontario from 1795–1900', *Ontario History* 75: 21–35. Provides a revealing history of midwifery in Ontario.

Reverby, Susan M. 1987. *Ordered to Care: The Dilemma of American Nursing*. Cambridge: Cambridge

University Press. A useful overview of the modern nurse's dilemma.

Romelis, Shelly. 1985. 'Struggle between Providers and Recipients: The Case of Birth Practices', in Ellen Lewin and Virginia Olesen, eds, *Women, Health and Healing*. London: Tavistock, 174–208. Examination of some of the politics of birth practices.

Stein, L. 1987. 'The Doctor-Nurse Game', in H.D. Schwartz, ed., *Dominant Issues in Medical Sociology*, 2nd edn. New York: Random House. Full of heuristic insights that can be applied outside of the particulars of the nurse-doctor situation described.

Chapter 15 *Complementary and Alternative Medicine*

Learning Objectives

- The acceptability of complementary and alternative medicine (CAM) is changing among Canadians.
- The views and practices of allopathic doctors with regard to CAM appear to be changing.
- Chiropractic, a major alternative to allopathic medicine, is based on a very different understanding of the nature and cause of disease.
- Chiropractors have a unique place in medicare in Canada.
- Naturopathy, too, has a different understanding of disease and its causes.
- Naturopathic practice is becoming increasingly legitimate in Canada.

Introduction

Have you ever been to a naturopathic doctor? Have you ever been to a chiropractor? Do you meditate or perform regular relaxation exercises? Do you or have you ever belonged to a support group? Do you make a point of regular exercise? Are you a vegetarian or do you follow a macrobiotic diet? Do you attend church and/or pray regularly? What do you know or believe about acupuncture? What do you know about probiotics and nutraceuticals? Such actions as these may be examples of complementary and alternative healing practices.

Alternative, Complementary, and Allopathic Medicine

As is often the case with a new concept, its definition can be amorphous and variable. There are debates about whether the descriptive term ought to be 'unconventional', 'alternative', 'unorthodox', or 'complementary' medicine or health care. Each term has its proponents. It is becoming conventional (as unconventional medicine becomes conventional) to use the term 'complementary and alternative medicine' (CAM) to describe the methods of treatment used both separately (alternatively) and often preventively, on the one hand,

Box 15.1   Holistic Health Care

Complementary and alternative medicines some-times arise out of a philosophy of holism that sees all parts of the universe and all parts of individuals as interdependent. Air, earth, water and body, mind, soul are all part of each other. Thus, complementary medicines tend to promote lifestyle, dietary, and exercise changes and relaxation exercises, as well as chiropractic adjustment or acupuncture or home-opathic remedies. The healer and the healee, too, are interdependent. And both are ultimately respon-sible for their own health. Thus, it is important for the CAM practitioner to 'practise what he/she preaches'. There is a tendency for CAM schools of thought to be anti-bureaucratic and anti-technology, and to date they have tended to be much less politically organ-ized and less likely to seek power and dominance in the medical system.

or in association with or complementary to allo-pathic medicine, on the other. Basically, CAMs are all those health-care practices that differ from allopathic medicine. They tend not to be taught at allopathic medical schools and are generally unavailable in North American hospitals. However, there are a growing number of excep-tions as well as courses offered at post-secondary institutions across both Canada and the United States. Various complementary and alternative treatments have been accepted and readily avail-able in a number of European countries and around the world in places where they may be seen as conventional.

Allopathic or conventional medicine is the subject matter of most of the second half of this text. It refers to the type of healing based on a theory of opposites, or on the assumption that opposites cure. Health is natural, not just the pre-ferred state of the body. Disease is an unwanted aberration caused by germs, bacteria, or such things as trauma from outside that attacks the equilibrium of the body. The germ theory of dis-ease provides some of the basic assumptions upon which allopathic medicine has developed. It is the root from which the monumental scien-tific and biomedical research industry has grown. Insofar as disease is fundamentally an unnatural, abnormal invasion into an otherwise healthy body, treatment involves an attack on the enemy—the disease. Such treatments as surgery, medication, and radiotherapy are the outcomes of this type of thinking.

A variety of criticisms of this medical model have been offered. Advocates of holistic health criticize the medical model for a reductionistic focus on, and limited mechanical and biomedical treatment of, the physical body. Instead, they advocate treating the whole person—body, mind, and spirit—through a combination of methods best suited to a particular individual. Among the methods chosen are massage, acupuncture, visu-alization (imaging a healthy body), meditation, prayer, psychic and faith healing, chiropractic, and naturopathy.

'Healers' who offer various services apart from or in competition with the allopathic physi-cian stand in differing relationships to the domi-nant medical profession (Wardell, 1988). The five types of relationships are: (1) *ancillary workers* whose work is controlled by the medical profes-sion, e.g., nurses; (2) *limited medical practitioners* who offer non-competing, limited, and parallel services, such as dentists; (3) *marginal practition-ers* who offer 'complete' or nearly 'complete' alter-natives to the medical profession but do not have widespread public and state support, e.g., natur-opaths and chiropractors; (4) *quasi-practitioners* who operate from a fundamentally different set of epistemological assumptions, e.g., psychic healers; and (5) *parallel professions* offering services considered almost equal to those of the allopathic practitioner, such as osteopaths.

Willis (1983) offers a critical analysis of the division of labour among health-care workers (see Chapter Thirteen). He sees the varying relationships to the medical profession as the result of the three different strategies used by allopathic practitioners to control the medical marketplace. He argues that in Australia, midwifery was subordinated to medicine, optometry was limited in the sorts of work that could be done, and chiropractic was excluded from the medical labour force (although over the years chiropractic has gained in numbers of practitioners and in perceived legitimacy).

It is clear today that these theories of the relationship between allopathic and CAM practitioners are undergoing radical change. In 1993 and again in 1998, David Eisenberg, a US physician, with a group of colleagues conducted a national representative survey of the US population to determine the patterns of practice, use, and cost of various unconventional therapies. The team selected the following 16 interventions for their questionnaire: relaxation techniques, chiropractic, massage, imagery, spiritual healing, commercial weight-loss programs, lifestyle diets (e.g., macrobiotics), herbal medicines, megavitamin therapy, self-help groups, energy healing, biofeedback, hypnosis, homeopathy, acupuncture, and folk remedies. Exercise and prayer were included as options, although they were considered to be too various and amorphous for follow-up study of a detailed sort. Approximately one in three of the 1,539 adults who took part in the telephone survey in 1990 had used at least one unconventional therapy in the previous year and a third of these had visited providers of alternative therapy as a part of their own regular health care. Those who did visit alternative providers made an average of 19 visits. Those who used unconventional medicines could be distinguished from others by their greater likelihood of

being non-black, between 25 and 49 years of age, and with relatively more education and income. Most people who used unconventional medical care also saw an allopathic physician (83 per cent). However, most people did not disclose to their allopathic doctors that they were using unconventional therapies.

When the study was replicated in 1997 (Eisenberg et al., 1998) the use of alternative therapies had increased from 33.8 per cent to 42.1 per cent. The likelihood of visiting a practitioner of these unconventional medicines had also increased, from 36.3 per cent to 38.5 per cent. The therapies that had grown in popularity most substantially included herbal medicine, massage, megavitamins, self-help groups, folk remedies, energy healing, and homeopathy. At both times, the alternative therapies were most likely to be used for chronic conditions such as back pain, anxiety, depression, and headaches. The use of both conventional and unconventional medicine at the same time was still common. In fact, 18.4 per cent of all people who reported that they used prescription drugs were also using megavitamins and/or herbal remedies. Eisenberg and colleagues estimated that the out-of-pocket expenses for American people (conservatively) were $12.2 billion and the total expenditures (again conservatively) were about $27 billion. This was comparable to the estimated out-of-pocket expenditures for physician services. Clearly, alternative medicine and therapy among basically 'well' American people are already substantial and growing. While this American survey is probably one of the most widely cited of such studies, it is clear from research in numerous other Western countries currently dominated by allopathic care that unconventional medicine is growing elsewhere, as well.

By 1996, according to a Statistics Canada survey, at least 3.3 million Canadians, spending at least $1 billion, had sought treatments outside of conventional medicine (Imman, 1996). There is some evidence that the number of alternative

Table 15.1   Percentage of Public Reporting Use of Complementary Medicine

Country	Any form of complementary medicine	Acupuncture	Homoeopathy	Manipulation (including osteopathy and chiropractic)	Phytotherapy or herbalism
Belgium	31	19	56	19	31
Denmark	23	12	28	23	nd
France	49	21	32	7	12
Germany	46	nd	nd	nd	nd
Netherlands	20	16	31	nd	nd
Sweden	25	12	15	48	nd
United Kingdom	26	16	16	36	24
United States	34	3	3	30	9

nd = data not available.

Source: Fisher and Ward (1994: 107).

practitioners is already growing at a faster rate than that of allopathic physicians, and it will continue to do so. Cooper and Stoflet (1996) predict that the per capita number of alternative medicine clinicians will grow by 88 per cent between 1994 and 2010, while the supply of physicians will grow by only 16 per cent. Whether these predictions are accurate or not is very difficult to know. In this context, it is worth noting that there was a time when referral by a physician to an alternative health provider was considered such a serious violation of medical practice that it resulted in loss of membership in medical societies and even the loss of medical licence. Indeed, one physician, in 1878, lost his life because he consulted with a homeopath (who was also his wife) (Rothouse, 1997).

Complementary medicine is booming worldwide. One study, as shown in Table 15.1, compared eight countries regarding their rates of use of complementary medicines and found significant minorities of the populations in Belgium, Denmark, France, Germany, Netherlands, Sweden, the United Kingdom, and the United States availed themselves of complementary measures (Fisher and Ward, 1994). The figures discussed so far are based on use by people who are well. However, the proportion of people using unconventional therapies increases significantly in studies of people with serious diagnoses. Estimated usage rates for people with cancer range from 10 per cent (Faw et al., 1977) to over 50 per cent (Cassileth et al., 1984). Moreover, these studies must be considered dated in the context of the rapid change in the use of CAM among the well.

Other signs indicate that unconventional medicine is moving into the mainstream. In 1992 Congress established an Office of Alternative Medicine at the US National Institutes of Health. As well, the National Library of Medicine in the US has increased access to research and other articles about complementary and alternative medicine. A number of medical schools and hospitals in the US have developed programs or departments for the study of alternative medicine. Beth Israel Hospital at Harvard University has raised millions of dollars for a Center for

Box 15.2   Evaluating Unconventional Therapies

In the absence of regulation and systematic evalua- tion of efficacy (which is also lacking in allopathic medicine to a significant extent, although because of its dominance it is not as overtly questioned or as widely recognized), Alastair Cunningham, a research scientist in psychology and immunology particularly as they pertain to cancer, has suggested three crite- ria for evaluating both conventional and unorthodox treatment: evidence, rationale, and consensus. His view follows. The strongest evidence for the effec- tiveness of a treatment is a randomized controlled trial (get out your methods books!) in which groups are selected so that they can be considered equiva- lent in all ways that might be pertinent to the disease state or its amelioration. One group (the experimen- tal group) receives the treatment and the other does not (the control group). The difference between the two groups is measured at some time after the treat- ment. This provides causal evidence because the difference between the two groups after the treat- ment is the result of the experimental intervention. This is the only model of research considered to pro- vide evidence of a causal relationship. The second

best type of evidence is correlative—for example, finding an improvement among people after they take a particular intervention. Anecdotal evidence, based on the story of one or a few people, cannot be considered conclusive.

Empirical evidence alone is not sufficient with- out a theoretical explanation or rationale of how the intervention works in the context of how we under- stand bodies to operate. Research evidence is never perfect. In fact, the growth of knowledge falls within the notion of a probabilistic definition of science. Hypotheses are never proven; they are either reject- ed or fail to be rejected by consensus, given certain parameters depending on sample size, measure- ments, measurement error, and the like. In the con- text of a probabilistic science, then, medical practice (allopathic or not) is never based on a perfect 100 per cent likelihood of a given result. Rather, particu- lar results can only be said to be likely to occur or not. If consensus between different practitioners is a useful measure of a probable diagnosis, prognosis, and treatment choice, then asking for a second opinion is often a wise course to take.

Source: Cunningham (1992).

Alternative Medicine and numerous medical schools, including Georgetown, Columbia, Harvard, Maryland, and Wayne State in the United States and a number of post-secondary schools in Canada offer courses in alternative medicine (see Table 15.2). At least five journals devoted to alternative medicine and intended for physicians and other health providers are in cir- culation. In addition, some insurance companies now provide coverage for the use of alternative health care. At least one, American Western Life, actually offers a 'wellness' plan that uses naturo- pathic rather than conventional physicians as

gatekeepers and offers naturopathic remedies as the first stage of treatment. Some insurers reim- burse for particular types of CAM only, such as acupuncture (which is among the most widely accepted of alternatives, especially for pain and substance abuse), and only when offered by allo- pathic doctors. Across Canada, naturopaths, acupuncturists, and Chinese medicine practition- ers are working towards inclusion in health prac- titioner regulatory legislation. The Vancouver Hospital has established an alternative medicine clinic to perform research on various CAMs. This hospital has also opened a Healing Touch Centre for energy-balancing therapies such as therapeutic touch. Therapeutic touch has become a recognized treatment and one found among the skills of nurses across Canada and the US. Finally, several schools that train CAM practitioners, such as the College of Naturopathic Medicine in Toronto, have recently expanded or are planning to expand (Imman, 1996: A3).

The use of unconventional medicine and healing is clearly increasing. As sociology students, we need to ask a number of questions about this phenomenon. Why are such approaches growing in popularity? Are people more and more dissatisfied with their allopathic doctors or with the medical treatments they provide? Are all of the various sorts of treatments effective? Are none of them effective? In what context are they effective or not? For what sorts of problems are they effective or not? Are there similarities and differences among them? Questions about medicalization and about the power of medical practitioners and medical science need to be considered.

First, let us look at the relationship between allopathic and unconventional practitioners and the attitudes of allopathic doctors to alternatives. A cross-sectional survey of a representative sample of general practitioners in Ontario and Alberta studied the reported beliefs and practice of allopathic doctors vis-à-vis unconventional medicine (Verhoef and Sutherland, 1995) and found that acupuncture, chiropractic, and hypnosis were considered the most useful, while reflexology, naturopathy, and homeopathy were considered to be the least useful. Still, the majority of doctors surveyed (54 per cent) believed that conventional medicine could benefit from some of the ideas and methods used by alternative medicine, and the same percentage said they sometimes refer their own patients to complementary and alternative practitioners. Forty-three per cent of the doctors disagreed with the notion that alternative medicine was a threat to public health; 23 per cent disagreed with the idea that

Table 15.2	Selected Alternative Health Programs Offered in Canadian Universities, Colleges, and Selected Complementary Health Institutions

Acupuncture

Chinese Medicine

Chiropractic

Complementary Care

Energy Healing Practitioner

Health Promotion

Holistic Health Practitioner

Homeopathic Medicine and Sciences Program

Massage Therapy

Midwifery

Music Therapy

Native Addictions Worker Diploma

Native Community Worker—Healing and Wellness

Naturopathy

Qigong Instruction

Reflexology

Reiki Practitioner

Shiatsu Therapy

Workplace Wellness and Health Promotion

Source: CIHI, *Canada's Health Care Providers*, 2002.

treatments not subject to scientific scrutiny should be discouraged; 25 per cent thought that alternative medicine is a useful supplement to allopathic medicine; and 24 per cent felt that its results were largely placebo effects. The Canadian Medical Association has no specific guidelines on alternative medicine, but there is some evidence of both historical and contemporary antipathy. Yet the findings of Verhoef and Sutherland reflect a fair amount of support for and open-mindedness towards alternative medicine, as Table 15.3 demonstrates. Sixteen per cent of those physi-

Box 15.3   Some Alternative Health-Care Methods

Acupressure: Use of finger pressure on acupuncture points on the body to stimulate the flow of energy and promote the body's ability to heal itself. No needles are used. The most widely known form is shiatsu.

Acupuncture: Includes use of herbs, tuina (Chinese massage), exercise, and diet. Refers to insertion of fine needles to various parts of body to stimulate the flow of energy (Qi). Points are located along 14 main meridian lines or channels through which the body's energy flows. Stimulates body's natural healing abilities, relieves pain, and restores internal regulation systems. There are two basic approaches. (1) Traditional Chinese medicine includes a holistic system of health care that aims to bring the body, mind, and spirit into balance, and includes such methods as moxibustion, i.e., application of heat, generated by burning dry moxa leaves on/near acupuncture point; Chinese herbology; tuina, i.e., massage of acupuncture points; nutritional counselling; and therapeutic exercises such as qi gong and tai chi. (2) Medical acupuncture or 'anatomical acupuncture' stimulates the body's production of endorphins. Electro-acupuncture uses needles with mild electrical impulses; laser may be used in place of needles.

Feldenkrais (Russian Method): System of retraining the body to improve its movement and reduce pain from disease or injury; relies on the interaction between the sensory pathways of the central nervous system carrying information to the brain, and the motor network carrying messages from the brain to the muscles. It may be particularly useful for accident victims, those with back problems, cerebral palsy, and multiple sclerosis, musicians, athletes, and others whose careers may benefit from improved body movement.

Herbalism: Plants for healing and preventive medicine. Suggested benefits: skin problems (psoriasis, acne, eczema), digestive disorders, heart and circulation problems, gynecological disorders, allergic responses.

Homeopathy: The use of highly diluted traces of botanical, mineral, and other natural substances to stimulate the body's self-healing abilities; 'like is cured by like'. A substance that would create symptoms of disease in a healthy person is said to trigger the immune system of the ill person; the homeopathic practitioner's skill lies in matching a person's symptoms and body type correctly with the hundreds of remedies available. It is believed to assist the body's process of healing, particularly in the case of chronic conditions, such as asthma, cold, and flu, and to alleviate certain emotional disorders and injuries, arthritis, hay fever, PMS, gout, constipation, headache, migraines, children's colic, earache. Homeopathy does not treat structural problems but works with the body's soft tissue, muscle, and ligaments to improve joint movement, back pain, spinal and joint problems, asthma, carpal tunnel syndrome, cramps, migraines, sciatica, respiratory disorders, chronic fatigue syndrome, allergies, digestive disorders, high blood pressure, and cardiac diseases.

Reflexology: Natural healing therapy based on the principle that there are 'reflex' points on the feet and hands that correspond to every part of the body. It is used to reduce stress and tension, and is considered an effective relaxation technique.

Rolfing: Manipulates the muscles and connective tissue to shift the body into alignment; pressure applied with the fingers and knuckles, etc. It is thought to be especially beneficial for athletes, dancers, students of yoga, musicians, and people suffering from chronic pain.

Shiatsu: Practitioner applies pressure to points on the body using fingers, palms, knees, or cushioned elbows to relax the body to promote its natural ability to heal.

Source: For further discussion of these and other CAMs, see Harden and Harden (1997).

Table 15.3   General Practitioners' Attitudes to Alternative Medicine

Attitude	Agree and strongly agree (%)	Neutral (%)	Disagree and strongly disagree (%)
Alternative medicine is a threat to public health	21	36	43
Treatments not tested in a scientifically recognized manner should be discouraged	47	30	23
Alternative medicine is a useful supplement to regular medicine	42	33	25
Alternative medicine's results are usually due to a placebo effect	38	38	24
Alternative medicine includes ideas and methods from which conventional medicine could benefit	56	28	16
Most alternative treatments stimulate the body's natural therapeutic powers	33	43	24

Source: Verhoef and Sutherland (1995: 1006).

cians surveyed indicated that they themselves practised some form of alternative medicine (ibid., 1008).

What explanation do people give for using alternative and complementary health care? Do people who are basically well have different beliefs about conventional and CAM practices than people who are ill? How do conventional doctors explain the use of unconventional therapies? The answers to these questions are myriad, contradictory, and confusing. Some people choose unconventional medicine in reaction to dissatisfaction with their own particular allopathic doctor or as a rejection of the whole class of allopathic medicine. For some, the use of CAM is an outcome of a serious, life-threatening or terminal illness. For others, it is part of an 'alternative' philosophy of life. One study of men and women with HIV/AIDS found that the decision to pursue an alternative approach was a predictable one, considering the whole ideology in which it was grounded (Pawlach et al., 1995), and that it was not an act of desperation but the product of patient, systematic, and thoughtful deliberation. Furthermore, it was consistent with the holistic

health movement as described in Box 15.1 and influenced by the gay rights and PHA (people with HIV/AIDS) movements. Another study, based on interviews with people terminally ill with cancer (Yates et al., 1993), found that those who chose CAM when terminally ill (40 per cent of the sample in this case) differed from those who did not use CAM, primarily with respect to a greater 'will to live', a greater desire for control over their treatment, and idiosyncratic views of the causes of cancer. Income and age were important, but these factors operated through the attitudes and beliefs noted above.

Sutherland and Verhoef (1994) studied the psychosocial determinants of alternative medicine use among people at a gastroenterology clinic in Calgary, 87 per cent of whom used CAM. The most popular CAM practitioners among these people were chiropractors, herbalists, homeopaths, and naturopaths. The reasons given in this case for CAM use were:

- Physicians' treatment did not help.
- Physicians could not diagnose the problems experienced.

- Physicians prescribed medications with serious side effects.

Consistent with other studies, Sutherland and Verhoef found that the desire for personal control was associated with choosing CAM. In addition, users of alternative medicine were more skeptical of traditional medicine, had symptoms over a longer period of time, and were less likely to see themselves as in excellent or good health or to be satisfied with the clinic physicians and with the answers given by clinic physicians.

Cassileth et al. (1984) and Furnham and Smith (1988) found that the desire to take control and responsibility in health care was frequently associated with use of CAM. Skepticism and criticism regarding allopathic medicine and its practitioners and treatments were also found to be important by Furnham and Smith (1988). Later, Furnham and Forey (1994) compared two groups of patients. One group was using conventional medicine and the other an alternative practitioner. The groups were not different with respect to sex, age, education level, marital status, occupational status, political views, newspaper readership, ethnicity, religion, or income. The major differences between the two groups seemed to relate to the tendency of those who used CAM to be skeptical and critical of allopathic medicine, to be more ecologically aware, and to have a greater belief in holism, more knowledge of the body, and a more optimistic view of health.

There are various ways of organizing and categorizing the many types of CAM. The US Office of Alternative Medicine organizes them into seven categories: diet and nutrition, mind/body techniques, bio-electromagnetics, traditional and folk remedies, pharmacologic and biologic remedies, manual healing, and herbal medicine. Muriel J. Montbriand, a nurse researcher and professor at the University of Saskatchewan, has organized CAM into three categories: spiritual, including prayer and psychic surgery (such as is practised in the Philippines); psychological,

including visualization, distraction, and cognitive strategies, e.g., adopting a positive attitude or a one-day-at-a-time philosophy; and physical (1994). Montbriand has found this, the physical, is the largest category of alternatives and includes as examples megavitamins (B complex, C, A, D), over-the-counter drugs (e.g., Aspirin, laxatives), old-time remedies (e.g., garlic and onion, cayenne pepper drinks), products from health-food stores (e.g., barley green, laetrile, lecithin), healers (e.g., massage, acupressure, and reflexology), herbs (e.g., red clover tea, aloe vera, arnica), and special diets (e.g., macrobiotic and metabolic). Montbriand, like Eisenberg et al. (1993, 1998), found that most cancer patients (75 per cent in a sample of 300) did not tell their doctors about the other remedies they were using.

Taking a proactive position, Montbriand advocates that nurses should encourage patients to reveal the alternative treatments in which they are engaging. She recognizes that this topic needs to be approached with caution because people may be reluctant to share the information. Such therapies often are recommended by a patient's significant others. Thus, debasing an alternative practice may be construed as an attack on the patient's loved ones and trusted friends. It may also be detrimental to the person's sense of hope (Montbriand, 1994: 1552). The fact that a large majority of people with the broader definitions employed by Montbriand used some CAMs suggests the importance of evaluating the effectiveness of such interventions, evaluating how such interventions interact with the interventions provided by allopathic practitioners, and perhaps regulating some alternative practitioners and practices (e.g., monitoring and standardizing vitamin supplements).

One study attempting to evaluate the effects of complementary and alternative medicine compared the length of time that people with cancer survived, depending on whether they received conventional or CAM treatment (Cassileth et al., 1991). This study matched 78 pairs of patients

Box 15.4   Evaluations of Unconventional Medicine

Ross Gray suggests that four perspectives are used in considering and evaluating unconventional medicine: biomedical, alternative, progressive, and postmodern. The dominant perspective is biomedical and its concern is with physiological disease and its diagnosis and cure. It has developed from the base of positivist research and has come to rely on a model of empiricism in which the 'best' type of research is the randomized clinical trial. Allopathic medical practice is regulated and thus practitioners 'have to meet educational standards and follow accepted professional practices' (Gray, 1998: 58). While conventional physicians have been antagonistic to alternative practitioners historically, a growing number of physicians practice alternative therapies on patients or on themselves (e.g., acupuncture) or refer patients to others who do provide alternative care.

The alternative perspective sees symptoms as evidence of underlying pathology, and disease prevention, health promotion, and health maintenance as important goals. Rather than relying on positivist science for the development of diagnostic and treatment strategies, alternative practitioners generally claim that clinical experience and a devotion to recognizing and treating each individual as unique are fundamental to practice. Lacking regulation, in some cases, the trustworthiness of some practitioners may be questionable.

Proponents of alternative medicine sometimes critique biomedicine because of the possibility of side effects, the aggressive character of treatment, and its frequent failure, particularly in the case of chronic illnesses. Others argue that biomedicine is not always empirically based. One article in the *British Medical Journal* suggested that only 'about 15 per cent of medical interventions are supported by solid scientific evidence' (Nelson, 1993: 1200, quoted in Gray, 1998: 62). Others have suggested that the actual practice of biomedicine is very infrequently affected by the results of the findings of clinical trials or published research. The argument that biomedicine is opposed to alternative medicine results from an interest in maintaining its political and economic ascendancy.

The progressive perspective is one that advocates neither conventional biomedicine nor alternative medicine per se but rather attempts to make decisions based on evidence. Proponents advocate even-handed scientific evaluation of all treatments and have supported the establishment of the Office of Alternative Medicine as a part of the National Institutes of Health in the US, thus subjecting alternatives to the research dictates of positivism.

The progressive perspective implicitly assumes that positivist empirical research has the potential to be value-free. In contrast, the postmodern perspective on health and medicine provides a critique of positivism and of science as the way to the truth. Knowledge is not objective in this view; rather, knowledge and approaches to knowledge are inherently the result of power relations. Postmodernists 'challenge the assumption that a universal standard for assessing the truth can be applied across the board' (Lovibond, 1989, quoted in Gray, 1998: 68). Outcome measures for allopathic medicine (e.g., life extension) may be quite different from those of alternative medicine, where quality of life may be a more important outcome measure. Postmodernism recognizes the multiple perspectives and some proponents have been especially keen to give voice to the relatively powerless/voiceless.

according to sex, race, age, diagnosis, and time from original diagnosis to metastatic disease (all patients had documented extensive malignant cancer and a predicted median survival time of less than one year). There was no difference in average length of survival between the two groups. Each lived about 15 more months. Interestingly, and surprisingly, given the ideology associated with CAM and the well-known side effects of chemotherapy and radiation for cancer, the quality-of-life scores were consistently higher among those who were treated conventionally.

The following sections describe the philosophies and the occupational status of each of two complementary/alternative practitioners: chiropractors, because they are the largest competing alternative health-care occupation in Canada and in the world; and naturopaths, because of their growing importance in Canadian society.

Chiropractic

Chiropractic has been frequently misunderstood. It is passionately supported by some and passionately repudiated by others. The central tenet of spinal manipulation is an ancient technique legitimated even by Hippocrates: 'look well to the spine, for many diseases have their origins in dislocations of the vertebral column' (cited in Caplan, 1984). In the beginning, American allopathic doctors vehemently opposed chiropractic. The American Medical Association (AMA) as late as the mid-1980s claimed that there was no scientific evidence for chiropractic and warned the public against the untold dangers of submitting to such treatment (ibid.). One chiropractor commented that when he first started to practise about 50 years ago, he was refused admittance to service clubs, and people would make a point of stopping him on the street to call him a quack (personal communication). Now chiropractic doctors may receive patients directly as primary-contact practitioners. They are trained to know when to refer patients to allopaths or others.

The founder of chiropractic, Daniel David Palmer, was born in Port Perry, Ontario, in 1845 and moved to Davenport, Iowa, when he was 20. His work as a healer was based at first on magnetic currents through the laying on of hands. His first success in spinal manipulation is said to have occurred in September 1895 when a deaf janitor

in Palmer's apartment building dropped by to be examined. After discovering that the man had been deaf for 17 years and that his deafness had begun when he had exerted himself and felt something give way in his back, Palmer manipulated the man's spine. This immediately restored his hearing (Langone, 1982). Encouraged by this remarkable healing, Palmer investigated the impact of vertebral displacements on human disease. He called the newly discovered technique 'chiropractic', from a combination of two Greek words: 'cheir' and 'practikas', meaning 'done by hand' (Salmon, 1984).

Palmer campaigned for the legitimation and popularization of this new method of healing. He founded the Palmer School of Chiropractic, whose only admission requirement was a $450 fee. In 1906 Palmer was charged with practising without a licence and put in jail. It was not until 1913 that the first state, Kansas, passed licensing laws to allow the practice of chiropractic.

Palmer's most important pupil was his own son, Bartlett Joshua, or B.J. For 50 years or so, B.J. was able to popularize chiropractic to such an extent that he died a multi-millionaire. He was a gifted salesman who developed mail-order diplomas and advertising strategies that spread chiropractic around the world. B.J. advertised extensively for students, emphasizing the lack of exams or other requirements, lectured on business psychology, and wrote books with titles such as *Radio Salesmanship*. He was fond of making up slogans and having them engraved on the school's walls. One such slogan was, 'Early to bed, early to rise; work like hell and advertise' (Weil, 1983: 130). B.J.'s sense of humour was also exhibited in the following question and answer, included in his book, *Questions and Answers About Chiropractic*, published in 1952. 'Q. What are the principal functions of the spine? A. (1) to support the head; (2) to support the ribs; (3) to support the chiropractor' (quoted ibid.).

B.J. Palmer believed that vertebral subluxation (misalignment) was the cause of all disease,

Box 15.5   The Case of a Chiropractor Who Adjusted the Neck of a Woman Who Later Died

A 45-year-old woman, Lana Dale Lewis, visited her chiropractor on 2 August 1996. Six days later she suffered a stroke as a result of a traumatic injury to a vertebral artery. On 12 September she died. This resulted in a $12 million lawsuit filed in 1999 by Mrs Lewis's son against Dr Philip Emanuele, the chiropractor who made the adjustment, and against representatives of the Canadian Memorial Chiropractic College in Toronto, the College of Chiropractors of Ontario, and the Canadian Chiropractic Protective Association. And, in 2001 an inquest was convened to examine the case, but then was adjourned. Reports noted that the dead woman had been a heavy cigarette smoker and was overweight (http://www.coca.com.au/newsletter/2002/jun0207a.htm).

Debates between those supporting and those opposing chiropractic treatment have resulted. On the one hand, the president of the Chiropractic College said that internationally published and peer-reviewed research on the risk of stroke after cervical manipulation indicates a very low rate of risk (one in a million). On the other hand, a spokesman from a network of about 100 doctors from the Stroke Consortium said that pulling the neck to get the body into proper alignment could tear an artery. This can result in an obstruction and a blockage of blood flow to the brain or even death. According to a study done by the consortium, one-third of 65 patients with torn neck arteries had been to a chiropractor prior to the tear (http:// www. canoe.ca/Health9911/02_neck.html).

What ideas do you have about how you might evaluate the sides to this debate and make a decision for yourself about chiropractic or any other treatment, including allopathic treatment?

and thus that chiropractic was a complete system that could cure everything. His belief that chiropractic was adequate to deal with all problems led to a major schism in 1924, when he introduced an expensive new piece of equipment—the neurocalometer—and insisted that all chiropractic offices rent one from the Palmer School at $2,500 per annum. The major dissenter was an Oklahoma City lawyer who had become a chiropractor. In response to the unilateral dictate to buy this equipment, he established his own school of chiropractic. Within a few years he developed the theory that chiropractors should use other methods, such as nutrition and physical therapy, as well as spinal adjustment. Such a combination is called 'mix', and this chiropractic philosophy is called 'Mixer'; B.J. Palmer's philosophy, in contrast, is called Straight. The schism continues today. However, Mixers are in the majority.

Chiropractic Theory and the Possible Future of Chiropractic

There are two patterns of practice based on spinal manipulation: osteopathy, founded in 1894 by Andrew Taylor Still, and chiropractic, founded by Daniel David Palmer in 1895. Osteopaths, who now include surgery and chemotherapy among their treatments, have achieved considerable legitimation, particularly in the United States. Chiropractic has now achieved a good deal of legitimation in Britain, Europe, and Canada. But as recently as 1971 the AMA established a Committee on Quackery whose purposes included the containment and eventual elimination of chiropractic (Wardell, 1988: 174–84). It had become a significant competitor to allopathic doctors. By the 1960s, 3 million Americans were visiting over 20,000 chiropractors and spending $300 million. In spite of the efforts of the AMA, today chiropractic has undisputed although limited legitimacy in the US and Canada. For instance, chiropractors are included (up to a limit) under medicare in Canada and medicaid in the US. Chiropractic education receives federal funds. Chiropractic is now the major healing occupation in competition with allopathic medicine throughout the world.

The theory of chiropractic is based on the idea that vertebral misalignment, by interfering with the patterns of the nervous system, can cause a wide variety of disorders, including peptic ulcers, diabetes, and high blood pressure. In fact, anything that can be said to result from or to develop out of the context of a depressed immune system can be treated or prevented by chiropractic.

Chiropractic theory has been distinguished from allopathic theory along three lines (Caplan, 1984). In the first place, allopathic medicine views the symptoms as evidence of the disease and as a result of a simultaneously occurring disease process. The removal of symptoms is tantamount to the removal of disease for the allopath. Chiropractic, on the other hand, theorizes that symptoms are the result of a long-term pathological functioning of the organism. Disease precedes symptoms for a long period of time, perhaps years. The correction of the spinal subluxation by chiropractic allows the body to heal itself.

The second distinction lies in the competing views of the role of pathogens in disease. The allopathic understanding is that pathogens of a specific type and frequency invade the body and begin any of a number of different disease processes. Killing the pathogens thus becomes a goal of treatment and the basis of scientific medicine. All practitioners not subscribing to this view are by definition 'unscientific' and have been derogatorily referred to as cultists and quacks (ibid., 84). Chiropractic says that pathogens are a necessary but not a sufficient condition for the initiation of a disease process. Before pathogens can take effect, the body must be vulnerable. While a number of factors can enervate the body, including genetic defects, poor nutrition, and stress, vertebral subluxation is also important.

The third distinction rests in the fact that allopathic doctors, even when they grant chiropractic some legitimacy, limit it to specific musculoskeletal conditions. Chiropractors, on the other hand, view their work as holistic, preventive care. The following statement of the philosophy of chiropractic from the Canadian Chiropractic Association explains this distinction:

> The human body has the natural power to heal itself, but sometimes it needs help in putting that power into action. Chiropractic assists the natural healing process by helping maintain, restore or enhance your health, and it does so without drugs or surgery. (www.ccachiro.org/cdninfo)

There are several alternative future scenarios for chiropractic. First, chiropractic could remain, as it is now, a marginal occupation only partially financed through medicare. Second, allopathic physicians could adopt chiropractic techniques to use themselves in addition to the traditional surgical and chemotherapeutic techniques. Third, chiropractors could be subjugated, as nurses and pharmacists have been, to work only under the jurisdiction of allopathic doctors. Fourth, chiropractic could increase in status and legitimacy and become an equal competitor with allopathic medicine for funding as an alternative to allopathy.

Current Status of Chiropractic in Canada

In Canada, the Canadian Chiropractic Association is an association of Mixers only, as its description of chiropractic indicates:

> Chiropractic is a healing discipline firmly grounded in science. Although its main focus is the relationship between the skeleton (particularly the spine) and the nervous system that runs through it, chiropractic is concerned with the care of the entire body. (www.ccachiro.org/ GENQA)

Table 15.4   Population/Chiropractor Ratio by Province

| Province | Population/Chiropractor Ratio, 31 December | | | | |
	1992	1993	1994	1995	1996
Newfoundland	48,442	36,363	29,080	29,055	29,101
Prince Edward Island	65,850	66,200	66,600	44,633	33,650
Nova Scotia	40,165	38,671	30,055	31,153	27,559
New Brunswick	24,252	22,188	22,247	22,300	20,527
Quebec	9,133	9,100	8,952	8,689	8,461
Ontario	6,145	5,978	6,019	5,640	5,610
Manitoba	7,986	7,533	7,082	6,970	6,820
Saskatchewan	8,230	7,601	7,536	7,528	7,146
Alberta	6,675	6,214	6,146	6,223	5,640
British Columbia	6,945	6,949	6,708	6,473	5,939
Yukon	16,000	16,550	11,300	17,350	8,825
Canada	7,684	7,541	7,297	6,958	6,753

Source: Papadopoulos (1998), using population estimates from Statistics Canada, *Population Projections for Canada, Provinces and Territories*, Catalogue no. 91–520, 125–9.

The number of chiropractors has grown from about 100 in 1906 to approximately 30,000 around the world today (Coburn and Biggs, 1987). There are approximately 20,000 chiropractors in the United States and 7,000 in Canada, of whom almost half are in Ontario (see Table 15.4). Chiropractors constitute the third largest group of primary medical care practitioners, after physicians and dentists. The number of chiropractors in Canada increased rapidly after World War II, when the Canadian Memorial Chiropractic College was established in 1945. The Department of Veterans Affairs gave an early impetus to the development of chiropractic in Canada when it funded the education of 250 veterans who desired training in chiropractic.

X-ray examinations, general examinations, and treatment by chiropractors have been funded under national medical insurance since 1970. However, only a limited number of visits per year are covered in every province where they are licensed, except in Saskatchewan, where the full services are covered by medicare, medicaid (the additional coverage, beyond basic medicare, for such things as drugs for the elderly, veterans, and other special groups), and most health insurance plans. Chiropractic services are covered under Workers' Compensation in seven provinces (Biggs, 1988). However, the relative cost of chiropractic services as a proportion of the total expenditures on health is negligible compared to the proportion of the health-care budget currently expended on allopathic practitioners.

The standards for admission to the Canadian Memorial Chiropractic College are comparable to those for other health occupations such as dentistry, pharmacy, optometry, and medicine. To enter, a student must have a minimum of three years of university in any discipline, preferably including a full course with labs in organic chemistry and biology, a half-course in introductory psychology, and at least one and a half courses in humanities or the social sciences (www.ccachiro.org/cdninfo). The four-year chiropractic program is based on studies of human anatomy and related basic sciences, including X-rays, diagnostic skills, and clinical studies. Graduates see themselves as part of a health-care team. They neither claim nor want to promote the view that their type of health care is the only useful model. In fact, according to Kelner et al. (1980: 80–1), they expect to refer at least a third of their patients to allopathic physicians.

The practice of chiropractic in Canada today is largely limited to musculoskeletal disorders such as headaches, neck and back pain, and soreness in the limbs. In addition, a wide range of functional and internal disorders are caused fully or in part by spinal dysfunction. Numerous recent studies have demonstrated but not explained the superiority of chiropractic in treating neck and back injuries. There is also evidence to suggest the efficacy of chiropractic in treating a broader spectrum of disorders, including epilepsy, asthma, and diabetes (Caplan, 1984). The future prospects for the development and spread of chiropractic look very promising.

Naturopathy

Naturopathy is a form of holistic health care considered by its practitioners to be relevant to all the disabilities and diseases that might bring a patient to a doctor's office. The term 'naturopath' was first adopted in 1901 at a convention of drugless practitioners in the US (Gort, 1986, cited in Boon, 1996: 16). It is based on the assumption that health and illness are both natural components of a total human being—spirit, body, and mind. Just as individuals are unique, this philosophy proposes, so, too, is each individual's sickness unique to him or her. Healing depends on the activation of the normal healing processes of the human body. The Canadian Naturopathic Association has defined naturopathy, based on these principles, as follows:

The human body possesses enormous power to heal itself. The principle known as the vis mediatrix naturae, or the healing power of nature is the foundation of naturopathic medical philosophy and practice. (Canadian College of Naturopathic Medicine, 1995: 6)

Naturopathy has its philosophic roots in Greek medicine and in the work of Hippocrates, who emphasized the body's own healing powers. One of its most important healing modalities is homeopathy. Homeopathy was first established by Samuel Hahnemann (1755–1843). A few years after he graduated from medical school in Vienna, because of disillusionment with the therapies available at the time, he left the practice of medicine to be a writer and translator of texts into German. It was the translation of a text by a Scottish physician, William Cullen, that led Hahnemann into developing the theory of homeopathy. What stimulated Hahnemann was Cullen's description of why the bark of the cinchona tree, containing quinine, was able to treat the fever and malaise of malaria. It was already known that quinine was a treatment for malaria. The explanation, however, was unknown. Cullen taught that it was due to its bitterness and astringent qualities. Hahnemann, having translated many other medical treatises, knew that many substances of greater bitterness and astringency were not effective against malaria. Thus began the homeopathic career of Hahnemann, the scientist who used the following method: (1) observation, (2) hypothesis, and (3) experiment. His first experiment was on himself. Knowing that quinine was not toxic in small doses, he ingested some. He developed the symptoms of malaria—chills, malaise, and headaches. He knew he did not have malaria and asked what had happened. Consulting Hippocrates, he found the idea that what causes a condition would also cure it. He rediscovered the old Hippocratic principle—'like cures like'. The substances that cause symptoms in a healthy person

Box 15.6   Homeopathy

The premier medical journal in Great Britain, read throughout the world, *The Lancet*, recently published a meta-analysis of 119 clinical trials that examined the efficacy of homeopathic medicine. The purpose of the analysis was to investigate the published research reports on homeopathy and its usefulness for particular conditions. In the eternally pessimistic language of the 'null hypothesis', the study found that 'the results of our meta-analysis are not compatible with the hypothesis that the clinical effects of homeopathy are completely due to placebo' (Linde et al., 1997: 834). In fact, the combined odds-ratio for the 89 studies entered into the main meta-analysis was 2.45 (95% CI 2.05–2.93) in favour of homeopathy. That is, homeopathy was approximately two and a half times as likely to work as not. This is contrary to the beliefs of some that the positive results from homeopathy can be explained by the fact that people believe in homeopathy—the placebo effect.

are able to relieve symptoms in an unwell person. Intuitively, this finding reminds us of the notion of balance—of a natural force. 'What homeopathy does is to treat the individual according to his or her own discomforts by pushing the organism in the same direction the vital force is trying to go' (Rothouse, 1997: 224). Homeopathy, from the Greek words 'homoios pathos', which mean 'similar sickness', is based on a number of principles that are in opposition to allopathic medicine. These include the following (Coulter, 1984):

1. The key to the cure of illness is embodied in the principle of similars, i.e., minute dosages of a natural substance known to cause similar symptoms to those indicative of the disease are administered as treatment.
2. Different people react differently to the same illness because each person is unique.
3. The body should receive only one remedy at a time; otherwise the body's healing powers will be divided. The physician looks for the 'most similar' remedy, not those that just seem superficially to be similar.
4. The physician should administer the minimum dosage required by the patient. This minimum dose will provide the same curative powers as a larger dose.

Sickness is thought of as a message rather than a biological pathology. Sickness provides a crisis through which the person can re-evaluate his or her own life (body, mind, and soul). Thus, symptoms are not viewed as signs of disease, nor is the goal to eradicate symptoms through heroic measures such as surgical removal or chemical destruction. Rather, symptoms are indications of a healing crisis to be enhanced by the administration of minimum doses of a substance that causes the same symptoms. Naturopathic diagnosis is based on knowledge, not of the disease's normal or standard course, effects, and treatment, but rather of the unique and idiosyncratic characteristics of the interaction of the individual person and the particular patterning of symptoms. Naturopathic medicine, therefore, does not treat diseases but stimulates the individual's vital healing force.

The goal of naturopathic medicine is to assist the body in creating the most suitable conditions under which it can heal itself. Naturopathic medical practice is very broad. It encompasses nutrition, botanicals, homeopathic medicines, physical therapies, hydrotherapy, acupuncture, and traditional Chinese medicine. Naturopathic medicine appears to have broadened its scope of practice and maintained licensing, in contrast to allopathic practitioners and alternative practi-

Box 15.7   Acupuncture

In surveys in the UK acupuncture is the most frequently used CAM: 7 per cent of the adult population in England has received acupuncture. Providers of acupuncture include allopathic doctors who have taken courses, Chinese medicine specialists, some of whom have specialized over five years in acupuncture, and physiotherapists. The estimated cost for acupuncture to the National Health Service is almost $26 million.

What is the evidence for its benefits? This review article found studies to support acupuncture for post-operative nausea and vomiting, chemotherapy-related nausea and vomiting, and post-operative dental pain. The evidence was ambiguous with respect to treatment for obesity, smoking cessation, and tinnitus.

The studies do not take into account the level of expertise or the amount of experience of the practitioner.

Source: A. Vickers, P. Wilson, and J. Kleijnen. 'Acupuncture', *Quality and Safety in Health Care* 11: 92–7.

tioners such as chiropractors. 'Naturopathic medicine' has become an umbrella term used by practitioners of a variety of unregulated alternative health occupations in Canada (Boon, 1996).

Homeopathy originated at a time when conventional medicine was 'primitive and brutal in form, and frequently lethal for the patient' (May and Sirur, 1998: 169). Treatments, which might involve the application of purgatives, bloodletting, or cupping, were basically the same as they had been for several centuries. However, because its development paralleled the therapeutic revolution founded on the highly visible reactions found in the chemistry lab, many saw its longer-term, less obvious effects as ineffectual. Because homeopaths, many of whom were also trained physicians, continued to focus on individual experiences of illness and invisible treatments and did not develop a theoretical foundation for their therapies that could compete with the 'supramolecular chemistry of the nineteenth century', they were unable to develop legitimacy in the competitive medical marketplace of North America.

Nevertheless, homeopathy is considered a legitimate alternative (and is evidently growing in legitimacy) in many Western countries. In Britain, for example, it has maintained a degree of acceptance among a minority. Four homeopathic hospitals, at Liverpool, London, Glasgow, and Bristol, were incorporated into the National Health Service in Britain at its inception in 1947. Indeed, some members of the British royal family have always preferred homeopathic medicines. More recently, adopting the blind randomized control trial, homeopathic remedies have been found to be effective in the treatment of respiratory disease (Ferley et al., 1989, cited in May and Sirur, 1998) and pollen allergies (Reilly et al., 1986, cited ibid.). At present, about 10,000 physicians in France practise homeopathy (Rothouse, 1997). Other European countries, too, have a history of greater open access to homeopathic medicine. In France, 25 per cent of pharmacies are homeopathic; in Britain, half of all conventional physicians use or recommend homeopathy. And in India, homeopathy is taught in almost all medical and pharmacy schools (ibid.).

Although there are numerous and complex methodological difficulties in comparing the efficacy of allopathic and homeopathic remedies, research has begun to confirm the value of homeopathy, for instance, in the treatment of rheumatoid arthritis (Gibson et al., 1980). The effectiveness of homeopathic hospitals as compared to regular hospitals was studied during the nineteenth-century cholera epidemics in

America, with the death rates in regular hospitals being five times greater than in homeopathic hospitals. Similarly, in London, England, in 1854, a Parliament-mandated study found that 59 per cent of those in regular hospitals died, while only 16 per cent died in homeopathic hospitals. Homeopathy treated cholera's symptoms of headache, malaise, diarrhea, anorexia, chills, convulsions, and so on with mild homeopathic remedies—camphora or veratrum album.

Current Status of Naturopathy and Homeopathy

Homeopathy arrived in the United States in 1825. By 1844, some of the most prominent allopathic physicians had adopted its principles and established the American Institute of Homeopathy, the country's first medical association (Coulter, 1984). The allopaths were threatened by this move and in 1846 founded a competing organization, the American Medical Association. Professional contact between allopaths and homeopaths was prohibited by the AMA's newly established Code of Ethics (Coulter, 1984).

The formal system of naturopathic treatment, which incorporated homeopathic medicine, was established by Benedict Lust (1872–1945), who founded the first naturopathic college in 1900 in New York City. Lust's primary method of treatment was hydrotherapy, but this was enhanced by a variety of other techniques, including homeopathy, botanical remedies, nutritional therapy, psychology, massage, and manipulation (Weil, 1983).

There was hostility between allopaths and naturopaths until around the turn of the twentieth century, when the number of naturopaths began to decline dramatically and they no longer posed a threat. Since then naturopathy has never constituted a well-organized occupational group, but rather a loose assortment of holistic practitioners providing a variety of healing modalities. Until recently most naturopaths were also chiropractors.

In Ontario, the Drugless Practitioners Act of 1925 can be seen as the starting point for the formal recognition by the province of naturopathy as a distinct healing occupation. By this Act a Board of Regents, composed of five appointees of the Lieutenant-Governor and made up of allopathic and chiropractic practitioners, was set up to regulate chiropractors and naturopaths. While naturopaths were allowed to practise, they were not formally included under this Act until 1944. In 1948, chiropractors were limited to 'hands only, spine only' (Gort, 1986: 87). In the following year, 1949, the Ontario Naturopathic Association was formed by chiropractors who had been deprived of the right to the full range of practice (i.e., including naturopathic medicines) by the 1948 decision. By 1952 each form of drugless therapy was allowed to govern itself because it had become increasingly difficult for one board to regulate practitioners with diverse education, training, and practice modalities.

Naturopathy in Canada

About 300 naturopaths practising in Canada today are registered with the Canadian Naturopathic Association (Boon, 1998). They are not covered by medicare. They are, however, licensed. Today, they are all trained at the only training institution in the country, the Ontario College of Naturopathic Medicine, which has trained two-thirds of the practising naturopaths in Canada. Homeopathic practitioners were once self-regulating in Canada. As early as 1845, homeopathic doctors began practising in Quebec and shortly after that in Toronto. They became regulated in Upper Canada in 1859 and in Montreal in 1865. They were also represented in the College of Physicians and Surgeons of Ontario from 1869 to 1960. In British Columbia regulation began in 1889. There was a homeopathic hospital in Montreal in 1894; in Toronto, a homeopathic dispensary opened in 1888 and a homeopathic hospital in 1890

In 1978 the Ontario College of Naturopathic

Medicine was opened; it at first offered a post-graduate program to allopaths, chiropractors, and naturopaths to help them upgrade their qualifications. In 1982 the Ontario Ministry of Health appointed a Health Professions Legislative Review Committee to determine which occupations needed regulation for the protection of the public interest. It was decided by this committee that naturopathy should not be regulated by the state but by its own members. The argument was that since (1) naturopathy was not scientific and (2) there was no standardization of practice, it posed a risk of harm to the patients and should not be regulated and thereby given official sanction.

The naturopaths responded in a brief titled *Naturopathic Medicine and Health Care in Ontario*, delivered in July 1983 to Keith Norton, the Minister of Health at the time. The brief justified the value and efficacy of naturopaths as well-educated and trained healers, and made it clear that they believed the allopaths were trying to exclude them from practice. It levied a series of sharp criticisms at the costliness and narrowness of allopathic medicine, its mechanistic fallacy, and its negative social consequences. The final statement highlighted and summarized their critique of allopathic medicine: 'We find little cause to applaud allopathy's near monopoly of the medical services of this province' (ONA, 1983: 21).

Among the naturopaths' recommendations were: the establishment of a separate Act to regulate naturopathic medicine; the right to use the title 'doctor'; the right to use the terms 'naturopathic medicine' and 'naturopathic physician'; the elimination of the term 'drugless practitioner' in favour of 'naturopathic physician'; the right to hospital privileges; the right to refer to various laboratory and X-ray services; and the right to authorize medical exemptions and to sign medical documents.

In the same year, 1983, the Ontario College of Naturopathic Medicine became the first Canadian institution to offer a complete education in naturopathy, having devoted the five years since its founding in 1978 to fundraising and offering single stand-alone courses. By 1986 the planned deregulation, in spite of the organized opposition of the Ontario Naturopathic Association, was passed by the Ontario government. Despite signs of the resurgence of naturopathy—rising numbers of practitioners and the presence of a college to provide training—it seems that naturopathy in Ontario is at a standstill because of deregulation.

One of the most difficult issues faced by naturopathic medicine in its struggle for legitimacy lies in the nature of its science. Allopathic medicine claims to be scientific because it is modelled on physics, the prototypical science of the nineteenth century. The goal of this model of research is the establishment of universally true causal laws. Individual differences are ignored in favour of generalizations. Homeopathy, on the other hand, is based on a different model of science. This assumes a universally true set of principles that are applied differentially to each individual. In contrast, allopathic scientific doctrine changes considerably over time as the result of new research findings (among other things). With each new discovery some part of allopathic medicine is often nullified.

In a study of all 296 licensed naturopathic practitioners in Canada, Boon (1998) observed two distinct paradigms of naturopathic practice. One she calls a 'scientific world view', the other, 'holistic'. Those in the first category appear to emphasize physical and structural treatments and to be more practical, concrete, reductionistic, and objective. Those in the second category are more subjective, spiritual, abstract, intuitive, and likely to emphasize treatment at an emotional level.

If the trend in the United States is any indication of the future for naturopathy, then it looks bright. From its heyday in the nineteenth century, when there were 15,000 practitioners, 14 medical schools, dozens of periodicals, and organized groups in every state and large city (Coulter, 1984: 72), naturopathy declined to a low of about

100 practitioners in 1950. In the 1960s, however, this trend was reversed, and today there are thousands of mainstream practitioners (allopaths, chiropractors, nurses, and clinical psychologists) who use at least some homeopathic methods. As well, a number of firms manufacture and export homeopathic remedies, and a number of governments have adopted licensing laws for the practice of naturopathic medicine.

In Canada, naturopathic doctors are highly trained after four years of naturopathic medicine. They have extensive scientific and clinical knowledge of natural remedies, including their use, contraindication, possible adverse reactions, and toxicities (www.naturopathicassoc.ca/dr.html). They are licensed to practise in British Columbia, Saskatchewan, Manitoba, and Ontario. As yet they are unlicensed in the other provinces. None, apparently, are currently practising in Newfoundland, the Northwest Territories, or Prince Edward Island. As the holistic health movement grows, naturopathy will likely become increasingly legitimate. Claims of malpractice against chiropractors, massage therapists, and acupuncturists for 1990–6 were compared with those made against conventional doctors (Studdert et al., 1998). CAM practitioners were sued less frequently than conventional doctors and when they were sued the injury was less severe. This might suggest that the safety records of CAM practitioners are better than those of allopathic practitioners. Nevertheless, there are sometimes serious and even fatal problems resulting from CAM practice, as there are in allopathic medicine, and more research needs to be done.

Therapeutic Touch

One other new and alternative healing modality is quickly being incorporated into the practice of allopathic medicine via the nursing profession. This is therapeutic touch. According to Michael Lerner in *Choices in Healing*, in which he critically reviews the research literature on the value of a wide variety of complementary and alternative medicines, therapeutic touch is a promising healing modality.

> The implications of therapeutic touch for medicine and science are—if the scientific studies of its efficacy are valid—truly awesome. Something is happening in these studies, if they are correct, that medicine should attend to and science cannot yet account for. (Lerner, 1994: 362)

Therapeutic touch has become established as a modern and empirically studied practice. It is now widely used in and out of hospitals, usually by nurses, across Canada and the US. It was started by Delores Kreiger, a nursing professor at New York University, and was based on her observations of and her collaboration with a renowned healer, Dora Kuntz, who believed that healing could be systematized, taught, and studied. Therapeutic touch does not involve touch (at least not primarily) but rather the movement of 'energy' along the outside of the body (for about 15–20 minutes) a number of inches from the body in order to balance and restore energy where it is lacking. Research on the efficacy of therapeutic touch has found it to: (a) raise hemoglobin levels, (b) elicit the relaxation response, and (c) heal wounds, among other benefits.

Summary

(1) Complementary and alternative medicines are growing in significance, rates of use, and public acceptance at a rapid pace. CAMs are even growing in legitimacy in the minds and referral practices of allopathic practitioners.
(2) Daniel David Palmer founded chiropractic in 1895. Attempts to legitimate and popularize this method of healing were stunted by allopathic practitioners. Distinguishing features of chiropractic are: through the corrective manipulation of spinal subluxation the body is able to heal itself; the goal is not to kill

germs but to make the body less vulnerable to germs; the work is viewed as holistic, preventive care. Although chiropractic in Canada today is limited to musculoskeletal disorders, its legitimacy continues to grow.

(3) Naturopathy is based on the assumption that health and illness are both natural components of a total but unique human being—spirit, body, and mind. Healing depends on the activation of the normal healing process-

es of the human body. Naturopathy was first introduced in the US in 1825. It was met with opposition by most allopaths. More and more mainstream practitioners use at least some naturopathic methods today.

Questions for Study and Discussion

1. Why is complementary and alternative medicine becoming more acceptable to Canadians?
2. Why are allopathic doctors changing their views regarding complementary and alternative medicine?
3. Assess the view that naturopathic and chiro-

practic medicines are non-scientific whereas allopathic medicine is based on science.
4. What do you think the medical marketplace will look like in 25 years?
5. Examine a popular magazine or newspaper for its coverage of CAM over a period of time.

Suggested Readings

Boon, Heather. 1995. 'The Making of a Naturopathic Practitioner: The Education of Alternative Practitioners in Canada', *Health and Canadian Society* 3, 1–2: 15–41. Compares different strands of naturopathic medicine.

Dossey, Larry. 1982. *Space, Time and Medicine*. Boston: New Science Library.

———. 1991. *Meaning and Medicine*. New York: Bantam Books. Popular interpretations of philosophical principles behind some complementary and alternative medicine.

Eisenberg, D.M., R.B. Davis, S.L. Appel, S. Wilkey, M. Van Rompay, and R.C. Kessler. 1998. 'Trends in Alternative Medicine Use in the United States, 1990–1997: Results of a Follow-up National Survey',

Journal of the American Medical Association 280, 18: 1569–75. Describes the survey to examine the prevalence of the use of complementary and alternative medicine in the United States of America.

Harden, Bonnie L., and Craig R. Harden. 1997. *Alternative Health Care: The Canadian Directory*. Toronto: Noble Ages Publishing. Provides basic information about a wide variety of CAMs.

Sutherland, Lloyd P., and M.J. Verhoef. 1994. 'Why Do Patients Seek a Second Opinion or Alternative Medicine?', *Journal of Clinical Gastroenterology* 19, 3: 194–7. Reports the results of a study examining the psychosocial determinants of alternative medicare use in Calgary.

Chapter 16

The Medical-Industrial Complex

Learning Objectives

- The medical-industrial complex includes many different organizations, products, and services.
- The pharmaceutical industry is one of the largest and most influential of these.
- Pharmaceutical use is affected by the socio-demographic characteristics of users.
- Pharmaceutical use is affected by the style of medical practice and the involvement of drug salespersons.
- Pharmacists' interests also affect drug-taking patterns.
- The pharmaceutical industry is one of the more profitable industries in Canada.
- The pharmaceutical industry retains its position through a number of powerful and effective marketing, pricing, and other business strategies.
- The cases of DES and thalidomide illustrate problems in the regulation of the drug industry in Canada.
- Similarly, there are many cases of the misuse by the pharmaceutical industry of drug markets in the developing world.
- The Health Protection Branch of the Canadian federal government has an ambiguous record with regard to protecting the health of Canadians.

Introduction

The medical-industrial complex is a large and growing network of private and public corporations engaged in the business of providing medical care and medical care products, supplies, and services for a profit. Included in the medical-industrial complex are proprietary hospitals and nursing homes, home-care services, diagnostic services, including the expensive CAT scanners and MRIs, hemodialysis supplies and equipment, the pharmaceutical companies, medical tools and technology, and even laundry and food-packaging companies that supply hospitals and other health-care organizations. The pharmaceutical industry, an important component of the medical-industrial complex, will be discussed in detail in this chapter.

When do you decide to go to the pharmacy for over-the-counter medication? Do you try to become aware of the side effects of various over-the-counter medications? When you have been prescribed a drug, do you generally ask the doctor about side effects? Do you take your medication exactly as directed—over the length of time suggested and at the prescribed intervals? Do you believe that all the drugs available in Canada have been adequately tested and are safe? What safety precautions are available in developing countries? Have you heard of thalidomide or DES? Do you know some of the devastating results of their use? To what extent are the pharmaceutical, medical device, and biotechnology companies reliant on making a profit and to what extent are these industries interested in serving those suffering sickness and pain? These are among the questions that will be addressed in this chapter.

Drug Use

Any discussion of the pharmaceutical industry and the use of drugs in contemporary Canadian society must be fairly wide-ranging because this topic involves a large number of sociological issues. The drug industry is a major actor in Canadian medical care, and its share of health spending in Canada grew from 9.8 per cent in 1983 to 12.6 per cent in 1990. Figure 16.1 illustrates the growth in expenditures on drugs as a percentage of all health spending. By 1996, Canadians spent $10.8 billion, or 14.4 per cent of total health expenditures, on pharmaceuticals (www.hc-sc.gc.ca/datapcb/datahesa/E_drugs.htm). In 1995 approximately 228 million prescriptions were written in Canada. Although not all prescriptions are filled, nor are all pills taken once the prescription is filled, this number indicates that, on average, eight prescriptions per Canadian were filled. The majority of Canadians have some form of coverage for pre-

scription drugs. In 1995 it was estimated that 88 per cent of Canadians had at least some coverage. Sixty-two per cent were covered under private plans, 19 per cent under provincial plans, and 7 per cent under both. Of the 12 per cent of Canadians without any drug coverage, more than half worked for employers who did not provide it, somewhat less than 4 per cent were self-employed, and the remaining 2 per cent were unemployed and lacked access even to government plans. The federal government covers Aboriginal Canadians and veterans. Most drug expenditures are for prescription drugs—70.7 per cent or about $256 per person. Most of the prescription drug expenditures are for patented drugs ($5 billion of the $7.7 billion total). Because of the relatively high cost of patented drugs, even though they represent only 10 per cent of all of the drugs available in Canada they accounted for 45.8 per cent of the drug spending (ibid.). It may be helpful to begin with a pictorial representation of the various levels of analysis that will be considered in our explanation and description of pharmaceutical use in Canada (see Figure 16.2).

At the first level the discussion will focus on how the socio-demographic characteristics of patients—age, gender, class—correlate with their drug-taking habits. The social characteristics of physicians, too, influence drug prescription—such as the form of medical practice (e.g., solo as compared with group practice), the amount of continuing education, and the size of the practice.

Pharmacists and the pharmaceutical industry are important forces in drug use as well. Cost, availability, advertising, and special pricing arrangements are among the factors known to influence physicians' decisions on what to prescribe and pharmacists' decisions on what to stock. Drug payment schemes—whether government-controlled, those offered by private insurance, or individual payment alternatives—affect drug use. Much of the recent sociological research on drug use in Canada has focused on

Figure 16.1   Spending on Drugs as a Percentage of Total Health-Care Expenditures, Canada, 1975–2000

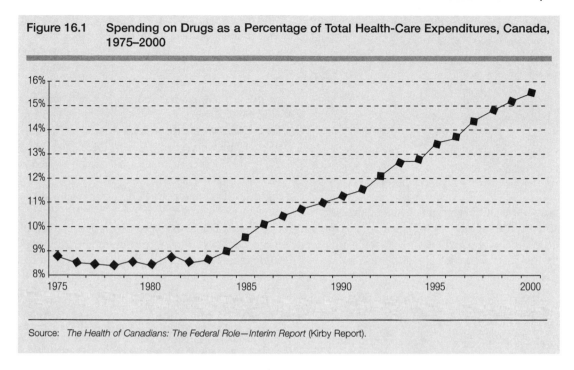

Source: *The Health of Canadians: The Federal Role—Interim Report* (Kirby Report).

Figure 16.2   Factors Affecting Drug Use in Canada

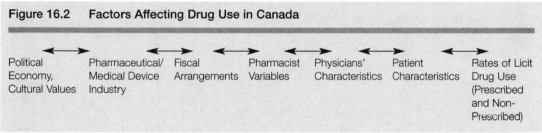

Political Economy, Cultural Values   ⟷   Pharmaceutical/ Medical Device Industry   ⟷   Fiscal Arrangements   ⟷   Pharmacist Variables   ⟷   Physicians' Characteristics   ⟷   Patient Characteristics   ⟷   Rates of Licit Drug Use (Prescribed and Non-Prescribed)

the pharmaceutical industry, its organization and structure, and especially on the fact that under capitalism it must be guided by the profit motive, which at times conflicts with the goal of promoting health.

Rates of Drug Use and Patient Variables: Age, Gender, and Class

Tables 16.1 and 16.2 show the extent of use and the money spent on licit drugs in Canada. Considerable evidence suggests that drugs are frequently over-prescribed in Canada. For example, it has been estimated that between one-third and two-thirds of the antibiotics used are unnecessary or inappropriate (Rachlis and Kushner, 1994). Between 5 per cent and 23 per cent of hospital admissions result from drug-related illnesses. On the basis of this estimate, inappropriate prescribing costs Canadians, via hospital costs, between $256 million and $1 billion annually (www.hc-sc.gc.ca/datapcb/datahesa/E_drugs.htm). Two groups, the elderly and women, are particularly vulnerable to misprescribing. One expert has estimated that one of the side effects of over-

Table 16.1	Utilization of Prescriptions, 2001	
Average family size		3.0
Prescriptions per person		10.1
Prescriptions per family		30.3
Average prescription price		$39.92
Consumption per family/year		$1,209.58

Source: Commission on the Future Health Care (2002: 192).

prescribing or misprescribing among the elderly is at least 200,000 illnesses due to bad reactions to drugs, many of which may not have been needed in the first place (Rachlis and Kushner, 1994).

Moreover, there is a long history of evidence that women are especially likely to be over- or misprescribed psychotropic drugs or sedatives (Harding, 1994b). In an analysis of the results of seven different surveys women and the elderly continue to be more likely to use tranquilizers and sleeping pills. Females are more likely than males to use these psychoactive drugs by a 3:2 ratio. That this 'overuse' by women may, in part, be explained by the greater degree of 'medicalization' of women is supported by the fact that their use of similarly acting over-the-counter drugs does not occur at the same rate. The extent to which a parallel explanation is plausible with respect to the age gradient of use is neither confirmed nor disconfirmed in this study (Graham and Vidal-Zeballos, 1998).

Table 16.2   Drug Expenditure Summary, by Province/Territory and Canada, 1999

	Total Drug Exp. ($)	Per cent Distribution	Total Drug Exp. per Capita	Total Drug Exp. as a % of Total Health Exp.	Drug Exp. Financed from Private Sources as a % of Total Private-Sector Health Expenditure	Prescribed Drug Exp. as a % of Total Drug Exp.	Proportion of Prescribed Drug Exp. Financed from Prov./Terr. Governments
	('000,000)	(%)	($)	(%)	(%)	(%)	(%)
Nfld	210.9	1.6	390.06	13.4	46.0	79.1	35.8
PEI	63.7	0.5	463.01	17.1	44.3	73.1	25.7
NS	430.0	3.2	457.56	15.6	39.5	74.8	34.3
NB	324.3	2.4	429.81	15.7	42.2	74.1	27.6
Que.	3,291.9	24.7	447.90	16.5	37.8	80.4	34.6
Ont.	5,555.3	41.7	482.12	15.9	33.1	74.6	40.4
Man.	426.7	3.2	373.47	11.7	30.8	74.8	33.1
Sask.	388.4	2.9	378.72	13.0	38.8	75.6	28.9
Alta	1,139.4	8.6	384.99	13.2	31.9	74.5	37.3
BC	1,459.0	11.0	362.20	11.9	28.0	72.3	48.2
Yukon	12.1	0.1	389.24	11.2	38.6	72.4	30.0
NWT	16.3	0.1	397.83	7.0	34.6	77.0	13.6
Nunavut	4.8	0.04	177.22	3.6	47.7	54.5	34.3
Canada	13,322.6	100.0	436.82	14.9	34.0	75.9	38.2

Sources: CIHI, at: <http://secure.cihi.ca/en/media_24apr2002_tab1_e.htm>.

There are strong relationships between gender, age, and drug use. Moreover, the incidence of multiple drug use among these populations is well substantiated in the literature (Lesage, 1991; Smith and Buckwalter, 1992). Although people over 65 comprise about 12 per cent of the population, they use approximately 40 per cent of all licit drugs. An elderly person uses an average of 13 prescriptions a year, and only 19 per cent of elderly Canadian men and women report using no prescription or over-the-counter drugs (Bergob, 1994). Moreover, multiple drug use increases as Canadians age. One-quarter of all potentially inappropriate drug combinations result from overlapping and similar prescriptions prescribed by two doctors for one patient. One study has estimated that the inappropriate use of pharmaceuticals costs the Canadian economy $3.5–$4.5 billion per year in direct health costs, which include hospitalization, visits to physicians, and laboratory expenses—and the total reaches $7–$9 billion when indirect costs such as premature death and absenteeism from work are added (ibid.).

Among seniors, the National Alcohol and Drug Survey found that multiple drug use was associated with perceived stress level and lack of help from family and friends, as well as with illness. Thus, social as well as medical explanations contribute to our understanding of drug use—including sleeping pills, tranquilizers, pain medication, heart and blood pressure medication, and stomach remedies and laxatives.

Drug interactions can affect the absorption rate, distribution throughout the body, metabolism, and the elimination of a drug, and one drug can diminish or exacerbate the pharmacological effects of another drug. Drug effects are known to be somewhat different among the elderly. Pharmaceuticals are routinely tested and prescribed on the basis that the average user is a male in his thirties. The elderly differ, on average, significantly from the average 30-year-old male. They are more likely to be female, to have slower metabolic rates, to weigh less, and to have some cognitive deficits. For those reasons, the elderly are twice as likely to experience drug reactions as younger adults. Some evidence suggests that as many as 77 per cent of the admissions of the elderly to hospital may result from drug overdoses or side effects (Pulliam et al., 1988).

Over-the-counter drug use may exacerbate the problems noted above. One study found that as many as 70 per cent of the elderly take over-the-counter medication without discussing this with their physicians. Incidences of medication errors by the elderly have been well documented. These include: forgetting to take medication, taking a smaller or larger dose than that prescribed, taking medication for the wrong reasons, inability to read labels, difficulty of opening containers, and impaired memory (ibid.). Consequences of such drug misuse include falls, dizziness, various illnesses, hospitalization, and even death.

If current trends continue, drug use will increase for the following reasons: (1) the rate of drug use for those over 65 is higher than for any other age group, and this is the part of the population that is growing most quickly; (2) the supply of physicians per population in Canada has been steadily growing since 1967; and (3) the ratio of pharmacists to the population is also increasing (Canada Year Book, 1988). This aging trend is typical throughout the Western industrialized world and in the total world population. Table 16.3 illustrates the significant increases in spending on six categories of drugs under the Quebec drug program over a period of just four years.

Females are consistently heavier prescription drug users than males. This pattern of greater use of prescription drugs among females is true of a wide variety of drugs. There are a few exceptions, chiefly in diagnostic and treatment drugs relevant to heart disease. Researchers have recently noted that there has been an overemphasis on diagnosing and treating heart disease in men, with the result that it has often been overlooked in women. At times this has been costly to women

Box 16.1   Halcion

A woman, Ilo Grundberg, shot her 83-year-old mother eight times in the face while being under the influence of the sleeping pill, Halcion. While taking Halcion, another woman stabbed her two sons. Despite her claims that Halcion was the cause, she was convicted twice of murder and eventually committed suicide.

Examining psychiatrists testified that Ilo Grundberg was involuntarily intoxicated from the effects of Halcion when she killed her mother. Halcion is intended only for short-term use, yet Grundberg's doctor had prescribed the drug to her for much longer. Grundberg had grown increasingly paranoid and agitated while on the drug. After being acquitted of murder, as there was no clear motive and Grundberg had little memory of it, Grundberg became involved in a $21 million civil suit against Upjohn, the Michigan-based manufacturer of Halcion. She charged that Halcion is a defective drug and Upjohn failed to warn the public about the sometimes severe reactions. Upjohn retaliated by stating that in no way was the company negligent and there was absolutely no connection between the murder and the drug.

Halcion, used by more than seven million Americans and sold in more than 90 countries, was Upjohn's second largest money-maker. Its annual sales were $250 million—$100 million in the United States. It is quite obviously liked by patients and doctors alike.

Since Halcion's arrival on the market, critics have debated whether or not Halcion is more dangerous than other benzodiazepine drugs. The critics claim that it is more likely to cause such nervous-system disturbances as amnesia, anxiety, delusions, and hostility. They state that Upjohn and the FDA have done very little to protect the pill-taking public. Upjohn responds by saying that Halcion is no more likely to cause adverse reactions than any other sleeping pill.

Since its entrance onto the market, Halcion has led a controversial life. When it first became available in the early 1970s, it appeared to be the answer to many problems with side effects resulting from the use of benzodiazepines. Clinical studies showed that while people fell asleep quickly, users experienced virtually no grogginess the next day as it cleared the system quickly. By 1979, however, there were reports of peculiar psychiatric changes in those using Halcion. These side effects included amnesia, hallucinations, paranoia, and verbal and physical aggression. Records show a long history of concern over the use of Halcion. In 1980, for example, a series of evaluations were written by the FDA recommending against its approval. The drug was eventually approved despite protests.

The FDA maintains a system of post-marketing surveillance. Doctors and drug companies file reports describing any adverse reactions to the drugs they prescribe or sell. Unfortunately, many adverse reactions never get reported. A drug's record can also be skewed by factors such as its manufacturer's reporting practices, the kinds of patients who happen to take it, and the amount of publicity it receives. In 1987, it was noted that during its first three years on the market, Halcion had collected approximately 8 to 30 times as many adverse reaction reports as other more popular drugs.

Upjohn may believe that adverse reactions to Halcion are no different from reactions gained from other benzodiazepines, but the company has never convincingly explained why Halcion has a record for generating strange stories. For instance, a 1987 doctor's report described episodes of delirium, sleepwalking, and amnesia in five elderly hospital patients who were receiving as little as an eighth of a milligram dose of Halcion. One man was found trying to turn somersaults in his room while others were trying to flee the hospital in their pyjamas. Not one of them remembered their adventures in the morning.

Halcion's critics feel that the drug poses risks other drugs may not have and therefore it should be taken off the market. Many people, however, prefer the periods of uneasiness to the heavy hangovers other sedatives can cause.

Sources: 'Sweet Dreams or Nightmare?' (1991); 'Horror Stories . . .' (1992).

Table 16.3   Increase in Spending for Six Categories of Pharmaceuticals in the Quebec Drug Insurance Program, 1997–2000

Categories	Cost ($ millions)				Growth, 1997–2000 (%)
	1997	1998	1999	2000	
Lipid reducing agents	105.7	131.0	158.4	189.6	79.3
Anti-hypertensives	111.9	135.2	161.7	193.5	73.0
Anti-inflammatories (analgesics)	60.0	61.3	71.4	119.0	98.3
Psychotropic	69.6	93.7	123.0	150.0	115.4
Gastrointestinal	89.6	108.1	129.7	150.6	68.0
Anti-infectives	82.1	97.9	111.0	120.8	47.2
Subtotal	518.9	627.2	755.2	923.5	78.0
Total drug costs	1,119.4	1,292.8	1,498.4	1,772.2	58.3
Proportion spent on six categories (%)	46.4	48.5	50.4	52.1	

Source: Commission on the Future of Health Care (2002: 193).

who have gone to the hospital with signs and symptoms of heart disease only to be sent home—to a fatal heart attack. Recently, policy-makers and researchers have turned their attention to some of the unique characteristics of heart disease in women in an attempt to reverse this growing rate.

Those in the lower income groups spend a greater percentage of their incomes on prescription drugs. They also spend a higher percentage of income on food and shelter. In regard to prescription drugs, however, this may be the result of more expensive drugs, as there is some evidence that prices for the same drug can vary up to 300 per cent, depending on the location. In Toronto, one study noted, the highest prices for drugs were charged in the areas of the city where people with the lowest incomes lived (*Globe and Mail*, 12 June 1970: 10). Indeed, more recent research has shown that those with less education and lower family income are more likely to be prescribed mood-altering drugs (Rawson and D'Arcy, 1991). As Harding (1994b: 171) says, 'a process of medicalization of the symptoms of poverty and other problems of lower socio-economic positions may be occurring.'

Nearly all provinces introduced drug programs to subsidize purchases by low-income families in the 1990s (Lexchin, 1996). These provincial plans coincided with large declines in drug expenditures as a percentage of total expenditures among people of low income, particularly with respect to prescription drugs. However, as a result of insurance programs of various sorts the decline was also evident among high-income people. Still, despite the introduction of programs for drugs for low-income people, per capita spending as a percentage of total family expenditure in the low-income group was almost twice as high as that of the high-income group both before and after the introduction of drug plans (Lexchin, 1996: 47). A significant portion of this increase certainly results from increases in drug costs. Figure 16.3 indicates these increases over the period 1990–7, while Figures 16.4 and 16.5 illustrate the proportion of drug costs as a percentage of total health-care spending for 1980 and 2001.

Figure 16.3   Contribution to Increases in Drug Costs by Major Components, 1990–1997

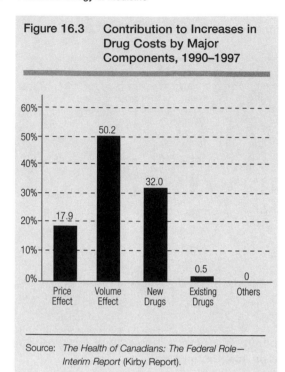

Source: *The Health of Canadians: The Federal Role—
Interim Report* (Kirby Report).

Physicians and Prescribing

There is a high correlation between the number of visits to a physician and the number of prescriptions. In Canada, general practitioners apparently prescribe drugs to from 21 per cent to 86 per cent of all patients who visit their offices (Lexchin, 1990; Williams et al., 1995), and on average, 6–10 prescriptions are given for every hospital admission (Borda et al., 1976). In Chapter Ten we saw that the number of physicians in a society affects the degree of medicalization. Physicians in general have a tendency towards medical intervention (e.g., to prescribe drugs) when confronted with a patient exhibiting a problem. But social characteristics and conditions affect the rates at which doctors prescribe drugs.

The Birmingham Research Unit of the Royal College of General Practitioners in Britain (1977) found a tenfold difference in the rate at which family practitioners prescribed psychotropic drugs, ranging from 40 per 1,000 patients to 415 per 1,000 patients. Doctors who have higher rates of writing prescriptions include males, gen-

Box 16.2   Effective Interaction To Aid Appropriate Prescribing by Physicians

A few strategies have been found to be somewhat effective in producing positive changes in physician prescribing: academic detailing and audit and feedback. The first, academic detailing, relies on pharmacists who are trained to visit doctors on an individual basis and to provide explicit educational information. Different studies have shown this to result in a reduction in inappropriate prescribing ranging from 12 to 49 per cent, effective for up to two years.

The second option is audit and feedback of the prescribing practices of physicians. Successful intervention depends on the willingness of a physician to

be audited (and to feel the need for improvement and to act on feedback fairly quickly).

Another intervention that appears to offer promise involves peer-review group discussions—in this case, physicians in groups discuss the results of audits and how they might change in response.

However, 'the high-volume practice that fee-for-service encourages makes it difficult for many physicians to spend time listening to their patients; without listening, it is hard to respect patients' choices. Moving to alternative forms of payment for physicians may help improve all four aspects of appropriate prescribing' (Lexchin, 1998: 264).

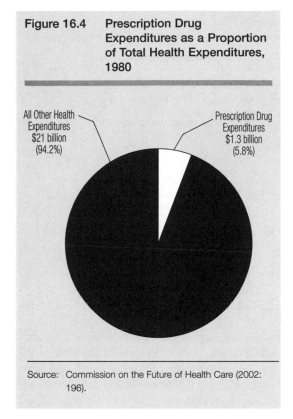

Figure 16.4   Prescription Drug Expenditures as a Proportion of Total Health Expenditures, 1980

All Other Health Expenditures $21 billion (94.2%)

Prescription Drug Expenditures $1.3 billion (5.8%)

Source: Commission on the Future of Health Care (2002: 196).

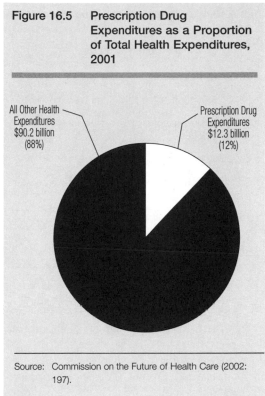

Figure 16.5   Prescription Drug Expenditures as a Proportion of Total Health Expenditures, 2001

All Other Health Expenditures $90.2 billion (88%)

Prescription Drug Expenditures $12.3 billion (12%)

Source: Commission on the Future of Health Care (2002: 197).

eral practitioners, isolated practitioners in rural areas and in solo practice, and possibly those from certain medical schools (www.hc-sc.gc.a/datapcb/datahesa/E_drugs.htm).

Research has documented significant deficiencies in doctors' knowledge about drugs. Lexchin (1984) reports that fully 27 per cent of the practising physicians in Ontario and 25 per cent of those in Nova Scotia had inadequate knowledge about the uses of antibiotics and sulphonamides. Only 41 per cent in Ontario and 12 per cent in Nova Scotia were skilled in their use; the remainder were in an intermediate position. Commercial sources of information, including drug advertising and salespersons, are significant influences on doctors' prescribing habits: the more heavily a drug is promoted the more it is prescribed, despite the fact that doctors

themselves believe that 'they used scientific sources and shunned commercial ones' (Lexchin, 1984: 122). One study, for example, found that more than 70 per cent of physicians made claims about particular drugs that reflected the claims made in drug advertisements even though these claims were diametrically opposite to those in the scientific literature (ibid.). Doctors have tended not to be critical of drug advertising. They have tended to trust it. In one study 82 per cent of physicians reported that the information they received from drug manufacturers was always or sometimes sufficient for making an informed decision about risks and benefits.

Good prescribing by physicians involves maximizing effectiveness, minimizing risks, minimizing costs, and respecting the choices of patients (Barber in Lexchin, 1998: 254). Even

Table 16.4	Inappropriate Drug Use and Inappropriate Prescribing

Inappropriate Drug Use	Inappropriate Prescribing
• Not having a prescription filled or refilled. • Taking too much or too little of the drug prescribed. • Erratic dosing, such as altering time intervals or omitting doses. • Stopping the drug too soon. • Combining prescription drugs with over-the-counter products or illicit drugs. • Combining prescription drugs with alcohol.	• Under-prescribing or not specifying sufficient quantities or correct intervals of dosage. • Over-prescribing or going beyond the maximum therapeutic dosage. • Prolonged use that results in iatrogenic effects and adverse reactions. • Prescribing that is contraindicated by the medical condition. • Contraindicated combinations that produced an undesirable effect.

Source: *The Health of Canadians: The Federal Role—Interim Report* (Kirby Report).

though there are very few studies of appropriate drug prescribing in Canada, those that do exist do not suggest that the values elucidated above are often realized. Overall, the rate of inappropriate prescribing ranges from 17 to 43 per cent. Eighteen per cent of the time drugs are prescribed when they are not needed. Thirty per cent of the inappropriate prescriptions relate to problems in drug administration such as dose, route of absorption, and duration. Studies of elderly people have examined and confirmed 'potentially undesirable prescribing'. For instance, a study of prescribing in Alberta found that over 2,600 of the elderly population (1.1 per cent) had prescriptions for two or more non-steroid anti-inflammatory drugs (NSAIDs) dispensed on the same day, despite the fact that there is little, if any, rationale for such a practice. In addition, with respect to one of the mood-altering drugs—diazepam—a detailed study found that 14,000 elderly people (3.7 per cent of the province's elderly) received a potentially inappropriate prescription—most (68 per cent) from a single physician, i.e., this over-prescription was not

entirely or largely the result of seniors visiting more than one doctor at a time for the same problem. According to Joel Lexchin (1998: 256) and based on the available published data, there is a 'substantial amount of inappropriate prescribing' (see Table 16.4).

Lexchin, a Canadian authority on the pharmaceutical industry, states that the causes of inappropriate prescribing are (1) the lack of knowledge on the part of physicians and (2) the patterns of practice of physicians. The typical Canadian doctor prescribes only a very limited number of the 5,000 drugs presently on the Canadian market: 50 per cent of all prescriptions written by GPs are for about 27 different medications, in spite of the fact that Canadian doctors are not inundated with new drugs. For instance, between 1991 and 1995 only 404 new drugs were patented in Canada and of these only 33 (about 8 per cent) were thought to be either breakthroughs or substantially better than existing drugs. Practising doctors, even though they know that reliable sources of information about prescribing include continuing medical education, peer-reviewed journals (many of which are now easily available on-line), and association meetings, rely largely on pharmaceutical company sales representatives, who do not 'disclose the side effects and contraindications of their products or the prices of their drugs in relation to other drugs, unless asked, and they frequently make incorrect statements about the drugs they are promoting' (ibid., 258).

Research has repeatedly confirmed the following correlations. The more frequently physicians saw drug sales representatives:

- the more likely they were to use drugs even when not using drugs was the best option;
- the more often they sympathized with a 'commercial' view of the value of a given drug;
- the more likely they were to prescribe antibiotics inappropriately;
- the less likely they were to prescribe generically;
- the more likely were they to use more expensive medications when equally effective but less costly drugs were available.

Pharmaceutical firms are a major source of information for doctors. Many doctors (28 per cent) say they learn much of what they know about medicines and their 'appropriate' use from drug firms (Wilson et al., 1963). There is no lack of evidence to document that the drug company representatives who call on physicians regularly with brochures, samples, and gifts are a major source of information about drugs for doctors (Hemminki, 1975). If expenditures by drug companies on promotion and advertising are any indication (twice as much as on research and development), then promotion and advertising have an important impact on prescribing (Rachlis and Kushner, 1994). In the United States, pharmaceutical companies spend more on advertising than do either the alcohol or the tobacco companies. Drug advertisements have repeatedly been

criticized as misleading and incomplete, and as portraying people in stereotypical ways. For instance, the elderly may be seen engaging in passive activities wearing depressed faces or acting childishly, playing with childish toys (Foster and Huffman, 1995). Advertisements recommend drugs for such a variety of everyday, 'normal' concerns that drugs seem to be suggested as useful to everyone at least some of the time. Drug prescribing, then, is often a symptom of the tendency towards the medicalization of social issues.

Another major source of information for most Canadian doctors is the *Compendium of Pharmaceuticals and Specialties* (*CPS*), a Canadian Pharmaceutical Association publication. Although the *Canadian Medical Association Journal* has recommended this as a source of information (Lexchin, 1984), there is no question that it is inadequate in a number of ways. It is not comprehensive, and it is known to have continued recommending certain drugs long after research documenting destructive side effects had been published in medical journals. The most thorough study of its value found that 46.3 per cent of the drugs listed by the *Compendium* were 'probably useless, obsolete, or irrational mixtures' (Bell and Osterman, 1983). Well-known risks and negative effects were ignored for over 60 per cent of the drugs listed. There were scientific errors regarding the biochemical effects of nearly 40 per cent of the entries. Bell and Osterman were led to conclude that that version of *CPS* was basically a tool to promote the interests of drug companies.

What other factors influence doctors' decisions about prescribing drugs? The few studies available indicate that the level of medical education has an effect. For example, Becker et al. (1982) studied the rate at which physicians prescribed chloramphenicol (because this drug has potentially fatal complications, lower rates of prescription were seen to indicate better prescribing): younger physicians who had more years of post-graduate education had lower and more appropriate rates for prescribing this drug.

Freidson (1975) distinguished between client-dependent and colleague-dependent forms of medical practice. His argument is that regulation is more effective in colleague-dependent than client-dependent practices. When doctors have to account to other doctors for the diagnoses they make and the treatments they choose, they are likely to exhibit higher medical standards than when primarily seeking to satisfy the patient. Following this line of reasoning, it can be predicted that doctors who are involved in medical networks or in some form of group practice are more likely to have appropriate prescribing habits.

Surprisingly, perhaps, especially as it contradicts the declarations made by many practising doctors, physicians who see fewer patients may spend more time with them but do prescribe more medications. A Canadian study compared a group of doctors who worked on the basis of fee-for-service with a group of doctors who worked on salary (Lexchin, 1988). Approximately one-half of the doctors in private clinics, as compared to one-quarter in community health centres, prescribed drugs inappropriately. Salaried physicians were also more likely to warn patients of side effects and other potential problems. The researchers explained that because salaried physicians had more time per patient, they were able to take the time to prescribe appropriately and to explain when and how to use the drug, as well as potential side effects.

Several studies have shown that both drug advertisements and drug detail men and women (pharmaceutical company representatives who visit doctors with samples and information about drugs) (Lexchin, 1994a) significantly affect the drug-prescribing habits of doctors. Lexchin (1994b) indicates that much of the over-prescription of antibiotics, ulcer medications, and anti-hypertensives results from drug advertising. The Canadian Medical Association and its journal (CMAJ) historically defend the pharma-ceutical industry and support its viewpoints (Lexchin, 1994a). Given the amount of money involved (see Figure 16.6), perhaps this is not surprising.

Pharmacists

Little sociological analysis exists of the role of pharmacists with respect to prescription and non-prescription drugs. There is no question, however, that they have considerable discretionary influence in making recommendations both to doctors and to individuals who shop for over-the-counter medical assistance. Consumers frequently ask the pharmacist to recommend 'something'—a non-prescription drug—for a cough, sleeplessness, pain, or anxiety. The pharmacist may suggest a particular brand-name drug or a range of suitable products of different brand names. A number of factors will affect the pharmacist's recommendation.

The cost of a particular drug varies greatly from pharmacy to pharmacy and even within the same pharmacy. One survey found that the prices of 15 of the most common drugs varied by as much as 89 per cent from one outlet to another. Even within the same outlet, price differences as great as 130 per cent over a two-week period have been noted (Allentuk, 1978: 68). In addition, pharmaceutical companies vary their drug costs from store to store and from situation to situation at times. Drug salespersons, advertising, and gifts given by pharmaceutical companies are all likely to have an effect on recommendations made by pharmacists. Pharmacists are sometimes owners of the drug stores or pharmacies in which they work. This being the case, they are most likely influenced in their decisions by the necessity of turning a profit. It is in the pharmacist's economic interest to recommend the drug that provides the greatest profit margin.

Pharmacists do have some discretionary power, too, when presented with a drug prescription. Unless the physician has written 'no substitution' on it, pharmacists are free to dispense any

Figure 16.6   Manufacturers' Sales ($ billions) of Patented and Non-Patented Drugs, 1990–2001

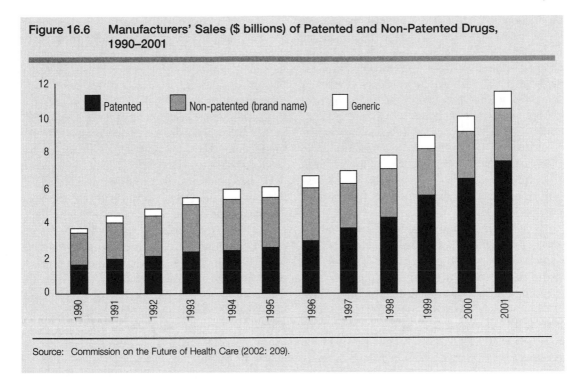

Source: Commission on the Future of Health Care (2002: 209).

company's brand of a particular drug. To encourage pharmacists to dispense their own brand of drug, pharmaceutical companies may discount the price on the given product. Discount pricing, in that it provides the pharmacists with the most room in which to make a profit, often encourages the pharmacist to use a particular drug. Discount pricing also affects provincial revenues in provinces with drug plans. Under discount pricing, a particular drug company will charge the pharmacist one price for the drug, e.g., $20 for 50 pills, and the pharmacist may charge the purchaser who may be reimbursed through a government or other drug plan a substantially different price, e.g., $100 for 50 pills. The pharmacist thereby realizes a profit of $80 on that particular drug company's product. The provincial government, the consumer, and the drug insurance plan are the losers. That this is not an insignificant cost to provincial governments is noted by Lexchin

(1988), who cites a news article estimating that discount pricing was costing provincial drug plans $40–$60 million annually across the country more than a decade ago.

The Pharmaceutical Industry

The Canadian drug industry has always been divided into domestically owned companies, the first one founded by E.B. Schuttleworth in Toronto in 1879, and foreign-owned subsidiaries, the first one established in Windsor by Parke, Davis and Company (Lexchin, 1984: 331). The industry grew slowly (the foreign-owned companies stayed in Canada because they could obtain tariff and tax advantages) until the 1940s. The antibiotic revolution and the development of medications to control patients in mental hospitals spurred the growth of the industry. Economies of scale became possible in the manufacture of these drugs, and production was centralized. This, plus the increasing openness of world trade (globalization), meant that the small Canadian companies could not compete with the larger foreign-owned companies. After World War II only one Canadian company of any consequence—Connaught Laboratories—was left. Today, subsidiaries of multinationals control 90 per cent of the Canadian market (Lexchin, 1984: 33). These large multinationals belong to the Pharmaceutical Manufacturers Association of Canada, a very effective lobby/pressure group headquartered in Ottawa (Rachlis and Kushner, 1994).

The pharmaceutical industry is one of the more profitable manufacturing activities in Canada. The use (and profitability) of drugs continues to increase. In Ontario, as one example, spending on the government-funded drug benefit plan, which provided funding for prescriptions to the elderly and those on social welfare, increased at an average annual rate of 19 per cent per year from 1981 to 1991—or from $180 million to $840 million (Taylor, 1992). By 1993, the cost was estimated at $1.1 billion (Williams et al., 1995). In New Brunswick, the cost of a similar program has increased 700 per cent since 1975 even though the eligible population only increased 16 per cent over the relevant time period (Davidson et al., 1995). High profitability and consistent growth due to long-term demographics (e.g., the aging of the population) provide reason for continuation of these trends. Furthermore, this appears to be a low-risk industry. A recent Canadian study indicated that the drug industry was ranked 67th in terms of risk, almost the lowest in Canada. What strategies do the drug companies use to maintain their profitability? What is the impact of the great financial success of the multinational drug companies on the health of Canadians and on the health of the people in less-developed countries? In what way do the profit-making strategies of the drug companies affect health negatively? These three questions will be discussed here.

The pharmaceutical industry is successful in maintaining its position as one of the most profitable industries through a variety of strategies, including: (1) the absence of a link between manufacturing cost and price; (2) patent protection; (3) competition and drug development focused on drugs with widespread potential for use (and thus profit) rather than drugs for rare conditions; (4) production of brand-name rather than generic products; (5) drug distribution (dumping) in less-developed countries; (6) advertising and providing select information to physicians and consumers.

First, one of the major reasons for the high profits in the drug industry is that *the selling price of drugs is not necessarily related to drug production costs* (Lexchin, 1984: 41–8). In the absence of price competition the manufacturer is free to determine prices in the interest of maximizing benefits to the company (i.e., profits). Thus, variations in cost bear little or no relationship to manufacturing costs. For example, Allentuck (1978: 66) points out that 'Carroll Labs simultaneously sold 400-milligram Meprobamate tranquillizer tablets at 3.15 per hundred and 200-milligram tablets of Meprobamate at 3.35 per hundred.' The development and introduction of 'new' drugs appears to have more to do with profitability than with medical value. 'From January 1988 to December 1991, a total of 271 new patented drug products were marketed in Canada for human use. Out of that number only 13, or less than 5 per cent, were felt to be either "break through" medications or substantial improvements over existing therapies, with the rest being line extensions (46 per cent) or moderate, little or no therapeutic improvements (41 per cent)' (Lexchin, 1991: 20). While high profitability is the case in the pharmaceutical industry worldwide, it appears to be particularly so in Canada. The Canadian Patented Medicine Prices Review Board examined prices for 195 drugs marketed between 1990 and 1992. Of the total, the Canadian price for 111 was above the average (median) price in the international market and in

30 per cent of the cases the Canadian price was the highest in the world (Lexchin, 1991). The wide variation in pricing for drugs from country to country is also reflected in the fact that some US citizens from border states cross the border to Canada to buy prescription drugs with Canadian dollars in order to save. Moreover, the future ability of individual countries to regulate drug costs and availability is threatened today by the accessibility of pharmaceuticals via the Internet.

Patent protection is the second technique used to maintain the high level of profits. Patents serve to limit competition. Once the company has invented a new drug, patent protection gives the company an exclusive right to manufacture and distribute the drug for a period of years. This period can be extended if the company takes out additional patents on associated drugs. Of 1,335 drugs listed in the Ontario Drug Benefit Formulary in July 1982, almost 75 per cent were available from only one manufacturer. Drug companies claim that patent protection allows them to pay for the research necessary for the invention of new drugs. However, this argument can be challenged because much of the research done in any drug company is directed towards developing imitative medicines that can compete with products already successfully developed and marketed. The pharmaceutical industry spends heavily on advertising, drug promotion, and lobbying.

The third strategy (Lexchin, 1988b) is that the *drug companies rarely do research or attempt to develop medicines in areas where there is unlikely to be a large market* or with a view to addressing the needs of people with less-than-common diseases. Rather, they tend to produce new drugs based on similar existing drugs, thus circumventing patent protection for large markets that have already been developed. As an example, there are numerous anti-inflammatory (anti-arthritis) and benzodiazepine (minor tranquilizer) drugs currently on the market in Canada (Lexchin, 1988a). Such a wide choice is of virtually no therapeutic or medical value. However, because there is a huge market, most every pharmaceutical company has a similar product. For instance, drugs introduced in Canada between 1982 and 1989 for three major therapeutic categories—arthritis, hypertension, and ulcers—were between 35 per cent and 67 per cent more expensive than existing drugs but provided only a little, if any, medical benefit (Lexchin, 1991). As a result there are 20,000 pharmaceutical products based on only 700 active ingredients.

Fourth, the *widespread use of brand-name rather than generic products contributes significantly to the profits of the pharmaceutical companies.* (The generic name is the scientific name for a particular drug, while the brand name is the name given to the drug by the pharmaceutical company that produces the drug in question.) On average, generics cost considerably less than the most expensive brand-name equivalents. It is clearly to the advantage of the pharmaceutical industry to promote brand-name products. Although brand-name products are usually prescribed, the pharmacist may substitute a generic if it is available (unless otherwise directed by a physician). Unfortunately, few are available. Of all the products listed in the 1982 Ontario Drug Benefit Formulary, generic equivalents were available for only 91. In 1980, only 8.7 million of 175 million prescriptions in Canada were filled by generics (Lexchin, 1984: 62).

Fifth, the history of the pharmaceutical industry is replete with stories of drug-related illness and death. The *'dumping' of out-of-date drugs in the developing countries* is one cause. The health-destroying side effects of many drugs, whether they are taken alone or in combination with other drugs, are another problem. The industry sometimes markets drugs for a wide variety of symptoms when they are only appropriate for a limited number of purposes.

The pharmaceutical industry is a prototypical global industry and its markets are growing. This is true with regard to distribution, marketing, intra-firm and international trade, acquisitions, mergers, and 'collaborative alliances in research and developmental marketing' (Tarabusi and Vickery, 1998: 68). World production and trade are concentrated on the OECD countries, where in 1993–4 the five largest countries accounted for more than 65 per cent of world markets, nearly 60 per cent of exports, and 40 per cent of imports.

There are three distinct categories of pharmaceuticals: (1) in-patent drugs; (2) out-of-patent and generic drugs; and (3) over-the-counter (OTC) drugs. The rapid growth in the pharmaceutical industry has been largely the result of in-patent drugs because it is here that the research and development (R&D) expenditures must pay off in high profitability. Once the drugs lose patent (after a varying number of years, depending on the country, with an average of 10 years), there is aggressive competition among firms to produce similar drugs of their own. Selling OTC drugs depends on marketing and advertising, but because they are generally not covered by drug insurance plans the pharmaceutical industry spends a considerable and growing proportion of its money on marketing. Canada's position is declining in this international market (ibid.).

Many countries in the developing world face serious problems in relation to pharmaceuticals. One problem is a lack of drugs, such as antibiotics, that have come to be essential in the developed North. Other drugs, known to extend or improve the quality of life in a chronic and potentially fatal disease such as AIDS, are much too expensive for the vast majority of the population. For instance, while protease inhibitors could lengthen the lifespan of people diagnosed with HIV/AIDS, they are completely out of financial reach for most people in many countries where people cannot even afford a condom. Aside from the lack of availability, there are other equally serious problems: at times drugs are used inappropriately because they lack directions for use or these directions are written in a foreign language, or the consumer lacks literacy, or they are to be

taken with water (which may be unsafe or lacking). Sometimes drugs banned in one country are shipped to and sold in a different country that lacks the regulatory infrastructure to protect its population (Ollila and Hemminki, 1997: 309).

As well, it is incorrect to assume that a drug licensed in one country is necessarily appropriate for another group because populations may differ in 'metabolism, weight, and nutrition— and these are known to affect the efficacy, safety, occurrence of side effects, and acceptability of a drug' (ibid., 323).

Drug licensing is important for ensuring safety and efficacy. Yet, according to the World Health Organization, only 5 per cent of less-developed countries have an effective drug regulatory administration (ibid.). Even in the industrialized world there are conflicts of interest faced by pharmaceutical companies and their scientists and the need for licensing and regulation. Because a patent gives a drug company the exclusive right to manufacture and sell a particular drug for a limited period of time—and because patented drugs are much more profitable to drug companies—it is in their interest to speed a newly patented drug through the approval and regulatory boards in order to have the longest time possible to gain from the patent status (Abraham, 1995).

The Dalkon Shield IUD (an intrauterine device for birth control) is one example of the great health costs of a profit-driven industry (Vavasour and Mennie, 1984). The Dalkon Shield went on the market in 1971 in the United States. By early 1972 there were numerous reports of adverse reactions, such as pelvic inflammatory disease, blood poisoning, and tubal pregnancies. By 1974, 17 people had died from its use. Because the US market began to look very poor, the manufacturer offered the Dalkon Shield to developing nations at a discounted price of 48 per cent of the original price. The shields were distributed to the developing nations even though they were unsterilized and nine out of ten

Box 16.3   Drug Promotion

At least 20 per cent of the sales revenue of the pharmaceutical industry is spent on drug promotion. Promotion includes traditional advertising in both medical journals and the mass media and outright gifts to physicians, ranging from a pen-and-pencil set to a Caribbean or European vacation for two. Sponsorship of medical and associated conferences and drug-related research are two other drug promotion strategies. Bribes by drug companies are sometimes used to help sell drugs. Drug promotion is excessive and puts pressure on physicians; in addition, it is also frequently false or partly false. According to an article in *The Times* (London), 'Promotional materials frequently exaggerate effectiveness and ignore dangers and the competition.'

In the developing world, the problems associated with drug promotion are even more acute, and the pressure greater. Drugs are sometimes promoted for diseases for which they are inappropriate, and no information is given about how they are to be used or what their hazards or side effects are. Anabolic steroids can, for example, stunt growth, cause liver tumours, and bring about irreversible masculinization in females. In Britain, anabolic steroids are cautiously recommended for osteoporosis, renal failure, terminal malignancies, and aplastic anemia. Yet, in the *African Monthly Index of Medical Specialties*, anabolic steroids have been suggested for such common conditions as malnutrition, weight loss, exhaustion, lack of appetite, and excessive fatigue in children.

lacked the necessary inserter. Furthermore, only one out of 1,000 was distributed with any instructions for insertion (and their insertion is a delicate and potentially dangerous procedure). In 1975 the United States banned the Dalkon Shield, but by 1979 they were still being sold in developing countries (Ehrenreich et al., 1979).

Clioquinol has long been promoted for the prevention and treatment of a wide variety of non-specific travellers' diarrheas. However, there is no adequate evidence that it is effective (Vavasour and Mennie, 1984). On the other hand, the dangers of clioquinol have been proven. Clioquinol has caused many thousands of cases of SMON—subacute myelo optic neuropathy—a condition that involves continuous pain, paralysis, blindness, and, in some cases, death. In 1977 a Japanese court determined that clioquinol had caused at least 10,000 cases of SMON. The manufacturer admitted responsibility for the tragedy and apologized to the victims and families. However, its concern did not prevent the company from marketing the drug in

Malaysia, Thailand, and Kenya as late as 1980 (Muller, 1982).

Chloramphenicol has been severely restricted in the US since 1961 because of its association with a severe and often fatal blood disease—aplastic anemia. As late as 1973 the manufacturer was still recommending chloramphenicol in Latin America for a wide variety of conditions, such as sore throats, ear infections, and pneumonia (ibid.).

The sixth profit strategy is to *provide select information to doctors and consumers about the efficiency and safety of various drugs.* On average, drug companies in Canada invest about $10,000 per physician to advertise (Williams et al., 1993). But they advertise in such a way as to seem to be educating doctors who report that they have inadequate knowledge about the effects and effectiveness of various pharmaceuticals and also that they are so busy that in the absence of adequate knowledge they are likely to 'try' something by prescribing drugs to a patient (Williams et al., 1995: 148). Drug industry contacts with physi-

Box 16.4   The Discovery of the DES Problem in Canada

In 1982, Harriet Simard was a healthy, 21-year-old philosophy student at McGill University in Montreal. Suddenly, after what was supposed to be a routine medical examination, Harriet was diagnosed with a rare cancer: clear cell adenocarcinoma of the cervix and vagina. Harriet had to have a hysterectomy. She was given an 85 per cent chance of survival after five years. Later she discovered that the cancer was linked to DES, a wonder drug marketed between 1941 and 1971 to prevent miscarriage. Harriet's mother had tried unsuccessfully to carry a baby to term eight years before becoming pregnant with Harriet. To prevent another miscarriage, the doctors prescribed DES.

At the time DES was prescribed for a variety of 'feminine conditions', including irregular bleeding and spotting, menopause, and as a 'morning-after pill' to prevent successful implantation after conception. In fact, it was prescribed as a 'morning-after pill' to numerous college and university students who had engaged in unprotected sexual intercourse and did not want to get pregnant.

Approximately one out of every thousand daughters of women prescribed DES will develop cancer. DES daughters also have an increased risk of contracting a precancerous condition called cervical dysplasia, of giving birth prematurely, of miscarriage during the second trimester, of ectopic pregnancy, of genital organ malformations, and perhaps of breast cancer. DES sons have an increased risk of undescended testicles, a condition sometimes related to testicular cancer. They may also have low sperm counts and abnormal sperm formation.

When Harriet Simard learned that she had this rare form of cancer, she began to read up on the subject and to ask questions. She discovered that American medical journals had already published a number of papers on some of the results of DES. Harriet was shocked to discover that the Canadian government was not taking action to inform people of the potential long-term intergenerational effects of DES, even though early screening is known to have beneficial effects on the outcome of the disease. Partly because of the lobbying efforts of women's groups in the US, the American federal government had sponsored screening clinics for DES daughters and sons, as well as a widespread information campaign. Doctors were encouraged to inform the government of patients who had ever been prescribed DES.

None of this had happened in Canada. Yet Harriet and her mother Shirley, working together, found DES-related cancers in Quebec and in Ontario, and discovered that approximately 100,000 people had been exposed to the drug.

In response, the Simards founded DES Action Canada. They set up an office and received a $50,000 annual grant from the federal government. Numerous newspaper and magazine stories have publicized their concerns. Many doctors have volunteered to help in screening DES daughters and in contacting patients who had taken the drug. The National Film Board has produced a film on the subject. DES Action Canada hosted an international conference. Nine chapters of the organization have been established across the country. About 30,000 Canadians have called DES Action Canada for advice and assistance.

This is one example of a highly successful grassroots movement. Harriet and Shirley Simard have shown what people can do to increase awareness and effect change.

cians are systematic and persistent and often include 'perks' such as meals, stationery, conference fees, travel expenses, and computer equipment (physicians who prescribe most are most likely to receive these additional perks) (ibid.).

Fifteen general practitioners in Australia

were asked to audiotape three encounters with pharmaceutical representatives (Roughead et al., 1998). Seven of these GPs agreed to take part. They asked 24 pharmaceutical representatives to participate; 16 agreed to do so. They were informed that they were being taped. A total of 64 medicines were described ('detailed') in the recordings. The interpretations averaged 2.75 minutes per drug. However the information provided by the pharmaceutical company representatives bore very little similarity to the Australian Approved Product Information categories. Thus, there was very little correspondence between the information provided by the drug company representatives and the views and position of the Australian government in respect to indications (for use), pharmacology, pharmacokinetics, side effects, precautions, warnings, interactions, use in special groups, dosage and administration, and availability. Despite the fact that the Australia Pharmaceutical Manufacturers' Code of Conduct is in place to regulate the marketing of drugs and 'includes standards for printed promotional material, pharmaceutical representatives' activities, competitions, gifts, samples, trade displays, and symposia' (ibid., 270), the results of this study indicate that pharmaceutical company representatives do not comply with standards outlined in their codes of conduct.

In its policy on 'Physicians and the Pharmaceutical Industry', updated in 1994, the Canadian Medical Association has expressed its concern about the conflict of interest that may confront physicians in their dealings with the pharmaceutical industry. The policy contains separate 'sections on research, surveillance studies, continuing medical education and clinical evaluation packages' (Lemmens and Singer, 1998). The Pharmaceutical Manufacturing Association of Canada has also developed a code similar to that of the CMA. The enforcement of the code, however, is still somewhat problematic.

The pharmaceutical industry invests in doctors because this has proven to be an effective strategy. 'For example, a publication for the drug market industry suggested that promotional dinners result in an 80 per cent increase in sales of the promoted drug' (ibid.). If the industry did not know from experience that marketing to doctors is effective, it would not have spent more than $5 billion in the US or $950 million in Canada annually in recent years.

The Case of Thalidomide

Just as the pharmaceutical companies have shown that their marketing strategies in developing countries take health less seriously than profits, so, too, have profits come first in Canada at times, and with deleterious consequences. Probably the incident with the most visibly tragic consequences was the thalidomide disaster, which resulted in the birth of over 100 babies in Canada with phocomelia (the absence of limbs and the presence of seal-like flippers instead).

A West German company developed thalidomide in 1954. It was called GRIPPEX, and was initially recommended for the treatment of respiratory infections, colds, coughs, flu, nervousness, and neuralgic and migraine headaches. It was widely available without prescription, quite cheap, and therefore very accessible. It was manufactured in West Germany, Canada, Great Britain, Italy, Sweden, and Switzerland under 37 different brand names (Klass, 1975: 92). Later it was marketed in Germany as the 'safest' sleeping pill available because it was impossible to take enough at any time to commit suicide. It was advertised in Great Britain (where it was called Distavel) as so safe that the picture accompanying an advertisement was of a little child in front of a medicine chest. The caption read, 'This child's life may depend on the safety of Distavel.'

By the summer of 1959 there were a number of reports in Germany, Australia, and Britain of serious side effects. These indicated that the drug caused nerve damage, affected balance, and caused tingling in the hands and feet. This should have been a warning about the potency of the

Box 16.5   Debate about New Reproductive Technologies

Among the most controversial of medical interventions available today are the new reproductive technologies. Largely unheard of, except in science fiction literature, before the birth of the first 'test-tube baby', Louise Brown, in 1978, these technologies fall roughly into four groups. They are (1) those concerned with fertility control (conception prevention); (2) labour and delivery 'management' (high-tech deliveries in hospital by obstetricians/gynecologists); (3) pre-conception and prenatal screening for abnormalities and sex selection (ultrasound, amniocentesis, genetic screening); and (4) reproductive technologies per se (conception, pregnancy, and birth management via technical, pharmaceutical, and medical intervention) (Eichler, 1988: 211). This discussion will be limited to the last category.

New reproductive technologies have separated gestational, genetic, and social parenthood for both men and woman; they have eliminated the need for intercourse between a man and a woman for reproducing; they enable men and women to reproduce without an opposite-sex, social parent through surrogate mothering arrangements or by sperm-bank utilization. With the new reproduction technologies, conception, gestation, and birth can be entirely separated from social parenting.

In 1985 the Canadian Medical Association decided that in vitro fertilization (IVF) was no longer experimental. This became a major factor in financial support of the procedure through public health insurance. The number of clinics for the treatment of the approximately 15 per cent of Canadians who are infertile grew, along with the numbers of specialists and researchers interested in treatment of this new 'disease'—infertility. Infertility was defined as one year of attempting to achieve pregnancy without success (Achilles, 1990: 287). While cost estimates are difficult to assess, one study suggested that

between 1985 and 1988 the Ontario government spent $77 million in directly funding IVF clinics. This is a significant underestimate of the overall costs to society because it does not include the expenditures on physicians, hospitals, drugs, medical devices, lost employment days, and other associated costs. By 1989 the Canadian federal government established the Royal Commission on New Reproductive Technologies to examine the medical and scientific developments related to IVF, as well as the social, ethical, research, legal, and economic implications. The government was responding to the increasingly widespread conviction that technological developments were outpacing society's ability to understand and control them.

This is an immensely complex issue with extensive ramifications. Sociologists have long been concerned to understand the relationships between technological innovation and social change. In particular, they have sought to understand the social organization and social control of technological innovation. To simplify, in this case the fundamental questions are: In whose interest are the new reproductive technological developments? Whose interests should they serve? To what extent has the availability of these new technologies reinforced and even exacerbated a pronatalist philosophy? What are the effects of such philosophy on men and women, particularly those who are infertile?

With respect to just one new intervention, in vitro fertilization, there are enormous costs for the 'mother', 'father', and the fetus/embryo. For the mother and the fetus/embryo, these costs include significant short- and long-term health effects. The treatments are very invasive and involve administration of hormonal drugs at extraordinary levels. In the short run, the 'mother's' body may experience pregnancy/non-pregnancy symptoms in turn, causing numerous minor side effects such as nausea, headaches, cramping, and the like. In the long run, these drugs (as DES before) may lead to a greater vulnerability to cancers—particularly of the reproductive system. As no long-term studies have yet been done, these effects are now only speculative.

In addition to the biological costs are the social and emotional costs of being preoccupied with bodily functioning, with motherhood, and with the experience of repeated failure to conceive. Estimates range from 0 to an 8.5 per cent success rate for conception (Burstyn, 1992: 13). Women have likened the experience of being involved with IVF to a roller coaster of emotions, including recurrent hope

and despair. Even when fertilization is successful, the offspring have higher than average neonatal and perinatal mortality rates; there are much higher incidences of multiple births (with all the attendant risks); 11 times the risk of low birth weight (associated with numerous long-term developmental problems); perhaps higher rates of childhood cancer (ibid., 14); five times the rate of spina bifida; and six times the rate of transposition (an unusual heart defect).

Given these side effects and the ethical issues, it is no wonder that new reproductive technologies have been the subject of widespread debate.

drug and its effects on the central nervous system (Winsor, 1973). But the manufacturer continued to market the drug in Germany and licensed another company to produce and market the drug in Canada and the US. The drug was tested briefly in the US and then samples were distributed. It was manufactured, beginning 1 April 1961, under the name KEVADON in Canada. A warning was included in the package about peripheral neuritis. It was distributed in Canada under a number of different names.

By 1 December 1961 two representatives of the German companies reported to Ottawa that a number of babies with congenital deformities had been born in Germany and that the mothers of these babies had taken thalidomide. Rather than contacting the research centres in Germany, England, and Australia directly, the Canadian government relied on the ambiguous and evasive reports presented by the pharmaceutical companies involved. It was not until three months later, on 2 March 1962, that the Food and Drug Directorate of National Health and Welfare decided to withdraw the drug, claiming that, until then, the evidence for its removal was 'only statistical' (ibid.). Removing the drug was compli-

cated. Unlike France, Belgium, the US, and Britain, Canada did not require the drug manufacturers to label the drug with its international name—thalidomide—under which its side effects were being publicized (*Kitchener-Waterloo Record*, 27 Sept. 1972). As a result, a number of pharmacists were not aware that their shelves contained the drug in question. By the time it was removed the damage had been done.

Approximately 115 babies were born in Canada with phocomelia. Other external defects included small ears, eye defects, depressed noses, and facial tumours. Internal problems were found in the cardiovascular system and the intestinal tract. There were several cases of missing organs, such as gall bladder or liver. These physical defects meant emotional traumas for those born with health and body-function problems, as well as for the mothers, fathers, siblings, other family members, and anyone who was involved with the 'thalidomide babies'. In some communities the birth of the deformed children made local newspaper headlines, and townspeople 'flocked' to the hospital to see for themselves. Some people blamed the mothers for having taken the drug. Whole families were stigmatized. There

Box 16.6   Premature Adoption of New Technology

There are a number of reasons that modern capitalist societies are prone to adopt technology prematurely. Butler (1993) documents three major forces: key societal values (e.g., placing a huge value on science and technology), federal government policies (e.g., policies that place the burden of responsibility for determining safety, quality, and efficacy of new technologies on their manufacturers), and reimbursement policies and economic incentives (policies that enable the costs of new technologies to be reimbursed adequately so as to ensure their profitability). These forces make it possible and even likely that new technologies are adopted prematurely even when this is at variance with physician opinion and of unproven medical benefit. Technological favouritism is characteristic of a variety of technologies (overuse of cardiac pacemakers, gastrointestinal endoscopy, and coronary bypass surgery have been estimated at 20 per cent, 17 per cent, and 15 per cent, respectively) and is especially prevalent in regard to child-bearing women (particularly with respect to electronic ultrasound, electronic fetal monitoring, and Caesarean section). It has been estimated, for instance, that the overuse of Caesarean sections is as high as 50 per cent (ibid.). Moreover, there are cases where women have been given Caesarean sections even against their will after obstetricians have asked for and received a court intervention (ibid.).

Box 16.7   Conflict of Interest: Doctors and the Pharmaceutical Industry

Do the relationships that physicians have with the pharmaceutical industry ever comprise a conflict of interest? There has been speculation that the support offered to doctors and medical students by the pharmaceutical industry may influence doctors unduly in their prescribing habits. One recent study in the New England Journal of Medicine reports on conflict of interest with respect to published articles about the safety of calcium blockers in the treatment of cardiovascular disorders. The researchers searched the English-language medical literature published from March 1995 through September 1996 for articles concerning the safety of calcium-channel antagonists. Articles were categorized as neutral, supportive, or critical with regard to using calcium blockers. The authors of the articles were surveyed about their financial relationships with the manufacturers of the calcium-channel blockers and with their competitors in the pharmaceutical marketplace. 'Pharmaceutical manufacturers were listed alphabetically; the nature of their products were not revealed. For each of the 40 manufacturers, authors were asked whether they had received any of five types of funding in the past five years: support to attend a symposium (i.e., funds for travel expenses), an honorarium to speak at a symposium, support to organize an educational program, support to perform research, and employment or consultation' (Stelfox et al., 1998: 102). The findings revealed that authors who supported the use of calcium-channel blockers were significantly more likely than neutral or critical authors to have financial relationships with manufacturers of these products.

were approximately 3,000 disabled babies in West Germany and 500 in Great Britain. When Belgium, Sweden, Portugal, and other European countries are included, the number of deformed babies reached 8,000 (Steacy, 1989).

Very few cases ever occurred in the US. Dr Frances Kelsey, the medical officer who reviewed safety data for the Food and Drug Administration, was skeptical and critical of the drug. She had, by chance, read a letter to the editor in a medical journal, which presented negative information about the drug (*Kitchener-Waterloo Record*, 17 Aug. 1972). She was dissatisfied with the available information on the safety of the product and did not allow it to be marketed. In particular, she was concerned that the drug could cross the placenta. Only the few samples of the drug given to doctors were ever used. Apparently, Dr Kelsey resisted extraordinary pressure from the drug company, which made 'no less than 50 approaches of submissions to the FDA' (Winsor, 1973).

The drug companies had used a number of tactics to increase the sales of thalidomide. One involved planting an article in the June 1961 issue of the *American Journal of Obstetrics and Gynecology*, allegedly written by Dr Ray Neilson of Cincinnati. The article said that the drug was safe for pregnant women (ibid.). Later, Dr Neilson admitted that the article had been written by the medical research director for the manufacturer and was based on incomplete evidence, i.e., on evidence only that the drug was harmless when taken in the last few months of pregnancy, when, of course, the limbs had already developed. Nevertheless, it was advertised as safe for pregnant women when it was clearly known to be unsafe if ingested in the early months. Canadians were reminded of this tragedy, and of the outcome for the people who suffered physical deformities and emotional and social scars as a result, when the Canadian Broadcasting Company aired a documentary, 'Broken Promises', on the events and their aftermath. This documentary revealed the culpability of the Canadian government in failing to keep the drug out of Canada. The *Globe and Mail* (15 Feb. 1989) reported on the program as follows: 'the most striking impression left by "Broken Promises" is that a number of pharmaceutical companies, druggists, doctors and prosthesis manufacturers have callously exploited the victims of thalidomide with the crudest and most obvious motive—profit.' In addition, the Canadian government was criticized for failing to provide compensation. It has subsequently compensated those who were directly affected by thalidomide. However, financial compensation cannot ever be a completely satisfactory conclusion to such a life-changing mishap.

The Case of DES

From the 1940s through the 1960s, many physicians prescribed the synthetic estrogen hormone DES (diethylstilbestrol, or simply stilbestrol) to pregnant women who had histories of miscarriage, diabetes, or toxemia of pregnancy. More than 4 million women worldwide took DES over this period. Approximately 2 million male and 2 million female children of these women had been exposed to DES in the US; there are approximately 400,000 children of 'DES mothers' in Canada. These children have developed a number of abnormalities, including a rare vaginal cancer, adenocarcinoma, and a variety of apparently benign structural changes of the uterus, cervix, and vagina. As many as 97 per cent of the DES daughters have cervical abnormalities. Adenosis, the most common problem, is estimated to occur in 43 to 95 per cent of the women. About one-half of DES daughters have had or may have problems with pregnancy, including primary infertility (difficulty in becoming pregnant), premature births, stillbirths, and ectopic pregnancies (gestation outside the uterus). Ectopic pregnancies, which may be dangerous to the mother-to-be as well as the fetus, appear to occur in five times as many DES daughters as in other women. Problems have been seen in DES sons as well.

Box 16.8   Antibiotic Resistance

Antibiotic resistance is growing (Branswell, 2002). The US Centers for Disease Control has recently confirmed that one of the most common and difficult of infections is becoming resistant to Vancomyecin, the strongest antibiotic presently available. Vancomyecin resistant staph areus (VRSA) may herald a day when there is no antibiotic solution for the many bacterial diseases whose treatments, since the 1940s, we have come to take for granted.

Why have so many people recently become allergic or resistant to different antibiotics? Have we chosen to overuse them? Have they been over-prescribed and prescribed when not absolutely necessary? Watch for new antibiotic-resistant strains of disease-causing microorganisms. Think critically about medicine and about the pharmaceutical industry as you decide whether or not to take any medication. Consider the side and long-term effects carefully.

Source: Helen Branswell, 'Superbug Genie is out of the Bottle', *National Post*, 8 July 2002, A4.

About 30 per cent have genital tract and semen abnormalities, including cysts and extremely small and undescended testicles. The impact of DES has become evident only over the past two decades or so. Thus, all of the long-term effects are not yet known.

Other Negative Effects of the Pharmaceutical Industry

Finally, the pharmaceutical industry must also be criticized for causing ill health in another way. As Harding (1987) suggests, 'the pharmaceutical industry is an outgrowth of the interlocking petrochemical industry, which also produces pesticides, herbicides and fertilizers.' Toxins from the petrochemical industry have been responsible for environmental health calamities. The public health dangers of this industry are therefore not confined to those that arise from the adverse effects of the drugs themselves.

Issues in Drug Regulation

Governments can have an important role in the regulation of the drug industry and ultimately in the drug-related health of their citizens. However, most government regulations are inadequate. As a result: (1) half the drugs now on the Canadian

market have never passed modern tests regarding safety or effectiveness; (2) even where regulations are in place in the industrialized world, substandard drugs are being marketed and distributed overseas; (3) drug companies seem to have a monopoly on the information available to doctors as well as on the side effects of various drugs. There are several reasons that the safety and effectiveness of drugs in Canada may even be declining. The responsibility for testing new drugs is increasingly being given over to the industry that manufactures and sells drugs for profit (Armstrong and Armstrong, 2003). The balance of power between the Health Products and Foods Branch and the industry has been moving towards the industry as Canadian government policies have generally moved towards the right, with an emphasis on market principles and globalization. The budget for the department of the government responsible for ensuring safety declined as independent government laboratories for testing drugs were closed (Armstrong and Armstrong, 2003).

However stringent the laws, the government cannot guarantee that any drug is safe for all the uses to which it may be put. It is not difficult to imagine a situation in which a drug is prescribed for one use or for one person, and is then used

Box 16.9   We All Have AIDS

According to a guest editorial in the *Washington Post* by Donald Berwick, we all have AIDS. AIDS, Berwick suggests, brings the Holocaust to mind. The only acceptable reaction to a crisis as severe as the imprisonment and slaughter of Jewish people in the concentration camps is the reported reaction of the Danes. The Danish king, followed by his people, said that if the Jews were forced to wear yellow stars of identification on their clothing, so would he. If the Nazis were to look for Jews to persecute in Denmark they would have to look at all Danes. Much worse in numerical terms than the Holocaust, AIDS has infected 36.1 million people already. In some countries more than one-third of the adults have AIDS. About 3 million people died of AIDS in the year 2000, 2.4 million of them in sub-Saharan Africa. This is the equivalent to a holocaust every two years. While prevention is the most important way to confront AIDS, there are some treatments available that extend life and improve its quality. These new treatments can also reduce the transmission of the virus from pregnant mother to child by two-thirds or more.

These treatments are costly. Berwick calls on the pharmaceutical companies and specifically the CEOs of some of the largest companies that currently produce anti-AIDS drugs to make their drugs available free or at cost for people around the world. 'Here is how it could happen', he says, 'the board chairs and executives of the world's leading drug companies decide to do it, period. To the anxious corporate lawyers, the incredulous stockholders, the cynical regulators and the suspicious public, they say together the same thing: the earth has AIDS, and therefore we all have AIDS' (Berwick, 2002).

What do you think? Is this possible? Is it desirable? Could it be effective?

Source: Donald Berwick, 'We All Have AIDS: the case for reducing the cost of HIV drugs to zero', *British Medical Journal* 324 (2002): 214–18.

again by the same person on another occasion when the symptoms seem to be similar or is passed on to a friend or a family member who seems to have the same problem. People often regulate their drug use, ignoring the specific directions given by the physician and/or the pharmacist. People have been known to develop drug allergies very suddenly.

While the government can insist that patients be told about drug interactions, it cannot regulate the actual mixture of drugs taken by any one individual. Some drugs react negatively when taken in conjunction with alcohol: 82 per cent of all Canadians drink (Canada's Health Promotion Survey, 1988). One characteristic of many alcoholics is that they try to keep their drinking habit secret—even from their doctor. Untold problems result from drug-alcohol interactions. In addition, a number of drug-related problems or side effects are only discovered after long-term use. For these and other reasons, the drug regulations established by the government can only be considered as partial protection.

The Canadian government is also in a weak position because of the Canadian branch-plant economy. Most drugs are developed and tested elsewhere. The Canadian government frequently relies on tests done abroad by other governmental bodies or by the drug firms' research departments. This raises complex problems of biased information from pharmaceutical companies and political problems of intergovernmental relations. Moreover, as Lexchin documents, in spite of the fact that Canadian drug laws are among the strictest in the world, there are still major gaps that may jeopardize people's health. These gaps,

Box 16.10   Patenting Genetic Material: What Are the Ethics?

The patenting of genetic material has been accepted in the US since 1980, when the US Supreme Court decided, in a five-four split, that it was legal to patent bacteria that had been modified to break down oil spills. This made the newly patented bacteria acceptable under the 1793 Patent Act because they involved a 'new composition of matter'. Since the mapping of the human genome this decision has become very controversial. One of the debates concerns the recently 'discovered' genes for breast cancer, the BRCA1 and BRCA2. They were discovered by a private laboratory, Myriad Genetics Laboratories, in the early 1990s.

Tests for the presence of the BRCA1 or BRCA2 are sometimes advised for or requested by women with a high risk of breast cancer because of family history. The presence or absence of one of the genes can help women decide what sorts of prophylactic action they might take. Because of the financial threats to Canada's health-care system

there have been many debates about whether or not women should be covered by medicare or should have to pay out of their own pockets for the test. Regardless of who was to pay, Myriad declared in 2001 that hospitals in several provinces were violating its patent on the genetic susceptibility to breast cancer. Myriad demanded that all tests were to be done in their US labs. This would cost about five times the current costs in Canada.

One province, Ontario, decided to challenge Myriad with respect to its right to control and to profit from diagnostic and medical tests using its patent. What do you think? Should human genes be able to be patented for the profit of the individual or company who discovers the gene? What are the possible consequences of this decision? For further discussion, see Commentary in the 6 Aug. 2002 *Canadian Medical Association Journal* and its references. (http://www.cmaj.ca/cgi/content/full/167/3/259)

Source: Donald J. Willison and Stuart M. MacLeod, 'Patenting of genetic material: Are the benefits to society being realized?', *Canadian Medical Association Journal* 167, 3 (2002).

Lexchin argues, are not accidents, nor are they idiosyncratic; rather, they are the result of the structure of the drug regulation body of the federal government—the Health Products and Foods Branch, formerly the Health Protection Branch—and its close ties with the international pharmaceutical industry and the Pharmaceutical Manufacturing Association of Canada. These two groups interact through an extensive system of liaison committees that allow the PMAC to participate at all stages in drug regulation, policy development, and implementation (Lexchin, 1990). It is not hard to imagine many situations involving a conflict of interest.

Medical Devices and Bioengineering

Companies that produce and sell various medical devices such as artificial heart valves, artificial limbs, kidney dialysis machines, anaesthesiology equipment, surgical equipment, and heart pacemakers are among the largest growth industries in the world. The regulations controlling the industry are uneven. Das Gupta, who was head of the Bureau of Radiation and Medical Devices, has said that he could document more than 200 deaths and 800 injuries caused by faulty technology and equipment simply from voluntarily sub-

Box 16.11   Direct-to-Patient Advertising

A new marketing tool appears to have opened up for the pharmaceutical industry—direct-to-patient advertising. It has already been shown to be effective in increasing the sales of particular drugs (Mintzes et al., 2002). According to a cross-sectional survey of primary-care physicians in Vancouver, British Columbia, and Sacramento, California, there is a significant likelihood, regardless of health status, drug payment method, gender, medical specialty, or number of years of practice that patients who request a particular drug will be given it. Furthermore, physicians indicated that in at least 40 per cent of the cases in which they prescribed a drug at the request of the patient they were ambivalent about the prescription of the particular drug. Clearly, patients' requests for certain drugs are a powerful factor in the prescribing habits of physicians despite their possible professional reluctance.

Source: Barbara Mintzes, Morris L. Barer, Richard L. Kravitz, Armine Kazanjian, Ken Basset, Joel Lexchin, Robert G. Evans, Richard Pan, and Stephen A. Marion, 'Influence of direct to consumer pharmaceutical advertising and patients' requests on prescribing decisions: two site cross-sectional survey', *British Medical Journal* 324 (2002): 278–9.

mitted reports from hospitals, doctors, and coroners. In fact, he estimated that if all the cases were known the numbers would be much higher. For instance, he suggested that anaesthesia equipment alone probably accounted for 200 deaths per year in Canada in the early to mid-eighties. Anaesthesia gas lines, he said, were simply patched together with masking tape in a number of major hospitals (ibid.).

> At present a manufacturer who wants to market a medical device in Canada has only to provide the bureau [Bureau of Radiation and Medical Devices] with a device notification in most cases—ten days after it is available for sale—detailing the directions for its use, its purpose, and its model number. (Ibid., 254)

The government does not generally require evidence concerning the potential for harm or benefit, or assuring the safety of the various devices. The exceptions are for tampons, condoms, contact (intra-ocular) lenses, and devices that are implanted for more than 30 days in the body. These are only accepted for marketing after the government has examined the evidence, provided by the manufacturing firm itself, as to the safety of the device.

The government, through the Bureau of Radiation and Medical Devices, has not developed its own safety standards in any systematic way. In fact, it has relied on the industry to police itself. Unfortunately, such policing has not always been adequate. There is evidence, for instance, that up to 50 per cent of all the medical devices delivered to hospitals have failed to meet the minimum standards for safety established by the independent Canadian Standards Association. Some of the inadequacies were minor, but some were potentially life threatening (ibid.). The case of the Même breast implants discussed earlier was perhaps the most widely publicized of recent health and safety hazards in the Canadian medical device marketplace.

Among the responsibilities of biomedical engineers are the evaluation and testing of equipment, the investigation and explanation of the causes of accidents, and the supervision of the repair of biomedical equipment. There is, however, a shortage of such personnel in Canada, owing in part to the lack of training programs. From what limited information is available, it is clear that the whole issue of medical devices and bio-engineering needs a great deal of research and more thorough and systematic regulation.

Summary

(1) There is a correlation between people's socio-demographic characteristics and their drug-taking habits. The heaviest users of drugs are those people under five and over 65 years of age. Females tend to use prescription drugs and visit doctors more frequently than males. Those in lower income groups spend a greater proportion of their income on pre-scription drugs than those in higher income groups.

(2) Psychoactive drugs are among the most heavily prescribed and often misprescribed drugs in Canada. Females, the elderly, and the unemployed are high users. Chronically ill patients are often prescribed two or more psychoactive drugs simultaneously. A good proportion of these mood-modifying drugs are given for social and personal reasons and not for medical problems.

(3) There are large differences in rates of pre-scription from doctor to doctor. Doctors receive much of their information about drugs from pharmaceutical companies. The drug promotion and advertising strategies used by these companies have an important impact on prescribing. Other factors in the rate at which doctors prescribe drugs include education, type of practice, and method of remuneration.

(4) Pharmacists tend to recommend non-pre-scription drugs that will maximize their prof-

it. Pharmacists may choose between a brand name (more expensive) and a generic drug for a customer when filling a prescription. Pharmaceutical companies offer incentives to ensure that the pharmacist will choose their brand.

(5) Multinationals control 90 per cent of the Canadian prescription drug market. Pharma-ceutical manufacturing is one of the more profitable manufacturing activities in Canada. Some of the reasons for this are: the absence of a link between manufacturing cost and price, the presence of patent protec-tion, price-fixing, discount pricing, advertis-ing, and drug distribution (dumping) in the less-developed countries.

(6) There are several instances where profits have come before health in Canada. One is the case of thalidomide, which resulted in the birth of 115 babies in Canada with pho-comelia. DES is another drug that was used by pregnant women with disastrous conse-quences. It is now known that it has caused many abnormalities in the reproductive sys-tems of the offspring of these mothers.

(7) The government is not able to regulate the use of drugs in Canada adequately. This means that half the drugs now on the Canadian market have never passed modern tests regarding safety or effectiveness. Drug companies seem to have a monopoly on the information available to doctors as well as on the side effects of various drugs.

(8) The medical devices industry is a profitable and growing industry. Except for devices to be used within the body, the government does not require evidence as to the harm or benefit or the safety of medical devices.

Questions for Study and Discussion

1. Explain the rates of prescription of antibiotics in Canada. What are the consequences of these rates?
2. Explain multiple drug use among seniors in Canada.
3. Why do doctors sometimes prescribe inappropriately?
4. What are some of the reasons for the high profitability of the pharmaceutical industry?
5. What are the problems in regard to drug promotion in the developing world?
6. Could a drug with the devastating effects of DES be marketed in Canada today?
7. What is the role of the Health Products and Foods Branch with respect to protecting the health of Canadians?

Suggested Readings

Harding, Jim. 1994. 'Social Basis of the Over Prescribing of Mood-Modifying Pharmaceuticals to Women', in Bolaria and Bolaria (1994b: 157–81). Analyzes aspects of the sociology of drug prescriptions of women.

Lexchin, Joel. 1984. *The Real Pushers: A Critical Analysis of the Canadian Drug Industry*. Vancouver: New Star Books. Offers an overview of the pharmaceutical industry. This author is one of the most important critical analysts of this industry.

_____. 1998. 'Improving the Appropriateness of Physician Prescribing', *International Journal of Health Services* 28, 2: 253–67. Describes one attempt at improving the appropriateness of physician prescribing.

Tarabusi, Claudio Casadio, and Graham Vickery. 1998. 'Globalization in the Pharmaceutical Industry Part 1', *International Journal of Health Services* 28, 1: 67–105. An empirical examination of globalization in the pharmaceutical industry.

Williams, Paul A., Rhonda Cockerill, and Frederick H. Lowy. 1995. 'The Physician as Prescriber: Relations between Knowledge about Prescription Drugs, Encounters with Patients and the Pharmaceutical Industry, and Prescription Volume', *Health and Canadian Society* 3, 1–2: 135–66. Offers a sociological look at prescribing drugs in Canada.

Appendix

Web Sites for Sociological Research on Health and Medicine

www.sosig.ac.uk/welcome.html

Social Science Information Gateway is a database of thousands of good Internet resources of relevance to social science researchers, academics, and practitioners. Based in the UK, it is funded by the Economic and Social Research Council and the Joint Information Systems Committee.

www.anu.edu.au/polsci/marx/marx.html

This site includes the Communist Manifesto as well as other classic Marxist texts and contemporary examples of Marxist materials.

www.cihi.ca/facts/canhe.html

This Canadian Institute for Health Information site is full of useful information for understanding health and medicine in Canada.

www.statcan.ca/start.html

The Statistics Canada Web site includes daily news, census materials, Canadian statistics, and so on.

www.hc-sc.gc.ca/ohih-bsi

This is the site for the Health Canada advisory council on issues related to health on the Web.

www.igc.org/igc

The goal of this site is 'connecting the people who are changing the world'. It provides international communication to link activists around the world via Peacenet, Econet, Labornet, Womensnet, Conflictnet, Anti-racism.net.

www.networklobby.org

The Catholic Social Justice Lobby promotes economic and social justice, including welfare reform, anti-poverty efforts, health-care reform.

www.worldbank.org/publications

This World Bank site includes ordering details for various timely publications related to international development, such as *World Development Indicators*, *World Bank Atlas*, and *Global Development Finance*, as well as complete text for such sources as the *World Bank Annual Report*.

www.who.org

The World Health Organization offers the biggest collection of current news stories about global health issues. The site includes information on diseases, the environment and lifestyle, family and reproductive health, health policies, statistics, and systems.

www.csih.org/
The Canadian Society for International Health is the leading Canadian health and development organization.

www.paho.org/
The Pan-American Health Organization's bilingual English/Spanish site contains lots of publications and links to useful documents.

www.globalpolicy.org
This site lists thousands of articles on the United Nations, the Security Council, the UN financial crisis, and NGO access.

www.idrc.ca
The International Development Resource Centre is Canadian-based.

www.healthconsultantsusa.com/health.htm
Occupational and Environmental Health Consultants tests workplaces for health and safety and offers programs designed to keep the workplace healthy. The site includes links to related organizations.

www.iwh.on.ca/
The mandate of the Institute for Work and Health, which is supported by the Workplace Safety and Insurance Board of Ontario, is to research the underlying factors that contribute to workplace health and disability.

www.ccohs.ca/
The Canadian Centre for Occupational Health and Safety promotes a safe and healthy working environment by providing information about workplace health and safety issues.

www.eohsi.rutgers.edu/guide.html
The Environmental and Occupational Health Sciences Institute sponsors research, education, and service programs related to environmental health, toxicology, occupational health, exposure assessment, public policy, and health assessment.

www.cdc.gov/niosh/homepage.html
The National Institute for Occupational Safety and Health is part of the Centers for Disease Control and Prevention in Atlanta.

www.iglhrc.org.
The International Gay and Lesbian Human Rights Commission seeks to protect and advance the human rights of all people and communities who experience discrimination and abuse on the basis of sexual orientation, gender identity, or HIV status.

www.hc-sc.gc.ca/seniors.aines
This Health Canada site provides resources related to aging issues such as health, medication, safety, and various government programs.

www.wilpf.org/
The Women's International League for Peace and Freedom, founded in 1915, works on issues including but not limited to women's rights, disarmament, ending US overseas intervention, and racial justice.

www.library.utoronto.ca///www/aging/depthome.html
This is the site for the Institute for Human Development, Life Course and Aging at the University of Toronto.

www.cwhn.ca/indexeng.html
The Canadian Women's Health Network includes both databases on women's health and links to other sources of information.

www.priory.com/med.htm
The *International Journal of Medicine* is a widely read on-line journal of timely medical research results and opinions.

www.feminist.com/health.htm
This Web site focuses on women and health. It includes links to American, Canadian, and international sites of relevance.

www.napo-onapa.ca
The National Anti-Poverty Organization site includes news, information about research, and activist advocacy.

www.ccsd.ca/facts.html
The Canadian Council on Social Development site includes information about poverty in Canada, child poverty in Canada, welfare, income.

www.hc-sc.ca
The Health Canada site includes information on Aboriginal health issues such as alcohol and drug use, HIV, AIDS, diabetes, Great Lakes environment, family violence, and other related health issues.

www.healthy.net/library/journals/self-carearchives/rnslfhgp.html
This site provides information about on-line support groups.

www.mentalhelp.net.selfhelp/
This is the site of the on-line self-help clearing house sponsored by the Mental Health Net. It also provides information about 'real-life' support groups and networks.

www.cfah.org/alliance/main.html
The Health and Behaviour Information Transfer offers a newsletter for the research community.

www.cma.cmaj/index.html
The Canadian Medical Association provides information about many different current issues facing the medical profession in Canada, as well as the *Canadian Medical Association Journal*. It includes its own internal search engine.

www.ama.assn.orgl
This is the site for the American Medical Association. It includes journal articles, links, and many timely, international medicine-related concerns. *JAMA*, one of the most influential of medical journals, is available on-line via this site.

www.nyu.edu/education/health/healthea/taub/hepr
Information on the International Union of Health Promoters and Educators is available at this site.

www.efn.org/~djz/birth/birthindex.html
The Online Birth Centre provides information on midwifery, breast-feeding, high-risk situations and complications, alternative health resources, and links to news groups and listservs.

www.martindalecenter.com/Nursing.html
This is the 'Virtual Nursing Centre—Martindales' Health Science Guide.

www.ajn.orgl
This is the site for issues related to nursing. It includes journals, continuing education, discussion groups, and nursing resources.

www.herbsplus.com/herbplus.html
This is the Web site for the Alternative Health e-mail directory, which includes information about herbs and their treatments, vitamins, fitness, organic food, nutraceuticals, retreats and seminars, and articles.

nccam.nih.goo/
The National Centre for Complementary and Alternative Medicine is associated with the National Institutes of Health in the US.

www.drweil.com
This is the Web site for one of America's most well-known natural health advocates, Dr Andrew Weil. It includes an interactive component in which the user can ask Dr Weil questions and it is updated daily. Dr Bernie Siegal also gives advice, tells survivor stories, and answers questions here.

www.ccachiro.org
The Canadian Chiropractic Association site.

www.naturspathicassoc.ca/alph_ac.html

The Canadian Naturopathic Association site includes links to related Canadian and international resources.

www.chiro.org

This site is organized and maintained by chiropractic volunteers. It includes numerous links regarding a wide variety of chiropractic practice from history to journals to listings of new doctors of chiropractic medicine.

www.homeopathyhome.coml

This homeopathy site includes a chat room, links, a directory, references to books and articles, and related issues.

www.views.vcu.edu/~gkrishna/PK/pk_company.html

This is an alphabetically organized and linked list of pharmaceutical companies on the Web.

www.pharminfo.com/

This is a descriptive database of pharmaceuticals and their effects, organized according to trade names. It includes links to a number of other sites, including disease-related sites and discussion groups. It serves as an entrance point to the Web for health-based information.

www.healthanswers.com/

This includes a drug database listing prescription drugs, side effects, precautions, drug interactions, doses, warnings, storage, what to do if a dose is missed, and so on.

www.hc-sc.gc.ca/hpb/lcdc

This is the site for the Health Protection Branch, Laboratory Centre for Disease Control, at Health Canada.

Bibliography

Abbott, Maude. 1931. *The History of Medicine in the Province of Quebec*. Montreal: McGill University Press.

Abel, U. 1990. *Chemotherapy of Advanced Epithelial Cancer: A Critical Survey*. Stuttgart: Hippocrates Verlag.

Abelson, J. Paddon, and C. Strohmenger. 1983. *Perspectives on Health*. Ottawa: Statistics Canada.

Abraham, John. 1995. *Science, Politics, and the Pharmaceutical Industry*. New York: St Martin's Press.

Academic American Encyclopedia. 1980. Princeton, NJ: Arete Publishing.

'Accessibility to Higher Education—New Trend Data'. 1988. *CAUT Bulletin* (June): 15.

Achilles, Rona. 1990. *Desperately Seeking Babies: New Technologies of Hope and Despair*. London: Routledge.

Achterberg, Jeanne. 1985. *Imagery in Healing*. Boston: Shambhala.

Ackerknect, E.H. 1968. *A Short History of Psychiatry*. New York: Haffner Press.

Ackerman-Ross, F.S., and N. Sochat. 1980. 'Close Encounters of the Medical Kind: Attitudes toward Male and Female Physicians', *Social Science and Medicine* 14A: 61–4.

Active Health Report—Perspective on Canada's Health Promotion Survey—1985. 1987. Ottawa: Minister of National Health and Welfare.

Adler, Nancy, and Karen Mathews. 1994. 'Health Psychology: Why Do Some People Get Sick and Some Stay Well', *American Review of Psychology* 45: 229–59.

Alford, R. 1971. 'The Political Economy of Health Care: Dynamics without Change', *Politics and Society* 2: 127–64.

Allentuck, Andrew. 1978. *Who Speaks for the Patient?* Toronto: Burns & MacEachern.

Alonzo, Angelo A. 1992. 'Health Behavior: Issues, Dilemmas and Explorations Toward a Paradigm', paper presented at the annual meeting of the American Sociological Association, Pittsburgh, Aug.

Altman, D. 1986. *AIDS in the Mind of America*. New York: Anchor Press/Doubleday.

Anderson, A. 1994. 'The Health of Aboriginal People in Saskatchewan: Recent Trends and Policy Implications', in Bolaria and Bolaria (1994a: 311–22).

Aneshensel, Carol, S. Leonard, and I. Pearlin. 1987. 'Structural Contexts of Sex Differences in Stress', in R.C. Barneth, L. Biener, and G.K. Baruch, eds, *Stress*. New York: Free Press, 75–95.

Angus, Douglas E. 1984. 'Health Care Costs: Past, Present, and (Can We Forecast?) the Future', working paper. Ottawa: University of Ottawa.

_____. 1987. 'Health Care Costs', in Coburn et al. (1987: 57–72).

_____ and P. Manga. 1985. *National Health Strategies:*

Time for a New Perspective. Ottawa: University of Ottawa, Faculty of Administration.

_____ and Manga Pran. 1990. 'Coop/consumer sponsored healthcare delivery effectiveness', *Canadian Cooperative Association* (Aug.).

Anstey, Kaarin J., Gary Andrews, and Mary A. Luszcz. 2001. 'Psychosocial factors, gender and late-life mortality', *Aging International* 27, 2: 73–89.

'Anti-Acne Drug Poses Dilemma for FDA (Accutane and Birth Defects)'. 1988. *Time* 131, 63 (2 May).

Antonovsky, A. 1967. 'Social Class, Life Expectancy and Overall Mortality', *Milbank Memorial Fund Quarterly* 45: 31–73.

_____. 1979. *Health, Stress and Coping*. San Francisco: Jossey Bass.

Appleby, Timothy. 1989. 'AIDS-Infected Prisoner's Treatment Cruel and Unusual, Judge Rules', *Globe and Mail*, 22 Feb., A11.

Armstrong, Liz, and Adrienne Scott. 1992. *Whitewash*. Toronto: HarperCollins.

Armstrong, Pat, and Hugh Armstrong. 2003. *Wasting Away: The Undermining of Canadian Health Care*, 2nd edn. Toronto: Oxford University Press.

_____, Jacqueline Choiniere, and Elaine Day. 1993. *Vital Signs: Nursing in Transition*. Toronto: Garamond Press.

Arney, William, et al. 1982. 'The Location of Pain in Childbirth: Natural Childbirth and the Transformation of Obstetrics', *Sociology of Health and Illness* 4, 1.

Aronowtz, Robert A. 1992. 'From Myalgic Encephalitis to Yuppie Flu: A History of Chronic Fatigue Syndrome', in Rosenberg and Golden (1992: 155–81).

Ashford, Nicholas A., and Claudia S. Miller. 1991. *Chemical Exposures*. New York: Van Nostrand Reinhold.

Ashworth, C.D., P. Williamson, and D. Montano. 1984. 'A Scale to Measure Physician Beliefs about Psychosocial Aspects of Patient Care', *Social Science and Medicine* 19: 1235–8.

Association of American Medical Colleges. 1984. *Physicians for the Twenty-first Century: Report of the Panel on the General Professional Education of the Physician and College Preparation for Medicine*. Washington: Anthon.

Bakwin, H. 1945. 'Pseudoxia Pediatricia', *New England Journal of Medicine* 232: 691–7.

Ballem, Penny. 1998. 'The Challenge of Diversity in the Delivery of Women's Health Care', *Canadian Medical Association Journal (CMAJ)* 159: 336–8.

Balshem, Martha. 1991. 'Cancer, Control and Causality: Talking about Cancer in a Working Class Community', *American Ethnologist* 18: 152–72.

Barber, N. 1995. 'What Constitutes Good Writing?', *British Medical Journal* 310: 923–5.

Bardossi, F. 1982. *Multiple Sclerosis: Grounds for Hope*. Toronto: Public Affairs Committee.

Barer, M.L., Robert G. Evans, Patrick Lewis, and Michael Rachlis. 2001. 'Rentalizing medicine: shared problems, public solutions', *Medical Reform* 21, 1: 4–6.

_____, R.G. Evans, and G.L. Stoddart. 1979. 'Controlling Health Care Costs by Direct Charges to Patients: Snare or Delusion?' Occasional Paper No. 10. Toronto: Ontario Economic Council.

_____, and G.L. Stoddart. 1999. *Improving Access to Needed Medical Services in Rural and Remote Canadian Communities: Recruitment and Retention Revisited*. Ottawa: Federal, Provincial, and Territorial Committee on Health Human Resources.

Barker-Benfield, G.L. 1976. *The Horrors of the Half-Known Life*. New York: Harper Colophon Books.

Barnes, Benjamin, et al. 1977. 'Evaluation of Surgical Therapy by Cost-Benefit Analysis', *Surgery* 82, 1: 21–3.

Baron, S.H., and S. Fisher. 1962. 'Use of Psychotropic Drug Prescriptions in a Prepaid Group Practice Plan', *Public Health Reports* 77: 871–81.

Barrington, E. 1985. *Midwifery Is Catching*. Toronto: NC Press.

Barsh, R. 1994. 'Canada's Aboriginal Peoples: Social Integration or Disintegration?', *Canadian Journal of Native Studies* 14: 1–46.

Barsky, Arthur J. 1981. 'Hidden Reasons Some Patients Visit Doctors', *Annals of Internal Medicine* 94: 492–8.

Batt, Sharon. 1994. *Patient No More: The Politics of Breast Cancer*. Charlottetown, PEI: Gynergy Books.

Battershell, Charles. 1994. 'Social Dimensions in the Production and Practice of Canadian Health Care Professionals', in Bolaria and Dickinson (1994: 135–57).

Baumgart, Alice J., and J. Larsen. 1988. *Canadian Nursing Faces the Future: Development and Change.* St Louis: Mosby.

Baxter, J., J. Eyles, and D. Willms. 1992. 'The Hagersville Tire Fire', *Qualitative Health Research* 2: 208–37.

Beardshaw, Virginia. 1983. *Prescription for Change: Health Action International's Guide to National Health Products.* The Hague: International Organization for Consumer Unions.

Beardwood, Barbara, and Vivienne Walters. 1999. 'Complaints against Nurses: A Reflection of the New Managerialism and Consumerism in Health Care?', *Social Science and Medicine* 48, 3: 363–74.

Becker, Gary, and Robert D. Nachtigall. 1992. 'Eager for Medicalization: The Social Production of Infertility as a Disease', *Sociology of Health and Illness* 14, 4: 456–71.

Becker, Howard S. 1963. *The Outsiders: Studies in the Sociology of Deviance.* New York: Free Press.

_____ et al. 1961. *Boys in White: Student Culture in Medical School.* Chicago: University of Chicago Press.

_____ et al. 1982. 'Union Activity in Hospitals: Past, Present, and Future', *Health Care Financing Review* 3: 1–110.

Beckman, L.F. 1977. 'Social Networks, Host Resistance and Mortality: A Follow-Up Study of Alameda County Residents', Ph.D. dissertation, University of California, Berkeley.

Been, V. 1994. 'Unpopular Neighbours: Are Dumps and Landfills Sited Equitably?', *Resources* 115: 16–19.

Belkin, Lisa. 1990. 'Seekers of Urban Living Head for Texas Hills', *New York Times*, 2 Dec., A1, A32.

Bell, C. 1971. 'Occupational Career, Family Cycle and Extended Family Relations', *Human Relations* 24 (Dec.): 463–75.

Bell, R.W., and J. Osterman. 1983. 'The Compendium of Pharmaceuticals and Specialties: A Critical Analysis', *International Journal of Health Services* 13: 107–18.

Bell, Susan E. 1989. 'Technology in Medicine: Development, Diffusion and Health Policy', in Howard E. Freeman and Sol Levine, eds, *Handbook of Medical Sociology*, 4th edn. Englewood Cliffs, NJ: Prentice-Hall, 185–204.

Belliveau, Jo-Anne, and Leslie Gaudette. 1995. 'Changes in Cancer Incidence', *Canadian Social Trends* (Winter): 2–7.

Benoit, Cecilia. 1995. 'Medical Dominance and Its Challenges', *Health and Canadian Society* 3, 1–2: 195–210.

Berger, Peter L., and Thomas Luckmann. 1966. *The Social Construction of Reality.* Garden City, NY: Doubleday.

Bergob, Michael. 1994. 'Drug Use among Senior Canadians', *Canadian Social Trends* (Summer): 25–9.

Berwick, Donald. 2002. 'We all have AIDS: The case for reducing the cost of HIV drugs to zero', *British Medical Journal* 324: 214–18.

Beyond Adjustment: Responding to the Health Crisis in Africa. 1993. Toronto: Inter-Church Coalition on Africa.

Bieliauskas, Linas A. 1982. *Stress and Its Relationship to Health and Illness.* Boulder, Colo.: Westview Press.

Biggs, C. Lesley. 1983. 'The Case of the Missing Midwives: A History of Midwifery in Ontario from 1795–1900', *Ontario History* 75: 21–35.

_____. 1988. 'The Professionalization of Chiropractic in Canada: Its Current Status and Future Prospects', in Bolaria and Dickinson (1988: 328–45).

Bilson, Geoffrey. 1980. *A Darkened House: Cholera in Nineteenth-Century Canada.* Toronto: University of Toronto Press.

Birnie, Lisa Hobbs, and Sue Rodriguez. 1994. *Uncommon Will: The Death and Life of Sue Rodriguez.* Toronto: Macmillan.

Black Report—DHSS Inequalities in Health: Report of Research Writing Group. 1982. London: Department of Health and Social Security.

Blane, David. 1985. 'An Assessment of the Black Report's Explanation of Health Inequalities', *Sociology of Health and Illness* 7 (Nov.): 423–45.

Blaxter, Mildred. 1978. 'Diagnosis as Category and Process: The Case of Alcoholism', *Social Science and Medicine* 12: 9–77.

Blishen, Bernard R. 1969. *Doctors and Doctrines: The Ideology of Medical Care in Canada.* Toronto: University of Toronto Press.

_____. 1991. *Doctors in Canada.* Toronto: University of Toronto Press.

Bliss, Michael. 1982. *The Discovery of Insulin.* Toronto: McClelland & Stewart.

_____. 1984. *Banting: A Biography*. Toronto: McClelland & Stewart.

Bloom, Joan, and Larry Kessler. 1994. 'Emotional Support Following Cancer: A Test of the Stigma and Social Activity Hypothesis', *Journal of Health and Social Behaviour* 35 (June): 118–33.

Bluebond-Langer, Myra. 1978. *The Private Worlds of Dying Children*. Princeton, NJ: Princeton University Press.

Bolaria, B. Singh, and Rosemary Bolaria, eds. 1994a. *Racial Minorities: Medicine and Health*. Halifax: Fernwood.

_____ and _____, eds. 1994b. *Women, Medicine and Health*. Halifax: Fernwood.

_____ and Harley D. Dickinson, eds. 1988. *Sociology of Health Care in Canada*. Toronto: Harcourt Brace Jovanovich.

_____ and _____, eds. 1994. *Health, Illness and Health Care in Canada*, 2nd edn. Toronto: Harcourt Brace & Company.

Boon, Heather. 1995. 'The Making of a Naturopathic Practitioner: The Education of "Alternative" Practitioners in Canada', *Health and Canadian Society* 3, 1–2: 15–41.

_____. 1998. 'Canadian Naturopathic Practitioners: Holistic and Scientific World Views', *Social Science and Medicine* 46, 9: 1213–25.

Boothroyd, Lucy J., Laurence J. Kirmayer, Sheila Spreng, Michael Malus, and Stephen Hodgins. 2001. 'Completed suicides among the Inuit of northern Quebec, 1982–1996: a case-control study', *Canadian Medical Association Journal* (18 Sept.): 165–6.

Borda, I.T., E. Napke, and C. Stapleton. 1976. 'Drug Surveillance in a Canadian Hospital', *CMAJ* 114: 517–22.

Bosk, Charles. 1979. *Forgive and Remember: Managing Medical Failure*. Chicago: University of Chicago Press.

Boston Women's Health Collective. 1996. *Our Bodies, Our Selves*, 25th Anniversary Edition. New York: Simon & Schuster.

Boughy, Howard. 1978. *Insights of Sociology: An Introduction*. Boston: Allyn and Bacon.

Bourbeau, R., J. Légare, and V. Edmond. 1997. *New Birth Cohort Life Tables for Canada and Quebec, 1801–1991*. Ottawa: Statistics Canada, Demography Division.

Bourgeault, Ivy Lynn, Jan Angus, and Mary Fynes. 1998. 'Gender, Medicine Dominance and the State: Nurse Practitioners and Midwives in Ontario', paper presented at International Sociological Association meeting.

'A Boycott over Infant Formula'. 1979. *Business Week*, 12 Apr., 137–40.

Brack, J., and Robert Collins. 1981. *One Thing for Tomorrow: A Woman's Personal Struggle with Multiple Sclerosis*. Saskatoon: Western Producer Prairie Books.

Braden, Charles Samuel. 1958. *Christian Science Today: Power, Policy, Practice*. Dallas: Southern Methodist University Press.

Bradshaw, York W., Rita Noonan, Laura Gash, and Claudia Buchmann Sershen. 1993. 'Borrowing Against the Future', *Social Forces* 71, 3: 629–56.

Bransen, Els. 1992. 'Has Menstruation Been Medicalized or Will It Never Happen?', *Sociology of Health and Illness* 14, 1: 98–110.

Branswell, Helen. 2002. 'Superbug genie is out of the bottle', *National Post*, 8 July, A4.

Bricker, Jon. 2002. 'Four killings bring horrors of war home', *National Post*, 27 July, A3.

Brook, R.H., C.J. Kanberg, A. Mayer Oakes, et al. 1989. *Appropriateness of Acute Medical Care for the Elderly*. Santa Monica, Calif.: Rand Corporation.

Broom, Dorothy H., and Roslyn Woodward. 1996. 'Medicalization Reconsidered: Toward a Collaborative Approach to Care', *Sociology of Health and Illness* 18, 3: 357–78.

Brown, Lester R., Michael Renner, and Christopher Flavin. 1998. *Vital Signs*. New York: W.W. Norton.

Brown, Phil. 1992. 'Popular Epidemiology and Toxic Waste Contamination: Lay and Professional Ways of Knowing', *Journal of Health and Social Behavior* 33 (Sept.): 267–8.

Brown, Richard E. 1979. *Rockefeller Medical Men: Medicine and Capitalism in America*. Berkeley: University of California Press.

Bryan, Larry. 1996. *A Design for the Future of Health Care*. Toronto: Key Porter Books.

Brym, R.J., and B.J. Fox. 1989. *From Culture to Power: The Sociology of English Canada*. Toronto: Oxford University Press.

Buckley, Richard E., and Peter H. Harasym. 1999. 'Level Symptoms and Causes of Surgical Residents' Stress', *Annals of the Royal College of*

Physicians and Surgeons of Canada 324 (June): 216–21.

Bull, Angela. 1985. *Florence Nightingale*. London: Hamish Hamilton.

Bullard, Robert D. 1983. 'Solid Waste Sites and the Black Houston Community', *Sociological Inquiry* 53: 273–88.

Bullough, Bonnie, and Vern Bullough. 1972. 'A Brief History of Medical Practice', in Judith Lorber and Eliot Freidson, eds, *Medical Men and Their Work: A Sociological Reader*. New York: Aldone Atherton, 86–101.

Bunker, J. 1970. 'Surgical Manpower: A Comparison of Operations and Surgeons in the United States and in England and Wales', *New England Journal of Medicine* 282, 3: 135–44.

_____. 1985. 'When Doctors Disagree', *New York Times Review of Books*, 25 Apr., 7–12.

_____, V.C. Donahue, P. Cole, and M.P. Knotman. 1976. 'Public Health Rounds at the Harvard School of Public Health. Elective Hysterectomy: Pro and Con', *New England Journal of Medicine* 295, 5: 264–8.

Burke, Mary Ann, Joan Lindsay, Ian McDowell, and Gerry Hill. 1997. 'Dementia Among Seniors', *Canadian Social Trends* (Summer): 24–7.

Burke, Mike, and H. Michael Stevenson. 1993. 'Fiscal Crises and Restructuring in Medicine: The Politics and Political Science of Health in Canada', *Health and Canadian Society* 1, 1: 51–80.

Burkett, Gary, and Kathleen Knaft. 1974. 'Judgement and Decision-Making in a Medical Specialty', *Sociology of Work and Occupations* 1: 82–109.

Burnett, Richard T., Sabit Cakmak, and Jeffrey R. Brook. 1998. 'The Effect of the Urban Ambient Air Pollution Mix on Daily Mortality Rates in 11 Canadian Cities', *Canadian Journal of Public Health* 89, 3: 152–5.

Burnfield, A. 1977. 'Multiple Sclerosis: A Doctor's Personal Experience', *British Medical Journal* 6058 (12 Feb.): 435–6.

Burstyn, Verna. 1992. 'Making Babies', *Canadian Forum* (Mar.): 12–17.

Burtch, Brian E. 1994. 'Promoting Midwifery, Prosecuting Midwives: The State and the Midwifery Movement in Canada', in Bolaria and Dickinson (1994: 504–23).

Bury, M.R. 1986. 'Social Constructionism and the Development of Medical Sociology', *Sociology of Health and Illness* 2: 137–69.

Buske, Lynda. 1999a. 'Our Incredible Shrinking Medical Schools', *CMAJ* 160: 772.

_____. 1999b. 'Canada's Informal Caregivers', *CMAJ* 160: 1427.

_____. 1999c. 'MDs Second on Honesty Scale, Lawyers and Politicians Lag', *CMAJ* 160: 1547.

———. 1999d. 'The Changing Face of AIDS in Canada', *CMAJ* 161: 124.

Butler, Irene. 1993. 'Premature Adoptions and Routinization of Medical Technology: Illustrations from Childbirth Technology', *Journal of Social Issues* 49, 2: 11–34.

Cadman, D., et al. 1986. 'Chronic Illness and Functional Limitation in Ontario Children: Findings of the Ontario Child Health Study', *CMAJ* 135 (Oct.): 761–7.

Calnan, Michael, and Simon Williams. 1992. 'Images of Scientific Medicine', *Sociology of Health and Illness* 14, 2: 233–54.

Cameron, Elaine, and John Bernardes. 1998. 'Gender and Disadvantages in Health', *Sociology of Health and Illness* 20, 5: 673–93.

Campbell, Marie. 1988. 'The Structure of Stress in Nurses' Work', in Bolaria and Dickinson (1988: 393–406).

Canada Health Act Annual Report 1992–1993. 1993. Ottawa.

Canada's Green Plan. 1994. Ottawa: Minister of Supply and Services.

Canada's Health Promotion Survey. 1988. *Technical Report*. Ottawa: Health and Welfare Canada.

Canada Year Book. Various years. Ottawa: Statistics Canada.

Canadian Advisory Council on the Status of Women. 1987. *Recommendations*. Ottawa.

_____. 1995. *What Women Prescribe: Report and Recommendations*. National Symposium on Women in Partnership: Working Towards Inclusive, Gender-Sensitive Health Policies. Ottawa, May.

Canadian Cancer Society. 1994. *Protecting Health and Revenue: An Action Plan to Control Contraband and Tax-Exempt Tobacco*. Ottawa.

Canadian College of Naturopathic Medicine. 1995. *The Power to Heal*. Toronto.

The Canadian Encyclopedia, 2nd edn. 1988. Edmonton: Hurtig.

Canadian Health Services Research Foundation (CHSRF). 2001. *Mythbusters* (pamphlet). Available at: <www.chsrf.ca>.

Canadian Institute for Health Information (CIHI). 2002. 'Health care in Canada'. Available at: <www.cihi.ca>.

Canadian Medical Association. 1999. *Code of Ethics*.

Canadian Social Trends. Various years and issue numbers. Ottawa: Statistics Canada, Cat. no. 11–008E.

Cannon, William B. 1932. *The Wisdom of the Body*. New York: W.W. Norton.

Capildeo, R., and A. Maxwell. 1982. *Progress in Rehabilitation: Multiple Sclerosis*. London: Macmillan.

Caplan, Elinor. 1989. 'Speaking Out'. Toronto: TVO, Winter.

Caplan, Ronald Lee. 1984. 'Chiropractic', in *Alternative Medicines: Popular and Policy Perspectives*. New York: Tavistock, 80–113.

Carlson, Rick. 1975. *The End of Medicine*. Toronto: Wiley.

Carpenter, M. 1980. 'Review Article: Medical Sociology and the Politics of Health', *Sociology of Health and Illness* 3: 104–12.

Cartwright, A. 1967. *Patients and Their Doctors*. London: Routledge & Kegan Paul.

_____ and R. Anderson. 1981. *General Practice Revisited: A Second Study of Patients and Their Doctors*. London: Tavistock.

Cassel, J. 1974. 'Psychological Processes and "Stress": Theoretical Formulation', *International Journal of Health Services* 4: 471–82.

Cassileth, Barrie R. 1986. 'Unorthodox Cancer Medicine', *Cancer Investigation* 4: 591–8.

_____, E.J. Lusk, D. Guerry, A.D. Blake, W. P. Walsh, L. Kascius, and D.J. Schultz. 1991. 'Survival and Quality of Life among Patients Receiving Unproven as Compared with Conventional Cancer Therapy', *New England Journal of Medicine* 324, 17: 1180–5.

_____, E.J. Lusk, T.B. Strouse, and B.J. Bodenheimer. 1984. 'Contemporary Unorthodox Treatments in Cancer Medicine: A Study of Patients, Treatments, and Practitioners', *Annals of International Medicine* 101: 105–12.

Castiglioni, Arturo. 1941. *A History of Medicine*. New York: Knopf.

Caudell, K.A. 1996. 'Psychoneuroimmunology and Innovative Behavioural Interventions in Patients with Leukemia', *Oncology Nursing Forum* 23, 3: 493–502.

Charles, Catherine A. 1976. 'The Medical Profession and Health Insurance: An Ottawa Case Study', *Social Science and Medicine* 10: 33–8.

Charmaz, Kathy. 1987. 'Struggling for a Self: Identity Levels of the Chronically Ill', *Research in the Sociology of Health Care* 6: 283–321.

Chen, Benjamin T.B. 2002. 'From perceived surplus to perceived shortage: What happened to Canada's physician work force in the 1990's?', *Canadian Institute for Health Information*.

Chivian, Eric, Michael McCally, Howard Hu, and Andrew Haines. 1993. *Critical Condition: Human Health and Environment*. Cambridge, Mass.: MIT Press.

Chopra, Deepak. 1987. *Creating Health*. Boston: Houghton Mifflin.

_____. 1989. *Quantum Healing: Exploring the Frontiers of Body Medicine*. New York: Bantam Books.

Chow, Sue. 1998. 'Specialty Group Differences Over Tonsillectomy: Pediatricians Versus Otolaryngologists', *Qualitative Health Research* 8, 1: 61–75.

Clark, Jack A., and Elliot G. Mishler. 1992. 'Attending to Patients' Stories: Reframing the Clinical Task', *Sociology of Health and Illness* 14, 3: 344–72.

_____, Deborah A. Potter, and John B. McKinlay. 1991. 'Bringing Social Structure Back Into Clinical Decision Making', *Social Science and Medicine* 32, 8: 853–63.

Clark, Warren. 1996. 'Youth smoking', *Canadian Social Trends* (Winter): 2–7.

_____. 1998. 'Exposure to Second Hand Smoke', *Canadian Social Trends* (Summer): 41.

_____. 2002. 'Time Alone', *Canadian Social Trends* (Autumn): 2–6.

Clarke, Juanne N. 1980. 'Medicalization in the Past Century in the Province of Ontario: The Physician as Moral Entrepreneur', Ph.D. dissertation, University of Waterloo.

_____. 1981. 'A Multiple Paradigm Approach to the Sociology of Medicine, Health and Illness', *Sociology of Health and Illness* 3, 1 (Mar.): 89–103.

_____. 1983. 'Sexism, Feminism and Medicalism: A Decade Review of the Literature on Gender and Illness', *Sociology of Health and Illness* 5 (Mar.): 62–82.

_____. 1984. 'Medicalization and Secularism in Selected English-Canadian Fiction', *Social Science and Medicine* 18, 3: 205–10.

_____. 1985. *It's Cancer: The Personal Experiences of Women Who Have Received a Cancer Diagnosis*. Toronto: IPI Publishing.

_____. 1987. 'The Paradoxical Effects of Aging on Health', *Journal of Gerontological Social Work* 10: 3–20.

_____. 1992a. 'Cancer, Heart Disease, and AIDS: What Do the Media Tell Us About These Diseases?', *Health Communication* 4, 2: 105–20.

_____. 1992b. 'Feminist Methods in Health Promotion Research', *Canadian Journal of Public Health*, Supp. 1 (Mar./Apr.): 554–7.

_____. 1995. 'Breast Cancer in Mothers: Impact on Adolescent Daughters', *Family Perspectives* 29, 3: 243–57.

_____. 1996. *Health, Illness, and Medicine in Canada*, 2nd edn. Toronto: Oxford University Press.

_____, with Lauren N. Clarke. 1999. *Finding Strength: A Mother and Daughter's Story of Childhood Cancer*. Toronto: Oxford University Press.

_____ and Ross Gray. 1997. 'The Prostate Cancer "Epidemic"', *Canadian Health Psychologist* 5, 2: 48–53.

_____ and L. Hoffman-Goetz. 1999. 'Information Technologies as a Source of Medical Information', paper presented to policy seminar. Ottawa.

Clements, F.E. 1932. 'Primitive Concepts of Disease', *Publications—American Archeology and Ethnology* 32, 2: 182–252.

Clendening, Logan, ed. 1960. *Source Book of Medical History*. New York: Dover.

'Clioquinol: Time to Act'. 1977. *Lancet* 1, 8022 (28 May): 1139.

Closson, Tom R., and Margaret Catt. 1996. 'Funding System Initiatives and the Restructuring of Health Care', *Canadian Journal of Public Health* 87, 2: 86–9.

Cobb, Sidney. 1976. 'Social Support as a Moderator of Life Stress', *Psychosomatic Medicine* 38: 301–14.

Coburn, David. 1998. 'State Authority, Medical Dominance, and Trends in the Regulation of the Health Professions: The Ontario Case', in Coburn et al. (1998: 332–46).

_____, Carl D'Arcy, and George Torrance, eds. 1998. *Health and Canadian Society: Sociological Perspec-*
tives, 3rd edn. Toronto: University of Toronto Press.

_____, _____, _____, and Peter New. 1987. *Health and Canadian Society: Sociological Perspectives*, 2nd edn. Markham, Ont.: Fitzhenry & Whiteside.

_____ and C. Lesley Biggs. 1987. 'Chiropractic: Legitimation or Medicalization?', in Coburn et al. (1987: 336–84).

_____ and J. Eakin. 1993. 'The Sociology of Health in Canada: First Impressions', *Health and Canadian Society* 1, 1: 83–112.

_____ and _____. 1998. 'The Sociology of Health in Canada', in Coburn et al. (1998: 619–34).

_____, Susan Rappolt, and Ivy Bourgeault. 1997. 'Decline vs. Retention of Medical Power Through Rest Ratification: An Examination of the Ontario Case', *Sociology of Health and Illness* 19, 1: 1–22.

_____, G.M. Torrance, and J.M. Kaufert. 1983. 'Medical Dominance in Canada in Historical Perspective: The Rise and Fall of Medicine', *International Journal of Health Services* 13, 3: 407–32.

Cohen, Donna. 2002. 'Ageism can be lethal: Undetected homicides in older people', *British Medical Journal* 325 (27 July): 181.

Cohen, Sheldon, and Tracy B. Herbert. 1996. 'Health Psychology: Psychological Factors and Physical Disease from the Perspective of Human Psycho Neuron Urology', *American Review of Psychology* 47: 113–42.

Colburn, Thea, Diane Dumanoski, and John Peterson Myers. 1996. *Our Stolen Future*. New York: Dutton.

Cole, Stephen, and Robert Lejeune. 1972. 'Illness and the Legitimation of Failure', *American Sociological Review* 37: 347–56.

Coleman, James, Elihu Katz, and Herbert Menzel. 1957. 'The Diffusion of Innovation Among Physicians', *Sociometry* 20: 253–69.

Colliers Encyclopedia. 1973. New York: Crowell-Collier.

Collishaw, N.E. 1982. 'Disability Attributable to Smoking—Canada, 1978–79', *Chronic Diseases in Canada* (Ottawa: Health and Welfare) 3 (Dec.): 61.

Colombo, John Robert. 1993. *The Canadian Global Almanac: A Book of Facts*. Toronto: Macmillan.

Colquitt, W., and C. Killian. 1991. 'Students Who Consider Medicine But Decide Against It',

Academic Medicine 66, 5: 273–8.

Commission on the Future of Health Care in Canada (Roy Romanow, chairman). 2002. *Final Report.* Ottawa.

Conger, Rand D., Frederick O. Lorenz, Glen Ceda Jr, Ronald L. Simons, and Xiojia Ge. 1993. 'Husband and Wife Differences in Response to Undesirable Life Events', *Journal of Health and Social Behavior* 32 (Mar.): 71–88.

Conley, M.C., and H.O. Maukasch. 1988. 'Registered Nurses, Gender and Commitment', in A. Statham, E.M. Miller, and H.O. Maukasch, eds, *The Worth of Women's Work: A Qualitative Synthesis.* Albany: State University of New York Press.

Conrad, Peter. 1975. 'The Discovery of Hyperkinesis: Notes on the Medicalization of Deviant Behaviour', *Social Problems* 23 (Oct.): 12–21.

———. 1987. 'The Experience of Illness: Recent and New Directions', in J. Roth and P. Conrad, eds, *Research in the Sociology of Health Care*, vol. 6. Greenwich, Conn.: JAI Press, 1–31.

———. 1998. 'Learning to Doctor: Reflections on Recent Accounts of the Medical School Years', in William C. Cockerham, Michael Glassen, and Linda S. Huess, eds, *Readings in Medical Sociology.* Upper Saddle River, NJ: Prentice-Hall, 335–45.

——— and Rochelle Kern, eds. 1990. *The Sociology of Health and Illness*, 3rd edn. New York: St Martin's Press.

——— and Joseph W. Schneider. 1980. *Deviance and Medicalization: From Badness to Sickness.* St Louis: Mosby.

Cooper, Lesley. 1997. 'Myalgic Encephalomyelitis and the Medical Encounter', *Sociology of Health and Illness* 19, 2: 186–207.

Cooper, R.A., and S.J. Stoflet. 1996. 'Trends in the Education and Practice of Alternative Medicine Clinicians', *Health Affairs* 15, 3: 226–38.

Cooperstock, Ruth, and Jessica Hill. 1982. *The Effects of Tranquilization: Benzodiazepine Use in Canada.* Ottawa: Health Promotion Directorate.

——— and Henry L. Lennard. 1987. 'Role Strains and Tranquilizer Use', in Coburn et al. (1987: 314–32).

Corbin, Juliet, and Anselm Strauss. 1987. 'Accompaniments of Chronic Illness: Changes in Body, Self, Biography and Biographical Time', *Research in the Sociology of Health Care* 6: 249–81.

Cornwell, Jocelyn. 1984. *Hard-Earned Lives: Accounts of Health and Illness from East London.* London: Tavistock.

Coulter, Harris L. 1984. 'Homeopathy', in *Alternative Medicines: Popular and Policy Perspectives.* New York: Tavistock, 57–9.

Cousins, Norman. 1979. *Anatomy of an Illness as Perceived by the Patient.* Toronto: Bantam Books.

———. 1983. *The Healing Heart.* New York: Norton.

———. 1989. *Head First: The Biology of Hope.* New York: E.P. Dutton.

Cowie, W. 1976. 'The Cardiac Patient's Perception of His Heart Attack', *Social Science and Medicine* 10: 87–96.

Crandall, Christian, and Dallie Moriarty. 1995. 'Physical Illness Stigma and Social Rejection', *British Journal of Social Psychology* 34: 67–83.

Crane, Diana. 1975. *The Sanctity of Social Life: Physicians' Treatment of Critically Ill Patients.* New York: Russell Sage Foundation.

Cranswick, Kelly. 1997. 'Canada's Caregivers', *Canadian Social Trends* (Winter): 2–6.

Crawford, Robert. 1984. 'A Cultural Account of Health: Control, Release, and the Social Body', in John B. McKinlay, ed., *Issues in the Political Economy of Health Care.* London: Tavistock.

Crichton, A., A. Robertson, C. Gordon, and W. Farrant. 1997. *Health Care: A Community Concern? Developments in the Organization of Canadian Health Services.* Calgary: University of Calgary Press.

Crompton, Susan. 2000. 'Health', *Canadian Social Trends* (Statistics Canada) 11, 8 (Winter): 12–15.

———. 2002. *The Daily* (Statistics Canada) (various dates).

Culane, Dara Speck. 1987. *An Error in Judgement: The Politics of Medical Care in an Indian/White Community.* Vancouver: Talon Books.

Cunningham, Alastair J. 1992. *The Healing Journey.* Toronto: Key Porter Books.

Cunningham, Rob. 1996. *Smoke and Mirrors: The Canadian Tobacco War.* International Development Research Centre.

Currie, Dawn. 1988a. 'Starvation Amidst Abundance: Female Adolescence and Anorexia', in Bolaria and Dickinson (1988: 198–216).

———. 1988b. 'Re-thinking What We Do and How We Do It: A Study of Reproductive Decisions', *Canadian Review of Sociology and Anthropology* 25, 2: 231–53.

_____ and Valerie Raoul, eds. 1992. *Anatomy of Gender: Women's Struggle for the Body*. Ottawa: Carleton University Press.

Daniels, Arlene Kaplan. 1975. 'Advisory and Coercive Functions in Psychiatry', *Sociology of Work and Occupations* 2, 1: 55–78.

D'Arcy, Carl. 1986. 'Unemployment and Health: Data and Implications', *Canadian Journal of Public Health* 77, Supp. 1: 124–31.

_____. 1987. 'Social Inequalities in Health: Implications for Priority Setting', paper presented at the Second Biennial Conference on Health Care in Canada: Setting Priorities. Waterloo, Ont.: Wilfrid Laurier University, Apr.–May.

_____. 1998. 'Health Status of Canadians', in Coburn et al. (1998: 43–68).

Davidson, W., W. Molloy, and M. Bedard. 1995. 'Physician Characteristics and Prescribing for Elderly People in New Brunswick: Relation to Patient Outcomes', *CMAJ* 152, 8: 1227–34.

Davis, D. 1979. 'Equal Treatment and Unequal Benefits: The Medical Program', in G.L. Albrecht and P.C. Higgins, eds, *Health, Illness, and Medicine*. Chicago: Rand McNally.

Davis, F. 1963. *Passage Through Crisis*. Indianapolis: Bobbs-Merrill.

Davison, Charlie, George Davey Smith, and Stephen Frankel. 1991. 'Lay Epidemiology and the Prevention Paradox: The Implication of Coronary Candidacy for Health Education', *Sociology of Health and Illness* 13, 1: 1–19.

Dema, D. 1993. 'Triple Jeopardy: Native Women with Disabilities', *Canadian Women's Studies* 113, 4: 53–5.

Demount, John. 2002. 'Growing up large', *Maclean's*, 5 Aug., 20–6.

Denscombe, Martyn. 2001. 'Uncertain identities and health-risking behaviour: The case of young people and smoking in late modernity', *British Journal of Sociology* 52, 1: 157–77.

Desai, N., E.J. Dole, S.T. Yeaton, and W.G. Troutman. 1997. 'Evaluation of Drug Information in an Internet Newsgroup', *Journal of the American Pharmaceutical Association* 37, 4: 391–4.

Devine, Carol. 1994. 'The Epidemic of HIV/AIDS in Women', *Canadian Women's Studies* 14, 3 (Summer): 17–18.

Devita, V.T., Jr, S. Hellman, and S.A. Rosenberg. 1985.

AIDS: Etiology, Diagnosis, Treatment, and Prevention. Philadelphia: J.B. Lippincott.

Devitt, Neil. 1977. 'The Transition from Home to Hospital Birth in the U.S. 1930–1960', *Birth and Family Journal* (Summer): 45–58.

Dickason, Olive Patricia. 2002. *Canada's First Nations: A History of Founding Peoples*, 3rd edn. Toronto: Oxford University Press.

Dickin McGinnis, Janice P. 1977. 'The Impact of Epidemic Influenza: Canada 1918–1919', Canadian Historical Association, *Historical Papers*.

Dickinson, Harley D., and David A. Hay. 1988. 'The Structure and Cost of Health Care in Canada', in Bolaria and Dickinson (1988: 51–74).

_____ and Mark Stobbe. 1988. 'Occupational Health and Safety in Canada', in Bolaria and Dickinson (1988: 426–38).

Dickson, Geri L. 1990. 'A Feminist Poststructural Analysis of the Knowledge of Menopause', *Advances in Nursing Science* (Apr.): 15–31.

Dimich-Ward, Helen, et al. 1988. 'Occupational Mortality among Bartenders and Waiters', *Canadian Journal of Public Health* 79 (May–June): 194–7.

Dobson, Roger. 2002. 'Number of people with diabetes will increase by 40% by 2023, says reports', *British Medical Journal* 324 (8 June): 1354.

Doll, R., and J. Peto. 1981. *The Causes of Cancer: Qualitative Estimates of Avoidable Risks of Cancer in the United States Today*. New York: Oxford University Press.

Doran, Chris. 1988. 'Canadian Workers' Compensation: Political, Medical and Health Issues', in Bolaria and Dickinson (1988: 460–72).

Dossey, Larry. 1982. *Space, Time and Medicine*. Boston: New Science Library.

_____. 1991. *Meaning and Medicine*. New York: Bantam Books.

Douglas, Mary. 1973. *Natural Symbols*. New York: Vintage Books.

Doyal, Lesley. 1979. *The Political Economy of Health*. London: Pluto Press.

Drass, Kriss. 1982. 'Negotiation and the Structure of Discourse in Medical Consultation', *Sociology of Health and Illness* 4, 3: 320–41.

Druzin, Paul, Ian Shrier, Mayer Yacowar, and Michael Rossignol. 1998. 'Discrimination Against Gay, Lesbian and Bisexual Family Physicians by Patients', *CMAJ* 158: 593–7.

Dubos, Rene. 1959. *The Mirage of Health*. Garden City, NY: Doubleday.

Dunbar, R. 1943. *Psychosomatic Diagnosis*. New York: Hoeber Press.

Dunkel-Schetter, C., and C. Wortman. 1982. 'Interpersonal Dynamics of Cancer: Problems in Social Relationships and Their Impact on the Patient', in Howard S.F. Friedman and M. Robin DeMatteo, eds, *Interpersonal Issues in Health Care*. New York: Academic Press, 69–117.

Durkheim, Émile. 1947 [1915]. *Elementary Forms of Religious Life*, trans. Joseph Ward Swain. New York: Free Press.

_____. 1951 [1879]. *Suicide*. Glencoe, Ill.: Free Press.

Dyer, Owen. 2002. 'Black twins are born to white parents after infertility treatment', *British Medical Journal* 325 (6 July): 64.

'Early Warnings: An Uproar over Accutane'. 1988. *Science* 240 (21 May): 714–15.

Eberts, Mary. 1987. *Report of the Task Force on the Implementation of Midwifery in Ontario*. Toronto: Ontario Ministry of Health.

Ebley, E.M., D.B. Hogan, and T.S. Fung. 1996. 'Correlates of Self-rated Health in Persons Aged 85 and Over: Results from the Canadian Study of Health and Aging', *Canadian Journal of Public Health* 87, 1: 28–31.

Economic and Ecological Interdependence: A Report on Selected Environment Resource Issues. 1982. Paris: Organization for Economic Co-operation and Development.

Eddy, Mary Baker. 1934. *Science and Health with a Key to the Scriptures*. Boston: Published by the Trustees under the Will of Mary Baker Eddy.

Edelstein, M.R. 1988. *Contaminated Communities*. Boulder, Colo.: Westview Press.

Educating Future Physicians for Ontario (EFPO). 1990. *Annual Report*. Hamilton: McMaster University, Faculty of Health Sciences.

_____. 1991. *Progress Report*. Hamilton: McMaster University, Faculty of Health Sciences, June.

Edwards, Nigel, Mary Jane Kornacki, and Jack Silverstein. 2002. 'Unhappy doctors: What are the causes and what can be done?', *British Medical Journal* 324: 835–8.

Ehrenreich, Barbara, M. Dowie, and S. Minkin. 1979. 'The Charge Genocide: The Accused the U.S. Government', *Mother Jones* (Nov.): 28–9.

_____ and Deirdre English. 1973a. *Witches, Midwives and Nurses: A History of Women Healers*. Old Westbury, NY: Feminist Press.

_____ and _____. 1973b. *Complaints and Disorders: The Sexual Politics of Sickness*. Old Westbury, NY: Feminist Press.

_____ and _____. 1978. *For Her Own Good: 150 Years of the Experts' Advice to Women*. New York: Anchor Press/Doubleday.

Eichler, Margrit. 1988. *Families in Canada Today*. Toronto: Gage.

Eisenberg, D.M., R.C. Kessler, C. Foster, F.E. Norlock, D.R. Calkins, T.L. Delbanco, et al. 1993. 'Unconventional Medicine in the United States: Prevalence, Costs and Patterns of Use', *New England Journal of Medicine* 328: 246–52.

_____, R.B. Davis, S.L. Appel, S. Wilkey, M. Van Rompay, and R.C. Kessler. 1998. 'Trends in Alternative Medicine Use in the United States, 1990–1997: Results of a Follow-up National Survey', *Journal of the American Medical Association (JAMA)* 280, 18: 1569–75.

Eisenberg, L. 1977. 'Disease and Illness: Distinctions between Professional and Popular Ideas of Sickness', *Culture, Medicine and Psychiatry* 1, 11: 9–23.

Elliott, S., et al. 1993. 'Modelling Psychological Effects of Exposure to Solid Waste Facilities', *Social Science and Medicine* 37, 6: 791–804.

Ellison, Christopher. 1991. 'Religious Involvement and Subjective Well-Being', *Journal of Health and Social Behavior* 32 (Mar.): 80–99.

Elstad, Jon Ivar. 1998. 'The Psych-social Perspective on Social Inequalities in Health', *Sociology of Health and Illness* 20, 5: 598–618.

Encyclopedia Britannica. 1976. Chicago: William Benton.

Engel, George L. 1971. 'Sudden and Rapid Death during Psychological Stress: Folklore or Folk Wisdom?', *Annals of Internal Medicine* 74: 771–82.

Engels, Friedrich. 1985 [1845]. *The Condition of the Working Class in England*. Stanford, Calif.: Stanford University Press.

Epp, Jake. 1986. *Achieving Health for All: A Framework for Health Promotion*. Ottawa: Minister of National Health and Welfare.

Epstein, Samuel S. 1979. *The Politics of Cancer*, rev. edn. New York: Doubleday.

_____. 1993. 'Evaluation of the National Cancer

Program and Proposed Responses', *International Journal of Health Services* 23, 1: 15–44.

———. 1994. 'Environmental and Occupational Pollutants Are Avoidable Causes of Breast Cancer', *International Journal of Health Services* 24, 1: 145–50.

———. 1998. *The Politics of Cancer Revisited*. Fremont Centre, NY: East Ridge Press.

'Everyday Carcinogens: Stopping Cancer Before It Starts'. 1999. Background paper, Workshop on Primary Cancer Prevention, 26–7 Mar., Hamilton, Ont., McMaster University.

Eyer, Joe. 1984. 'Capitalism, Health and Illness', in John B. McKinley, ed., *Issues in the Political Economy of Health Care*. New York: Tavistock, 23–59.

Eyles, John. 1993. 'From Disease Ecology and Spatial Analysis to . . . ?: The Challenges of Medical Geography in Canada', *Health and Canadian Society* 1, 1: 113–46.

———, D. Snider, J. Baxter, S.M. Taylor, and D. Willms. 1990. 'The Impacts and Effects of the Hagersville Tire Fire', *Environment Ontario: The Challenge of a New Decade* (Toronto: Environment Ontario), 2.

Fabrega, Horatio. 1973. 'Toward a Model of Illness Behaviour', *Medical Care* 11, 6: 470–84.

———. 1974. *Disease and Social Behaviour: An Interdisciplinary Perspective*. Cambridge, Mass.: MIT Press.

Facts about Chiropractic. n.d. Toronto: Ontario Chiropractic Association.

Faw, C., et al. 1977. 'Unproven Cancer Remedies', *JAMA* 238: 1536–8.

Ferguson, Eamonn, David James, and Laura Madely. 2002. 'Factors associated with success in medical school: Systematic review of the literature', *British Medical Journal* 324: 952–7.

Ferguson, J.A. 1990. 'Patient Age as a Factor in Drug Prescribing Practices', *Canadian Journal of Aging* 9: 278–95.

Fife, Betsy. 1994. 'The Conceptualization of Meaning in Illness', *Social Science and Medicine* 38, 2: 309–16.

Findlay, Deborah. 1993. 'The Good, the Normal and the Healthy: The Social Construction of Medical Knowledge about Women', *Canadian Journal of Sociology* 18, 2: 115–33.

Finlayson, Ann. 1988. 'Blood on the Coal', *Maclean's* (Oct.): N1–N4.

Firth, Matthew, James Brophy, and Margaret Keith. 1997. *Workplace Roulette: Gambling with Cancer*. Toronto: Between the Lines

Fisher, Jeffrey A. 1992. 'RX 2000: Breakthroughs in health, medicine, and longevity by the year 2000 and beyond', *Healthwatch* (Fall): 17.

Fisher, Peter, and Adam Ward. 1994. 'Complementary Medicine in Europe', *British Medical Journal* (July): 309–10.

Fisher, Sue. 1986. *In the Patient's Best Interest: Women and the Politics of Medical Decisions*. New Brunswick, NJ: Rutgers University Press.

——— and Alexandra Dundas Todd, eds. 1963. *The Social Organization of the Doctor-Patient Communication*. Washington: Center for Applied Linguistics.

Fitzpatrick, Roy, et al. 1984. *The Experience of Illness*. London: Tavistock.

Flexner, Abraham. 1910. *Medical Education in the United States and Canada. A Report to the Carnegie Foundation for the Advancement of Teaching*. Bulletin No. 4. New York: Carnegie Foundation.

Forget, Evelyn L., Raisa Deber, and Leslie L. Roos. 2002. 'Medical savings accounts: Will they reduce costs?', *Canadian Medical Association Journal* 167, 2 (23 July): 143.

Foster, Michelle, and Elizabeth Huffman. 1995. 'The Portrayal of the Elderly in Medical Journals', paper written for Qualitative Methods sociology course at Wilfrid Laurier University.

Foucault, Michel. 1973. *The Birth of Illness*, trans. A.M. Sheridan Smith. New York: Pantheon Books.

———. 1975. *The Birth of the Clinic: An Archeology of Medical Perception*, trans. A.M. Sheridan Smith. New York: Vintage Books.

Fox, Nicholas J. 1993. 'Discourse, Organization and the Surgical Ward Round', *Sociology of Health and Illness* 15, 1.

———. 1994a. 'Anaesthetists, the Discourse on Patient Fitness and the Organization of Surgery', *Sociology of Health and Illness* 16, 1: 1–18.

———. 1994b. *Postmodernism, Sociology and Health*. Toronto: University of Toronto Press.

Fox, Renee C. 1957. 'Training for Uncertainty', in Merton, Reader, and Kendall (1957: 207–18, 228–41).

_____. 1976. 'Advanced Medical Technology: Social and Ethical Implications', *Annual Review of Sociology* 2: 231–68.

_____. 1977. 'The Medicalization and Demedicalization of American Society', in John H. Knowles, ed., *Doing Better and Feeling Worse: Health in the United States*. New York: W.W. Norton, 9–22.

Frank, Arthur. 1991. *At the Will of the Body*. Boston: Houghton Mifflin.

_____. 1993. 'The Rhetoric of Self-change: Illness Experience as Narrative', *Sociological Quarterly* 32, 1: 39–52.

Frank, Jeffrey. 1996. '15 Years of AIDS in Canada', *Canadian Social Trends* (Summer): 4–7.

Frankel, Gail B., Mark Speechley, and Terence Wade. 1996. *Sociology of Health and Health Care: A Canadian Perspective*. Toronto: Copp Clark.

Frankl, V. 1965. *Man's Search for Meaning*, trans. I. Lasch. Boston: Beacon Press.

Frankenberg, Ronald. 1974. 'Functionalism and After: Theory and Development in Science Applied to the Health Field', *International Journal of Health Services* 4, 3: 411–27.

Frederick, Judith, and Janet E. Fast. 1999. 'Eldercare in Canada: Who does how much?', *Canadian Social Trends*: 26–30.

Freeland, M.S., and C.E. Schendler. 1981. 'National Health Expenditures: Short-term Outlook and Long-term Projections', *Health Care Financing Review* 2: 97–126.

Freidson, Eliot. 1970. *Professional Dominance: The Social Structure of Medical Care*. New York: Atherton Press.

_____. 1975. *The Profession of Medicine: Study in the Sociology of Applied Knowledge*. New York: Dodd Mead.

Freund, Peter, and Meredith B. McGuire. 1991. *Health, Illness and the Social Body*. Englewood Cliffs, NJ: Prentice-Hall.

Frideres, J. 1994. 'Health Promotion and Indian Communities: Social Support or Social Disorganization', in Bolaria and Bolaria (1994a: 269–96).

Fried, Peter, Barbara Watkinson, Deborah James, and Robert Gray. 2002. 'Current and former marijuana use: Preliminary findings of a longitudinal study of effects on IQ in young adults', *Canadian Medical Association Journal* 166, 7 (2 Apr.).

Friedman, Meyer, and Ray H. Rosenman. 1974. *Type A Behaviors and Your Heart*. New York: Alfred A. Knopf.

_____ et al. 1982. 'Feasibility of Altering Type A Behavior Pattern after Myocardial Infarction', *Circulation* 66, 1: 83–92.

Fries, J.F. 1980. 'Aging, Natural Death and Compression of Morbidity', *New England Journal of Medicine* 303: 130–5.

Fry, H. 1987. 'Ontario Task Force Disagrees with CMA about Need for Midwives', *CMAJ* 137, 11 (1 Dec.): 1032.

Fuchs, M. 1974. 'Health Care Patterns of Urbanized Native Americans', Ph.D. dissertation, University of Michigan.

Fuller, Colleen. 1998. *Caring for Profit: How Corporations Are Taking Over Canada's Health Care System*. Vancouver. New Star Books.

Furnham, Adrian, and Julie Forey. 1994. 'The Attitudes, Behaviours and Beliefs of Patients of Conventional vs. Complementary (Alternative) Medicine', *Journal of Clinical Psychology* 50, 3: 458–69.

_____ and Chris Smith. 1988. 'Choosing Alternative Medicine: A Comparison of the Beliefs of Patients Visiting a General Practitioner and a Homeopath', *Social Science and Medicine* 26, 7: 685–9.

Gabe, J., and M. Calnan. 1989. 'The Limits of Medicine: Women's Perception of Medical Technology', *Social Science and Medicine* 28: 223–31.

Gagnon, Louise. 2002. 'Montreal physicians protest poverty', *Canadian Medical Association Journal* 167, 1 (9 July).

Galabuzi, G.E. 2001. 'Canada's creeping economic apartheid', CSJ Foundation for Research and Education. Available at: <www.socialjustice.org>.

Gallagher, Eugene B., and C. Maureen Searle. 1989. 'Content and Context in Health Professional Education', in Howard E. Freeman and Sol Levine, eds, *Handbook of Medical Sociology*, 4th edn. Englewood Cliffs, NJ: Prentice-Hall, 437–55.

Garland, L.H. 1959. 'Studies in the Accuracy of Diagnostic Procedures', *American Journal of Roentgenology* 82: 25–38.

Gasner, Douglas. 1982. *The American Medical Association Book of Heart Disease*. New York: Random House.

General Social Survey Analysis Series. 1987. Ottawa: Statistics Canada.

Gentleman, Jane F., and Judy Lee. 1997. 'Who Doesn't Get a Mammogram', *Health Reports* 9, 1 (Summer): 19–30.

Geran, L. 1992. 'Occupational Stress', *Canadian Social Trends* (Autumn): 14–17.

Gerber, L.A. 1983. *Married to Their Careers: Career and Family Dilemmas in Doctors' Lives*. New York: Tavistock.

Ghosh, Sabitri. 2002. 'HIV/AIDS: One Generation's Story', *Voices* 9: 10.

Giacomini, M., P. Rozee-Koker, and F. Pepitone-Arreola-Rockwell. 1986. 'Gender Bias in Human Anatomy Textbook Illustrations', *Psychology of Women Quarterly* 10: 413–20.

Gibson, R.G., S.L.M. Gibson, A.D. MacNeill, W. Watson, and W. Buchanan. 1980. 'Homeopathic Therapy in Rheumatoid Arthritis: Evaluation of Double-Blind Clinical Therapeutic Trial', *British Journal of Clinical Pharmacology* 9: 453–9.

Gidney, R.D., and W.P.S. Millar. 1984. 'Origins of Organized Medicine, Ontario, 1850–1869', in Charles G. Roland, ed., *Health, Disease and Medicine: Essays in Canadian History*. Toronto: Hannah Institute for the History of Medicine, 72–95.

Gilman, Charlotte Perkins. 1973 [1899]. *The Yellow Wallpaper*. Old Westbury, NY: Feminist Press.

Glaser, Barney G., and Anselm L. Strauss. 1967. *The Discovery of Grounded Theory*. Chicago: Aldine.

_____ and _____. 1968. *Time for Dying*. Chicago: Aldine.

Globe and Mail. 12 June 1970; 5, 14 Feb. 1989.

Godon, D., J.P. Thouez, and P. Lajoie. 1989. 'Analyse géographique de l'incidence des concer au Québec en function de l'utilisation des pesticides en agriculture', *Canadian Geographer* 33: 204–17.

Goffman, Erving. 1959. 'The Moral Career of the Mental Patient', *Psychiatry* 22: 123–35.

_____. 1961. *Asylums: Essays on the Situation of Mental Patients and Other Inmates*. New York: Anchor Press/Doubleday.

_____. 1963. *Stigma: Notes on the Management of Spoiled Identity*. Englewood Cliffs, NJ: Prentice-Hall.

Goldman, Brian. 1998. 'The News on the Street: Prescription Drugs on the Black Market', *CMAJ* 159: 149–50.

Goldscheider, C. 1971. *Population, Modernization and Social Structure*. Boston: Little, Brown.

Goldstein, Jeffrey, C. Chao, E. Valentine, B. Chabon, and L. Davis. 1991. 'Use of Improved Cancer Treatments by Patients in a Radiation Oncology Department: A Survey', *Journal of Psychosocial Oncology* 9, 3: 59–66.

Good, Mary Jo, Byron J. Good, and Paul D. Cleary. 1987. 'Do Patient Attitudes Influence Physician Recognition of Psychosocial Problems in Primary Care?', *Journal of Family Practice* 25: 53–9.

Goodall, Alan. 1992. 'Motor Vehicles and Air Pollution', *Canadian Social Trends* (Spring): 21–6.

Goode, William J. 1956. 'Community within a Community: The Professions', *American Sociological Review* 22 (Apr.): 194–200.

_____. 1960. 'Encroachment, Charlatanism and the Emerging Profession: Psychology', *Sociology Review* 25, 6: 902–14.

_____. 1969. 'The Theoretical Limits of Professionalization', in Amitai Ezioni, ed., *The Semi-Professions and Their Organizations: Teachers, Nurses, Social Workers*. New York: Free Press.

Gordon, Deborah R. 1988. 'Tenacious Assumptions in Western Medicine', in M. Locke and D.R. Gordon, eds, *Biomedicine Examined*. Dordrecht, Netherlands: Kluwer, 19–56.

Gordon, Sidney, and Ted Allan. 1952. *The Scalpel, The Sword*. Toronto: McClelland & Stewart.

Gorey, Kevin M., Eric J. Holowaty, Ethan Lauckkanen, Gordon Fehringer, and Nancy L. Richter. 1998a. 'Association between Socioeconomic Status and Cancer Incidence in Toronto, Ontario: Possible Confounding of Cancer Mortality by Incidence and Survival', *Cancer Prevention and Control* 2: 236–41.

_____, _____, _____, _____, and _____. 1998b. 'An International Comparison of Cancer Survival: Advantages of Toronto's Poor over the Near Poor of Detroit', *Canadian Journal of Public Health* 89, 2: 102–4.

Gort, Elaine. 1986. 'A Social History of Naturopathy in Ontario: The Formation of an Occupation', MA thesis, University of Toronto.

Gouldner, Alvin W. 1970. *The Coming Crisis in Western Sociology*. New York: Basic Books.

Gove, N.R. 1973. 'Sex, Marital Status and Mortality', *American Journal of Sociology* 79: 45–67.

Graham, Hilary. 1984. *Women, Health and the Family*.

Brighton, Sussex: Wheatsheaf Books.

———. 1985. 'Providers, Negotiators, Mediators: Women as the Hidden Carers', in Ellen Lewis and Virginia Olesen, eds, *Women, Health and Healing: Toward a New Perspective*. New York: Tavistock, 25–52.

Graham, Kathryn, and David Vidal-Zeballos. 1998. 'Analysis of Use of Tranquilizers and Sleeping Pills Across Five Surveys of the Same Population (1985–1991): The Relationship with Gender, Age, and Use of Other Substances', *Social Science and Medicine* 46, 3: 381–95.

Graham, Wendy. 1994. 'Sexual Harassment of Physicians', *Women's Health Office Newsletter* (14 Apr).

Gray, Charlotte. 1998. 'The Private Sector Invades Medical's Home-Town', *CMAJ* 15, 9: 165–7.

———. 2002. 'MDs still the key to eliminating unfit drivers, jury decides', *Canadian Medical Association Journal* 166, 9 (30 Apr.).

Gray, David. 1993. 'Perceptions of Stigma: The Parents of Autistic Children', *Sociology of Health and Illness* 15, 1.

Gray, Gwen. 1998. 'Access to Medical Law Under Strain: New Pressures in Canada and Australia', *Journal of Health Politics, Policy and Law* 23, 6: 905–47.

Gray, Ross. 1998. 'Four Perspectives on Unconventional Therapies', *Health* 2, 1: 55–74.

——— et al. 1990. 'Empowerment and Persons with Cancer: Politics in Cancer Medicine', *Journal of Palliative Care* 6, 2: 33–45.

Grimes, David A. 1993. 'Editorial: Over-the-Counter Oral Contraceptives—An Immodest Proposal', *American Journal of Public Health* 83, 8: 1092–3.

Grippando, Gloria M. 1986. *Nursing Perspectives and Issues*, 3rd edn. Albany, NY: Delmar.

Gross, M.J., and C.W. Schwenger. 1981. *Health Care for the Elderly in Ontario*. Toronto: Ontario Economic Council.

Growe, S.J. 1991. 'The Nature and Type of Doctors' Cultural Assumptions about Patients as Men', *Sociological Focus* 24, 3: 211–23.

Grymonpre, R.E., P.A. Metenko, et al. 1988. 'Drug Associated Hospital Admission in Older Medical Patients', *Journal of American Geriatric Society* 36: 1092–8.

Guyatt, Gordon, Armine Yalnizyan, and P.J. Devereaux.

2002. 'Solving the public healthcare sustainability puzzle', *Canadian Medical Association Journal* 167, 1 (9 July).

Hacker, Charlotta. 1974. *The Indomitable Lady Doctors*. Toronto: Clarke, Irwin.

Hall, Edward T. 1977. *Beyond Culture*. Garden City, NY: Anchor Press/Doubleday.

Hall, Emmett M. 1980. *Canadian National-Provincial Health Program for the 1980's: A Commitment for Renewal*. Ottawa: National Health and Welfare.

Hall, Oswald. 1946. 'Some Organizational Consideration in Professional-Organizational Relationship', *Administrative Science Quarterly* 12, 3: 461–78.

———. 1948. 'The Stages of a Medical Career', *American Journal of Sociology* 53 (Mar.): 328–36.

Ham, Chris, and K.G.M.M. Alberti. 2002. 'The medical profession, the public and the government', *British Medical Journal* 324 (6 Apr.): 838–42.

Hamilton, J.T. 1995. 'Testing for Environmental Racism: Prejudice, Profits, Political Power?', *Journal of Policy Analysis and Management* 14: 104–32.

Hamilton, Vivian, and Barton Hamilton. 1993. 'Does Universal Health Insurance Equalize Access to Care?: A Canadian-U.S. Comparison', paper presented at Northwestern University Fourth Annual Health Economics Workshop, Aug.

Hamilton, V. Lee, Clifford L. Broman, William S. Hoffman, and Deborah S. Renner. 1990. 'Hard Times and Vulnerable People: Initial Effects of Plant Closings on Auto Workers' Mental Health', *Journal of Health and Social Behavior* 31 (June): 123–40.

Hammer, Vicki. 1981. 'So Many Like Her', *World Health* (Geneva: World Health Organization).

Hamowy, Ronald. 1984. *Canadian Medicine: A Study in Restricted Entry*. Vancouver: Fraser Institute.

Hanvey, Louise, Denise Avard, Ian Graham, Kristen Underwood, Joan Campbell, and Carrie Kelly. 1994. *The Health of Canada's Children: A CICH Profile*, 2nd edn. Ottawa: Canadian Institute of Child Health.

Harden, Bonnie L., and Craig R. Harden. 1997. *Alternative Health Care: The Canadian Directory*. Toronto: Noble Ages Publishing.

Hardey, M. 1998. *The Social Context of Health*. Milton Keynes: Open University Press.

Harding, Jim. 1987. 'The Pharmaceutical Industry as a

Public Health Hazard and an Institution of Social Control', in Coburn et al. (1987: 314–32).

_____. 1994a. 'Environmental Degradation and Rising Cancer Rates: Exploring the Links in Cancer', in Bolaria and Dickinson (1994: 649–67).

_____. 1994b. 'Social Basis of the Over Prescribing of Mood-Modifying Pharmaceuticals to Women', in Bolaria and Bolaria (1994b: 157–81).

Harding, T.W., and W. Curran. 1978. *The Law and Mental Health: Harmonizing Objectives*. Geneva: World Health Organization.

Harpur, Tom. 1994. *Uncommon Touch*. Toronto: McClelland & Stewart.

Harrison, Michelle. 1982. *A Woman in Residence*. New York: Random House.

Heacock, Helen Jane, and Jason Keller Rivers. 1986. 'Occupational Diseases of Hairdressers', *Canadian Journal of Public Health* 77 (Mar.–Apr.): 109–13.

Heagerty, John J. 1928. *Four Centuries of Medical History in Canada*, 2 vols. Toronto: Macmillan.

Health and Social Support 1985. 1987. Series No. 1 of General Social Survey Analysis Series. Ottawa: Statistics Canada.

Health and the Status of Women. 1980. Geneva: World Health Organization.

Health and Welfare Canada. 1982, 1984. *National Health Expenditures in Canada 1970–1982*. Ottawa.

_____. 1986. *Issues for Health Promotion in Family and Child Health: A Sourcebook*. Ottawa: Medical Service Branch, Indian and Inuit Services.

_____, Mental Health Division. 1984. *Alzheimer's Disease: A Family Information Handbook*. Ottawa: Published in Co-operation with the Alzheimer Society.

_____ and Statistics Canada. 1981. *The Health of Canadians: Report of the Canada Health Survey*. Cat. no. 82–538E. Ottawa: Minister of Supply and Services and the Ministry of National Health and Welfare.

Health, Health Care and Medicine: A Report to the National Council of Welfare. 1990. Ottawa.

Health Promotion. 1987, 1988. Ottawa: Health and Welfare Canada.

'The "Heart of Ontario": The Where, Why and Who of Cardiovascular Disease', *Informed* 5, 2: 1–3.

Hemminki, Elina. 1975. 'Review of Literature on the Factors Affecting Drug Prescribing', *Social Science and Medicine* 9: 111–15.

Hilfiker, David. 1985. *Healing the Wounds: A Physician Looks at His Work*. New York: Pantheon Books.

Hoffman-Goetz, Laurie, and Juanne N. Clarke. 2000. 'Quality of breast cancer sites on the World Wide Web', *Canadian Journal of Public Health* 91: 281–4.

Holling, S.A. 1981. 'Primitive Medicine among the Indians of Ontario', in Holling et al., eds, *Medicine for Heroes*. Mississauga, Ont.: Mississauga Historical Society.

Holmes, T.H., and M. Masuda. 1974. 'Life Change and Illness Susceptibility', in B.S. and B.P. Dohrenwend, eds, *Stressful Life Events: Their Nature and Effect*. New York: Wiley.

_____ and R.H. Rahe. 1967. 'The Social Readjustment Rating Scale', *Journal of Psychosomatic Research* 11: 213–18.

Hopkins, Janne Janice. 2002. 'High level of resources for neonatal intensive care do not give better outcome', *British Medical Journal* 324: 1353.

Horn, Joshua. 1969. *Away With All Pests: An English Surgeon in People's China, 1954–1969*. New York: Monthly Review Press.

Horowitz, Lawrence C. 1988. *Taking Charge of Your Medical Fate*. New York: Random House.

'Horror Stories Start with Pill, End in Murder'. 1992. *Winnipeg Free Press*, 20 Dec., A11.

House, J., K.R. Landis, and D. Umberson. 1988. 'Social Relationships and Health', *Science* 241: 540–5.

Howson, Alexandra. 1998. 'Surveillance, Knowledge and Risk: The Embodied Experience of Cervical Screening', *Health* 2, 2: 195–215.

Hughes, C.C. 1967. 'Ethnomedicine', in David Gills, ed., *International Encyclopedia of Social Sciences*, vol. 10. New York: Macmillan and Free Press, 87–92.

Hughes, David. 1989. 'Paper and People: The Work of the Casual Receptions Clerk', *Sociology of Health and Illness* 11, 4: 382–408.

Hughes, Everett C. 1971. *The Sociological Eye*. Chicago: Aldine-Atherton.

Hunt, Charles W. 1989. 'Migrant Labour and Sexually Transmitted Disease: AIDS in Africa', *Journal of Health and Social Behavior*.

Hunt, L., B. Jordan, S. Irwin, and C.H. Browner. 1989. 'Compliance and the Patient's Perspective: Controlling Symptoms in Everyday Life', *Culture, Medicine and Psychiatry* 13: 315–34.

Hutchinson, James M., and Robert N. Foley. 1999. 'Method of Physician Renumeration and Rates of Antibiotic Prescription' *CMAJ* 160: 1013–17.

Hutten-Czapski, Peter. 2000. 'Primary care reform: A rural perspective discussion paper'. Society of Rural Physicians of Canada, available at: <www.srpc.org>.

Ideas. 1983. 'We Know Best: Experts' Advice to Women'. Toronto: Canadian Broadcasting Corporation, 2–23 Jan., broadcast transcript.

Illich, Ivan. 1976. *Limits to Medicine*. Toronto: McClelland & Stewart.

'Ill-planned cuts hurt SARS fight'. 2003. *Toronto Star*, 9 May, A30.

Imbert, Lorrie. 1993. 'Ayurveda: Ancient Medicine for Modern Times', *Health Naturally* (Oct.–Nov.): 5–7.

Imman, Wallace. 1996. 'Alternate Treatments Gaining Ground', *Globe and Mail*, 28 Dec., A3.

Impicciatore, P., C. Pandolfini, N. Casella, and M. Bonati. 1994. 'Reliability of Health Information for the Public on the World Wide Web. Systematic Survey of Advice on Managing Fever in Children at Home', *British Medical Journal* 314: 1875–81.

Indian Conditions—A Survey. 1980. Ottawa: Minister of Indian Affairs and Northern Development.

Jackson, Marni. 2002. 'Smoke out of politicians', *Globe and Mail*, 26 Aug., A11.

James, W.J., and S. Lieberman. 1975. 'What the American Public Knows About Cancer and Cancer Tests,' in Patricia Hubbs, ed., *Public Education About Cancer*. Geneva: International Union Against Cancer.

Jarvis, G.K., and M. Boldt. 1982. 'Death Styles Among Canada's Indians', *Social Science and Medicine* 16: 1345–52.

Jeffcoate, Thomas N.A. 1957. *Principles of Gynecology*. London: Butterworth and Co.

Jefferis, Barbara J.M.H., Chris Power, and Clyde Hertzman. 2002. 'Birth weight, childhood socio-economic environment, and cognitive development in the 1958 British cohort study', *British Medical Journal* 325 (10 Aug.): 305.

Jennett, P.A., M. Cooper, S. Edworthy, et al. 1991. 'Consumer Use of Official Health Care: Facts and Implications', Proceedings of the 5th ACMC Conference on Physician Manpower, Association of Canadian Medical Colleges, Ottawa, 28 Apr.

Jensen, Phyllis Marie. 1988. 'Nursing', in *The Canadian Encyclopedia*, vol. 3. Edmonton: Hurtig, 1546.

Jerrett, Michael, John Eyles, and Donald Cole. 1998. 'Socio-economic and Environmental Covariates of Premature Mortality in Ontario', *Social Science and Medicine* 47, 1: 33–49.

Jin, Robert L., Chandrekant P. Shah, and Tonislav J. Svoboda. 1994. 'The Health Impact of Unemployment', unpublished paper, available from Dr C.P. Shah, Faculty of Medicine, University of Toronto.

Johnson, H. 1996. *Osler's Web*. New York: Crown Publishers.

Johnson, M. 1975. 'Medical Sociology and Sociological Theory', *Social Science and Medicine* 9: 227–32.

Johnson, Robert J., and Frederic D. Wolinsky. 1990. 'The Legacy of Stress Research: The Course and Impact of This Journal', *Journal of Health and Social Behavior* 32 (Sept.): 217–25.

Johnson, Terence. 1972. *The Professions and Power*. London: Macmillan

———. 1977. 'Industrial Society: Class, Change and Control', in R. Scase, ed., *The Professions in the Class Structure*. London: Allen and Unwin, 93–110.

———. 1982. 'Social Class and the Division of Labour', in A. Giddens and G. Mackenzie, eds, *The State and the Professions: Peculiarities of the British*. Cambridge: Cambridge University Press, 182–208.

Johnstone, Tracey, and Julie Robinson. 1995. '*Shape* versus *Men's Fitness*: Are Fitness Magazines Different for Each Sex?', paper for Qualitative Research Methods course, Wilfred Laurier University.

Jonas, H.A., and J. Lunly. 1993. 'Triplets and Quadruplets Born in Victoria between 1982 and 1990: The Impact of IUF and GIFT in Rising Birthrates', *Medical Journal of Australia* 17, 5: 158; 17, 10: 659–63.

Jones, K., and G. Moon. 1987. *Health, Disease and Society*. London: Routledge & Kegan Paul.

Jones, W.H.S. 1943. *Hippocrates*, vol. 2. London: Heinemann.

Jossa, Diana. 1985. *Smoking Behaviour of Canadians 1983*. Ottawa: National Health and Welfare.

Judd, Charles M., Eliot R. Smith, and Louise H. Kidder.

1991. *Research Methods in Social Relations*, 6th edn. Fort Worth, Texas: Holt, Rinehart and Winston.

Justice, Blair. 1987. *Who Gets Sick: Thinking and Health*. Houston: Peak Press.

Kanter, Rosabeth Moss. 1977. *Men and Women of the Corporation*. New York: Basic Books.

Kaperski, Janet M. 2001. 'Where have all the doctors gone? Responses to the George Panel on health professional human resources report'. Toronto: Ontario College of Family Physicians.

Kaplan, Howard B. 1991. 'Social Psychology and the Immune System: A Conceptual Framework and Review of the Literature', *Social Science and Medicine*: 909–23.

Karliner, Joshua. 1994. 'Toxin Town', *New Statesman and Society* 7, 2 (2 Dec.): 18.

Kassulke, Desley, Karen Stenner-Day, Michael Coory, and Ian Ring. 1993. 'Information-seeking Behaviour and Sources of Health Information: Associations with Risk Factor Status in an Analysis of Three Queensland Electorates', *Australian Journal of Public Health* 17, 1.

Katzmarzyk, Peter T. 2002. 'The Canadian obesity epidemic, 1985–1998', *Canadian Medical Association Journal* 166 (16 Apr.): 8.

Kaufert, Patricia. 1988. 'Through Women's Eyes: The Case for Feminist Epidemiology', *Healthsharing*: 10–13.

———. 1992. 'Mammography and the Misplacement of Faith', paper presented at the American Anthropological Association annual meeting, San Francisco.

——— and P. Gilbert. 1987. 'Medicalization and the Menopause', in Coburn et al. (1987).

Keating, M. 1986. *To the Last Drop: Canada and the World's Water Crisis*. Toronto. Macmillan.

Kelly, Ken. 1962. 'Baby-Deforming Drug Sold First as Sleeping Pill', *Kitchener-Waterloo Record*, 17 Aug., 27.

Kelly, O. 1979. *Until Tomorrow Comes*. New York: Everest House.

Kelner, Merrijoy, Oswald Hall, and Jan Coultner. 1980. *Chiropractors: Do They Help?* Toronto: Fitzhenry & Whiteside.

Kemery, Anna. 2002. 'Driven to Excel: A Portrait of Canada's Workaholics', *Canadian Social Trends* (Spring): 2–6.

Kendall. P.P., and G.G. Reader. 1988. 'Innovations in Medical Education of the 1950's Contrasted with Those of the Early 1970's and 1980's', *Journal of Health and Social Behavior* 29, 4: 279–93.

Kidder, Louise H. 1986. *Research Methods in Social Relations*. New York: Holt, Rinehart and Winston.

Kim, Kwang Kee, and Phillip M. Moody. 1992. 'More Resources, Better Health? A Cross-National Perspective', *Social Science and Medicine* 34, 8: 837–42.

Kirk, Jo-Ann. 1994. 'A Feminist Analysis of Women in Medical School', in Bolaria and Dickinson (1994: 158–83).

Kirkby, Pat. 1986. *Education for Excellence 1986/1987*. Toronto: Registered Nurses Association of Ontario.

Kirkmayer, Laurence J. 1988. 'Mind and Body as Metaphor: Hidden Values in Biomedicine', in M. Lock and E.R. Gordon, eds, *Biomedicine Examined*. Dordrecht, Netherlands: Kluwer, 57–93.

Klass, Alan. 1975. *There's Gold in Them Thar Pills*. London: Penguin Books.

Klein, J.D., et al. 1993. 'Adolescents' Risky Behavior and Mass Media Use', *Pediatrics* 92, 1 (July): 24–31.

Kleinman, Arthur. 1988. *The Illness Narratives: Suffering, Healing and the Human Condition*. New York: Basic Books.

Koblinsky, M., J. Timyan, and J. Gay. 1993. *The Health of Women: A Global Perspective*. Boulder, Colo.: Westview Press.

Koss, Mary P., Lori Heise, and Nancy F. Russo. 1994. 'The Global Health Burden of Rape', *Psychology of Women Quarterly* 18: 509–37.

Kowser, Omer Hashi, and Joan Silver. 1994. 'No Words Can Express: Two Voices on Female Genital Mutilation', *Canadian Women's Studies* 14, 3: 62–5.

Kramer, Peter D. 1993. *Listening to Prozac*. New York: Penguin Books.

Krause, Elliot A. 1978. *Power and Illness: The Political Sociology of Health and Medical Care*. New York: Elsevier.

Kroll-Smith, Steve, and Anthony E. Ladd. 1993. 'Environmental Illness and Biomedicine: Anomalies, Exemplars and the Politics of the Body', Visiting Fellow Centre for Disaster Management, University of New England, Armidale NSW, Australia.

Kronenfeld, Jennie Jacobs, Mark Reiser, Deborah C. Glik, Carlos Alatorre, and Kirby Jackson. 1997. 'Safety Behaviours of Mothers of Young Children: Impact of Cognitive, Stress and Background Factors', *Health* 1, 2: 205–25.

Kuhn, Thomas. 1962. *The Structure of Scientific Revolutions*. Chicago: University of Chicago Press.

LaFlamme, Lucie, and Karin Engstom. 2002. 'Socio-economic differences in Swedish children and adolescents injured in road traffic incidents: A cross-sectional study', *British Medical Journal* 324: 396–7.

Lalonde, Marc. 1974. *A New Perspective on the Health of Canadians*. Ottawa: Information Canada.

Langlois, Stéphanie, and Peter Morrison. 2002. 'Suicide Deaths and Attempts', *Canadian Social Trends* (Autumn): 20–5.

Langone, John. 1982. *Chiropractors*. New York: Addison-Wesley.

Last, J. 1963. 'The Iceberg: Completing the Clinical Picture in General Practice', *Lancet* 2, 729: 28–31.

'Last Gasp'. 1992. *Equinox* (May–June): 85–98.

LaVeist, Thomas A. 1992. 'The Political Empowerment and Health Status of African-Americans: Mapping a New Territory', *American Journal of Sociology* 97, 4: 1080–95.

Lawton, R., and D. Parker. 2002. 'Barriers to incident reporting in a healthcare system', *Quality and Safety in Health Care* 11: 15–18.

Lazarus, Ellen S. 1997. 'Politicizing Abortion: Personal Morality and Professional Responsibility of Residents Training in the United States', *Social Science and Medicine* 44, 9: 1417–25.

Lazarus, R.S., and A. Delongis. 1983. 'Psychological Stress and Coping in Aging', *American Psychologist* 38: 245–54.

Lee, Charles. 1987. *Toxic Waste and Race in the U.S.* New York Commission for Racial Justice, United Church of Christ.

Lemmens, Trudo, and L. Peter Singer. 1998. 'Bioethics for Clinicians: Conflict of Interest in Research, Education, and Patient Care', *CMAJ* 159: 960–5.

Lerner, Michael. 1994. *Choices in Healing*. Cambridge, Mass.: MIT Press.

Lesage, J. 1991. 'Polypharmacy in Geriatric Patients', *Nursing Clinics of North America* 26: 273–90.

LeShan, Larry. 1978. *You Can Fight for Your Life*. New York: M. Evans.

Levin, J.S. 1993. 'Esoteric vs. Exoteric Explanations for Findings Linking Spirituality and Health', *Advances* 9, 4: 54–6.

_____ and P.L. Schiller. 1987. 'Is There a Religious Factor in Health?', *Journal of Religion and Health* 26, 1: 9–36.

_____ and H.Y. Vanderpool. 1989. 'Is Religion Therapeutically Significant for Hypertension?', *Social Science and Medicine* 29, 1: 69–78.

Levin, Lowell S., and Ellen L. Idler. 1981. *The Hidden Health Care System*. Cambridge, Mass.: Ballinger.

Levine, Mitchell A.H., and Ashish Pradhan. 1999. 'Can the Health Care System Buy Better Antibiotic Prescribing Behaviour?', *CMAJ* 160: 1023–4.

Lewinsohn, Rachel. 1998. 'Medical Theories, Science and the Practice of Medicine', *Social Science and Medicine* 46, 10: 1261–70.

Lewis, Charles E., and Mary Anne Lewis. 1977. 'The Potential Impact of Sexual Inequality on Health', *New England Journal of Medicine* 297 (Oct.): 863–9.

Lexchin, Joel. 1984. *The Real Pushers: A Critical Analysis of the Canadian Drug Industry*. Vancouver: New Star Books.

_____. 1988a. 'Profits First: The Pharmaceutical Industry in Canada', in Bolaria and Dickinson (1988: 497–513).

_____. 1988b. 'Pushing Pills: Who's to Blame for So Much Poor Prescribing?', *Globe and Mail*, 13 Dec., A7.

_____. 1988c. 'Pharmaceutical Industry', in *The Canadian Encyclopedia*, vol. 3. Edmonton: Hurtig, 1653–4.

_____. 1990. 'Drug Makers and Drug Regulators: Too Close for Comfort: A Study of the Canadian Situation', *Social Science and Medicine* 31, 11: 1257–63.

_____. 1991. 'Adverse Drug Reaction: Review of the Canadian Literature', *Canadian Family Physician* 37: 109–18.

_____. 1994a. 'Profits First: The Pharmaceutical Industry in Canada', in Bolaria and Dickinson (1994: 700–20).

_____. 1994b. 'Canadian Marketing Codes: How Well Are They Controlling Pharmaceutical Promotion', *International Journal of Health Services* 24, 1: 91–104.

_____. 1996. 'Cost-Effective Pharmaceutical Care for the Elderly and the Formulation of

Pharmaceutical Policy in Canada', *Health and Canadian Society* 3, 1–2: 119–33.

———. 1998. 'Improving the Appropriateness of Physician Prescribing', *International Journal of Health Services* 28, 2: 253–67.

Liang, B.A. 2002. 'A system of medical error disclosure', *Quality and Safety in Health Care* 11: 64–8.

Liang, M.H., et al. 1973. 'Chinese Health Care: Determinants of the System', *American Journal of Public Health* 63, 2: 102–10.

Light, Donald W., and Grace Budrys. 1992. 'Health Care Technology: Social Construction of Reality', unpublished paper, Rutgers University and DePaul University.

Linde, Klaus, Nicola Clasius, Gilbert Ramirez, Dieter Melchart, Florian Eitel, Larry V. Hedges, and Wayne B. Toras. 1997. 'Are the Clinical Effects of Homeopathy Placebo Effects? A Meta-analysis of Placebo-controlled Trials', *Lancet* 350 (20 Sept.): 834–41.

Litoff, J. 1978. *American Midwives: 1860 to the Present.* Westport, Conn.: Greenwood Press.

Lock, Margaret, and Gilles Bibeau. 1993. 'Healthy Disputes: Some Reflections on the Practice of Medical Anthropology in Canada', *Health and Canadian Society* 1, 6: 147–76.

Locke, Michael, and Joel G. Ray. 1999. 'Higher Neonatal Morbidity After Routine Early Hospital Discharge: Are We Sending Newborns Home Too Early?', *CMAJ* 161: 249–53.

Lorber, J. 1975. 'Women and Medical Sociology: Invisible Professionals and Ubiquitous Patients', in M. Millman and R. Kanter, eds, *Another Voice.* New York: Anchor Books, 75–105.

———. 1984. *Women Physicians, Careers, Statuses and Power.* New York: Tavistock.

Loring, Marti, and Brian Powell. 1988. 'Gender, Race and DSM-III: A Study of the Objectivity of Psychiatric Diagnostic Behaviours', *Journal of Health and Social Behavior* 29 (Mar.): 1–22.

Lupton, Deborah. 1993. 'Risk as Moral Danger: The Social Political Functions of Risk Discourse in Public Health', *International Journal of Health Services* 23, 3: 425–35.

———. 1994. 'Femininity, Responsibility and the Technological Imperative: Discourses on Breast Cancer in the Australian Press', *International Journal of Health Services* 24, 1: 73–89.

Lynch, James L. 1977. *The Broken Heart: The Medical Consequences of Loneliness.* New York: Basic Books.

McAndrew, Brian. 1999. 'Innu Suicide Rate Highest in World', *Toronto Star*, 8 Nov., A1, A14.

McCormack, Thelma. 1991. 'Public Policies and Reproductive Technology: A Feminist Critique', *Research in the Sociology of Health Care* 9: 105–24.

McCormick, Rod, Richard Nedan, Paul McNicoll, and Judith Lynam. 1997. 'Taking Back the Wisdom: Moving Forward to Recovery and Action', *Canadian Journal of Community Mental Health* 16, 2: 5–8.

McCrea, F.B. 1983. 'The Politics of Menopause: The Discovery of a Deficiency Disease', *Social Problems* 31, 1: 111–23.

McDaniel, Susan. 1988. 'Women's Roles. Reproduction and the New Reproductive Technologies: A New Stork Rising', in Nancy Mandell and Ann Duffy, eds, *Reconstructing the Canadian Family: Feminist Perspectives.* Toronto: Butterworths, 175–207.

McDonough, Peggy. 1997. 'Income Dynamics and Mortality', *Institute for Social Research Newsletter* 12, 3: 1–3.

MacIntyre, S., and D. Oldman. 1984. 'Coping with Migraine', in N. Black et al., eds, *Health and Disease, A Reader.* Milton Keynes: Open University Press, 271–5.

Macionis, John T., et al. 1994. *Sociology*, Canadian edn. Englewood Cliffs, NJ: Prentice-Hall.

McKeown, T. 1976. *The Role of Medicine: Dream, Mirage or Nemesis.* London: Neufeld Provincial Hospitals Trust.

——— and R.G. Record. 1975. 'An Interpretation of the Decline of Mortality in England and Wales during the Twentieth Century', *Population Studies* 29: 391–422.

McKinlay, John B. 1982. 'Toward the Proletarianization of Physicians', in C. Derber, ed., *Professionals as Workers.* Boston: Hall, 37–62.

———. 1996. 'Some Contribution from the Social System to Gender Inequality in Heart Disease', *Journal of Health and Social Behavior* 37, 1: 1–26.

——— and Sonja M. McKinlay. 1977. 'The Questionable Contribution of Medical Measures to the Decline of Mortality in the United States in the Twentieth Century', *Milbank Memorial Fund Quarterly* (Summer): 405–28.

——— and ———. 1981. 'From Promising Report to

Standard Procedure: Seven Stages in the Career of a Medical Innovation', *Milbank Memorial Fund Quarterly* 59: 374–411.

_____ and _____. 1987. 'Medical Measures and the Decline of Mortality', in Howard D. Schwartz, ed., *Dominant Issues in Medical Sociology*, 2nd edn. New York: Random House.

McKinlay, Sonja M. 1971. 'Some Approaches and Problems in the Study of the Use of Services: An Overview', *Journal of Health and Social Behavior* 13: 115–52.

McLaughlin, John R., Anthony Fields, Jane Gentleman, Isra Levy, Barbara Wylie, Heather Whittaker, Rod Riley, Judy Lee, B. Ann Coombs, and Leslie Gaudette. 1997. 'Cancer Incidence and Mortality', *Health Reports* 8, 4 (Spring): 41–52.

MacLeod, L. 1987. *Wife Battering in Canada: The Vicious Circle*. Report of the Canadian Advisory Council on the Status of Women. Ottawa: Ministry of Supply and Services.

McLeod, Thomas H., and Ina McLeod. 1987. *Tommy Douglas: The Road to Jerusalem*. Edmonton: Hurtig

McNab, E. 1970. *A Legal History of Health Professions in Ontario*. Committee on the Healing Arts. Toronto: Queen's Printer.

Major, Ralph H. 1954. *A History of Medicine*, 2 vols. Springfield, Ill.: Thomas.

Makdessian, Frances. 1987. *Occupational Health and Safety Management Book*. Don Mills, Ont.: Corpus Information Services.

Manga, Pran. 1993. 'Health Economics and the Current Health Care Cost Crisis: Contributions and Controversies', *Health and Canadian Society* 1, 1: 177–203.

Manning, Peter K., and Horatio Fabrega. 1973. 'The Experience of Self and Body: Health and Illness in the Chiapas Highlands', in George Psathas, ed., *Phenomenological Sociology*. New York: John Wiley and Sons, 251–301.

Mansour, Valerie. 1995. 'Judge Ends Trial in N.S. Mine Deaths', *Toronto Star*, 10 June, A3.

Mao, Y., H. Morrison, R. Semenciw, and D. Wigle. 1986. 'Mortality on Canadian Indian Reserves, 1977–1982', *Canadian Journal of Public Health* 77: 263–8.

Marchak, Patricia, 1975. *Ideological Perspectives on Canada*. Toronto: McGraw-Hill.

Markowitz, Fred, E. 1998. 'The Effects of Stigma on the Psychological Well-Being and Life Satisfaction of Persons with Mental Illness', *Journal of Health and Social Behavior* 39, 4: 335–47.

Marks, Geoffrey, and William K. Beatty. 1976. *Epidemics*. New York: Charles Scribner's.

Marshall, V.W. 1980. *Last Chapters: A Sociology of Aging and Dying*. Monterey Calif.: Brooks/Cole Publishing.

Martin, Emily. 1987. *The Woman in the Body: A Cultural Analysis of Reproduction*. Boston: Beacon Press.

Martin, Peter. 2001. 'Individual and social resources predicting well-being and functioning in the later years: Conceptual models, research and practice', *Aging International* 27, 2: 3–29.

Martindale, Don. 1960. *The Nature and Types of Sociological Theory*. Boston: Houghton Mifflin.

Marx, Karl. 1964. *The Economic and Philosophic Manuscripts of 1844*, trans. M. Milligan. New York: International Publishers.

May, Carl, and Deepak Sirur. 1998. 'Art, Science and Placebo: Incorporating Homeopathy in General Practice', *Sociology of Health and Illness* 20, 2: 168–90.

May, J., and J. Wasserman. 1984. 'Selected Results from an Evaluation of the New Jersey Diagnosis-related Group System', *Health Services Research* 19, 5 (Dec.): 548.

Meador, Clifton. 1965. 'The Art and Science of Non-Disease', *New England Journal of Medicine* 235: 424–45.

Mechanic, David. 1978. *Medical Sociology: A Comprehensive Text*. New York: Free Press.

_____. 1993. 'Sociological Research in Health and the American Socio-political Context', *Social Science and Medicine* 36, 2: 95–102.

Meddison, D., and W.L. Walker. 1967. 'Factors Affecting the Outcome of Conjugal Bereavement', *British Journal of Psychiatry* 113: 1057–67.

Meichenbaum, Donald. 1983. *Coping with Stress*. Toronto: Wiley.

Merton, Robert K., George Reader, and Patricia Kendall, eds. 1957. *The Student Physician: Introductory Studies in the Sociology of Medical Education*. Cambridge, Mass.: Harvard University Press.

Mhatra, Sharmila, and Raisa B. Deber. 1992. 'From Equal Access to Health Care to Equitable Access to Health: A Review of Canadian Provincial Health Commissions and Reports', *International Journal of Health Services* 22, 4: 645–68.

Milgram, Stanley. 1974. *Obedience to Authority*. New York: Harper & Row.

Millar, Wayne. 1992. 'A Trend to a Healthier Lifestyle', *Canadian Social Trends* (Spring).

———, Jill Strachan, and Surinder Wadhera. 1993. 'Trends in Low Birthweight', *Canadian Social Trends* 28 (Spring): 26–9.

Millman, Marcia. 1977. *The Unkindest Cut*. New York: William Morrow.

Mills, C. Wright. 1959. *The Sociological Imagination*. New York: Oxford University Press.

Mills, Donald, 1964. *Royal Commission on Health Services Study of Chiropractors, Osteopaths, and Naturopaths in Canada*. Ottawa: Queen's Printer.

Min, Simon T., and Donald A. Redelmeier. 1998. 'Car Phones and Car Crashes: An Ecologic Analysis', *Canadian Journal of Public Health* (May–June): 157–61.

Mintzes, Barbara, Morris L. Barer, Richard L. Kravitz, et al. 2002. 'Influence of direct to consumer pharmaceutical advertising and patients' requests on prescribing decisions: Two site cross-sectional survey', *British Medical Journal* 324: 278–9.

Mishler, Elliot. 1984. *The Discourse of Medicine: Dialectics of Medical Interviews*. Norwood, NJ: Ablex.

Mitchinson, Wendy. 1987. 'Medical Perceptions of Healthy Women: The Case of Nineteenth Century Canada', *Canadian Women's Studies* 8, 4: 42–3.

Montbriand, J.J. 1994. 'An Overview of Alternate Therapies Chosen by Patients with Cancer', *Oncology Nursing Forum* 21, 9: 1547–54.

———. 1995. 'Decision Tree Model Describing Alternative Health Care Choices Made by Oncology Patients', *Cancer Nursing* 18, 4: 104–17.

Montini, Theresa, and Kathleen Slobin. 1991. 'Tensions Between Good Science and Good Practice: Lagging Behind and Leapfrogging Ahead Along the Cancer Care Continuum', *Research in the Sociology of Health Care* 9: 127–40.

Morbidity and Mortality Weekly Report. 1981. Atlanta Centers for Disease Control. Atlanta, Georgia (5 June, 3 July).

Morgan, P.P. 1984. 'Pharmaceutical Advertising in Medical Journals', *CMAJ*: 130–42.

Moss, Nancy E. 2001. 'Mythbuster-Myth: Canadian doctors are leaving for the United States in droves', Canadian Health Services Research Foundation, available at: <www.cich.ca>.

———. 2002. 'Gender equity and socio-economic inequality: A framework for the patterning of women's health', *Social Science and Medicine* 54: 649–61.

———. 2002. 'National Council of Welfare Reports', *Poverty Profile* (Summer).

Moyer, Anne, Susan Grenner, John Beavis, and Peter Salovey. 1994. 'Accuracy of Health Research Reported in the Popular Press: Breast Cancer and Mammography', *Health Communication* 7, 1: 147–61.

Moynihan, Ray, Iona Heath, and David Henry. 2002. 'Selling sickness: The pharmaceutical industry and disease mongering', *British Medical Journal* 324: 886–91.

Mular, Wayne, and Marie P. Beaudet. 1996. 'Health Facts from the 1994 National Population Health Survey', *Canadian Social Trends* (Spring): 24–7.

Muller, M. 1982. *The Health of Nations*. London: Faber and Faber.

Mumford, Emily. 1983. *Medical Sociology: Patients, Providers and Policies*. New York: Random House.

Mustard, Fraser. 1987. 'Health in a Post-Industrial Society', in J. Clarke et al., eds, *Health Care in Canada: Looking Ahead*. Ottawa: Canadian Public Health Association.

Muzzin, Linda J., Gregory P. Brown, and Roy W. Hornosty. 1993. 'Professional Ideology in Canadian Pharmacy', *Health and Canadian Society* 1, 2: 319–46.

'NAFTA Gives Tobacco Companies Power to Block Plain Packaging'. 1994. *CCPA Monitor* (Canadian Centre for Policy Alternatives) 1, 2 (3 June).

Nathanson, C.A. 1977. 'Sex, Illness and Medical Care: A Review of Data, Theory and Method', *Social Science and Medicine* 11: 13–25.

National Council of Welfare. 1991. *Funding Health and Higher Education: Danger Looming*. Ottawa: Minister of Supply and Services.

———. 2002. 'National Council of Welfare Reports', *Poverty Profile* (Summer). Ottawa: National Council of Welfare.

Nault, Francois. 1997. 'Narrowing Mortality Gaps 1978 to 1995', *Health Reports* 9, 1 (Summer):

35–41.

Navarro, Vincente. 1975a. 'The Industrialization of Fetishism or the Fetishism of Industrialization: A Critique of Ivan Illich', *Social Science and Medicine* 9, 7: 351–63.

_____. 1975b. 'Women in Health Care', *New England Journal of Medicine* 202: 398–402.

_____. 1976. 'Social Class, Political Power and the State and Their Implications for Medicine', *Social Science and Medicine* 10: 437–57.

_____. 1992. 'Has Socialism Failed? An Analysis of Health Indicators under Socialism', *International Journal of Health Services* 22, 4: 585–601.

Naylor, C.D. 1982. 'In Defense of Medicare: Are Canadian Doctors Threatening the Health Care System?', *Canadian Forum* 62 (Apr.): 12–16.

Nelson, Melvin D. 1992. 'Socio-economic Status and Childhood Mortality in North Carolina', *American Journal of Public Health* 82, 8: 1131–3.

Neidhardt, J., M.S. Weinstein, and Robert R. Coury. 1985. *No-gimmick Guide to Managing Stress.* Vancouver: Self-Counsel Press.

Newbold, B. 1998. 'Problems in Search of Solution: Health and Canadian Aboriginals', *Journal of Community Health* 23, 1 (Feb.): 59–73.

Ng, Edward. 1996. 'Disability among Canada's Aboriginal Peoples in 1991', *Health Reports* 8, 1 (Summer): 25–31.

Nicholson, G.W.L. 1967. *The White Cross in Canada.* Montreal: Harvest House.

_____. 1975. *Canada's Nursing Sisters.* Toronto: Hakkert.

Nicholson, Malcolm, and Cathleen McLaughlin. 1987. 'Social Constructionism and Medical Sociology: A Reply to M.R. Bury', *Sociology of Health and Illness* 9, 2: 107–26.

Nikiforuk, Andrew. 1991. 'The Great Fire', *Equinox* 59 (Sept.–Oct.).

Noh, J., and R.J. Turner. 1983. 'Class and Psychological Vulnerabilities Among Women: The Significance of Social Support and Personal Control', *Journal of Health and Social Behavior* 24: 2–15.

'Nursing Shortage Looming', *The Canadian Nurse* 8, 1: 15.

Oakley, A. 1984. *The Captured Womb: A History of the Medical Care of Pregnant Women.* Oxford: Basil Blackwell.

Oberg, Gary R. 1990. *An Overview of the Philosophy of the American Academy of Environmental Medicine.* Denver: American Academy of Environmental Medicine.

O'Brien, Patricia. 1987. 'All a Woman's Life Can Bring: The Domestic Roots of Nursing in Philadelphia, 1830–1885', *Nursing Research* 36, 1: 12–17.

Occupational Health and Safety: A Training Manual. 1982. Toronto: Copp Clark.

O'Connor, J. 1973. *The Fiscal Crisis of the State.* New York: St Martin's Press.

Ollila, Eeva, and Elina Hemminki. 1997. 'Does Licensing of Drugs in Industrialized Countries Guarantee Drug Quality and Safety for Third World Countries? The Case of Norplant Licensing in Finland', *International Journal of Health Services* 27, 2: 309–25.

Olsen, Gregg M. 1998. 'Locating the Canadian Welfare State: Family Policy and Health Care in Canada, Sweden and the United States', in Coburn et al. (1998: 580–97).

Olson, E. 1984. *No Place to Hide.* Wheaton, Ill.: Tyndale House.

Omran, Abdel R. 1979. 'Changing Patterns of Health and Disease During the Process of National Development', in G. Albrecht and P.C. Higgins, eds, *Health, Illness and Medicine.* Chicago: Rand McNally, 81–93.

Ontario Ministry of Health. *Good Nursing, Good Health: An Investment for the 21st Century.* www.gov.on.ca/health/english/pub/ministry/nurs-erep99/finance.html

Ontario Naturopathic Association (ONA). 1983. *Naturopathic Medicine and Health Care in Ontario. A Brief Prepared by the ONA and the Board of Directors of Drugless Therapy for the Honorable Keith Norton, Minister of Health.* Toronto (July).

Oppenheimer, J. 1983. 'Childbirth in Ontario: The Transition from Home to Hospital in the Early Twentieth Century', *Ontario History* 75 (Mar.): 36–60.

Orbach, Susie. 1986. *Hunger Strike: An Anorexic's Struggle as a Metaphor for Our Age.* New York: W.W. Norton.

Osler, W. 1910. 'The Lumleian Lectures on Angina Pectoris: Delivered Before the Royal College of Physicians of London', *Lancet*: 839–44.

Paget, Marianne A. 1988. *The Unity of Mistakes: A Phenomenological Interpretation of Medical Work.*

Philadelphia: Temple University Press.

_____. 1993. *A Complex Sorrow: Reflections on Cancer and an Abbreviated Life*, ed. Marjorie L. Devault. Philadelphia: Temple University Press.

Pampel, Fred. 2002. 'Inequality, diffusion, and the status gradient in smoking', *Social Problems* 49, 1: 35–57.

Papadopoulous, Costa. 1998. *Opportunities in Chiropractic*. Toronto: Canadian Chiropractic Association.

Parsons, Evelyn, and Paul Atkinson. 1992. 'Lay Constructions of Genetic Risk', *Sociology of Health and Illness* 14, 4: 437–55.

Parsons, Talcott. 1951. *The Social System*. Glencoe, Ill.: Free Press.

_____. 1954. 'The Professions and the Social Structure', in *Essays in Sociological Theory*, rev. edn. Glencoe, Ill.: Free Press, 428–47.

Patterns of Growth: Seventh Annual Review. 1970. Ottawa: Queen's Printer.

Pawluch, Dorothy, R. Cain, and J. Gilbert. 1995. 'Ideology and Alternative Therapy Use among People Living with HIV/AIDS', *Health and Canadian Society* (Summer): 63–84.

Payne-Jackson, Arvilla. 1999. 'Biomedical and Folk Medical Concepts of Adult Onset Diabetes in Jamaica: Implications for Treatment', *Health* 3, 1: 5–46.

Payer, Lynn. 1988. *Medicine and Culture: Varieties of Treatment in the United States, England, West Germany and France*. New York: Holt.

Peters-Golden, Holly. 1982. 'Breast Cancer: Varied Perceptions of Social Support in the Illness Experience', *Social Science and Medicine* 16: 483–91.

Pettigrew, Eileen. 1983. *The Silent Enemy: Canada and the Deadly Flu of 1918*. Saskatoon: Western Producer Prairie Books.

Phifer, James F., Z. Kryzsztof, and Fran H. Norris. 1988. 'The Impact of Natural Disaster on the Health of Older Adults: A Multiwave Prospective Study', *Journal of Health and Social Behavior* 29 (Mar.): 65–78.

Phillips, D.P., and R.A. Feldman. 1973. 'A Dip in Deaths Before Ceremonial Occasions: Some New Relationships Between Social Integration and Mortality', *American Sociological Review* 38: 678–96.

Phlanz, Manfred. 1975a. 'A Critique of Anglo-American Medical Sociology', *International Journal of Health Services* 4, 3: 565–74.

_____. 1975b. 'Relations Between Social Scientists, Physicians and Medical Organizations in Health Research', *Social Science and Medicine* 9: 7–13.

Picard, André. 2002. 'Alzheimer's taking huge economic toll, study says', *Globe and Mail*, 25 July, A6.

_____. 2002. 'Wine lifestyle touted as promoting health', *Globe and Mail*, 25 July, A3.

Pilnick, Alison. 1998. 'Why Didn't You Say Just That? Dealing with Issues of Asymmetry, Knowledge and Competence in the Pharmacist/Client Encounter', *Sociology of Health and Illness* 20, 1: 29–51.

Pinquart, Martin. 2001. 'Creating and maintaining purpose in life in old age: A meta-analysis', *Aging International* 27, 2: 90–114.

Pirie, Marion. 1988. 'Women and the Illness Role: Rethinking Feminist Theory', *Canadian Review of Sociology and Anthropology* 25, 4: 628–48.

Pollard, John. 1994. 'Attitudes toward Euthanasia in Metropolitan Toronto', *Institute for Social Research Newsletter* 9, 2 (Summer): 3–4.

Porter, John. 1989. *Health for Sale*. New York: Manchester University Press.

Priest, Lisa. 1993. 'Thalidomide Survivors Have Tackled Life with Gusto', *Calgary Herald*, 21 Feb., B8.

_____. 1996. 'Mothers-to-be Are Turned Away as Demand Swamps Midwives', *Toronto Star*, 10 Mar., A6.

_____. 1997a. 'Wake-up Call on Medicare', *Toronto Star*, 20 Sept., A33.

_____. 1997b. 'The Health Police', *Toronto Star*, 26 Sept., A26.

Pulliam, C., J. Hanlon, and S. Moore. 1988. 'Medication and Geriatics', in F. Abellah and S. Moore, eds, *Surgeon General's Workshop: Health Promotion and Aging. Background Papers*. Menlo Park, Calif.: Henry J. Kaiser Foundation.

Punnet, Laura. 1976. 'Women-Controlled Medicine—Theory and Practice in 19th Century Boston', *Women and Health* 1, 4 (July–Aug.): 3–10.

Purvis, Trevor, and Alan Hunt. 1993. 'Discourse, Ideology, Discourse, Ideology', *British Journal of Sociology* 44, 3: 499.

Quine, Lyn. 2002. 'Workplace bullying in junior doctors: Questionnaire survey', *British Medical Journal* 324: 878–9.

Quinn, K., M.J. Baker, and B. Evan. 1992. 'A Population-wide Profile of Prescription Drug Use in Saskatchewan, 1989', *CMAJ* 146: 2177–86.

Rabe, Barry G. 1992. 'When Citing Works, Canada Style', *Journal of Health Politics, Policy and Law* 17, 1 (Spring).

Rachlis, Michael, and Carol Kushner. 1989. *Second Opinion: What's Wrong with Canada's Health Care System*. Toronto: HarperCollins.

_____ and _____. 1994. *Strong Medicine: How to Save Canada's Health Care System*. Toronto: HarperCollins.

Radley, Alan. 1999. 'Abhorrence, Compassion and the Social Response to Suffering', *Health* 3, 2 (Apr.): 167–88.

Radway, Scott. 2002. 'Soldiers easing back to normal life', *Globe and Mail*, 27 July, A7.

Raffel, S. 1979. *Matters of Fact: A Sociological Inquiry*. London: Routledge & Kegan Paul.

Rahe, R.H., J.J. Mahan, and R.J. Arthur. 1970. 'Prediction of Near-Future Health Changes from Subjects' Preceding Life Changes', *Journal of Psychosomatic Research* 14: 401–6.

_____ and J. Paasikivi. 1971. 'Psychosocial Factors and Myocardial Infarction, II: An Outpatient Study in Sweden', *Journal of Psychosomatic Research* 15: 33–9.

Ranzijn, Rob. 2001. 'The potential of older adults to enhance community quality of life: Links between positive psychology and productive aging', *Aging International* 27, 2: 30–55.

Raphael, Dennis. 1999. 'Health effects of economic inequality: Overview and purpose', *Canadian Review of Social Policy* 44: 25–40.

_____. 2001. 'Inequality is bad for our hearts: Why low income and social exclusion are major causes of heart disease in Canada'. New York: New York Health Network.

Ratcliff, Kathryn Strother. 1994. 'Midwifery in East London: Responding to the Challenges', *Women and Health* 21, 1: 49–78.

Raven, Peter H., Linda R. Berg, and George B. Johnson. 1993. *Environment*. Toronto: Saunders.

Rawson, Nigel S.B., and Carl D'Arcy. 1991. 'Sedative-Hypnotic Drug Use in Canada', *Health Reports* 3, 1: 33–57.

Raymond, Chris. 1989. 'Distrust, Rage May Be "Toxic Core" That Puts Type A at Personal Risk', *JAMA* 261, 6: 813.

Reasons, C.E., L.E. Ross, and Craig Patterson. 1981. *Assault on the Worker: Occupational Health and Safety in Canada*. Toronto: Butterworths.

Registered Nurses Association of Ontario. 1987. *The RNAO Responds: A Nursing Perspective on the Events at the Hospital for Sick Children and the Grange Inquiry*. Toronto: RNAO, Apr.

Regush, Nicholas. 1987. *Canada's Health Care System: Condition Critical*. Toronto: Macmillan.

_____. 1993. *Safety Last: The Failure of the Consumer Health Protection System in Canada*. Toronto: Key Porter Books.

Reif, L. 1975. 'Ulcerative Colitis: Strategies for Managing Life', in Strauss and Glaser (1975: 81–8).

Reinharz, Shulamit. 1992. *Feminist Methods in Social Research*. Oxford: Oxford University Press.

Reissman, Catherine Kohler. 1987. 'Women and Medicalization: A New Perspective', in Howard D. Schwartz, ed., *Dominant Issues in Medical Sociology*, 2nd edn. New York: Random House, 101–21.

Reitz, J.G. 1980. *The Survival of Ethnic Groups*. Toronto: McGraw-Hill Ryerson.

Relman, Arnold S. 1987. 'The New Medical-Industrial Complex', in Howard D. Schwartz, ed., *Dominant Issues in Medical Sociology*, 2nd edn. New York: Random House, 597–607.

Report to the OMA Board of Directors from the Ad Hoc Committee on Women's Health Issues. 1987. Toronto: Ontario Medical Association.

Reuters. 2002. 'Week-old infant raped in S. Africa', *Toronto Star*, 31 July, A2.

Reverby, Susan M. 1987. *Ordered to Care: The Dilemma of American Nursing*. Cambridge: Cambridge University Press.

Richardson, Astrid H., and Ronald J. Burke. 1991. 'Occupational Stress and Job Satisfaction Among Physicians: Sex Differences', *Social Science and Medicine* 33, 10: 1179–87.

Richardson, Diane, and Victoria Robinson. 1993. *Thinking Feminist: Key Concepts in Women's Studies*. New York: Guilford Press.

Rieff, P. 1966. *Triumph of the Therapeutic*. New York: Harper and Row.

Ritzer, George. 1975. 'Sociology: A Multiple Paradigm Science', *American Sociologist* 10: 156–67.

Roberts, Paul William. 1992. 'Feud', *Saturday Night* (Dec.): 52–7, 96–106.

Rochon-Ford, Anne. 1986. 'In Poor Health', *Healthsharing* 7 (Winter): 8–10.

———. 1990. *Working Together for Women's Health: A Framework for the Development of Policies and Programs.* n.p.: Federal/Provincial/Territorial Working Group on Women's Health.

Rogers, Karen. 1994. 'Wife Assault in Canada', *Canadian Social Trends*: 2–8.

Roland, Charles. 1988. 'Medicine, History of', in *The Canadian Encyclopedia*, vol. 2. Edmonton: Hurtig, 1330.

Romelis, Shelly. 1985. 'Struggle between Providers and Recipients: The Case of Birth Practices', in Ellen Lewin and Virginia Olesen, eds, *Women, Health and Healing*. London: Tavistock, 174–208.

Rosen, George. 1963. 'The Evolution of Social Medicine', in Howard E. Freeman, Sol Levine, and Leo G. Reader, eds, *Handbook of Medical Sociology*. Englewood Cliffs, NJ: Prentice-Hall, 23–50.

Rosenberg, Charles E., and Janet Golden, eds. 1992. *Framing Disease: Studies in Cultural History.* New Brunswick, NJ: Rutgers University Press.

Roth, Julius. 1962. 'Management Bias in Social Science Research', *Human Organization* 21: 47–50.

———. 1963. *Timetables: Structuring the Passage of Time in Hospital Treatment and Other Careers.* Indianapolis: Bobbs-Merrill.

Rothouse, Herbert. 1997. 'History of Homeopathy Reveals Discipline's Excellence', *Alternative and Complementary Therapies* (June): 223–7.

Rotter, J.B. 1966. 'Generalized Expectation for Internal versus External Control of Reinforcement', *Psychological Monographs* 80: 1–28.

Roughead, Elizabeth E., Andrew L. Gilbert, and Ken J. Harvey. 1998. 'Self-Regulatory Codes of Conduct: Are They Effective in Controlling Pharmaceutical Representatives' Presentation to General Practitioners?', *International Journal of Health Services* 282: 269–79.

Rutherford, R.D. 1975. *The Changing Sex Differential in Mortality.* International Population and Urban Research, University of California, Berkeley, Studies in Population of Urban Demography No. 1. Westport, Conn.: Greenwood Press.

Sajan, Amin, Trevor Corneil, and Stefan Grzybowski. 1998. 'The Street Value of Prescription Drugs', *CMAJ* 159: 139–42.

Salmon, J. Warren. 1984. *Alternative Medicines: Popular and Policy Perspectives.* New York: Tavistock.

Samson, Colin. 2003. *A Way of Life That Does Not Exist: Canada and the Extinguishment of the Innu.* St John's: ISER Books.

———, James Wilson, and Jonathan Mazower. 1999. *Canada's Tibet: The Killing of the Innu.* London: Survival.

Sarick, Lila. 1994. 'Childbirth's Ancients Are Reborn as a Profession', *Globe and Mail*, 14 May, A1, A6.

Schacter, S. 1975. 'Cognition and Peripheralist-Centralist Controversies in Motivation and Emotion', in M.S. Gazzaniga and C. Blakemore, eds, *Handbook of Psychobiology.* London: Academic Press, 529–62.

Scheff, Thomas J. 1963. 'The Role of the Mentally Ill and the Dynamics of Mental Disorder', *Sociometry* 26 (June): 463–83.

Schneider, Joseph, and Peter Conrad. 1980. 'In the Closet with Illness: Epilepsy, Stigma Potential and Information Control', *Social Problems* 28, 1 (Oct.): 32–44.

——— and ———. 1983. *Having Epilepsy: The Experience and Control of Illness.* Philadelphia: Temple University Press.

Schwabe, Arlette M. 1995. 'International Dependency and Health: A Comparative Case Study of Cuba and the Dominican Republic', in Eugene Gallagher and Janardan Subedi, eds, *Global Perspectives on Health Care.* Englewood Cliffs, NJ: Prentice-Hall, 292–310.

Schwendinger, Julia, and Herman Schwendinger. 1971. 'Sociology's Founding Fathers: Sexist to a Man', *Journal of Marriage and the Family* 334: 783–9.

Scientific American. 1995. 272, 2 (June): 16.

Scott, James C. 1985. *Weapons of the Weak: Everyday Forms of Peasant Resistance.* New Haven: Yale University Press.

Scrambler, G. 1998. *Modernity, Medicine and Health.* London: Routledge.

Scully, Diana. 1980. *Men Who Control Women's Health: The Miseducation of Obstetrician-Gynecologists.* Boston: Houghton Mifflin.

Scutt, Jocelynne. 1983. *Even in the Best of Homes:*

Violence in the Family. Sydney: Penguin Books Australia.

Sechzer, Jeri A., Anne Griffin, and Sheila M. Pfafflin. 1994. *Forging a Women's Health Research Agenda: Policy Issues for the 1990s*. New York: Annals of the New York Academy of Science.

Segall, Alexander, Michael J. Mahon, Judith G. Chipperfield, and Daniel S. Bailis. 1997. *Understanding the Relationship Between Perceived Control, Personal Health Practices, and Health Status*. Final Report. Winnipeg: University of Manitoba, Max Bell Centre.

Selye, H. 1956. *The Stress of Life*. New York: McGraw-Hill.

Shackleton, Doris French. 1975. *Tommy Douglas*. Toronto: McClelland & Stewart.

Shaffir, William B., Robert A. Stebbins, and Allan Tarowetz. 1980. *Fieldwork Experience: Qualitative Approaches to Social Research*. New York: St Martin's Press.

Shannon, H., et al. 1988. 'Lung Cancer and Air Pollution in an Industrial City: A Geographical Analysis', *Canadian Journal of Public Health* 79: 255–9.

Shapiro, Martin. 1978. *Getting Doctored: Critical Reflections on Becoming a Physician*. Toronto: Between the Lines.

Shephard, D.A., ed. 1982. *Norman Bethune—His Times and Legacy*. Ottawa: Canadian Public Health Association.

Shkilyk, Anastasia. 1985. *A Poison Stronger than Love*. New Haven: Yale University Press.

Shorr, R.I., S.F. Bauwens, and C.S. Landefeld. 1990. 'Failure to Limit Quantities of Benzodiazepine Hypnotic Drugs for Outpatients: Placing the Elderly at Risk', *American Journal of Medicine* 89: 725–32.

Shorter, Edward. 1992. *From Paralysis to Fatigue: A History of Psychosomatic Illness in the Modern Era*. New York: Free Press.

Shortt, Samuel E.D. 2002. 'Medical savings accounts in publicly funded health care systems: Enthusiasm versus evidence', *Canadian Medical Association Journal* 167, 2 (23 July): 159.

Sibbald, Barbara. 1998. 'In Your Face: A New Wave of Militant Doctors Lashes Out', *CMAJ* 158: 1505–9.

Siggner, A.J. 1979. *An Overview of Demographic, Social and Economic Conditions Among Canada's Registered Indian Population*. Ottawa: Research Branch, DIAND.

Siirla, Aarne. 1981. *The Voice of Illness: A Study in Therapy and Prophecy*, 2nd edn. New York: Edwin Mellen Press.

Simkin, J. 1998. 'Not All Your Patients Are Strongest', *CMAJ* 159: 370–5.

Simonton, Carl O., Stephanie Matthews Simonton, and James L. Creighton. 1978. *Getting Well Again*. Toronto: Bantam Books.

Single, Eric, Lynda Robson, Xiaodi Xie, Jurgen Rehm, et al. 1996. *The Cost of Substance Abuse in Canada*. Ottawa: Canadian Centre for Substance Abuse.

Smith, Dorothy E. 1987. *The Everyday World As Problematic: A Feminist Sociology*. Toronto: University of Toronto Press.

_____. 1993. *Texts, Facts, and Femininity: Exploring the Relations of Ruling*. London: Routledge.

Smith, Marianne, and Kathleen Burkwalter. 1992. 'Medication Management, Anti-depressant Drugs, and the Elderly: An Overview', *Journal of Psychosocial Nursing* 30, 10: 30–6.

Smith, Murray E.G. 1992. 'The Burznyski Controversy in the United States and in Canada: A Comparative Case Study in the Sociology of Alternative Medicine', *Canadian Journal of Sociology* 17, 2: 133–60.

Smith, Richard. 2002. 'In search of "non-disease"', *British Medical Journal* 324 (13 Apr.): 883–5.

Soderstrom, Lee. 1978. *The Canadian Health System*. London: Croom Helm.

Sontag, Susan. 1978. *Illness as a Metaphor*. New York: Random House.

_____. 1989. *AIDS and Its Metaphors*. Markham, Ont.: Penguin Books.

Speedling, E.J. 1982. *Heart Attack: The Family Response and the Hospital*. New York: Tavistock.

Spiegel, D., J. Bloom, H. Kraemer, and E. Gotheil. 1989. 'Effects of Psychosocial Treatment on Survival of Patients with Metastatic Breast Cancer', *Lancet* (Oct.): 15.

Squires, B.P. 1987. 'In Whose Service?', *CMAJ* 137: 983.

Stanley, E.M.G., and M.P. Ramage. 1984. 'Sexual Problems and Urological Symptoms', in S.L. Stanton, ed., *Clinical Gynecological Urology*. St Louis: Mosby, 398–405.

Stanley, Liz, and Sue Wise. 1993. *Breaking Out Again:*

Feminist Ontology and Epistemology. London: Routledge.

Starr, Paul. 1982. *The Social Transformation of American Medicine*. New York: Basic Books.

Statistics Canada. n.d. *Corporate Financial Statistics: Detailed Income and Retained Earnings Statistics for 182 Industries*. Ottawa.

——. Various years. *Census of Canada*. Ottawa.

——. 1977. *Vital Statistics 1977*, vol. 3. Ottawa.

——. 1981. *Health of Canadians. Report of the Canada Health Survey*. Ottawa.

——. 1982. *Medicare: The Public Good and Private Practice*. Ottawa: National Council on the Welfare of Canada's Health Insurance System (May).

——. 1983. *Health of Canadians*. Report of the Canada Health Survey. Ottawa.

——. 1984. *Life Tables, Canada and the Provinces*. Ottawa (May).

——. 1985. *Health and Social Support*. General Social Survey Analysis Series. Ottawa.

——. 1986. *Mortality and Vital Statistics*, vol. 3. Ottawa.

——. 1987. *Active Health Report: Perspectives on Canada's Health Promotion Survey*. Ottawa: Ministry of Supply and Services.

——. 1988. *Work Injuries, 1985–87*. Ottawa: Statistics Canada, Labour Division.

——. 1990. *Selected Infant Mortality, 1921–1990*. Ottawa: Statistics Canada.

——. 1991. *Accidents in Canada*. Ottawa.

——. 1993a. 'The Violence Against Women Survey', *The Daily*, 18 Nov.

——. 1993b. *Work Injuries, 1990–92*. Cat. no. 72–208. Ottawa.

——. 1995. *Births and Deaths*. Ottawa: Statistics Canada.

——. 1997. *National Population Health Survey. Overview 1996–1997*. Cat. no. 82–567-XPB. Ottawa: Statistics Canada.

——. 1998. Cat. no. 82–221–XDE. Ottawa: Statistics Canada.

——. 2002. 'Unmet health care needs', *The Daily*, 24 Jan.

Steacy, Anne. 1989. 'Facing the Future: Thalidomide Victims Seek Compensation', *Maclean's*, 20 Feb.

Stein, Howard F. 1990. *American Medicine as Culture*. Boulder, Colo.: Westview Press.

Stein, L. 1987. 'The Doctor-Nurse Game', in H.D. Schwartz, ed., *Dominant Issues in Medical Sociology*, 2nd edn. New York: Random House.

Steinem, Gloria. 1983. *Outrageous Acts and Everyday Rebellions*. New York: Holt, Rinehart and Winston.

Stelfox, Henry Thomas, Grace Chua, Keith O'Rourke, and Allan S. Detsky. 1998. 'Conflict of Interest in the Debate Over Calcium—Channel Antagonists', *New England Journal of Medicine* 338, 2: 101–6.

Stelling, Joan. 1994. 'Staff Nurses' Perceptions of Nursing: Issues in a Women's Occupation', in Bolaria and Dickinson (1994: 609–26).

Sternglass, Ernest J., and Jay M. Gould. 1993. 'Breast Cancer: Evidence for a Relation to Fission Products in the Diet', *International Journal of Health Sciences* 23, 4: 783–804.

Stevenson, Lloyd. 1946. *Sir Frederick Banting*. Toronto: Ryerson Press.

Stewart, David C., and Thomas J. Sullivan. 1982. 'Illness Behaviour and the Sick Role in Chronic Disease: The Case of Multiple Sclerosis', *Social Science and Medicine* 16: 1307–1404.

Stewart, Roderick. 1977. *The Mind of Norman Bethune*. Westport, Conn.: Lawrence Hill.

Stoddart, Greg L., and Roberta J. Labelle. 1985. *Privatization in the Canadian Health Care System: Assertions, Evidence, Ideology and Options*. Ottawa: Health and Welfare Canada.

Stone, Deborah S. 1986. 'The Resistible Rise of Preventative Medicine', *Journal of Health Politics, Policy, and Law* 11: 671–96.

Stones, Ilene. 1987. 'Rotational Shiftwork: A Summary of the Adverse Effects and Improvement Strategies'. Hamilton, Ont.: Canadian Centre for Occupational and Health Safety.

Stoppard, Janet M. 1992. 'A Suitable Case for Treatment: Premenstrual Syndrome and the Medicalization of Women's Bodies', in Currie and Raoul (1992: 119–29).

Strauss, Anselm L., and Barney G. Glaser. 1975. *Chronic Illness and the Quality of Life*. St Louis: Mosby.

Strauss, Arlene. 1987. 'Alzheimer's Disease and the Family Care Provider', supervised research project, Sociology and Anthropology Department, Wilfrid Laurier University.

Strauss, Robert. 1957. 'The Nature and Status of Medical Sociology', *American Sociological Review* 22: 200–4.

Strauss, Stephen. 1994. 'Arctic Pollution', *Globe and Mail*, 19 Nov.

_____. 2002. 'Global warming may not be so bad', *Globe and Mail*, 18 May, F7.

Strike, Carol. 1995. 'Women Assaulted by Strangers', *Canadian Social Trends* (Spring): 2–6.

Strong, P.M. 1979. 'Sociological Imperialism and the Profession of Medicine: A Critical Examination of the Thesis of Medical Imperialism', *Social Science and Medicine* 13, 2: 194–215.

Stronk, Karien, and H. Dike van de Mheen. 1996. 'Behavioural and Structural Factors in the Explanation of Socio-economic Inequalities in Health: An Empirical Analysis', *Sociology of Health and Illness* 18, 5: 653–74.

Studdert, D.M., D.M. Eisenberg, F.H. Miller, D.A. Curto, T.J. Kaptchuk, and T.A. Brennan. 1998. 'Medical Malpractice Implications of Alternative Medicine', *JAMA* 280, 18: 1610–15.

Sudnow, D. 1967. *Passing On: The Social Organization of Dying*. Englewood Cliffs, NJ: Prentice-Hall.

Sutherland, Lloyd P., and M.J. Verhoef. 1994. 'Why Do Patients Seek a Second Opinion or Alternative Medicine?', *Journal of Clinical Gastroenterology* 19, 3: 194–7.

'Sweet Dreams or Nightmares?'. 1991. *Newsweek*, 19 Aug.

Syre, Thomas R. 1997. 'Alcohol and other drug use at a university in the southeastern United States: Survey findings and implications', *The College Student Journal* 31, 3: 272–381.

Szasz, T.S. 1974. *The Myth of Mental Illness*. New York: Harper and Row.

_____ and M.H. Hollender. 1956. 'A Contribution to the Philosophy of Medicine: The Basic Models of Doctor-Patient Relationship', *Archives of International Medicine* 97: 585–92.

Tamblyn, R.M., Peter J. MacLeod, et al. 1994. 'Questionable Prescribing for Elderly Patients in Quebec', *CMAJ* 151: 1808–9.

Tan, Lisa, Jennifer Wing, Larry DeGusseme, and Raymond Roch. 1996. 'Worksafe Focus Report on the Health Care Industry'. Research and Evaluation Section, Prevention Division of the Government of British Columbia.

Task Force on Sexual Abuse of Patients. 1991. *Final Report*. Toronto: College of Physicians and Surgeons of Ontario.

Tarabusi, Claudio Casadio, and Graham Vickery. 1998. 'Globalization in the Pharmaceutical Industry Part 1', *International Journal of Health Services* 28, 1: 67–105.

Targ, Elisabeth. 1997. 'Evaluating Distant Healing: A Research Review', *Alternative Therapies* 3, 6: 74–8.

Tataryn, Lloyd. 1979. *Dying for a Living*. Ottawa: Deneau and Greenberg.

Taunton, R.L., S.V.M. Klienbeck, R. Stafford, C. Woods, and M. Bott. 1994. 'Patient Outcomes: Are They Linked to Registered Nurse Absenteeism, Separation or Workload?', *Journal of Nursing Administration* 24, 45: 48–55.

Taylor, Paul. 1992. 'Prescriptive Plan Skyrockets in Cost', *Globe and Mail*, 10 Mar., A11.

_____. 1993. 'Why the Rich Live Longer, Healthier', *Globe and Mail*, 16 Oct., 1–2.

Taylor, William. 1985. *Hormonal Manipulation: A New Era of Monstrous Athletes*. Jefferson, NC: McFarland & Company.

_____. 1991. *Macho Medicine: A History of the Anabolic Steroid Epidemic*. Jefferson, NC: McFarland & Company.

Terris, M. 1980. 'Preventative Services and Medical Care: The Costs and Benefits of Basic Change', *Bulletin of the New York Academy of Medicine* 56: 180–9.

Terry, Edith. 1991. 'The Work Place As Killing Field', *Globe and Mail*, 21 Sept., D2.

Tesh, Sylvia Noble. 1988. *Hidden Arguments, Political Ideology and Disease Prevention Policy*. New Brunswick, NJ: Rutgers University Press.

'Thalidomide's After-Effects Today'. 1989. *Globe and Mail*, 14 Feb.

'Thalidomide Tragedy, Labelling Snag Linked'. 1972. *Kitchener-Waterloo Record*, 27 Sept.

Theorell, T., and R.H. Rahe. 1971. 'Psychosocial Factors and Myocardial Infarction, I: An Inpatient Study in Sweden', *Journal of Psychosomatic Research* 15: 25–31.

Thoits, Peggy A. 1982. 'Conceptual, Methodological and Theoretical Problems in Studying Social Support as a Buffer Against Life Stress', *Journal of Health and Social Behavior* 23: 145–59.

_____. 1983. 'Dimensions of Life Events that Influence Psychological Distress: An Evaluation and Synthesis of the Literature', in H.B. Kaplan, ed., *Psychosocial Stress: Trends in Theory and*

Research. New York: Academic Press.

_____. 1991. 'On Merging Identity Theory and Stress Research', *Social Psychology Quarterly* 54: 101–12.

_____. 1994. 'Stressors and Problem-Solving: The Individual as Psychological Activist', *Journal of Health and Social Behavior* 35 (June): 145–59.

Thomas, D.J. 1982. *The Experience of Handicap*. London: Methuen.

Thomas, Lewis. 1985. *The Youngest Science: Notes of a Medicine-Watcher*. London: Oxford University Press.

Thomas, Lewis H., ed. 1982. *The Making of a Socialist: The Recollections of T.C. Douglas*. Edmonton: University of Alberta Press.

Thompson, Joanne Emily. 1974. *The Influence of Dr Emily Howard Stowe on the Women Suffrage Movement in Canada*. Waterloo, Ont.: Waterloo Lutheran University Press.

Tierney, D., P. Romita, and K. Messing. 1990. 'She Ate Not the Bread of Idleness: Exhaustion Is Related to Domestic and Salaried Working Conditions Among 539 Quebec Hospital Workers', *Women and Health* 16, 1: 21–42.

Timmermans, Stefan. 1998. 'Social Death No Self-fulfilling Prophecy: David Sudnow's Passing On Revisited', *Sociological Quarterly* 39, 3: 453–72.

Toombs, S. Kay. 1995. 'The Lived Experience of Disability', *Human Studies* 18: 9–23.

Torrance, G. 1987. 'Socio-Historical Overview: The Development of the Canadian Health System', in Coburn et al. (1987: 6–32).

Trovato, Frank, and Carl F. Grindstaff, eds. 1994. *Perspectives on Canada's Population: An Introduction to Concepts and Issues*. Toronto: Oxford University Press.

Trudeau, Richard. 1995. 'Male Registered Nurses', *Health Reports* 8, 2: 13–15.

Trussell, James, Felicia Stewart, Malcolm Potts, Felicia Guest, and Charlotte Ellertson. 1993. 'Should Oral Contraceptives Be Available Without Prescription?', *American Journal of Public Health* 83, 8: 1094–7.

Trypuc, Joann M. 1988. 'Women's Health', in Bolaria and Dickinson (1988: 154–66).

Tuckett, David, ed., 1976. *An Introduction to Medical Sociology*. London: Tavistock.

Tuohy, Carolyn J. 1976. 'Medical Politics after Medicare: The Ontario Case', *Canadian Public Policy* 2 (Spring): 192–210.

Turner, B.S. 1987. *Medical Power and Social Knowledge*. London: Sage.

Turner, R. Jay, and William R. Avison. 1992. 'Innovation in the Measurement of Life Stress: Crisis Theory and the Significance of Event Resolution', *Journal of Health and Social Behavior* 33, 1 (Mar.): 36–50.

_____, B.G. Frankel, and D. Levin. 1983. 'Social Support, Conceptualization, Measurement and Implication for Mental Health', in J.R. Greenly, ed., *Research in Community Mental Health*, vol. 3. Greenwich, Conn.: JAI, 27–67.

_____, C.F. Grindstaff, and N. Phillips. 1990. 'Social Support and Outcomes in Teenage Pregnancy', *Journal of Health and Social Behavior* 31, 1 (Mar.): 43–57.

Tully, Patricia, and Etienne Pierre. 1997. 'Downsizing Canada's Hospitals, 1986/7 to 1994/5', *Health Reports* 8, 4 (Spring).

Twaddle, A.C. 1982. 'From Medical Sociology to Sociology of Health: Some Changing Concerns in the Sociological Study of Sickness and Treatment', in T. Bottomore et al., eds, *Sociology: The State of the Art*. London: Sage, 324–58.

_____ and R.M. Hessler. 1977. *A Sociology of Health*. St Louis: Mosby.

Tyre, Robert. 1982. *Douglas in Saskatchewan: The Story of a Socialist Experiment*. Vancouver: Mitchell Press.

UNICEF. 1990. *The State of the World's Children*. Oxford: Oxford University Press.

United Nations. 1982. *Demographic Indicators of Countries: Estimates and Projections as Assessed in 1980*. New York: UN.

United Nations Development Program (UNDP). 1999. *Human Development Report 1999*. New York: United Nations.

Valpy, Michael. 1994. 'A Fine Mythology Up in Smoke', *Globe and Mail*, 11 Feb., A2.

Vavasour, M., and Y. Mennie. 1984. *For Health or Profit*. Ottawa: World Inter-Action Ottawa and Inter-Paris.

Vayda, Eugene, Robert G. Evans, and William R. Mindell. 1979. 'Universal Health Insurance in Canada', *Journal of Community Health* 4, 3 (Spring): 217–31.

Verbrugge, Lois M. 1985. 'Gender and Health: An Update on Hypothesis and Evidence', *Journal of Health and Social Behavior* 26: 156–82.

_____. 1989. 'The Twain Meet: Empirical Explanations of Sex Differences in Health and Mortality', *Journal of Health and Social Behavior* 31, 3: 282–304.

_____ and Deborah Wingard. 1987. 'Sex Differentials in Health and Mortality', *Women and Health* 12, 2: 103–45.

Verhoef, M.J., and L.R. Sutherland. 1995. 'Alternative Medicine and General Practitioners', *Canadian Family Physician* 41: 1005.

_____, _____, and L. Brkich. 1990. 'Use of Alternative Medicine by Patients Attending a Gastroenterology Clinic', *CMAJ* 142, 2: 121–5.

Verrengia, Joseph B. 2002. 'Pollution blamed for African drought', *Toronto Star*, 22 July, A3.

Verrilli, D.K., Robert Berenson, and Steven J. Katz. 1998. 'A Comparison of Cardiovascular Procedure Use Between the United States and Canada', *Health Reports* 3 (Aug.): 467–87.

Vickers, A., P. Wilson, and J. Kleijnen. 2002. 'Acupuncture', *Quality and Safety in Healthcare* 11: 92–7.

Villeneuve, Paul J., and Howard I. Morrison. 1995. 'Trends in Mortality from Smoking Related Cancers, 1950–1971', *Canadian Social Trends* (Winter): 8–11.

Vincent, C.A., and A. Coulter. 2002. 'Patient safety: What about the patient?', *Quality and Safety in Health Care* 11: 76–80.

Wade, S., and W. Schramm. 1969. 'The Mass Media as Sources of Public Affairs, Science and Health Knowledge', *Public Opinion Quarterly* 33: 197–209.

Wahn, Michael. 1987. 'The Decline of Medical Dominance in Hospitals', in Coburn et al. (1987: 422–41).

Waitzkin, Howard. 1989. 'A Critical Theory on Medical Discourse: Ideology, Social Control, and the Processing of Social Context in Medical Encounters', *Journal of Health and Social Behavior* 30 (June): 220–39.

_____ and Theron Brett. 1989. 'Changing the Structure of Medical Discourse: Implications of Cross-National Comparisons', *Journal of Health and Social Behavior* 30, 4 (Dec.): 436–49.

Waldron, Ingrid. 1977. 'Increased Prescribing of Valium, Librium and Other Drugs—An Example of the Influence of Economic and Social Factors on the Practice of Medicine', *International Journal of Health Services* 7: 37–62.

_____. 1981. 'Why Do Women Live Longer than Men?', *Journal of Human Stress* 2: 19–30.

_____ and Susan Johnston. 1981. 'Why Do Women Live Longer than Men Part II', *Journal of Human Stress* 2.

Walsh, Kiri, Robert Blizard, Louise Jones, Michael King, and Adrian Tookman. 2002. 'Spiritual beliefs may affect outcome of bereavement: Prospective study', *British Medical Journal* 324 (29 June): 1551.

Walters, Vivienne. 1982. 'State, Capital and Labour: The Introduction of Federal-Provincial Insurance for Physician Care in Canada', *Canadian Review of Sociology and Anthropology* 19: 157–72.

_____. 1991. 'Beyond Medical and Academic Agendas: Lay Perspectives and Priorities', *Atlantis* 17, 1: 28–35.

_____. 1992. 'Women's Views of Their Main Health Problem', *Canadian Journal of Public Health* 83, 5: 371–4.

_____. 1994a. 'Women's Perceptions Regarding Health and Illness', in Bolaria and Dickinson (1994: 317–25).

_____. 1994b. 'The Social Construction of Risk in Nursing: Nurses' Responses to Hazards in Their Work', in Bolaria and Dickinson (1994: 627–43).

_____ and J. Haines. 1989. 'Workload and Occupational Stress in Nursing', *Canadian Journal of Nursing Research* 21, 3: 49–58.

Wanke, Margaret I., Duncan L. Sanders, Raymond W. Pong, and John B. Church. 1996. 'Building a stronger foundation: A framework for planning and evaluating community based health services in Canada', *Health Sources in Canada*. Ottawa: Health Canada, Health Promotion Programs.

Warburton, Rennie, and W. Carroll. 1988. 'Class and Gender in Nursing Work', in Bolaria and Dickinson (1988: 364–75).

Wardell, Walter. 1980a. 'Limited and Marginal Practitioners', in H. Freeman, S. Levine, and L. Reader, eds, *Handbook of Medical Sociology*, 3rd edn. Englewood Cliffs, NJ: Prentice-Hall.

_____. 1980b. 'The Present and Future Role of the Chiropractor', in S. Halderman, ed., *Modern Developments in the Principles and Practice of Chiropractic*. Englewood Cliffs, NJ: Prentice-Hall.

_____. 1988. 'Chiropractors: Evolution to Acceptance', in Norman Gentz, ed., *Other Healers: Unorthodox Medicine in America*. Baltimore: Johns Hopkins University Press, 174–84.

Watson, Rory. 2002. 'More women in the workforce reduces mortality', *British Medical Journal* 324 (8 June): 1352.

Weber, Max. 1947. *The Theory of Social and Economic Organization*, trans. A.M. Henderson and Talcott Parsons. New York: Free Press

_____. 1968. *Economy and Society: An Outline of Interpretive Sociology*, trans. Ephraim Fischoff; eds G. Roth and C. Witlich. New York: Bedminster Press.

Weiger, Charles. 1995. 'Our Bodies, Our Science', *The Sciences* (May–June).

Weigts, Wies, Hannecke Hontkoop, and Patricia Mullen. 1993. 'Talking Delicately: Speaking About Sexuality During Gynecological Consultation', *Sociology of Health and Illness* 15, 4.

Weil, Andrew. 1983. *Health and Healing: Understanding Conventional and Alternative Medicine*. Boston: Houghton Mifflin.

Weisman, D.K., and J.W. Worden. 1975. 'Psychological Analysis of Cancer Deaths', *Omega* 6: 61–75.

Weiss, Gregory L., and Lynne E. Lonnquist. 1992. 'Dissecting the Medical Encounter: A Model of the Physician-Patient Relationship', paper presented at the 87th meeting of the American Sociology Association, Pittsburgh.

Weitz, Rose. 1999. 'Watching Brian Die: The Rhetoric and Reality of Informed Consent', *Health* 3, 2: 209–27.

Welch, W.P., D.K. Verrilli, S.J. Katz, and E. Latmer. 1996. 'A Detailed Comparison of Physician Services in the United States and Canada', *JAMA* 225, 18: 1410–16.

Weller, G. 1986. 'Health Care Delivery in the Canadian North: The Case of Northwestern Ontario', paper presented at the annual meeting of the Western Association of Sociology and Anthropology, Thunder Bay, 13–15 Feb.

Wellman, Beverly. 1994. 'Lay Referral Networks: Using Conventional Medicine and Alternative Therapies for Low Back Pain', *ASA: Sociological Abstracts*.

Wennberg, John E. 1984. 'Dealing with Medical Practice Variations: A Proposal for Action', *Health Affairs* 4 (Summer): 6–32.

_____, John P. Buncker, and Benjamin Barnes. 1980. 'The Need for Assessing the Outcomes of Common Medical Practice', *Annual Review of Public Health* 1: 277–95.

Wennemo, Irene. 1993. 'Infant Mortality, Public Policy and Inequality—A Comparison of 18 Industrialized Countries, 1950–1985', *Sociology of Health and Illness* 15, 4: 429–46.

Wertz, Richard W., and Dorothy C. Wertz. 1977. *Lying-In: A History of Childbirth in America*. New York: Free Press.

_____ and _____. 1986. 'Notes on the Decline of Midwives and the Rise of Medical Obstetricians', in Peter Conrad and Rochelle Kern, eds, *The Sociology of Health and Illness: Critical Perspectives*. New York: St Martin's Press.

Weston, Marianne, and Bonnie Jeffrey. 1994. 'AIDS: The Politicizing of a Public Health Issue', in Bolaria and Dickinson (1994: 721–39).

'Westray Probe's Scope Curbed'. 1995. *Toronto Star*, 17 Nov., A12.

White, Kevin. 1991. 'Trend Report: The Sociology of Health and Illness', *Current Sociology* 39, 2: 1–115.

Widman, L., and D.A. Tong. 1997. 'Requests for Medical Advice from Patients and Families to Health Care Providers Who Publish on the World Wide Web', *Archives of Internal Medicine* 157: 209–12.

Wilensky, Harold L. 1964. 'The Professionalization of Everyone', *American Journal of Sociology* 70: 137–58.

Wilkins, Kaibryn. 1996. 'Causes of Death: How the Sexes Differ', *Canadian Social Trends* (Summer): 11–15.

Wilkins, R., and O. Adams. 1993. *Healthfulness of Life: A Unified View of Mortality, Institutionalization and Non-institutionalized Disability in Canada, 1978*. Montreal: Institute for Research on Public Policy.

Wilkinson, Richard G. 1990. 'Income Distribution and Mortality: A "Natural" Experiment', *Sociology of Health and Illness* 12, 4: 391–412.

Williams, A.P., Karin Dominick, and Eugene Vayda. 1993. 'Women in Medicine: Toward a Conceptual Understanding of the Potential for Change', *Journal of the American Medical Women's Association* 48, 4: 115–23.

Williams, P., and D.R. Rush. 1986. 'Geriatric

Polypharmacy', *Hospital Practice* 21: 109–20.

Williams, Paul A., Rhonda Cockerill, and Frederick H. Lowy. 1995. 'The Physician as Prescriber: Relations between Knowledge about Prescription Drugs, Encounters with Patients and the Pharmaceutical Industry, and Prescription Volume', *Health and Canadian Society* 3, 1–2: 135–66.

Williams, Simon J. 1998. 'Health as Moral Performance: Ritual, Transgression and Taboo', *Health* 2, 4: 435–58.

_____ and Michael Calnan. 1996. 'The Limits of Medicalization?: Modern Medicine and the Lay Population in "Late" Modernity', *Social Science and Medicine* 42, 12: 1609–20.

Williamson, Deana L., and Janet E. Fast. 1998. 'Poverty and Medical Treatment: When Public Policy Compromises Accessibility', *Canadian Journal of Public Health* 89, 2: 120–4.

Willis, Evan. 1983. *Medical Dominance: The Division of Labour in Australian Health Care*. Sydney: George Allen and Unwin.

Wilson, Bryan R. 1961. *Sects and Society: A Sociological Study of Three Religious Groups in Britain*. London: Heinemann.

Wilson, C.W.M., J.A Banks, R.E.A. Mapes, and S.M.T. Korte. 1963. 'Influence of Different Sources of Therapeutic Information on Prescribing by General Practitioners', *British Medical Journal* 3: 599.

Wilson, Edward O. 1991. 'Biodiversity, Prosperity and Value', in Herbert F. Brohman and Stephan R. Kellert, eds, 'Ecology, Economics and Ethics: The Broken Circle', special issue of *Society* 30, 1 (Nov.–Dec.): 90–3.

Wilson, Jane. 1987. 'Why Nurses Leave Nursing', *The Canadian Nurse* 83 (Mar.): 20–3.

Wilson S.J. 1982. *Women, the Family and the Economy*. Toronto: McGraw-Hill.

Winsor, Hugh. 1973. 'Thalidomide', *Globe and Mail*, 10 Mar.

Wnuk-Lipinski, Edmund, and Raymond Illsley. 1990. 'International Comparative Analysis: Main Findings and Conclusions', *Social Science and Medicine* 31, 8: 879–89.

Wohl, Stanley. 1984. *The Medical Industrial Complex*. New York: Harmony Books.

Wolf, Naomi. 1990. *The Beauty Myth*. Toronto: Vintage Books.

Wolfe, Morris. 1993. 'Dental Flaws', *Saturday Night* (Nov.): 15–16, 20–4.

Wolfson, Michael C. 1996. 'Health Adjusted Life Expectancy', *Health Reports* 8, 1: 41–4.

Wolgelerenter, Daniel. 1998. 'Controversy Lingers over Role of Midwife', *Toronto Star*, 29 June, E1, E3.

Women in Canada, 3rd edn. Ottawa: Statistics Canada. Cat. no. 89–503E.

Women's Health Office Newsletter. 1994. Hamilton, Ont.: McMaster University, Apr.

Wood, S. 1980. *WHO International Classifications of Impairments, Disabilities in Preventable Deaths and Handicaps*. Geneva: World Health Organization.

Woodward, Christel A. 1999. 'Medical Students' Attitudes toward Women: Are Medical Schools Microcosms of Society?', *CMAJ* 160: 347–8.

Woolhandler, Steffie, David U. Himmelstein, Ralph Silba, Michael Bader, M. Narnley, and Alice A. Jones. 1985. 'Medical Care and Mortality: Racial Differences in Preventable Deaths', *International Journal of Health Services* 15, 1: 1–11.

World Development Report. 1992. *Development and the Environment*. Oxford: Oxford University Press.

World Health Organization. 1983. *International Code* (May 1981, Article 1). Geneva: WHO.

_____. 1997. *The World Health Report*. Geneva: WHO.

_____. 1998. *The World Health Report. Life in the 21st Century: A Vision for All*. Report of the Director General. Geneva: WHO.

_____. 1999. *The World Health Report: Making a Difference*. Geneva: WHO.

Wotherspoon, T. 1994. 'Colonization, Self-determination and the Health of Canada's First Nations Peoples', in Bolaria and Bolaria (1994a: 247–68).

Wysong, Peggy. 1986. 'Health Profession Legislation Review', *RNAO News* 9 (Spring): 18–19.

Yates, Patsy M., G. Beadle, A. Clavarino, J.M. Najman, D. Thomson, G. Williams, L. Kenny, S. Roberts, B. Mason, and D. Schlect. 1993. 'Patients with Terminal Cancer Who Use Alternative Therapies: Their Beliefs and Practices', *Sociology of Health and Illness* 15: 199–216.

Yeaton, W.H., D. Smith, and K. Rogers. 1990. 'Evaluating Understanding of Popular Press Reports of Health Research', *Health Education Quarterly* 17: 223–34.

Yudkin, J.S. 1978. 'Provisions of Medicines in a Developing Country', *Lancet* (Apr.).

Zabolai-Csekme, Eva. 1983. *Women, Health and Development*. Geneva: World Health Organization.

Zborowski, Mark. 1952. 'Cultural Components in Response to Pain', in E. Jaco, ed., *Patients, Physicians and Illness*. Glencoe, Ill.: Free Press, 256–68.

_____. 1969. *People in Pain*. San Francisco: Jossey Bass.

Zelek, B., S. Phillips, and Y. Lefebre. 1997. 'Gender Sensitivity in Medical Curricula', *CMAJ* 156, 9: 1297–300.

Zimmerman, Mark, 1983. 'Methodological Issues in the Assessment of Life Events: A Review of Issues and Research', *Clinical Psychology Review* 3: 339–70.

Zola, Irving. 1972. 'Medicine as an Institution of Social Control', *Sociological Review* 20: 487–504.

_____. 1973. 'Pathways to the Doctor: From Person to Patient', *Social Science and Medicine* 7, 9: 677–89.

_____. 1975. 'In the Name of Health and Illness: On Some Socio-Political Consequences of Medical Influence', *Social Science and Medicine* 9: 83–7.

Index

Italics indicate illustrations, figures, and boxes.